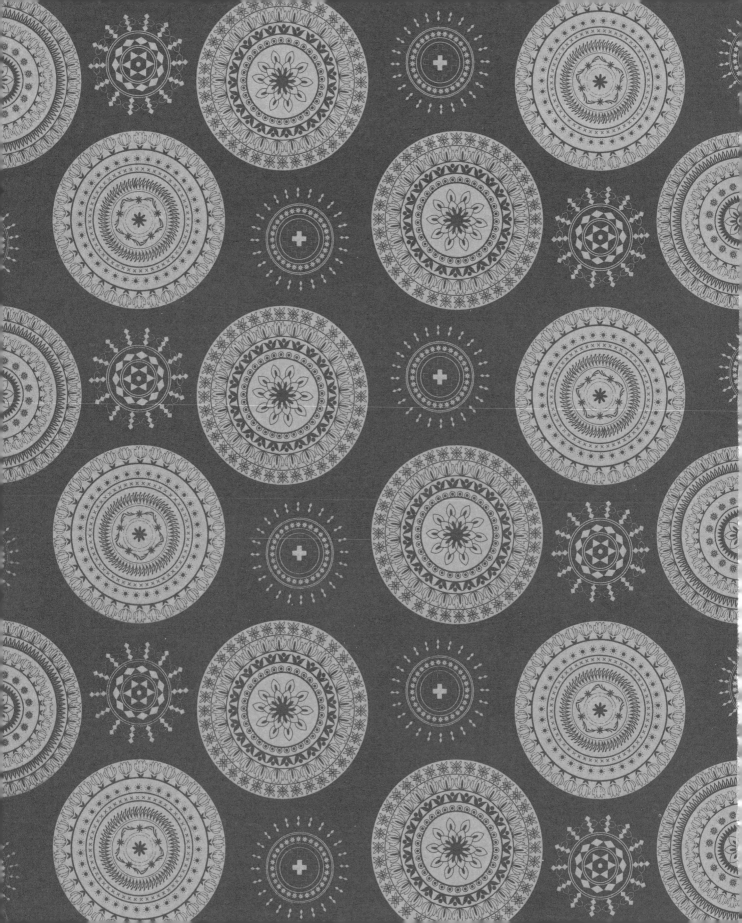

2,100
ASANAS

Cover design by Christopher Lin
Jacket photograph by Daniel Lacerda
Cover copyright © 2018 by Hachette Book Group, Inc.

Black Dog & Leventhal Publishers
Hachette Book Group
1290 Avenue of the Americas
New York, NY 10104

www.hachettebookgroup.com
www.blackdogandleventhal.com
First Edition: October 2015

Black Dog & Leventhal Publishers is an imprint of Hachette Books, a division of Hachette Book Group. The Black Dog & Leventhal Publishers name and logo are trademarks of Hachette Book Group, Inc.

The Hachette Speakers Bureau provides a wide range of authors for speaking events. To find out more, go to www.HachetteSpeakersBureau.com or call (866) 376-6591.

Management of layout and design by Tatiana Usova
Additional proofreading by: Aggie Metford, Victoria Bergin, Susan Marchese

Print book interior design by Sheila Hart Design, Inc.

Library of Congress Cataloging-in-Publication Data

Lacerda, Daniel (Yoga teacher)
    2,100 Asanas : the complete yoga poses / Daniel Lacerda, Founder of Mr. Yoga, Inc.
       pages cm
    Includes index.
    ISBN 978-1-63191-010-4 (hardback)
    1. Hatha yoga.   2. Yoga.   3. Exercise.   I. Title.   II. Title: Twenty-one hundred Asanas.   III. Title: Two thousand and one hundred Asanas.
    RA781.7.L33 2015
    613.7'046—dc23

ISBNs: 978-1-63191-010-4 (hardcover), 978-0-316-27062-5 (ebook)

Printed in China

IM

10 9 8 7 6 5 4

2,100 ASANAS

The Complete Yoga Poses

Daniel Lacerda

FOUNDER OF MR. YOGA, INC.

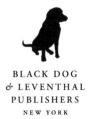

BLACK DOG
& LEVENTHAL
PUBLISHERS
NEW YORK

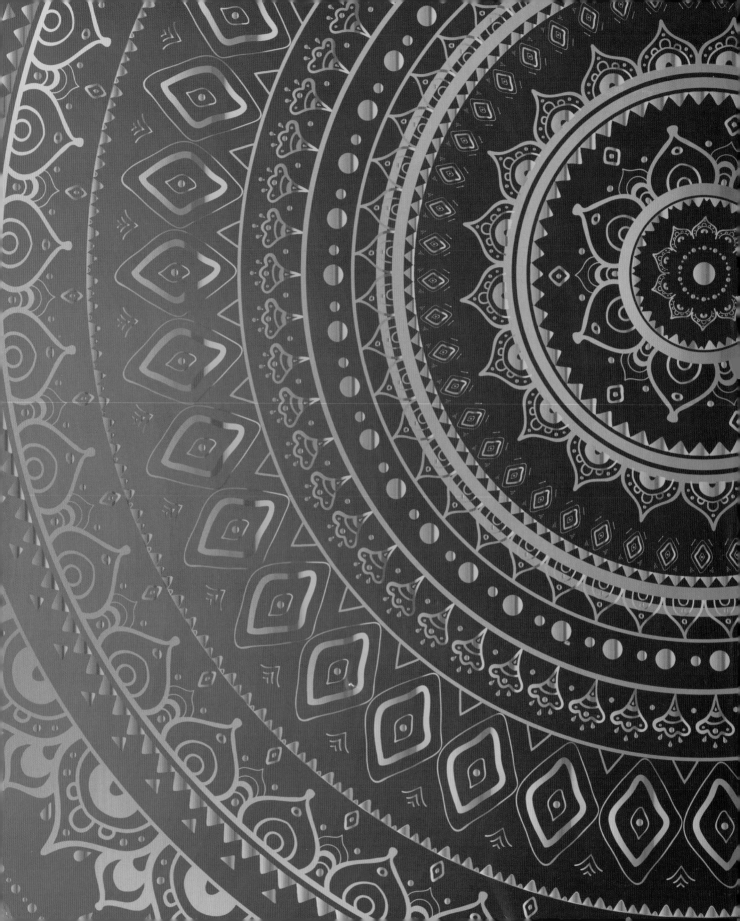

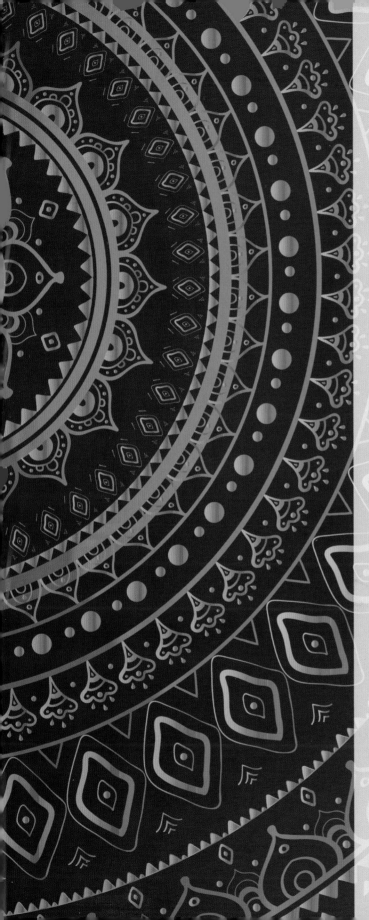

CONTENTS

A MESSAGE FROM MR. YOGA

Opening Prayer

Om

For the peaceful resolution
From the illusionary nature of dualistic
    existence,
I ground myself before the lotus feet of
    the gurus,
Who remind me that the light I search for
    is within me
Bringing stillness to the whirling of the
    cascading ego mind
I behold the awakened joy of my own
    Soul
Realizing the truth of pure radiance
That we are in fact the same
To the self-awakened gurus of the past,
    present, and future,
I salute

Om

Daniel Lacerda, Mr. Yoga

The ultimate goal of yoga is self-realization. You do not need to go to the mountaintop to find it or pay a teacher to show you the way. There are currencies that we exchange with one another that are much more valuable than money: kindness, selflessness, being one part of the greater good. Nor do you need to look outside yourself. If you have an open mind, a sincere desire to learn and to apply that knowledge on a daily basis, and the commitment to follow through on what you've begun, you can achieve self-realization.

Self-realization is the knowledge that we sentient beings are interconnected and that what we think, say, and do affects those around us. Burdened by the pressures and demands that exist outside of ourselves—of our jobs, bills, desire for status and for material possessions—we forget this. Self-realization is the ability to achieve freedom from these demands and to know that true happiness comes from fulfilling our own potential and from lifting up those around us without the thought of self-gain. Dedicating yourself to the regular practice of yoga can help bring you back to this place.

Yoga is, indeed, an excellent form of exercise that carries with it many immediate and long-term physical benefits from improved flexibility to stronger muscles and bones. However, yoga is not just about moving through the poses. Mindfulness plays an essential part in any dedicated yoga practice. If performed properly, yoga quiets the mind of all distracting thoughts from the outside world (*chittavritti*, meaning mind chatter), bringing you to a place of peace within. In turn, being mindful of your thoughts will allow you to be mindful of, and truly connected with, your body, thus completing the cycle of mental and physical health that will allow you to enjoy all the wonderful things that life has to offer.

For the past eleven years, I have dedicated my life to yoga, teaching an average of twenty-five classes seven days a week. I have done this to make a difference in the lives of my students. Now it's my pleasure to share this passion and dedication with you.

Namaste!

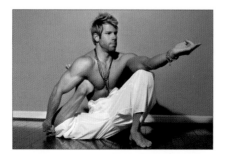

A HISTORY OF YOGA

Most of us know yoga as a set of poses performed in a gym or yoga studio setting. The majority of yoga styles practiced today were invented in the last quarter of the 20th century and are either a far cry from yoga's roots or have no authentic lineage.

If we really want to examine the roots of yoga, we need to go back to the Harrapan culture, dating back 3,500 years, when yoga was a meditative practice. According to some, around 1500 BCE, Harrapan culture was diminished due to Aryan invasion. Barbarians from Normandy introduced the caste system and enforced a set of religious rituals that involved blood sacrifice practices. Along with these religious practices came sacred scriptures called the Vedas, a large body of spiritual texts originating in India. The word "yoga" was first mentioned in the oldest of the Vedas, *Rig Veda*. It referred to the concept of discipline.

Fast forward to 800 BCE. The Upanishads, a collection of texts that contain some of the earliest concepts of Hinduism, prescribed the method of achieving enlightenment by studying under a teacher and dedicating one's life to a yoga practice. The Upanishads outlined two paths to enlightenment: Karma Yoga (selfless dedication to the service of others) and Jnana Yoga (intense study of spiritual writings). Around the 3rd century BCE, the

Maitrayaniya Upanishad prescribed a six-step process to enlightenment, which included mastering *pranayama* (breath control), *pratyaharia* (sense withdrawal), *dhyana* (meditation), *dharana* (one-pointed concentration), *tarka* (self-reflection), and *samadhi* (absolute absorption) in order to unite the Atman (individual's spirit) and Brahman (universal spirit or source of creation). The sacred syllable *om* appeared in this particular Upanishad as a symbol of union between mind and breath.

At around the same time that *Maitrayaniya Upanishad* was introduced, *Bhagavad Gita* gained prominence. This scripture combined and mythological tales that later made their way into a celebrated collection of tales, *Mahabharata*. Three methods of devotion were outlined in *Bhagavad Gita*: Karma Yoga, Jnana Yoga, and Bhakti Yoga (devotion).

Compiled around 400 CE by Patanjali, *The Yoga Sutras* introduced the eight-fold path to yoga practice, which is considered to be the classical yoga manual and the foundation of many of today's yoga practices, particularly Ashtanga Yoga. We will hear more about this eight-fold path in The Eight Limbs of Yoga (page 8), which include *yama* (self-restraint) *niyama* (self-purification by self-restraint and discipline), *asana* (seat or posture), *pranayama* (control of breath), *pratyahara* (sense withdrawal), *dharana* (one-pointed concentration), *dhyana* (meditation), and *samadhi* (total absorption).

Around the 4th century CE, Tantra Yoga emerged. This new form of yoga celebrated the physical body as a vehicle to enlightenment. The philosophy behind Tantra Yoga can be summarized by the idea of uniting all the dualities within a human body (e.g., male and female; good and evil), which gave Tantra a very sexual reputation. This is, however, a common misunderstanding, since Tantra practices extend far beyond sexuality.

Hatha Yoga was introduced in the 10th century CE. It combined the physicality and conscious intent of using bodily postures, or *asana* practice, and *pranayama* breath control for the goal of self-realization.

In 14th century CE, the Yoga Upanishads were introduced. One of these sacred texts, *Tejo Bindu Upanishad*, added seven more important parts of yoga practice on top of Patanjali's eight. They were as follows: *mula bandha* (root lock), balance, undisturbed vision, *tyaga* (abandonment), *mauua* (quiet), *desha* (space), and *kala* (time).

It was not until the 20th century that yoga gained any kind of popularity in Western Europe and North America. Swami Sivananda Saraswati was one of the first yogis to travel outside of India to spread the teachings of yoga to the West. He established yoga centers in North America at the time Swami Satchidananda also delivered an opening speech at the Woodstock Festival in 1969. However, T. Krishnamacharya is arguably the father of the yoga practice with which Westerners are familiar today. In the 1930s, he began teaching his students the Mysore vigorous sequences of yoga poses that emphasize strength and athletic ability. Students were only allowed to learn the next and more challenging pose after they had grasped the previous one. His three most prominent and influential students are Pattabhi Jois, Iyengar, and Indra Devi. Pattabhi Jois established Ashtanga yoga. It is one of the most popular types of yoga practiced in the West. Iyengar became successful by creating his own sequences of yoga poses, which were characterized by a focus on the alignment of the body and the use of various props. Indra Devi is considered the first famous yogini (female yoga master). Krishnamacharya also educated his son Desikachar in yoga. An engineer by training, Desikachar saw great value in studying yoga only when he was already a college graduate. Desikachar developed Vinyoga, which is a more therapeutic and less intense approach to physical practice, as compared to Ashtanga.

The 21st century presents us with an endless variety of yoga "styles" or "brands," such as Bikram Yoga, Power Yoga, Kundalini Yoga, and countless more. It is important to be open-minded, try as many styles and approaches as possible, and figure out what gives you the best results in terms of achieving both your physical and spiritual goals. There is no wrong way to achieve self-realization. Just make sure you are mindful, patient, practical, and consistent in your practice.

A Note on the Naming of Poses:

One of the ways that the distance from yoga's roots expresses itself in Western culture is in the naming of the poses. "Seated forward bend," "eagle pose," and "dolphin pose," for example, are all imprecise translations of the original Sanskrit name. *Garudasana*, for example, is widely known as eagle pose, but traditionally this pose was named in dedication to Garuda, who is a Hindu deity, portrayed as half-man and half-eagle. He is the charioteer of Lord Vishnu, who is part of the Holy Trinity in Hinduism. Knowing this history adds a whole new dimension to our understanding of the significance, philosophical depth, and essence of the pose, and can in turn enrich our practice.

The poses throughout this book are identified by both their English and Sanskrit names. The English name is a direct translation of the Sanskrit, which sometimes differs from the more common Western name, also provided in the notes. For a literal translation of each part of the Sanskrit name, you may consult the glossary at the back of the book. The intention is to provide you with as much information about the name of the pose and its history as possible, so no matter what style of yoga you practice, you will have the most complete understanding of the names of the poses.

THE EIGHT LIMBS OF YOGA

The Yoga Sutras, also known as *The Eight Limbs (Ashtanga) of Raja (King) Yoga*, was the first fully developed and recorded system of yoga. Created by Patanjali around 400 CE, this system influences much of the yoga that is practiced today. Although most of the sutras were originally focused on mindfulness, the yoga practiced in the West today seems to focus more on the body. Somewhere along the way, it seems, we began to practice the movement of yoga in isolation from its original philosophies.

For those interested in truly integrating the mindfulness of yoga with its movement, I recommend that you read *The Eight Limbs of Yoga* in its entirety and digest it very slowly. Take time to reflect on it piece by piece so you can implement it into both your practice and your daily life. Wisdom is in the doing. The following, however, is a useful summary of *The Eight Limbs of Yoga*, which will introduce you to the basic concepts of the philosophy. A deep understanding of yoga philosophy and history will greatly enhance the benefits of your practice and put you on the path to mindfulness and self-realization.

There is a wonderful lesson in Buddhism that applies here:

Once, a very old king went to see an old hermit who lived in a bird's nest in the top of a tree. He asked the hermit, "What is the most important Buddhist teaching?" The hermit answered, "Do no evil, do only good. Purify your heart." The king expected to hear a long and detailed explanation. He protested, "Even a five-year-old child can understand that!" "Yes," replied the wise sage, "but even an eighty-year-old man cannot do it."

Your biggest obstacle to self-realization is you. As it says in the *Bhagavad Gita*, "The mind is restless and hard to control, but it can be trained by constant practice (*abhyasa*) and freedom from desire (*vairagya*). A man who cannot control his mind will find it difficult to attain this divine communion; but the self-controlled man can attain it if he tries hard and directs his energy by the right means."

Pantanjali's *Eight Limbs of Yoga* will help you form the necessary groundwork to get on the right track, but you must decide to confront your problems at their roots. Reading and intellectualizing is not enough. If you want to reap the full benefits of the yoga experience, implement the Eight Limbs into every aspect of your life. You must live it, breathe it, and engage this planet and its inhabitants with the lessons below.

The first and second limbs, *Yama* and *Niyama*, form your foundation. Here, awareness and realization is established. *Yama* and *Niyama*

lay the footing for everything to come. A serious student should be mindful of every limb, as each of these limbs need constant reflection. As you commit yourself to their study and practice, your depth of understanding for each limb will get deeper over time. In our world that perpetuates instant gratification, many people will take shortcuts and go straight to the yoga poses. Others will go straight to meditation and neglect physical health. I highly recommend starting with Pantanjali's first two limbs. Your practice will be at its deepest and most fulfilling if the first two limbs are practiced at a high level. If the first two limbs are not practiced at a proficient level, the rest of the limbs will be performed at a more superficial and less effective level.

FIRST LIMB **Yama** (Self-Restraint)

The focus of the first limb is on being an ethical and moral person, and on improving your relationship with the outer world. These values are as important today as they were centuries ago. The *Yamas*, as they are referred to, are not meant to be a moral straitjacket, but instead are meant to help develop a greater awareness of one's place in the world. It is not a coincidence that this is the first limb of the practice. When taking steps to transform our inner world, our outer world becomes a total reflection of this effort. There are five *Yamas*:

1. *Ahimsa:* **Non-violence**
   Replace harmful thoughts, speech, and actions with that of loving kindness toward yourself and others.

2. *Satya:* **Truth to be expressed in thought, word, and action**
   Be honest in your thoughts, words, and actions toward yourself and others.

3. *Asteya:* **Non-stealing and non-covetousness**
   Curb desires for things that are not your own. Share the beauty of your thoughts, speech, actions, and material belongings to uplift others instead of stealing and hoarding them for yourself.

4. *Brahmacharya:* **Abstinence from sexual intercourse when not married, practicing monogamy and not having sexual thoughts about another person who is not your spouse**
   It is believed that a life built on celibacy and spiritual studies done by free will increases energy and zest for life. Celibacy may sound like an unrealistic goal today, but it may help to remember that brahmacharya is also about monogamy. When brahmacharya is fully realized in marriage, the sex lives of both partners improve because the level of trust and devotion deepens their connection. It is important that the sexual activity is an expression based on the highest level of mutual respect, love, selflessness, and wisdom.

5. *Aparigraha:* **Non-possessiveness or non-greediness**
   Replace the habit of hoarding with sharing. Do not take without giving back. If you want something, work for it. This builds appreciation

for what you have. This will help minimize the insatiable desire to constantly consume. An appetite that is not wisely disciplined leads to personal ill health, financial debt or poor credit, and destruction of the planet's natural resources. The Greek god Apollo's motto, "Nothing in excess. All things in moderation," is a great way to describe *aparigraha*.

SECOND LIMB **Niyama**
(Self-Purification by Self-Restraint and Discipline)

The second limb helps refine your spiritual path. Discipline and self-restraint lead to a more orderly and productive life. From the perspective of ancient yoga texts, life is extremely short and we need to make the most of it while we can. This limb gives us guidance. There are five Niyamas:

1. *Shaucha:* **Purity of body and mind**
When you develop *shaucha* (cleanliness), unwholesome thoughts that lead to foul speech and a sick body are cleared. Purity starts with your mind. Speech and action follow. So, the second limb directs you to make a habit of consuming both food and mental stimuli that support well-being for yourself and the environment (humanity and the planet). This will allow destructive habits (hatred, greed, and delusion) to dissolve.

2. *Santosha:* **Contentment with what one has**
When you achieve *santosha* (contentment), bonds to the material world are broken and authentic peace and happiness are established within. A lack of contentment is often based on a distorted perception of what one has versus what others have. You advance on the path to self-realization when you can be content with your lot, whether you sit on a throne of dirt or gold.

3. *Tapas:* **Self-discipline, sometimes associated with austerity, and being able to conquer the body and mind through mental control**
Tapas literally means "heat" or "glow." This refers to a burning desire to accomplish one's goal despite what obstacles may appear. The commitment to achieving a goal, no matter how challenging it becomes, builds character. However, note that the highest level of *tapas* is to complete one's goal without a selfish motivation. When *tapas* is attained, laziness is overcome and willpower is developed for future use.

4. *Svadhyaya:* **Self-study that leads to introspection and a greater awakening of the soul and the source of creation; traditionally studied through Vedic scriptures**
Svadhyaya (self-study) leads to a greater awakening of your true potential, the root of one's place in this world and how to live in harmony with the Earth and all its inhabitants.

5. *Ishvara pranidhana:* **The surrender to God**
When you accept that all things come from a higher power, pride and egocentric behavior are turned into humility and devotion. This strengthens your practice of all the limbs leading up to *samadhi* (the eighth limb).

Asana and *Pranayama* are the third and fourth limbs, and they relate to health and longevity, which allow us more time to achieve the ultimate goal of yoga, Self-Realization or Enlightenment. The third and fourth limbs are important, as they prepare the body for meditation, which will be the key to calming your mind and discovering your true potential.

THIRD LIMB **Asana**
(Seat or Posture)

Here is a question: If Gandhi is one of the greatest yogis of our time, does that mean he can touch his toes or bring his foot behind his head? The answer is that it doesn't matter. Gandhi's ability to perform the *asanas* had very little to do with what he contributed to the world as a great yogi. The same applies to you. The practice of *asanas* is as much about training the mind as it is the body. How you approach your *asana* practice is often a reflection of how you approach life. Do you keep a sense of peace and calm when a challenge presents itself? Do you break down the impossible into smaller tasks, making the whole possible through commitment to and reflection on each of the parts? Do you overcome self-perceived limitations on your own or do you accept support from others?

Your practice of yoga poses should be characterized by two components: steadiness (*sthira*) and ease (*sukha*). Concentrating on the sound of your breath (*ujjayi*, the most commonly practiced breathing technique in yoga, see page 710), can provide the steadiness. If you lose your breath, it is most likely because you are pushing too hard; ease off the pose and let the pose cater to the breath.

There is no such thing as a perfect pose; let the poses come like the steps of a dance. Just like in dance, when we focus too much on the mechanics, we let go of the ability to enjoy the music. While the mechanics of alignment are important to prevent injury, never forget the final goal. Feel the music of life flow through you as you do each pose and your body will learn the moves naturally. There are more than enough postures to keep you busy for the rest of your life, so allow yourself to let go of ambition and enjoy the journey. Incorporating a combination of forward bends, backbends, twists, and inversions in your yoga session is optimal for health.

Remember, too, that *asanas* help prepare the mind and body for meditation, relieving tension and protecting the body from disturbances by purifying the nervous system.

FOURTH LIMB **Pranayama** (Control of Breath)

The English word "spirit" comes from the Latin *spiritus*, meaning "breath."

The breath and the mind are interconnected. Deep, rhythmic, and fluid breathing will energize yet calm the mind and body. Rapid, irregular, and strained breathing produces a chaotic and disturbed mind. A calm mind will give you the mental space to make better decisions and a life in which you take control instead of feeling like a victim of circumstances.

Breathing properly is fundamental to our very existence. Your brain feeds on oxygenated blood, which is supplied with every inhalation. If you are unable to draw oxygen into your body, you will become brain dead after a few minutes. On the other hand, proper exhaling helps expel carbon dioxide. If your ability to exhale were impaired, you would most likely die due to the toxic buildup of carbon dioxide and poison. Stress tends to negatively affect breathing patterns, which contributes to a chain of effects that cause wear and tear on both your body's nervous and immune systems. In fact, 90 percent of illness is stress-related and, for this reason, attention to breathing properly is, indeed, a matter of life and death.

FIFTH LIMB **Pratyahara** (Sense Withdrawal)

Our perception of reality is predominantly influenced by our sensory experience—what we see, feel, hear, touch, and taste. *Pratyahara* refers to the withdrawal of the senses from external objects and our modern-day need for constant gratification from sensory stimuli. Our minds are constantly being pulled outward to evaluate all the information the senses bring in. Evaluation involves categorizing what has been perceived; often, we hold on to what we believe is desirable, push away what we believe is undesirable, and ignore what we believe to be neutral. *Pratyahara* gives our minds a moment to rest and teaches us to be free of the grasping and clinging to the things we enjoy and avoiding the undesirable.

When you throw a pebble into a pond, your reflection becomes distorted by the resulting ripples. Your mind works in very much the same way: Every thought creates a ripple that distorts the ability to see your true self clearly. Constantly disrupted by these ripples, you begin to believe that the distorted reflection is who you really are. Practicing *pratyahara* calms the mind, allowing you to see yourself clearly.

SIXTH LIMB **Dharana** (One-Pointed Concentration)

Asanas, *pranayamas*, and *pratyahara* help prepare us for meditation.

When the mind moves from experiencing random scattered thoughts to single one-pointed concentration, it can then find complete absorption in the present moment. By practicing one-pointed concentration, we clear the mind of all distracting thoughts. This can be achieved by focusing on your breath, counting, reciting mantras, or observing a candle flame or an image. Because we are constantly entangled in reliving past memories or living in anticipation of what is to come, it is very seldom that we live in the present moment. It is even less common to be mindful of the present moment with a calm and focused mind. However, this is crucial when trying to achieve self-realization. The power is in the now!

SEVENTH LIMB **Dhyana** (Meditation)

Just as there are many different types of yoga poses, there are many ways of meditating. Meditation is a form of inner contemplation that allows you to access a state of mind that has transcended the ego. This is a state of pure awareness of the present moment that is free of judgment. All meditation leads to a state of full awareness that does not discriminate or categorize things in a dualistic manner, which is to say the perception of what is good versus what is bad, beautiful versus ugly, pleasant versus unpleasant, etc. When we examine reasons behind such judgments, we find many of these beliefs are based on learned behavior, may vary from one culture to another, and have no fixed or concrete reality. With consistent reflection and an open mind, we can correct our biased perceptions. You will develop that part of you called "the Observer." Once grounded in a regular seated mediation, it is important to take it into a moving mediation throughout your daily life.

EIGHTH LIMB **Samadhi** (Total Absorption)

Samadhi occurs when the analytical mind becomes absent and at one with the object of meditation. The object of meditation can be whatever you are focusing on in your meditation that is used to achieve one-pointed concentration. The word *om*, a deity, or a candle flame are all examples of objects of meditation. Total absorption involves the feeling of oneness with all creation, dissolving all lines between the act of meditation and the object being meditated upon.

It is the absorption in the present moment (*amanaska*) where dualistic thinking is transcended. Many are mistaken in believing *samadhi* is the final goal of yoga. It is but a temporary state of mind that we enter based on the conditions that we have nurtured to support it.

It's useful to remember that every moment in your life gives you an opportunity to practice the eight limbs. Learn at your own pace, but stay focused, be consistent, and enjoy the journey!

THE *UJJAYI* BREATH

Breath is an essential staple of every yoga practice. By focusing on the breath, a yogi is able to stay in the present moment. Since the breath is neutral, a yogi neither seeks to avoid it, nor is she eager to chase it. Proper and continuous breath helps clear the mind of distracting thoughts and to remain in the present moment with one-pointed concentration.

Deep, conscious breathing also slows down the heartbeat and activates the parasympathetic nervous response, which soothes the nervous system, and allows the muscles to relax into the stretches and stay strong in the strength-based yoga poses. Maintaining deep, fluid breathing will help transform your yoga practice into a moving meditation.

Ujjayi pranayama is one of the most commonly used breathing techniques in every yoga practice. *Ujjayi* means "victorious" in Sanskrit. When practicing this breathing technique, a yogi creates what can be described as the "ocean sound" in the back of the throat by gently squeezing the glottis (the opening between the vocal cords in the throat). You're aiming to create a breathy and whispery sound at the back of the throat. The sound is often compared to the sound Darth Vader makes when breathing! In order to practice *ujjayi* breath, first sit in a comfortable position. Inhale through the nose and, as you exhale, imagine you are trying to fog up a glass. Try to inhale with the same sound. Once you feel like you have an understanding of the *ujjayi* breath technique, seal your lips in order to prevent the throat from drying out. (A dry throat usually leads to coughing and drinking water, which distracts you from your yoga practice.) Inhale and exhale through the nose, while still maintaining the sensation in the throat of trying to fog up a glass.

Using breath to facilitate poses:

- Keep your breath deep and rhythmic.

- If your breathing becomes restricted or choppy, there is a good chance that you are pushing yourself unnecessarily. In this case, you should ease off the pose and return to a place that promotes smooth and fluid breathing.

- The body lifts up and lengthens on the inhale. For example, lift up from a forward bend into a mountain pose on the inhale, using the inhale to lengthen the limbs of the body and the spine. Use the exhales to go deeper into the pose.

THE BANDHAS

Bandha means "lock." *Bandhas* were traditionally believed to regulate the flow of life energy (*prana*) throughout the body. In contemporary yoga practice, *bandhas* serve a more practical purpose. They are contractions, or "body locks," that you can implement to help correct your posture or aid you in proper alignment.

There are three major *bandhas*: *mula bandha, uddiyana bandha,* and *jalandhara bandha.* The combination of all three *bandhas* is called *maha bandha,* or "the great lock."

Mula bandha refers to the triggering of the perineum muscle that is located between the genitals and the anus. *Mula* means "root," therefore *mula bandha* translates as "root lock." When this *bandha* is engaged, you will feel a slight pull on the inside of the thighs, similar to what you feel when trying to stop the flow of urine.

Uddiyana bandha means "flying/moving up." To engage this *bandha,* place three fingers below the belly button and pull your lower abdominal muscles slightly in and up. This will cause your pelvis to tilt forward slightly with an upward action, protecting the lower back and strengthening the lower abdominals.

Mula and *uddiyana bandhas* should be engaged throughout the yoga practice. Together they help correct the posture and create proper alignment, which will reduce the chance of injury.

Jalandara bandha is a chin lock. To practice this lock, bring the chin toward the clavicle bone while keeping your spine upright and moving your shoulder blades down the back. This *bandha* is rarely used, but can be found when engaged in *Dandasana*, Staff Pose.

THE *DRISHTIS*

Drishtis are the meditation gazing points to focus on while performing the poses. They are designed to aid with proper alignment, as well as to strengthen the focus on the present moment. While practicing we tend to look around, compare ourselves to others in the room, or look at the clock. This takes away from the focus on the internal aspects of the practice. *Drishtis* are meant help you look inward.

They are as follows:
1. *Nasagrai* or *Nasagre* (nose)
2. *Bhrumadhye* or *Ajna Chakra* (third eye, between the eyebrows)
3. *Nabhi, Nabhicakre,* or *Nabi Chakra* (belly button)
4. *Hastagrai* or *Hastagre* (hands)
5. *Padayoragrai* or *Padayoragre* (toes/feet)
6. *Parshva Drishti* (to the right)
7. *Parshva Drishti* (to the left)
8. *Angushtamadhye* or *Angushta Ma Dyai* (thumbs)
9. *Urdhva* or *Antara Drishti* (up to the sky)

Drishtis can be complicated to grasp at first. However, there are general guidelines for the gaze. It comes down to letting your eyes follow the direction of the stretch. For example, in backbends we look at our third eye in order to let the head roll back and deepen the backbend. Similarly, in seated forward bends, such as *Paschimottanasana* (Western Intense Stretch Pose), we gaze at the toes to lengthen the spine. The purpose of *drishtis* is not for you to become cross-eyed; they are a way to softly focus without intensely staring.

HOW TO APPROACH YOGA POSES

Yoga poses provide much more than a physical workout. Performing them builds character. Facing your fears and challenges that extend beyond your comfort zone with a sense of peace, calmness, and psychological equanimity will help you overcome your self-perceived limitations.

I find it helpful to think of every yoga pose as a prayer you do with your body. While you perform the pose, focus on what is good in your life with a feeling of gratitude. Being at one with your mind and body in this place of grace helps you transcend the ego, which helps you get closer to the ultimate goal of yoga, which is enlightenment.

Universal Alignment Cues

- Engage *mula* and *uddhiyana bandhas*.

- Engage the *ujjayi* breath and maintain deep conscious breathing all throughout the yoga session. If your breath is suffering, then back off a bit.

- Keep the chest open and shoulder blades down the back.

- Lengthen the body and limbs on the inhale, deepen the pose on the exhale.

- Avoid jerky and uncontrolled movements during the poses that are based on flexibility.

- Square your hips.

- Don't let your knee go past your ankle when doing any kind of lunge.

- In Plank and the majority of arm balances, shoulders should be just over the fingertips.

- Even if you are intermediate or advanced, start with the beginner modifications in order to ensure proper form and get the blood into the targeted muscle as a warm-up.

Universal Flexibility Cues

- Hold flexibility for a minimum of 30 to 90 seconds.

- Stretch to the edge of comfort and stimulation without straining.

- Don't overstretch to the point of pain; your muscles will tighten up in order to protect themselves and your flexibility will decrease.

RELAXATION AND MEDITATION

Relaxation
Corpse Pose (Shavasana)
(Shava in Sanskrit means "corpse")

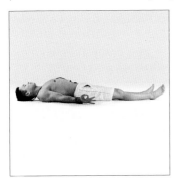

After an intensive *asana* practice, the final resting yoga pose, Corpse Pose or *Shavasana,* helps deepen the connection between our physical body and mind and helps prepare both for meditation. *Shavasana* can be thought of as an awakening, giving us the time to contemplate the question "If I died today, would I be fully satisfied and content with what I accomplished in this lifetime?" Have you lived up to your full potential? Have you fully acknowledged the people in your life that are of great importance to you? Would you be able to pass on with no regrets?

1. Lie down on your back, shoulder blades tucked in, legs apart. Relax your arms and let your palms face the ceiling. Let your fingers naturally curl. Relax your body into a neutral, comfortable position.

2. Close your eyes. Let your jaw naturally separate as you relax your whole body as if it were sinking down to the floor. Release all tension from your body.

3. Without letting the mind wander, concentrate on your breathing to reach a deep state of conscious relaxation, both physically and mentally.

Meditation
Easy Pose (Sukhasana), Seated Lotus Pose (Padmasana)

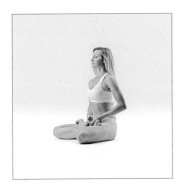

1. Start in Staff Pose (*Dandasana*), both legs extended in front of you. Grab onto your sitting bones and pull back the flesh to lengthen your legs and spine.

2. Sit in a cross-legged position that is comfortable. You can sit on a chair, in Easy Pose (*Sukhasana*), in Half Lotus (*Ardha Padmasana*), or Full Lotus (*Padmasana*). Press your sitting bones into the ground as you extend up through the spine. Lift the crown of your head up to the sky. Place one hand on top of the other and have the thumbs lightly touch. Gently close your eyes. Perform the 1:4:2 Healing Breath Zen Meditation as follows:

   Inhale for a count of 4 and feel your lower abdomen expand as you push it out. Hold and retain the air in your lungs for the count of 16. Exhale for a count of 8 as you squeeze the belly button back to the spine. Visualize the numbers as you count throughout the set. This will help develop what is called "one-pointed concentration." Your breathing must be so fine that it would not ruffle a feather. Each count should be one second long.

   After 10 breath cycles are performed, the exercise is finished. In an authentic yoga practice, the ego may not be permitted to intrude into the process. Don't "perform" the exercises as if you had an appreciative audience. This is your personal journey. Explore and express yourself while you gain the wonderful physical and mental benefits. This breathing technique is called Abdominal Breathing and should be maintained during the entire yoga practice.

A BRIEF SUMMARY OF *CHAKRAS*

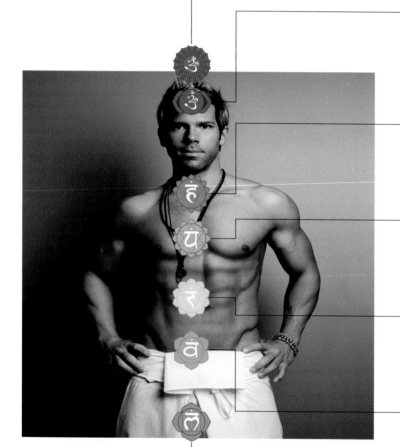

7th **Crown Chakra**/Thousand Petal or Spoked Wheel/*Sahasrara Chakra*
Location: just above the crown of the head
Color: encompasses all colors
Mantra Seed Syllable: encompasses all sounds

6th **Third Eye Chakra**/Rule or Command Wheel/*Ajna Chakra*
Location: in the middle of the forehead, between the eyebrows
Color: indigo
Mantra Seed Syllable: *om*

5th **Throat Chakra**/Especially Pure Wheel/ *Vishuddha Chakra*
Location: throat
Color: turquoise or blue
Mantra Seed Syllable: *ham*

4th **Heart Chakra**/Wheel of the Unstruck or Singular Sound/*Anahata Chakra*
Location: within the center of the chest
Color: green
Mantra Seed Syllable: *yam*

3rd **Solar Plexus or Navel Chakra**/Wheel of the Jewel City/*Manipura Chakra*
Location: solar plexus
Color: yellow
Mantra Seed Syllable: *ram*

2nd **Sacral Chakra**/One's Own Self-Based Wheel/*Svadhisthana Chakra*
Location: sacrum
Color: orange
Mantra Seed Syllable: *vam*

1st **Root Chakra or Root Wheel**/*Muladhara Chakra*
Location: base of the spine
Color: crimson
Mantra Seed Syllable: *lam*

Element: the ultimate reality of all truth
Number of Petals: 1000
(symbolic for unlimited)
Focus: detachment from ego and illusory nature of the material world, attaining the goal of yoga (self-realization).

Element: the universal mind
Number of Petals: 12
Focus: intuition, decision-making, and the surrendering of egocentric intellect in favor of attaining nondualistic wisdom

Element: ether/space
Number of Petals: 16
Focus: self-expression and communication

Element: air
Number of Petals: 12
Focus: peace, love, and empathy

Element: fire
Number of Petals: 10
Focus: power, will, and self-esteem

Element: water
Number of Petals: 6
Focus: emotions, desires, and creativity

Element: earth
Number of Petals: 4
Focus: physical survival, self-preservation, and security

In Sanskrit the word *chakra* can be translated into "wheel" or "turning." In the yogic interpretation, the *chakras* are based on the concept of a vortex and are visually portrayed as a lotus flower.

According to various Eastern yogic spiritual practices such as Hinduism and Tantric Buddhism, *chakras* are described as wheels or rings of energy found in the subtle (non-physical) body; the culmination of the mind, intelligence, and ego, which influences the gross physical body. Within this subtle body there are energy channels called *nadis* that carry the life force or vital energy (*prana*). The main *nadi* that runs through the *chakras* is called the *sushumna* (*brahma*) *nadi*. The *sushumna* joins two other important *nadis* (*ida* and *pingala*) together at the first and seventh *chakras*. The diameter of a singular *nadi* is believed to be no thicker than a thousandth of a hair's width and is located along the spine.

There are various opinions on how many *chakras* there are, but it is generally agreed that *chakras* spin in a "wheel-like" motion to draw in vital energy that creates a balance between the spiritual and physical body.

The earliest known recording of *chakras* dates back to the ancient Vedas (1700 BCE). The most popular *chakra* model used today is based on two Indian texts: *Shat-Cakra-Nirupana*, written by a Bengali yogi named Purnananda Swami in 1577, and the *Padaka-Panchaka*, written in the 10th century.

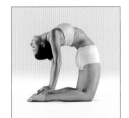

Chakras are activated in the following ways:

By stretching open the area where the *chakra* is located. For example, the throat *chakra* can be activated in Camel Pose (*Ushtrasana*). The head is rolled back so there is a stretch in the front of the throat.

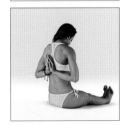

By applying physical pressure on the area where the *chakra* is located. Throat *chakra*, for example, can be activated in Staff Pose (*Dandasana*). The Chin Lock (*Jaladhara Bandha*) is engaged by bringing the chin to the clavicle bone, therefore applying pressure to the throat area.

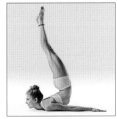

By combining the two methods above, throat *chakra* is activated in full version of Inverted Locust Pose (*Viparita Shalabhasana*). The head is rolling back, creating a stretch in the front of the throat. At the same time, the throat area is pressed to the floor, so there is physical pressure on that area.

BENEFITS AND CAUTIONS FOR 8 CONDITIONS

CONDITION	BENEFICIAL POSES	POSES TO APPROACH WITH CAUTION

1. Headache & Migraine
Many headaches are caused by tension and stress. In yoga we breathe deeply and relax. The yoga practice stretches the tight muscles in the upper body, releases endorphins (a "feel good" hormone) and relaxes the mind. It helps release tension by increasing blood flow to the muscles, making the nervous system less agitated and reducing a chance of a headache or migraine.

Poses that put weight or pressure on the head and neck should be avoided. If you suffer from migraines, avoid poses that dramatically increase blood flow to the head. If your migraines are severe, avoid practicing yoga poses and lie down in a dark room.

Seated forward bends – Ex. Both Hands to Ankle Head to Knee Pose (*Dwi Hasta Kulpa Janu Shirshasana*) pg. 328. Seated forward bends release tension in the hamstrings and lower back and help prevent headaches caused by tension in the legs and lower back.

Seated twists – Ex. Half Root Lord of the Fishes Pose (*Ardha Mula Matsyendrasana*) pg. 283. Seated twisting poses can help prevent headaches caused by tension in the upper and lower back.

Hand position of the pose dedicated to Garuda – Ex. Hand Position of the Pose Dedicated to Garuda in Child's Pose (*Hasta Garudasana in Balasana*) pg. 417. Any pose with this hand position helps stretch the upper back and back shoulder heads and can help prevent headaches caused by tension in the muscles of the upper back.

Hand position of Cow Face Pose – Ex. Hand Position of Cow Face Pose in Bound Angle Pose (*Hasta Garudasana in Baddha Konasana*) pg. 286. Any pose with this hand position helps stretch the triceps, front shoulder heads, and rotator cuffs and can help prevent headaches caused by tension in the arms and shoulder muscles.

Inversions – Ex. Peacock Feather Pose (*Picha Mayurasana*) pg. 526, Leg Position of One-Legged King Pigeon 1 Version B in Headstand 5 (*Pada Eka Pada Raja Kapotasana 1 B in Shirshasana 5*) pg. 542, and Leg Position of the Pose Dedicated to Garuda in Hands Bound Supported Whole Body Pose (*Pada Garudasana in Baddha Hasta Salamba Sarvangasana*), also known as Shoulderstand pg. 555. Avoid any intense inversions that require a lot of strength, as they increase the heart rate and blood flow to the head and may trigger headaches or migraines.

Backbends with feet and head on the floor – Ex. Bridge Pose (*Setu Bandhasana*) pg. 677. Avoid poses that put pressure on the head and neck, as they may trigger headaches or migraines.

---

2. Carpal Tunnel
To help prevent or alleviate carpal tunnel syndrome with yoga, you'll need to practice poses that strengthen and stretch the flexor muscles of the forearm, which are the muscles on the palm side of the forearm. Depending on the severity of your condition, you may want to start with poses that bear less weight on the wrist joint.

Poses that strengthen the wrist without straining it – Ex. Staff Pose (*Dandasana*) pg 303. Stretching and gently strengthening the wrist and muscles of the forearm can help prevent or reduce carpal tunnel syndrome.

Poses with hands in the reverse prayer position – Ex. Hidden Lotus Pose (*Gupta Padmasana*) pg. 570 and Reverse Prayer Mountain Pose (*Viparita Namaskar Tadasana*) pg. 25. These poses help stretch out the wrists, forearms, front shoulder heads, chest, and rotator cuffs. Releasing tension from these areas is helpful because muscles in the upper body are interconnected and carpal tunnel can be caused or worsened by a chain reaction of tense muscles.

Poses that have hands in prayer (Anjali Mudra) – Ex. Revolved Prayer Standing Rising Wind Relieving Pose (*Parivritta Namaskar Stiti Utthita Vayu Muktyasana*) pg. 46. Stretching the wrists and forearm muscles can promote blood flow and lessen tension in the area.

Poses with bound hands, palms facing out – Ex. Mountain Pose—Raised Bound Hands (*Tadasana Urdhva Baddha Hastasana*) pg. 26 These poses help stretch the forearm muscles that are strained and tight in most people who have carpal tunnel syndrome.

Arm balances with both feet off the floor – Ex. Crane Pose (*Bakasana*) pg. 510. These poses have the entire body weight resting on the wrists, which puts a great amount of strain on the carpal tunnel and may drastically worsen its symptoms.

Backbends with hands and feet on the floor – Ex. Upward Bow Pose (*Urdhva Dhanurasana*) pg. 496 and Wild Thing Pose (*Chamatkarasana*) pg. 498. These poses are very hard on the wrists.

Backbends with straight arms – Ex. Upward Facing Dog (*Urdhva Mukha Shvanasana*) pg. 587. These poses put strain on the wrist joints because most of the upper body weight rests on the hands.

ADDITIONAL NOTES: There are some options to avoid pressure on the wrist while practicing Upward Facing Dog Pose (*Urdhva Mukha Shvanasana*) pg. 587 or Downward Facing Dog (*Adho Mukha Shvanasana*) pg. 116. If you feel that these poses irritate the carpal tunnel, drop the knees to the floor and rotate the hands 45 degrees to the outside to take the pressure off the nerve. You may also experiment with placing props (rolled-up yoga mat, thin book, or slant board) under the heels of the palms to shift the weight to the knuckles and fingers to reduce the compression of the wrist.

Benefits and Cautions for 8 Conditions

3. Asthma

Yoga can help bring awareness to your breathing patterns and release tension from the neck, upper back, chest, and shoulders. Focus on developing full and complete breaths through seated mediation sitting in Easy Pose (*Sukhasana*) pg. 257. Since a symptom of asthma is short shallow breaths, developing control of the breath will help the body obtain the oxygen needed and help calm the body, preventing future attacks.

Some yoga poses may be strenuous to the respiratory system and could cause asthma attacks. It's recommended that you pace yourself, gradually raising your body temperature and gradually cooling down. Cold air can cause bronchi to contract and cause an asthma attack. Hot and humid air can cause dehydration and can also cause an asthma attack. Find a room with a comfortable temperature.

Poses on hands and knees – Ex. Going from Tiger Pose (*Vyaghrasana*) pg. 427 to Unsupported Tiger Pose (*Niralamba Vyaghrasana*) pg. 432. Many people who suffer from asthma have tension in the upper back and chest from coughing during asthma attacks. Combining mild backbends with mild forward bends gently stretches the chest, upper back, and the neck, which can help reduce the symptoms of asthma worsened by tension in those areas.

Mild backbends – Ex. Fish Pose (*Matsyasana*) pg. 672. Mild backbends help open the chest and front shoulder heads and improve the quality of breathing.

Lion's Pose variations – Ex. Lion Pose Dedicated to an Avatar of Lord Vishnu in Garland Pose (*Narasimhasana in Malasana*) pg. 238. Lion's Pose variations can help release tension in the throat, neck, and jaw because you "roar" like a lion in these poses. They also can help push the stale air out of your lungs.

Seated meditation focusing on breathing – Ex. Lotus Pose (*Padmasana*) pg. 263. Bringing awareness to your breath and developing control can be useful during an asthma attack. It can also help prevent an attack from happening.

Inversions – Ex. Headstand 5 (*Shirshasana 5*), also known as Tripod Headstand pg. 541. Inversions help promote proper movement of the diaphragm during an exhalation. Since the majority of the body is upside down, gravity works with the exhalation, not against it.

Inversions on the shoulders – Ex. Ear Pressure Pose (*Karnapidasana*) pg. 562. Inversions on the shoulders compress the neck and chest, especially when the knees are bent toward the head. This compression restricts your breathing and may cause an asthma attack.

Backbends on the chin and chest – Ex. Inverted Locust Pose (*Viparita Shalabhasana*) pg. 612. These poses compress the throat and restrict your breathing, and may cause an asthma attack.

Seated forward bends – Ex. Western Intense Stretch Pose (*Paschimottanasana*) pg. 304. These poses compress the lungs and restrict your breathing, and may cause an asthma attack.

Cardio-intense poses – Ex. Crocodile Pose (*Nakrasana*) pg. 451. Poses that require a lot of strength and that are demanding on the cardiovascular system can cause shortness and shallowness of breath, and may cause an asthma attack.

Intense backbends – Ex. Little Thunderbolt Pose (*Laghuvajrasana*) pg. 480. These poses can be stimulating and cause shortness of breath if you have asthma. It is recommended to start with mild backbends and progress into deeper ones slowly, according to how your body feels.

Arm balances with both feet off the floor – Ex. Uneven Half Repose Pose Dedicated to Ashtavakra (*Vishama Ardha Shayana Ashtavakrasana*) pg. 518. These types of poses require a lot of strength and endurance and may cause shortness of breath.

4. Neck Pain

Yoga practice can help prevent and relieve neck pain. The combination of gentle stretches and strengthening movements can open up tight muscles in the body, increasing neck flexibility and rebalancing postural muscles. Simple and slow movements will lubricate the neck and increase its range of movement. Hold each pose for 30 to 90 seconds.

While it's important to strengthen and stretch the neck muscles in order to help prevent neck injury, if you already have a neck concern it's best not to aggravate it. Poses that are most strenuous for the neck are the ones that bear the majority of the body's weight on the head or neck.

Seated neck stretches – Ex. Easy Pose with Neck Stretch (*Sukhasana*) pg. 258. Neck pain can be caused by tension in the neck muscles. Stretching these muscles can help prevent or reduce neck pain.

Seated twists – Ex. Pose Dedicated to Bharadvaja 1 (*Bharadvajasana 1*) pg. 343. Muscles in the neck are connected to the muscles in the upper back. Seated twists increase the range of motion in the upper back and neck and can help prevent or reduce neck pain caused by tension in these areas.

Poses on hands and knees – Ex. Going from Tiger Pose (*Vyaghrasana*), modification knee to the forehead, pg. 429 to Tiger Pose (*Vyaghrasana*), also known as Cat Tilt pg. 432, top. Rounding the back and then going into a mild backbend can help strengthen the neck muscles and stretch the front of the neck (in Dog Tilt) and the back of the neck (in Cat Tilt).

Hand position of the pose dedicated to Garuda – Ex. Hand Position of the Pose Dedicated to Garuda in Hero Pose (*Hasta Garudasana in Virasana*) pg. 338. Any pose with this hand position helps stretch the upper back and back shoulder heads and can help prevent neck pain caused by tension in the muscles of the upper back.

Full inversions – Ex. Revolved Leg Position of One-Legged King Pigeon 1 Version B in Headstand 5 (*Parivritta Pada Eka Pada Raja Kapotasana 1 B in Shirshasana 5*) pg. 542, One-Legged Unsupported Whole Body Pose (*Eka Pada Niralamba Sarvangasana*), also known as Shoulderstand pg. 554 Full inversions with the head on the floor put strain on the neck since the majority of the body weight tends to rest on the head or neck. If you have a neck injury, it's best to avoid these.

Backbends with feet and head on the floor – Ex. Inverted Tip Toe Bow Pose (*Viparita Prapada Dhanurasana*), also known as Headstand Bow Pose (*Shirsha Dhanurasana*) pg. 489. Backbends with head and feet on the floor require a lot of neck strength and should be avoided if you have a neck concern.

5. High Blood Pressure

If you think you may be at risk or have already been diagnosed with high blood pressure, it is advisable to speak with your health care provider. Practicing yoga may help with blood pressure management since it combines the benefits of meditation, muscle relaxation, and strength training exercise. When practicing yoga poses, ensure that you are able to breathe comfortably and deeply. If you have any difficulty breathing, come out of the pose and rest or perform an easier version of the pose. If difficulty breathing persists, then consult your health care provider immediately.

Seated backbends – Ex. Hands Bound Lotus Pose (*Baddha Hasta Padmasana*) pg. 264. Seated backbends gently open the chest and improve the flow of oxygen to the lungs. They release tension in the chest and front shoulder heads often caused by stress and hunching over a computer on a daily basis. This can help lower high blood pressure that is a result of stress.

Seated twists – Ex. Revolved Easy Pose (*Parivritta Sukhasana*) pg. 258. Seated twists help release tension from the upper back and detoxify the body. This can help lower high blood pressure that is a result of tension in the upper back.

Supine forward bends – Ex. Reclining Both Hands to the Leg Pose (*Supta Dwi Hasta Padasana*) pg. 695. Supine forward bends stretch the hamstrings without increasing blood pressure, as opposed to standing forward bends where the head is below the heart. This can help lower high blood pressure that is a result of muscle tension of the lower back and legs.

Inversions – Ex. Feet Spread Out Intense Stretch Pose 2 (*Prasarita Padottanasana 2*) pg. 111 and Crane Pose in Headstand 5 Prep. (*Bakasana in Shirshasana 5 Prep.*) pg. 543. Inversions should be avoided if you have high blood pressure that is not controlled. They are very stimulating postures since the head is below the heart, which causes an increased demand for oxygen. These increase blood flow and heart rate, generating pressure to the blood vessels of the brain, and may cause blood pressure to rise dramatically.

Lunges with back knee off the floor – Ex. Revolved Son of Anjani (Lord Hanuman) Lunge Pose with Hands in Prayer (*Parivritta Anjaneyasana Namaskar*) pg. 190. These poses can require a lot of lower body strength if you are not used to practicing them. They can raise the heart rate and increase blood pressure.

Arm balances with both feet off the floor – Ex. Leg Position of Cow Face Pose in Pendant Pose (*Pada Gomukhasana in Lolasana*) pg. 508. These poses are demanding on the upper body and may increase heart rate, which can increase blood pressure.

Backbends with hands and feet on the floor – Ex. Elevated Both Legs Inverted Staff Pose (*Utthita Dwi Pada Viparita Dandasana*) pg. 497. Poses such as these can be demanding on the upper body and can elevate blood pressure by increasing heart rate.

6. Menstruation

During a period, uterine contractions can cause painful cramps in the lower abdomen and lower back. Yoga can help release endorphins to relax the body. Stretch out the lower body and back to help release the pain. Forward bends, inside hip openers, and gentle twists can help relieve the symptoms of menstruation.

Some are of the opinion that inversions can cause engorgement in the blood vessels of the uterus, which may increase blood flow, and should be avoided during a period. On the other hand, B.K.S. Iyengar's book *The Path to Holistic Health* recommends inversions during a period to reduce blood flow. You should listen to your own body and judge accordingly. If you are not feeling strong, engage in a slower-paced yoga pose practice.

Supine hip openers – Ex. Universal All-Encompassing Diamond Pose (*Vishvavajrasana*) pg. 680. Poses such as this open up the hips and groin and allow the lumbar spine to rest, which can help relieve the menstrual discomfort.

Low squats – Ex. One Leg Bound Garland Pose (*Eka Pada Baddha Malasana*) pg. 239. Practice poses such as this to stretch out the groin, the chest, and front shoulders. Releasing tension from those areas can help relieve menstrual discomfort.

Seated hip openers – Ex. One Legged King Pigeon Pose 1 Prep. (*Eka Pada Raja Kapotasana 1 Prep.*) pg. 370. Poses such as this help open up the hip and stretch the lower abdomen, which can help relieve menstrual discomfort due to tension in that area.

Backbends on the knees – Ex. Camel Pose (*Ushtrasana*) pg. 475. Poses such as this can help stretch out the lower abdomen and release tension from that region, which can help relieve menstrual discomfort.

Gentle seated twists – Ex. Easy Lord of The Fishes Pose Prep. (*Sukha Matsyendrasana Prep.*) pg. 309. Seated twists stimulate internal organs and can help relieve the symptoms of menstruation by gently encouraging the natural blood flow during menstruation.

Arm balances with hands and feet on the floor – Ex. Four Limbed Staff Pose (*Chaturanga Dandasana*) pg. 451. Poses such as this are very demanding on the upper body and core, and may worsen the symptoms of menstruation due to overstraining.

Arm balances with both feet off the floor – Ex. Pose Dedicated to Galava, One-Legged Variation (*Eka Pada Galavasana*) pg. 514. These poses demand a lot of strength and may worsen the symptoms of menstruation due to overstraining.

High squats – Ex. Tip Toe Fierce Pose (*Prapada Utkatasana*) pg. 209. Poses such as this are demanding on the legs and core, and may worsen the symptoms of menstruation due to overstraining.

Backbends on hands and feet – Ex. Partridge Pose (*Kapinjalasana*) pg. 462. Intense backbends put a lot of strain on the body, because they engage the entire body. They may worsen the symptoms of menstruation due to overstraining.

7. Pregnancy

Don't engage in a vigorous yoga practice with jump-through and jump-back *Vinyasas*. Jumping is dangerous during pregnancy. Avoid hot yoga classes that can dangerously elevate your core temperature or cause dehydration. After giving birth, be mindful when going into deep stretches. The levels of relaxin (the hormone that loosens the muscles and joints to accommodate birth) in the body may still be high, increasing the danger of injury due to overstretching. If you had a C-section, make sure the wound heals properly. Avoid doing any intense twists or backbends, as they may interfere with healing of the wound.

Seated inner hip openers – Ex. Knees Spread Wide Hero Pose (*Prasarita Janu Virasana*) pg. 343. Poses such as this stretch out the inner hips without compressing the abdomen.

Wide-legged squats – Ex. Lotus Hand Seal in Upward Hands Pose Dedicated to Goddess Kali (*Padma Mudra Urdhva Hasta Kalyasana*) pg. 99. Wide-legged squats strengthen quadriceps (front of the thighs), hamstrings (back of the thighs), and glutes (buttocks) without putting pressure onto the abdomen.

Standing side bends – Ex. Extended Side Angle Pose (*Utthita Parshva Konasana*) pg. 135. Standing side bends stretch out the side of the torso and lower back while strengthening the legs without putting pressure onto the abdomen.

Poses on hands and knees – Ex. Tiger Pose (*Vyaghrasana*) pg. 427. Poses on hands and knees can be done during pregnancy because they do not compress the abdomen.

Mild backbends on the knees – Ex. Half Camel Pose (*Ardha Ushtrasana*) pg. 476. Mild backbends can be practiced during pregnancy since they don't compress the abdomen.

Inversions – Ex. Repose Pose (*Shayanasana*) pg. 528. Don't do any inversions where your heart is above your head beyond the first trimester. Turning your body upside down creates pressure on your internal organs and may be damaging to the developing fetus.

Forward bend twists – Ex. Two Hands Revolved Western Intense Stretch Pose (*Dwi Hasta Parivritta Paschimottanasana*) pg. 306. Don't do any forward bends or twists that compress the abdomen and squeeze the fetus and placenta.

Core poses – Ex. Revolved Boat Pose (*Parivritta Navasana*) pg. 397. Don't do strenuous core poses that compress the abdomen.

Prone poses – Ex. One-Legged Pose Dedicated to Siddhar Konganar (*Eka Pada Konganarasana*) pg. 597. Avoid prone poses since they put a lot of pressure on the abdomen.

Supine poses where the back is flat on the floor – Ex. Reclined Leg Position of Cow Face Pose (*Supta Pada Gomukhasana*) pg. 679. Supine poses with the back flat on the floor take out the natural curve in the lumbar spine that is present during pregnancy and can compress the fetus and placenta.

Intense backbends – Ex. One-Legged Pigeon Pose (*Eka Pada Kapotasana*) pg. 483. Intense backbends create too much stretch in the abdomen and should be avoided during pregnancy.

8. Menopause

Common symptoms of menopause such as hot flashes and mood swings can be alleviated with regular yoga pose practice. Focus on poses that open up the pelvic area as well as mediation to help control stress.

Avoid practicing hot yoga and avoid overexertion. Both can trigger menopause symptoms. It is recommended to avoid vigorous Sun Salutes, as they can increase body temperature and cause hot flashes.

Mild supine backbends – Ex. Bridge Whole Body Pose (*Setu Bandha Sarvangasana*) pg. 658. Mild backbends open up the chest and heart area. They can help balance blood pressure and hormonal secretions as well as help relieve mood swings and hot flashes.

Supine hip openers – Ex. Reclined Bound Angle Pose (*Supta Baddha Konasana*) pg. 674. These poses open up the chest, heart and pelvic areas. Blood flow is increased into the pelvic area and reproductive organs and that can help balance hormonal functions. These poses can help relieve high blood pressure, headaches, and breathing problems.

Supine thigh openers – Ex. Reclined Hero Pose (*Supta Virasana*) pg. 692. Poses such as this can help improve blood circulation in the ovarian region and stimulate the pelvic organs, which can help balance hormonal functions and relieve the symptoms of menopause.

Backbends on hands and feet – Ex. Tip Toe One Hand Upward Bow Pose (*Prapada Eka Hasta Urdhva Dhanurasana*) pg. 497. Poses such as these can be too strenuous on the upper body (arms and shoulders). They can raise the body temperature and cause hot flashes.

Core poses – Ex. Boat Pose (*Navasana*) pg. 391. Avoid any vigorous core yoga poses, as it creates too much tension around the abdominal organs and may worsen the menopause symptoms.

Standing twists – Ex. Revolved Side Angle (*Parivritta Parshvakonasana*) pg. 141. Avoid any intense twists, as it creates too much compression around the internal organs of the torso, which may worsen the menopause symptoms.

Inversions – Ex. Headstand 1 (*Shirshasana 1*) pg. 534. Avoid any full inversions, as they increase blood flow to the internal organs of the torso and raise heart rate which may cause hot flashes.

Standing Poses

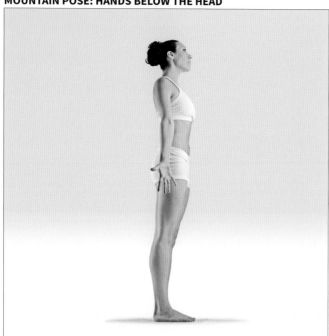

Mountain Pose

Tadasana

(tuh-DAHS-uh-nuh)

Also Known As: Equal Steady Standing, State of Balance (Samasthiti)

Modification: palms rotated forward

Pose Type: standing

Drishti Point: Nasagrai or Nasagre (nose)

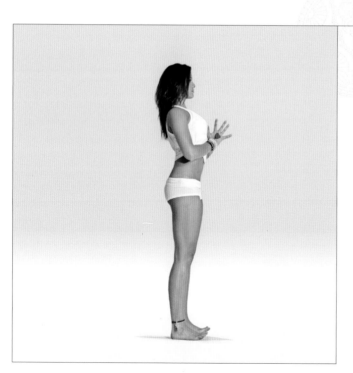

Mountain Pose with Hands in Prayer

Tadasana Namaskar

(tuh-DAHS-uh-nuh nuh-muhs-KAHR)

Modification: hands in Anjali Mudra (Hands in Prayer); feet to the front, toes lifted

Pose Type: standing

Drishti Point: Nasagrai or Nasagre (nose)

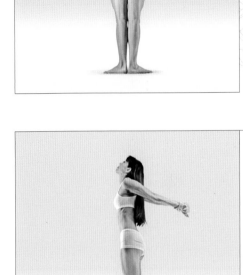

Reverse Prayer Mountain Pose

Viparita Namaskar Tadasana

(vi-puh-REE-tuh nuh-muhs-KAR tuh-DAHS-uh-nuh)

Also Known As: Penguin Pose, Back of the Body Prayer Mountain Pose
(Paschima Namaskara Tadasana)

Modification: feet rotated out

Pose Type: standing

Drishti Point: Nasagrai or Nasagre (nose)

Hands Bound Mountain Pose

Baddha Hasta Tadasana

(BUH-duh HUH-stuh tuh-DAHS-uh-nuh)

Pose Type: standing

Drishti Point: Bhrumadhye or Ajna Chakra (third eye, between the eyebrows)

MOUNTAIN POSE: HANDS ABOVE THE HEAD & TANDAVA AND LASYA DANCE MODIFICATIONS

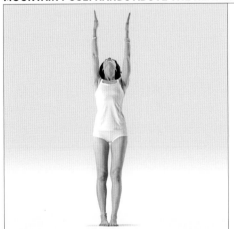

Upward Salute Pose

Urdhva Hastasana

(OORD-vuh huh-STAHS-uh-nuh)

Also Known As: Volcano Pose

Modification: arms shoulder width apart

Pose Type: standing, mild backbend

Drishti Point: Angushtamadhye or Angushta Ma Dyai (thumbs)

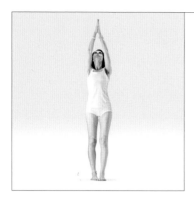

Upward Salute Pose

Urdhva Hastasana

(OORD-vuh huh-STAHS-uh-nuh)

Also Known As: Volcano Pose
Modification: palms pressed together
Pose Type: standing, mild backbend
Drishti Point: Angushtamadhye or Angushta Ma Dyai (thumbs)

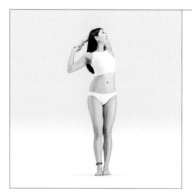

Mountain Pose—Raised Bound Hands

Tadasana Urdhva Baddha Hastasana

(tuh-DAHS-uh-nuh OORD-vuh BUH-duh huh-STAHS-uh-nuh)

Also Known As: Mountain Pose (Parvatasana)
Pose Type: standing
Drishti Point: Nasagrai or Nasagre (nose)

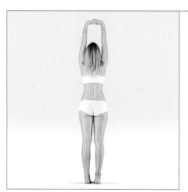

Mountain Pose

Tadasana

(tuh-DAHS-uh-nuh)

Modification: shoulder opener, intense version
Pose Type: standing
Drishti Point: Parshva Drishti (to the right), Parshva Drishti (to the left)

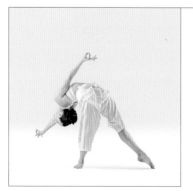

Pose Inspired by Parvati's Graceful Dance

Lasyasana

(lahs-YAHS-uh-nuh)

Modification: both legs straight; one leg extended to the front, heel up; one arm up over the head reaching to the floor, other arm reaching up to the sky; deep backbend
Pose Type: standing, backbend
Drishti Point: Bhrumadhye or Ajna Chakra (third eye, between the eyebrows)

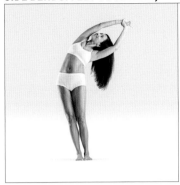

Standing Crescent Pose

Indudalasana

(in-doo-duh-LAHS-uh-nuh)

Modification: grabbing onto the wrist of the top hand
Pose Type: standing, side bend
Drishti Point: Urdhva or Antara Drishti (up to the sky)

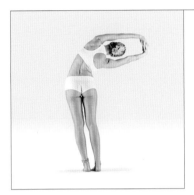

Sideways Mountain Pose— Raised Bound Hands

Parshva Tadasana Urdhva Baddha Hastasana

(PAHRSH-vuh tuh-DAHS-uh-nuh OORD-vuh BUH-duh HUH-STAHS-uh-nuh)

Also Known As: Side Bending Pose (Parshva Bhangi)
Pose Type: standing, side bend
Drishti Point: Nasagrai or Nasagre (nose)

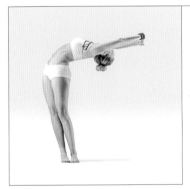

Revolved Upward Mountain Pose— Raised Bound Hands

Parivritta Urdhva Tadasana Urdhva Baddha Hastasana

(puh-ri-VRIT-tuh OORD-vuh tuh-DAHS-uh-nuh OORD-vuh BUH-duh HUH-STAHS-uh-nuh)

Also Known As: Side Bending Pose (Parshva Bhangi)
Pose Type: standing, side bend, backbend
Drishti Point: Angushtamadhye or Angushta Ma Dyai (thumbs)

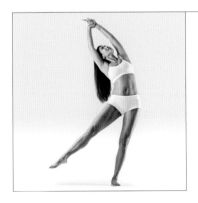

One-Legged Standing Crescent Pose

Eka Pada Indudalasana

(EY-kuh PUH-duh in-doo-LAHS-uh-nuh)

Modification: grabbing onto the wrist
Pose Type: standing one-legged balance, side bend
Drishti Point: Urdhva or Antara Drishti (up to the sky)

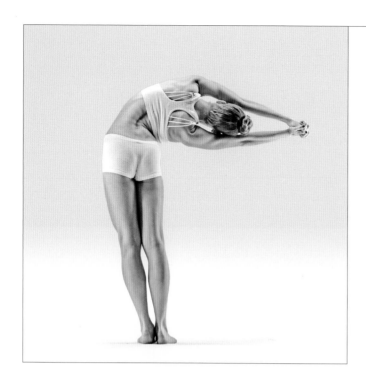

Side Stretch Pose

Parshvasana
(pahrsh-VAH-suh-nuh)

Modification: fingers interlocked, palms pressed together
Pose Type: standing, side bend
Drishti Point: Nasagrai or Nasagre (nose), Urdhva or Antara Drishti (up to the sky)

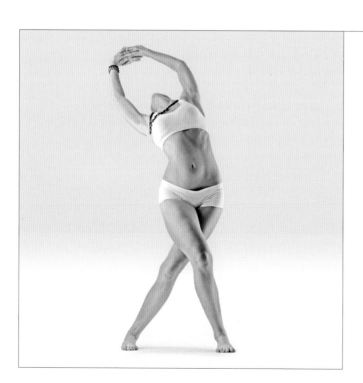

Pose Inspired by Shiva's Vigorous Cycle of Life Dance

Tandavasana
(tahn-duh-VAHS-suh-nuh)

Modification: heels down, legs crossed, arms up over the head
Pose Type: standing, side bend, backbend
Drishti Point: Angushtamadhye or Angushta Ma Dyai (thumbs)

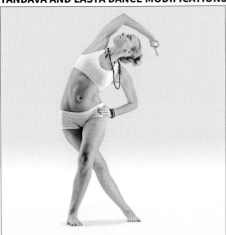

Pose Inspired by Parvati's Graceful Dance

Lasyasana

(lahs-YAHS-uh-nuh)

Modification: legs crossed, knees bent; one hand on the hip, one arm over the head

Pose Type: standing, side bend

Drishti Point: Urdhva or Antara Drishti (up to the sky)

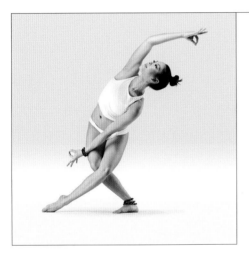

Pose Inspired by Parvati's Graceful Dance

Lasyasana

(lahs-YAHS-uh-nuh)

Modification: front leg ankle stretch, both knees bent, legs crossed, one arm toward the opposite knee, other arm up over the head

Pose Type: standing, side bend

Drishti Point: Urdhva or Antara Drishti (up to the sky)

SIDE BENDS: ONE ARM UP OVER THE HEAD, OTHER ARM ALONG THE SIDE OF TORSO

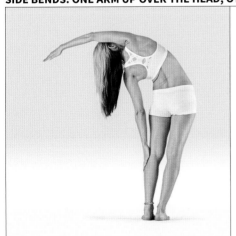

One Hand Side Stretch Pose

Eka Hasta Parshvasana

(EY-kuh HUH-stuh pahrsh-VAH-suh-nuh)

Modification: one arm up over the head, other hand sliding down the leg

Pose Type: standing, side bend

Drishti Point: Urdhva or Antara Drishti (up to the sky)

1.

Swaying Palm Tree Pose

Tiryak Tala-Vrikshasana

(TIR-yuhk TAHL-uh-vrik-SHAHS-uh-nuh)
Pose Type: standing, side bend
Drishti Point: Hastagrai or Hastagre (hands)

Modification: elbow of the top arm bent
1. mild version
2. intense version

tiryak = horizontally, sideways, obliquely, across
tala-vrikshasana = palm tree

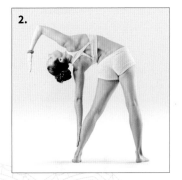

2.

How to Perform the Pose:

1. Begin by standing in Mountain Pose (*Tadasana*). Engage your *mula bandha*, *uddhiyana bandha*, and *ujjayi* breathing.

2. Inhale; step your feet slightly wider than shoulder-distance apart with toes facing forward and feet parallel to each other. Expand your chest and hold your arms straight out to the sides, parallel to the floor.

3. Exhale as you side bend to the left, dropping your left hand either to the side of the left thigh or the left shin. (Avoid putting pressure on the knee joint.) Bring your right arm over head and bend it at the elbow.

4. Inhale as you rotate your chest up to the sky; do not collapse it forward. Feel the deep stretch on the right side of your torso as you look toward your right hand (Pose #1).

5. On your next exhale, try to reach your right arm over your head with fingertips pointing toward the floor (Pose #2).

6. Hold the pose for at least 30, and up to 90, seconds in order to receive the full benefits of the stretch. Exhale as you release the pose. Inhale as you press strongly into both feet to come up.

7. Exhale, come back to Mountain Pose (*Tadasana*), and repeat on the left side.

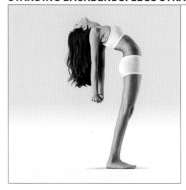

Hands Bound Rising Standing Locust Pose

Baddha Hasta Utthita Stiti Shalabhasana

(BUH-duh HUH-stuh UT-ti-tuh STI-ti shuh-luh-BAHS-uh-nuh)

Also Known As: Baddha Hasta Utthita Nindra Shalabhasana

Pose Type: standing, backbend

Drishti Point: Bhrumadhye or Ajna Chakra (third eye, between the eyebrows)

Sun Salutation Pose—Raised Bound Hands

Surya Namaskarasana Urdhva Baddha Hastasana

SOOR-yuh nuh-muhs-kahr-AHS-uh-nuh OORD-vuh BUH-duh huh-STAHS-uh-nuh)

Pose Type: standing, backbend

Drishti Point: Angushtamadhye or Angushta Ma Dyai (thumbs)

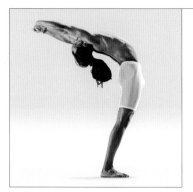

Rising Standing Cobra Pose

Utthita Stiti Bhujangasana

(UT-ti-tuh STI-ti bu-juhng-AHS-uh-nuh)

Also Known As: Utthita Nindra Bhujangasana

Modification: toes down, hands on the front of the knees

Pose Type: standing, backbend

Drishti Point: Bhrumadhye or Ajna Chakra (third eye, between the eyebrows)

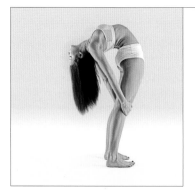

Sun Salutation Pose

Surya Namaskarasana

(SOOR-yuh nuh-muhs-kahr-AHS-uh-nuh)

Modification: palms facing up

Pose Type: standing, backbend

Drishti Point: Angushtamadhye or Angushta Ma Dyai (thumbs)

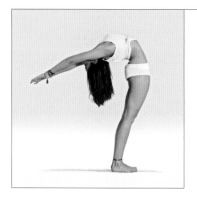

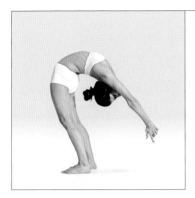

Sun Salutation Pose

Surya Namaskarasana

(SOOR-yuh nuh-muhs-kahr-AHS-uh-nuh-uh-nuh)

Modification: fingers interlocked, pointer fingers out

Pose Type: standing, backbend

Drishti Point: Angushtamadhye or Angushta Ma Dyai (thumbs)

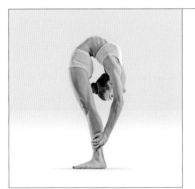

Reverse Facing Intense Stretch Pose

Tiryang Mukhottanasana

(TEER-yuhng mu-ko-tahn-AHS-uh-nuh)

Also Known As: Full Wheel Pose (Purna Chakrasana)

Modification: grabbing onto the shins

Pose Type: standing, backbend

Drishti Point: Bhrumadhye or Ajna Chakra (third eye, between the eyebrows)

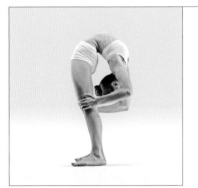

Reverse Facing Intense Stretch Pose

Tiryang Mukhottanasana

(TEER-yuhng mu-ko-tahn-AHS-uh-nuh)

Modification: grabbing onto the front of the knees

Pose Type: standing, backbend

Drishti Point: Bhrumadhye or Ajna Chakra (third eye, between the eyebrows)

STANDING BACKBENDS: KNEES BENT

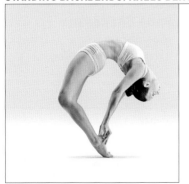

Standing Upward Facing Intense Ankle Stretch Bow Pose

Stiti Urdhva Mukgattana Kulpa Dhanurasana

(STI-ti OORD-vuh mu-ko-TAH-nuh KUL-puh duh-nur-AHS-uh-nuh)

Also Known As: Nindra Urdhva Mukgattana Kulpa Dhanurasana

Modification: hands to the heels

Pose Type: standing, backbend, balance

Drishti Point: Bhrumadhye or Ajna Chakra (third eye, between the eyebrows)

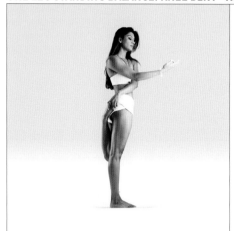

One Hand to Foot Rising Standing One-Legged Frog Pose

Eka Hasta Pada Utthita Stiti Eka Pada Bhekasana

(EY-kuh HUH-stuh PUH-duh UT-ti-tuh STI-ti EY-kuh PUH-duh bey-KAHS-uh-nuh)

Also Known As: Eka Hasta Pada Utthita Nindra Eka Pada Bhekasana

Modification: grabbing onto the foot, arm crossed in front; foot toward the glutes

Pose Type: standing one-legged balance, binding

Drishti Point: Hastagrai or Hastagre (hands)

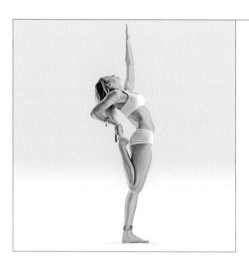

Lord of the Dance Pose

Natarajasana

(NAH-tuh-rahj-AHS-uh-nuh)

Modification: one hand to foot, foot toward the glutes

Pose Type: standing one-legged balance, backbend

Drishti Point: Hastagrai or Hastagre (hands)

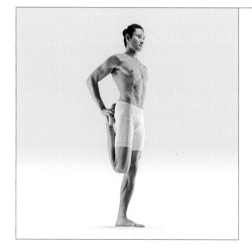

Both Hands to Foot Rising Standing One-Legged Frog Pose

Dwi Hasta Pada Utthita Stiti Eka Pada Bhekasana

(dwi -huh-stuh PUH-duh UT-ti-tuh STI-ti EY-kuh PUH-duh bey-KAHS uh-nuh)

Also Known As: Dwi Hasta Pada Utthita Nindra Eka Pada Bhekasana

Pose Type: standing one-legged balance

Drishti Point: Nasagrai or Nasagre (nose)

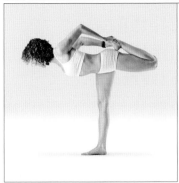

Bowing with Respect
Lord of the Dance Pose

Nantum Natarajasana
(NUHN-tum NAH-tuh-rahj-AHS-uh-nuh)
Modification: half forward bend, both hands to the back foot, foot toward the glutes
Pose Type: standing one-legged balance, forward bend
Drishti Point: Nasagrai or Nasagre (nose)

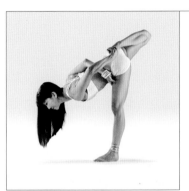

Half Bound Bowing with Respect
Lord of the Dance Pose

Ardha Baddha Nantum Natarajasana
(UHR-duh BUH-duh NUHN-tum NAH-tuh-rahj-AHS-uh-nuh)
Modification: grabbing onto the back foot with opposite hand
Pose Type: standing one-legged balance, forward bend, binding
Drishti Point: Nasagrai or Nasagre (nose)

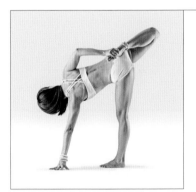

Half Moon Bow Pose Prep.

Ardha Chandrachapasana Prep.
(UHR-duh CHUHN-druh-chahp-AHS-uh-nuh)
Modification: grabbing onto the back foot with the hand on the same side
Pose Type: standing one-legged balance, forward bend, twist
Drishti Point: Urdhva or Antara Drishti (up to the sky)

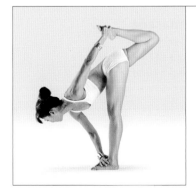

Hand to Foot Revolved Half Moon Bow Pose

Hasta Pada Parivritta Ardha Chandrachapasana
(HUH-stuh PUH-duh puh-ri-VRIT-tuh UHR-duh CHUHN-druh-chahp-AHS-uh-nuh)
Also Known As: Lord of the Dance Pose Modification (Natarajasana)
Pose Type: standing one-legged balance, forward bend, twist
Drishti Point: Parshva Drishti (to the right), Parshva Drishti (to the left)

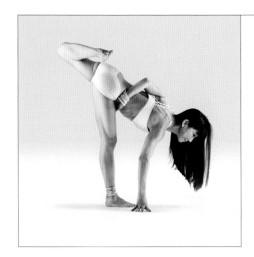

Half Bound Unsupported Bound One-Legged Intense Stretch Pose Prep.

Ardha Baddha Niralamba Baddha Eka Pada Uttanasana Prep.

(UHR-duh BUH-duh nir-ah-LUHM-buh BUH-duh EY-kuh PUH-duh ut-tahn-AHS-uh-nuh)

Also Known As: Lord of the Dance Pose Prep. Modification (Natarajasana Prep.) and Half Bound Unsupported Bound One-Legged Forward Bend Prep.

Modification: one hand to the floor

Pose Type: standing one-legged balance, forward bend, binding

Drishti Point: Hastagrai or Hastagre (hands), Nasagrai or Nasagre (nose)

ONE LEG STANDING BALANCE: KNEE BENT—HEEL TO THE SITTING BONES—FORWARD BEND

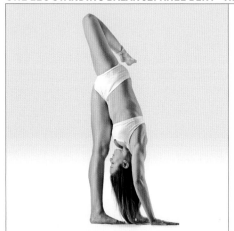

One Leg Stretched Upward Pose Prep.

Urdhva Prasarita Ekapadasana Prep.

(OORD-vuh pruh-SAH-ri-tuh EY-kuh-puh-DAHS-uh-nuh)

Modification: top leg bent, heel toward the glutes; both palms to the floor

Pose Type: standing one-legged balance, forward bend

Drishti Point: Padayoragrai or Padayoragre (toes/feet), Nasagrai or Nasagre (nose)

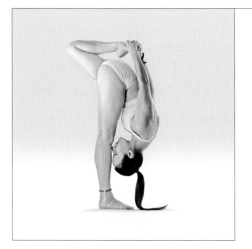

Unsupported Bound One Foot Intense Stretch Pose

Niralamba Baddha Eka Pada Uttanasana

(nir-ah-LUHM-buh BUH-duh EY-kuh PUH-duh ut-TAHS-uh-nuh)

Also Known As: Unsupported Bound One Foot Full Forward Bend

Pose Type: standing one-legged balance, forward bend

Drishti Point: Nasagrai or Nasagre (nose)

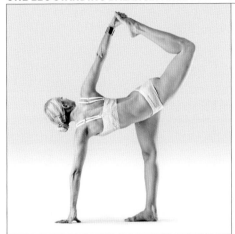

Revolved Half Moon Bow Pose

Parivritta Ardha Chandrachapasana

(puh-ri-VRIT-tuh UHR-duh CHUHN-druh-chahp-AHS-uh-nuh)

Pose Type: standing one-legged balance, backbend, forward bend, twist

Drishti Point: Urdhva or Antara Drishti (up to the sky), Padhayoragrai or Padayoragre (toes/feet), Hastagrai or Hastagre (hands)

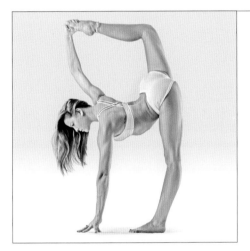

Pose Dedicated to Yogi Gitananda

Gitanandasana

(geet-ah-nuhn-DAHS-uh-nuh)

Also Known As: Lord of the Dance Pose Modification (Natarajasana)

Modification: foot away from the head

Pose Type: standing one-legged balance, backbend, forward bend

Drishti Point: Hastagrai or Hastagre (hands)

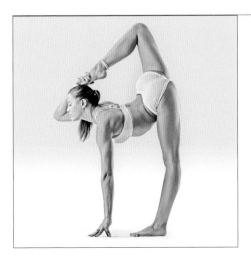

Pose Dedicated to Yogi Gitananda

Gitanandasana

(geet-ah-nuhn-DAHS-uh-nuh)

Also Known As: Lord of the Dance Pose Modification (Natarajasana)

Modification: foot to the head

Pose Type: standing one-legged balance, backbend, forward bend

Drishti Point: Bhrumadhye or Ajna Chakra (third eye, between the eyebrows)

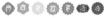

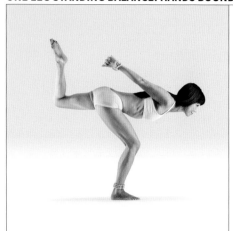

Toppling Tree Pose

Patan Vrikshasana

(PUH-tuhn vrik-SHAHS-uh-nuh)

Modification: both knees bent

Pose Type: standing one-legged balance, forward bend

Drishti Point: Nasagrai or Nasagre (nose), Bhrumadhye or Ajna Chakra (third eye, between the eyebrows)

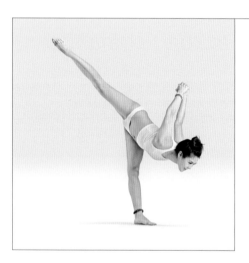

Toppling Tree Pose

Patan Vrikshasana

(PUH-tuhn vrik-SHAHS-uh-nuh)

Modification: both legs straight

Pose Type: standing one-legged balance, forward bend

Drishti Point: Nasagrai or Nasagre (nose), Bhrumadhye or Ajna Chakra (third eye, between the eyebrows)

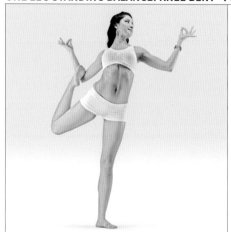

Lord of the Dance Pose Prep.

Natarajasana Prep.

(NAH-tuh-rahj-AHS-uh-nuh)

Modification: foot to the elbow crease, arms open to the sides, elbows bent

Pose Type: standing one-legged balance, backbend

Drishti Point: Hastagrai or Hastagre (hands)

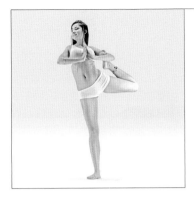

Prayer Lord of the Dance Pose

Namaskar Natarajasana

(nuh-muhs-KAHR NAH-tuh-rahj-AHS-uh-nuh)
Modification: foot to the elbow crease
Pose Type: standing one-legged balance, backbend
Drishti Point: Parshva Drishti (to the right), Parshva Drishti (to the left)

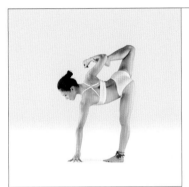

Half Moon Bow Pose Prep.

Ardha Chandrachapasana Prep.

(URH-duh chuhn-druh-chahp-AHS-uh-nuh)
Modification: foot to the elbow crease
Pose Type: standing one-legged balance, backbend, forward bend
Drishti Point: Hastagrai or Hastagre (hands)

ONE LEG STANDING BALANCE: KNEE BENT BEHIND

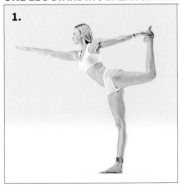

1.

Lord of the Dance Pose

Natarajasana

(NAH-tuh-rahj-AHS-uh-nuh)
Also Known As: Baby Dancer's Pose (Bala Natarajasana)
Modification: hand to the foot on the same side using an under-head grip, back knee bent
1. thigh parallel to the floor
2. thigh 45 degrees to the floor, half forward bend
Pose Type: standing one-legged balance, backbend
Drishti Point: Hastagrai or Hastagre (hands)

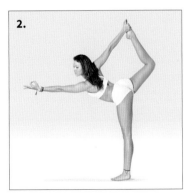

2.

1.

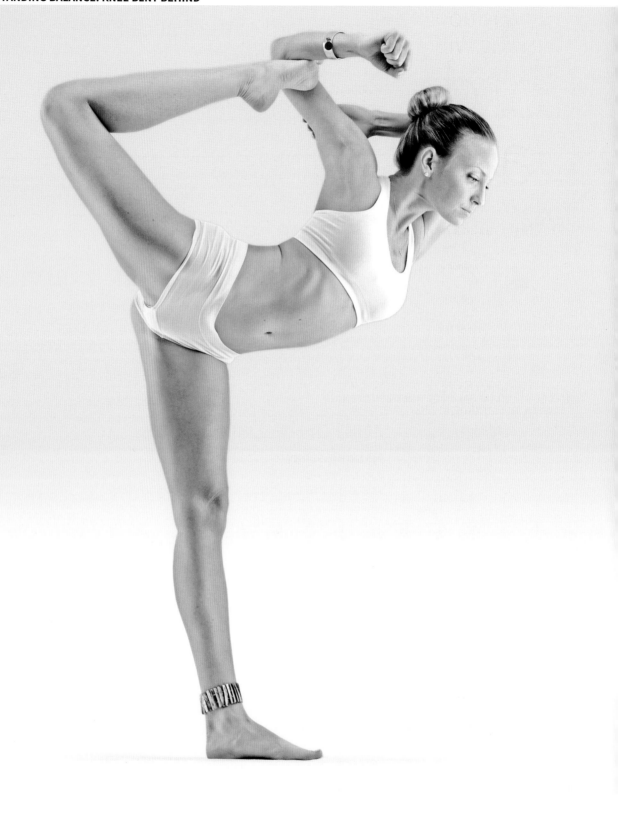

Hand Position of Mermaid Pose
in Bowing With Respect

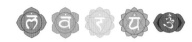

Lord of the Dance Pose

Hasta Naginyasana in Nantum Natarajasana

(HUH-stuh nuh-gin-YAHS-uh-nuh in nan-toom NAH-tuh-rahj-AHS-uh-nuh)

Pose Type: standing one legged balance, backbend, forward bend

Drishti Point: Nasagrai or Nasagre (nose) or Bhrumadhye or Ajna Chakra (third eye, between the eyebrows)

hasta = hand
naga = great mythological snake
nantum = to bow with respect
Nataraj = name of Shiva as a cosmic dancer

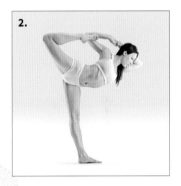

2.

How to Perform the Pose:

1. Begin by standing in Mountain Pose (*Tadasana*). Engage your *mula bandha*, *uddhiyana bandha*, and *ujjayi* breathing.

2. Inhale and bring your weight onto the left foot. Exhale as you bend your right knee, grab onto the right foot with your right hand, and bring your right heel to your right sitting bone. Keep your standing leg strong and straight by pulling the knee cap up and engaging the front thigh muscles (quadriceps). Keep your knees together.

3. On the next exhale, start pushing your right foot back and up to the sky, while tipping your torso forward.

4. Exhale as you bring the right foot to the right elbow crease and bend your right arm to keep the foot in place.

5. Inhale as you reach your left arm out in front of you. Exhale, bend the left elbow, and grab onto the right hand with your left hand (Pose #2). This is the arm position of Mermaid Pose (*Hasta Naginyasana*).

6. To deepen the shoulder stretch, on the next exhale start walking your left hand down your left forearm. Grab first onto the left elbow and then to your left tricep (Pose #1).

7. Hold the pose for at least 30, and up to 90, seconds in order to receive the full benefits of the stretch. Exhale as you release the pose, come back to Mountain Pose (*Tadasana*), and repeat on the right side.

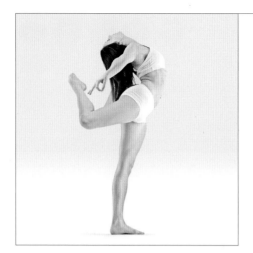

Open Heart Lord of the Dance Pose

Anahata Chakra Natarajasana

(uhn-AH-huh-tuh CHUHK-ruh NAH-tuh-rahj-AHS-uh-nuh)

Modification: back knee bent, arms open to the sides, foot working toward the head

Pose Type: standing one-legged balance, backbend

Drishti Point: Bhrumadhye or Ajna Chakra (third eye, between the eyebrows)

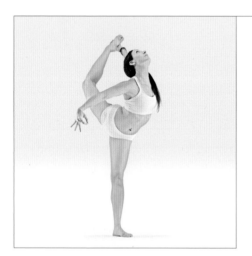

Lord of the Dance Pose

Natarajasana

(NAH-tuh-rahj-AHS-uh-nuh)

Modification: hand to opposite foot using an under-head grip, back knee bent

Pose Type: standing one-legged balance, backbend

Drishti Point: Bhrumadhye or Ajna Chakra (third eye, between the eyebrows)

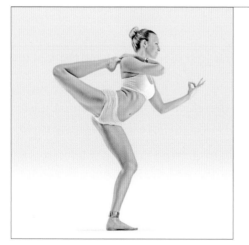

Lord of the Dance Pose

Natarajasana

(NAH-tuh-rahj-AHS-uh-nuh)

Modification: standing leg bent, heel to the floor; hand to the foot on the same side using an overhead grip, foot to the shoulder

Pose Type: standing one-legged balance, backbend

Drishti Point: Hastagrai or Hastagre (hands)

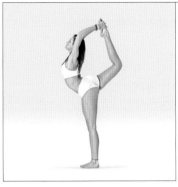

Lord of the Dance Pose

Natarajasana

(NAH-tuh-rahj-AHS-uh-nuh)

Also Known As: Lord of the Dance Pose 1 (Natarajasana 1)

Modification: both hands grabbing onto the back foot with overhead grip, foot away from the head

Pose Type: standing one-legged balance, backbend

Drishti Point: Bhrumadhye or Ajna Chakra (third eye, between the eyebrows)

ONE LEG STANDING BALANCE: GRABBING ONTO THE BACK KNEE

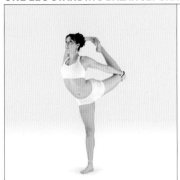

Bound Lord of the Dance Pose

Baddha Natarajasana

(BUH-duh NAH-tuh-rahj-AHS-uh-nuh)

Also Known As: Yogi Yogananda Pose (Yoganandasana)

Modification: hand binding to the knee on the same side of the body; back foot away from the head

Pose Type: standing one-legged balance, backbend

Drishti Point: Bhrumadhye or Ajna Chakra (third eye, between the eyebrows)

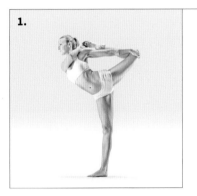
1.

Bound Lord of the Dance Pose

Baddha Natarajasana

(BUH-duh NAH-tuh-rahj-AHS-uh-nuh)

Modification: one hand binding to the knee on the same side of the body, other arm crossed in front of the neck

1. left side view
2. right side view

Pose Type: standing one-legged balance, backbend

Drishti Point: Bhrumadhye or Ajna Chakra (third eye, between the eyebrows), Nasagrai or Nasagre (nose)

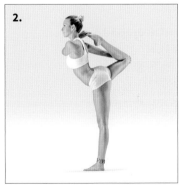
2.

Standing Poses

43

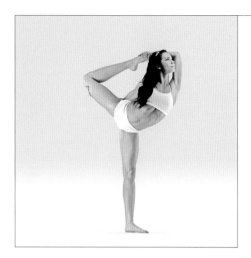

Bound Lord of the Dance Pose

Baddha Natarajasana
(BUH-duh NAH-tuh-rahj-AHS-uh-nuh)

Also Known As: Yogi Yogananda Pose (Yoganandasana)
Modification: hand binding to the inside of the thigh on the same side of the body, back foot away from the head
Pose Type: standing one-legged balance, backbend
Drishti Point: Bhrumadhye or Ajna Chakra (third eye, between the eyebrows)

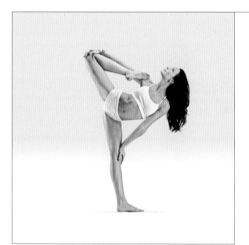

Supported Sideways Hand to Knee Lord of the Dance Pose

Salamba Parshva Hasta Janu Natarajasana
(sah-LUHM--buh PAHRSH-vuh HUH-stuh JAH-nu NAH-tuh-rahj-AHS-uh-nuh)

Pose Type: standing one-legged balance, forward bend, twist
Drishti Point: Urdhva or Antara Drishti (up to the sky)

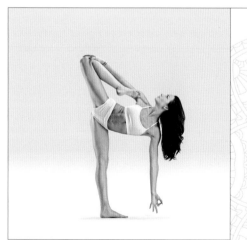

Unsupported Sideways Hand to Knee Lord of the Dance Pose

Niralamba Parshva Hasta Janu Natarajasana
(nir-ah-LUHM-buh-nuh PAHRSH-vuh HUH-stuh JAH-nu NAH-tuh-rahj-AHS-uh-nuh)

Pose Type: standing one-legged balance, forward bend, twist
Drishti Point: Urdhva or Antara Drishti (up to the sky)

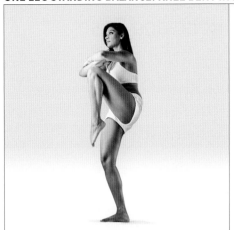

Hand Bound Rising Standing Wind Relieving Pose Prep.

Baddha Hasta Utthita Stiti Vayu Muktyasana Prep.

(BUH-duh HUH-stuh UT-ti-tuh STI-ti VAH-yu muk-TYAHS-uh-nuh)

Also Known As: Baddha Hasta Utthita Nindra Vayu Muktyasana Prep.

Modification: knee of the standing leg bent; fingertips to elbows, arms parallel to the floor, knee of the lifted leg to the forearm

Pose Type: standing one-legged balance

Drishti Point: Nasagrai or Nasagre (nose)

1.

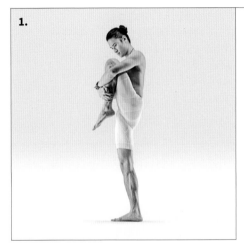

Standing Rising One-Legged Chin to Knee Pose Prep.

Stiti Utthita Eka Pada Chibi Janu Shirshasana Prep.

(STI-ti UT-ti-tuh EY-kuh PUH-duh CHI-bi JAH-nu sheer-SHAHS-uh-nuh)

Also Known As: Nindra Utthita Eka Pada Chibi Janu Shirshasana Prep.

Modification: 1. arms wrapped around the shin

2. fingers interlocked over the shin

Pose Type: standing one-legged balance, forward bend

Drishti Point: Nasagrai or Nasagre (nose)

2.

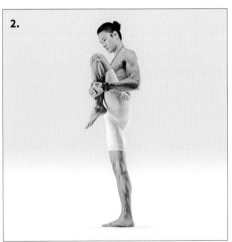

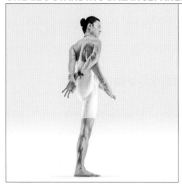

Standing Rising Wind Relieving Pose

Stiti Utthita Vayu Muktyasana

(STI-ti UT-ti-tuh VAH-yu muk-TYAHS-uh-nuh)

Also Known As: Nindra Utthita Vayu Muktyasana; Standing Pose Dedicated to Marichi (Nindra Marichyasana)

Modification: standing up straight

Pose Type: standing one-legged balance, forward bend, binding

Drishti Point: Nasagrai or Nasagre (nose)

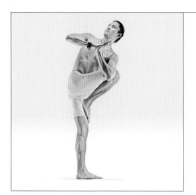

Revolved Prayer Standing Rising Wind Relieving Pose

Parivritta Namaskar Stiti Utthita Vayu Muktyasana

(puh-ri-VRIT-tuh nuh-muhs-KAHR STI-ti UT-ti-tuh VAH-yu mukTYAHS-uh-nuh)

Also Known As: Parivritta Namaskar Nindra Utthita Vayu Muktyasana

Modification: hands in Anjali Mudra (Hands in Prayer)

Pose Type: standing one-legged balance, forward bend, twist

Drishti Point: Urdhva or Antara Drishti (up to the sky)

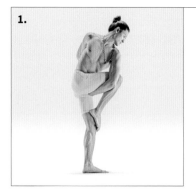

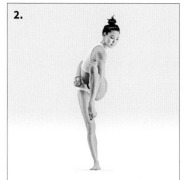

Revolved Bound Standing Rising Wind Relieving Pose

Parivritta Baddha Stiti Utthita Vayu Muktyasana

(puh-ri-VRIT-tuh BUH-duh STI-ti UT-ti-tuh VAH-yu muk-TYAHS-uh-nuh)

Also Known As: Parivritta Baddha Nindra Utthita Vayu Muktyasana

Modification: binding around the back of the thigh

1. foot on the knee
2. foot away from the knee

Pose Type: standing one-legged balance, forward bend, twist, binding

Drishti Point: Nasagrai or Nasagre (nose)

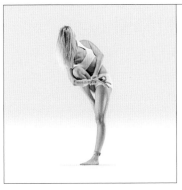

Revolved Bound Standing Rising Wind Relieving Pose

Parivritta Baddha Stiti Utthita Vayu Muktyasana

(puh-ri-VRIT-tuh BUH-duh STI-ti UT-ti-tuh VAH-yu muk-TYAHS-uh-nuh)

Also Known As: Parivritta Baddha Nindra Utthita Vayu Muktyasana

Modification: binding around the shin

Pose Type: standing one-legged balance, forward bend, twist, binding

Drishti Point: Urdhva or Antara Drishti (up to the sky)

ONE LEG STANDING BALANCE: BOTH KNEES BENT—BINDING & TWISTS

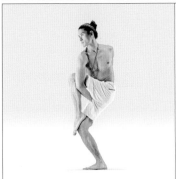

Revolved Bound Standing Rising Wind Relieving Pose Prep.

Parivritta Baddha Stiti Utthita Vayu Muktyasana Prep.

(puh-ri-VRIT-tuh BUH-duh STI-ti UT-ti-tuh VAH-yu muk-TYAHS-uh-nuh)

Also Known As: Parivritta Baddha Nindra Utthita Vayu Muktyasana Prep.

Modification: foot resting on the knee, standing leg bent

Pose Type: standing one-legged balance, forward bend, twist, binding

Drishti Point: Bhrumadhye or Ajna Chakra (third eye, between the eyebrows)

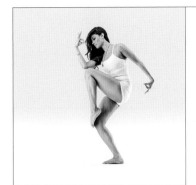

Pose Inspired by Shiva's Vigorous Cycle of Life Dance

Tandavasana

(tahn-duh-VAHS-uh-nuh)

Modification: knee to the opposite elbow, foot resting on the knee, standing leg bent, heel down

Pose Type: standing one-legged balance, forward bend, twist

Drishti Point: Nasagrai or Nasagre (nose), Hastagrai or Hastagre (hands)

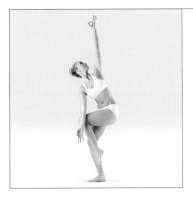

Pose Inspired by Shiva's Vigorous Cycle of Life Dance

Tandavasana

(tahn-duh-VAHS-uh-nuh)

Modification: both arms straight, one forearm to the opposite knee, other arm straight up to the sky, both knees bent

Pose Type: standing one-legged balance, forward bend, twist

Drishti Point: Hastagrai or Hastagre (hands)

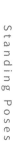

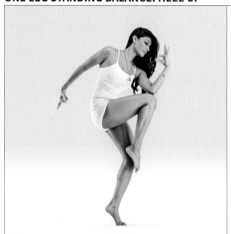

Tip Toe Pose Inspired by Shiva's Vigorous Cycle of Life Dance

Prapada Tandavasana

(PRUH-puh-duh tahn-duh-VAHS-uh-nuh)

Modification: knee to the opposite elbow, foot resting on the knee, standing leg bent

Pose Type: standing one-legged balance, forward bend, twist

Drishti Point: Nasagrai or Nasagre (nose), Hastagrai or Hastagre (hands)

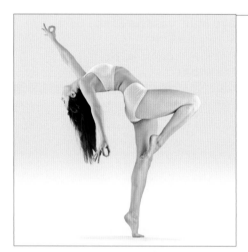

Tip Toe Pose Inspired by Parvati's Graceful Dance

Prapada Lasyasana

(PRUH-puh-duh lahs-YAHS-uh-nuh)

Modification: deep backbend, one arm reaching up to the sky, other arm reaching down to the floor; standing leg straight, other knee bent; foot to the inside of the knee of the opposite leg

Pose Type: standing one-legged balance, backbend

Drishti Point: Bhrumadhye or Ajna Chakra (third eye, between the eyebrows), Hastagrai or Hastagre (hands)

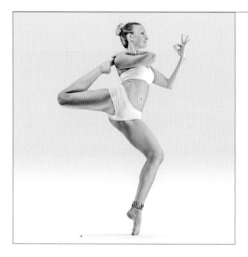

Intense Ankle Stretch Tip Toe Lord of the Dance Pose

Uttana Kulpa Prapada Natarajasana

(ut-TAHN-uh KUL-puh PRUH-puh-duh NAH-tuh-rahj-AHS-uh-nuh)

Also Known As: Tip Toe Pose Inspired by Parvati's Graceful Dance (Prapada Lasyasana)

Modification: standing leg bent, toes curled under, overhead grip, foot to the shoulder

Pose Type: standing one-legged balance, backbend

Drishti Point: Hastagrai or Hastagre (hands)

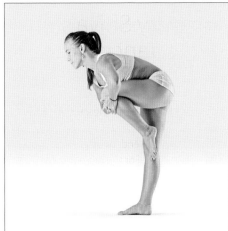

Half Standing Wind Relieving Intense Stretch Pose 1 & 2 Prep.

Ardha Stiti Vayu Muktyuttonasana 1 & 2 Prep.

(UHR-duh STI-ti VAH-yu muk-tew-ton-AHS-uh-nuh)

Also Known As: Ardha Nindra Vayu Muktyuttonasana; Standing Wind Relieving Half Forward Bend

Modification: fingers interlocked on the knee, half forward bend

Pose Type: standing one-legged balance, forward bend

Drishti Point: Nasagrai or Nasagre (nose)

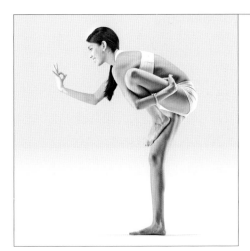

One Hand Bound Half Standing Wind Relieving Intense Stretch Pose

Eka Hasta Baddha Ardha Stiti Vayu Muktyuttonasana

(EY-kuh HUH-stuh BUH-duh UHR-duh STI-ti VAH-yu muk-tew-ton-AHS-uh-nuh)

Also Known As: Eka Hasta Baddha Ardha Nindra Vayu Muktyuttonasana; One Hand Bound Standing Wind Relieving Half Forward Bend

Modification: binding around the shin, palm to the rib cage, foot resting on the thigh of the standing leg

Pose Type: standing one-legged balance, forward bend, binding

Drishti Point: Hastagrai or Hastagre (hands)

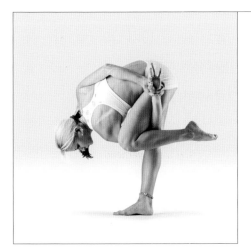

Standing Wind Relieving Intense Stretch Pose 1

Stiti Vayu Muktyuttonasana 1

(STI-ti VAH-yu muk-tew-ton-AHS-uh-nuh)

Also Known As: Nindra Vayu Muktyuttonasana; Standing Wind Relieving Half Forward Bend 1

Modification: chin away from the shin, binding on the inside of the thigh

Pose Type: standing one-legged balance, forward bend, binding

Drishti Point: Padayoragrai or Padayoragre (toes/feet)

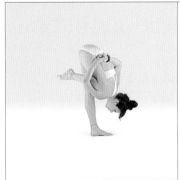

Standing Wind Relieving Intense Stretch Pose 2

Stiti Vayu Muktyuttonasana 2

(STI-ti VAH-yu muk-tew-ton-AHS-uh-nuh)

Also Known As: Nindra Vayu Muktyuttonasana; Standing Pose Dedicated to Sage Marichi (Nindra Marichyasana) and Standing Wind Relieving Full Forward Bend

Modification: chin away from the shin, binding around the shin

Pose Type: standing one-legged balance, forward bend, binding

Drishti Point: Padhayoragrai or Padayoragre (toes/feet)

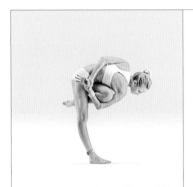

Revolved Half Standing Wind Relieving Intense Stretch Pose

Parivritta Ardha Stiti Vayu Muktyuttonasana

(puh-ri-VRIT-tuh UHR-duh STI-ti VAH-yu muk-tew-ton-AHS-uh-nuh)

Also Known As: Parivritta Ardha Nindra Vayu Muktyuttonasana; Revolved Standing Wind Relieving Half Forward Bend

Pose Type: standing one-legged balance, forward bend, twist, binding

Drishti Point: Padayoragrai or Padayoragre (toes/feet)

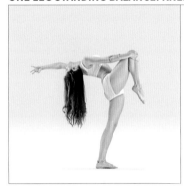

Hand to Knee Pose Inspired by Parvati's Graceful Dance

Hasta Janu Lasyasana

(HUH-stuh JAH-nu lahs-YAHS-uh-nuh)

Modification: arm up over the head and parallel to the floor

Pose Type: standing one-legged balance, backbend

Drishti Point: Bhrumadhye or Ajna Chakra (third eye, between the eyebrows), Hastagrai or Hastagre (hands)

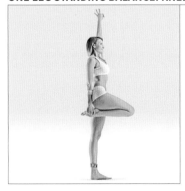

Standing One-Legged Hero Pose

Stiti Eka Pada Virasana

(STI-ti EY-kuh PUH-duh veer-AHS-uh-nuh)

Also Known As: Nindra Eka Pada Virasana; Standing One-Legged Thunderbolt Pose (Nindra Eka Pada Vajrasana)

Modification: hand grabbing onto the foot, heel toward the glutes, shin parallel to the floor, other arm up to the sky

Pose Type: standing one-legged balance

Drishti Point: Nasagrai or Nasagre (nose)

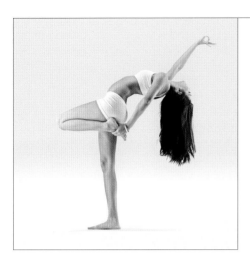

Hand to Foot Pose Inspired by Parvati's Graceful Dance

Hasta Pada Lasyasana

(HUH-stuh PUH-duh lahs-YAHS-uh-nuh)

Modification: arm up over the head reaching to the sky
Pose Type: standing one-legged balance, backbend
Drishti Point: Bhrumadhye or Ajna Chakra (third eye, between the eyebrows), Hastagrai or Hastagre (hands)

ONE LEG STANDING BALANCE: KNEE BENT, KNEES IN LINE, FORWARD BENDS

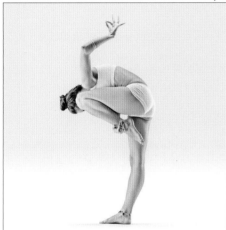

Hand to Ankle Half Standing Wind Relieving Intense Stretch Pose

Hasta Kulpha Ardha Stiti Vayu Muktyuttonasana

(HUH-stuh kul-puh UHR-duh STI-ti VAH-yu muk-tew-ton-AHS-uh-nuh)

Also Known As: Hasta Kulpha Ardha Nindra Vayu Muktyuttonasana; Knee to Ear Half Standing Wind Relieving Intense Stretch Pose (Janu Karna Ardha Nindra Vayu Muktyuttonasana) and Hand to Ankle Standing Wind Relieving Half Forward Bend
Modification: one hand grabbing onto the ankle, knee to the temple; other arm up to the sky, elbow bent
Pose Type: standing one-legged balance, forward bend
Drishti Point: Nasagrai or Nasagre (nose)

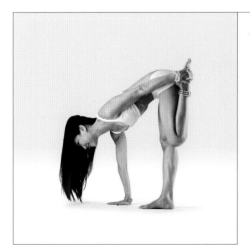

Hand to Foot One-Legged Half Intense Stretch Pose

Hasta Pada Eka Pada Ardha Uttanasana

(HUH-stuh PUH-duh EY-kuh PUH-duh UHR-duh ut-tahn-AHS-uh-nuh)

Also Known As: Hand to Foot One-Legged Half Forward Bend
Modification: hand to the foot from the same side, heel to the sitting bone, other palm to the floor
Pose Type: standing one-legged balance, forward bend
Drishti Point: Nasagrai or Nasagre (nose), Bhrumadhye or Ajna Chakra (third eye, between the eyebrows)

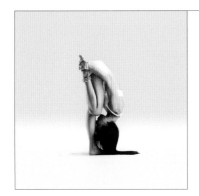

Hand to Foot One-Legged Intense Stretch Pose

Hasta Pada Eka Pada Uttanasana

(HUH-stuh PUH-duh EY-kuh PUH-duh ut-tahn-AHS-uh-nuh)

Also Known As: Hand to Foot One-Legged Full Forward Bend
Modification: hand to the foot on the same side, heel to the sitting bone; other palm to the floor
Pose Type: standing one-legged balance, forward bend
Drishti Point: Nasagrai or Nasagre (nose)

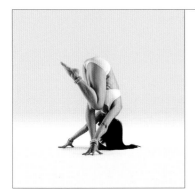

One-Legged Intense Stretch Pose 1

Eka Pada Uttanasana 1

(EY-kuh PUH-du ut-tahn-AHS-uh-nuh)

Also Known As: One-Legged Full Forward Bend 1
Modification: leg bent, heel to the sitting bone, knees together; fingertips to the floor, arms extended behind the foot
Pose Type: standing one-legged balance, forward bend
Drishti Point: Nasagrai or Nasagre (nose)

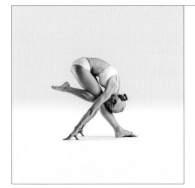

One-Legged Intense Stretch Pose 2

Eka Pada Uttanasana 2

(EY-kuh PUH-du ut-tahn-AHS-uh-nuh)

Also Known As: One-Legged Full Forward Bend 2
Modification: leg bent, heel to the sitting bone, knees together; fingertips to the floor, arms extended behind the foot
Pose Type: standing one-legged balance, forward bend
Drishti Point: Nasagrai or Nasagre (nose)

ONE LEG STANDING BALANCE: BOTH KNEES BENT & SHIVA DANCE IN THE RING OF FIRE

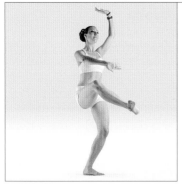

Pose Inspired by Shiva's Vigorous Cycle of Life Dance

Tandavasana

(tahn-duh-VAHS-uh-nuh)

Modification: both knees bent, both elbows bent
Pose Type: standing one-legged balance
Drishti Point: Nasagrai or Nasagre (nose)

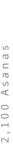

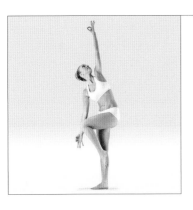

Pose Inspired by Shiva's Vigorous Cycle of Life Dance

Tandavasana
(tahn-duh-VAHS-uh-nuh)

Modification: standing leg straight; other knee bent, foot to the inside of the knee; one forearm to the opposite knee, other arm extended up to the sky

Pose Type: standing one-legged balance, twist

Drishti Point: Hastagrai or Hastagre (hands)

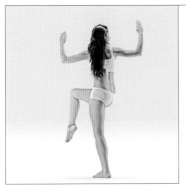

Pose Inspired by Shiva's Vigorous Cycle of Life Dance

Tandavasana
(tahn-duh-VAHS-uh-nuh)

Modification: standing leg straight, other knee bent at 90 degrees; both elbows bent, fingertips reaching to the sky; twisting to the outside of the body

Pose Type: standing one-legged balance, twist

Drishti Point: Parshva Drishti (to the right), Parshva Drishti (to the left)

ONE LEG STANDING BALANCE: KNEE BENT TO THE SIDE

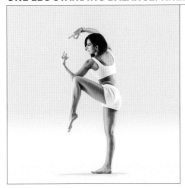

Pose Inspired by Shiva's Vigorous Cycle of Life Dance

Tandavasana
(tahn-duh-VAHS-uh-nuh)

Modification: knee to the tricep on the same side; both elbows bent, one arm up over the head

Pose Type: standing one-legged balance, side bend

Drishti Point: Hastagrai or Hastagre (hands)

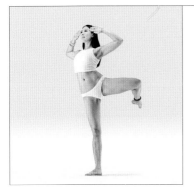

Pose Inspired by Shiva's Vigorous Cycle of Life Dance

Tandavasana
(tahn-duh-VAHS-uh-nuh)

Modification: standing leg straight, other knee bent, toes pointing away from the head; fingertips to the temples

Pose Type: standing one-legged balance

Drishti Point: Nasagrai or Nasagre (nose)

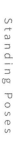

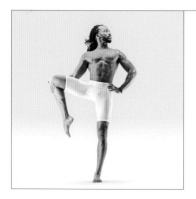

Extended Hand to Big Toe Pose 2 Prep.

Utthita Hasta Padangushtasana 2 Prep.

(UT-ti-tuh HUH-stuh puh-DAHNG-goosh-tahn-AHS-uh-nuh)

Also Known As: Extended Hand to Big Toe Pose B Prep. (Utthita Hasta Padangushtasana B Prep.)
Modification: knee bent
Pose Type: standing one-legged balance
Drishti Point: Parshva Drishti (to the right), Parshva Drishti (to the left)

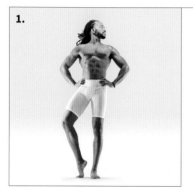

1.

Easy Tree Pose Modification

Sukha Vrikshasana

(SOOK-uh vrik-SHAHS-uh-nuh)

Modification: hands on the hips
1. toes to the floor
2. foot to the calf muscle
Pose Type: standing one-legged balance
Drishti Point: Parshva Drishti (to the right), Parshva Drishti (to the left)

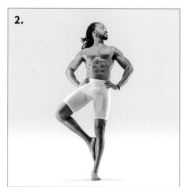

2.

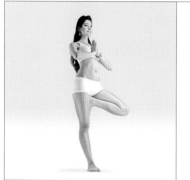

Tree Pose with Hands in Prayer

Vrikshasana Namaskar

(vrik-SHAHS-uh-nuh nuh-muhs-KAHR)

Pose Type: standing one-legged balance
Drishti Point: Angushtamadhye or Angushta Ma Dyai (thumbs), Nasagrai or Nasagre (nose)

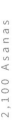

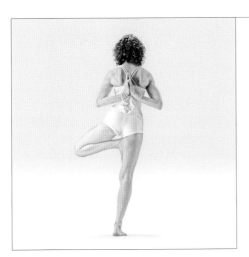

Reverse Prayer Tree Pose

Viparita Namaskar Vrikshasana
(vi-puh-REE-tuh nuh-muhs-KAHR vrik-SHAHS-uh-nuh)
Also Known As: Back of the Body Prayer Tree Pose (Paschima Namaskara Vrikshasana)
Pose Type: standing one-legged balance
Drishti Point: Nasagrai or Nasagre (nose)

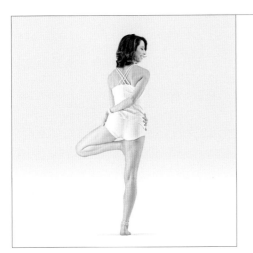

Revolved Half Bound Tree Pose

Parivritta Ardha Baddha Vrikshasana
(puh-ri-VRIT-tuh UHR-duh BUH-duh vrik-SHAHS-uh-nuh)
Pose Type: standing one-legged balance, twist
Drishti Point: Parshva Drishti (to the right), Parshva Drishti (to the left)

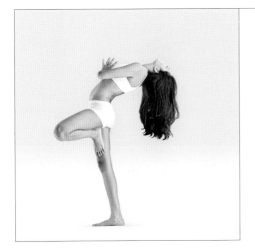

Tree Pose with Hands in Prayer

Vrikshasana Namaskar
(vrik-SHAHS-uh-nuh nuh-muhs-KAHR)
Modification: backbend
Pose Type: standing one-legged balance, backbend
Drishti Point: Bhrumadhye or Ajna Chakra (third eye, between the eyebrows)

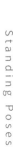

1.

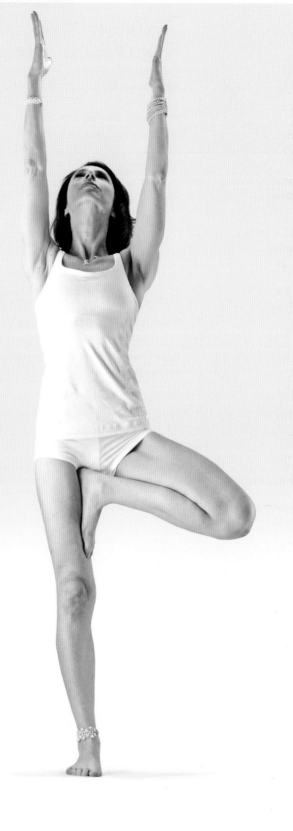

Tree Pose

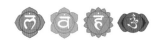

Vrikshasana

(vrik-SHAHS-uh-nuh)

Also Known As: Upward Hands Tree Pose (Urdhva Hasta Vrikshasana) or Pose Dedicated to Royal Sage Bhagiratha (Bhagirathasana)

Pose Type: standing one-legged balance, mild backbend

Drishti Point: Angusthamadhye or Angustha Ma Dyai (thumbs)

Modification: arms extended up over the head
1. arms shoulder width
2. arms shoulder width, head rolling back
3. palms together
4. palms together, head rolling back

vriksha = tree

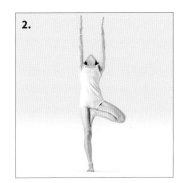

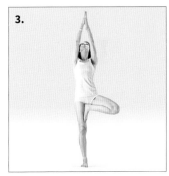

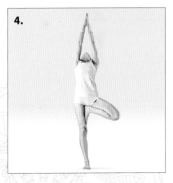

How to Perform the Pose:

1. Begin by standing in Mountain Pose (*Tadasana*). Engage your *mula bandha*, *uddhiyana bandha*, and *ujjayi* breathing. Find a still point on the floor to keep your gaze on. This will help you find and keep your balance.

2. Inhale and bring your weight onto the right foot. Exhale as you bend your left knee, and bring it out to the left side, opening the inside of your left hip. Keep your hips leveled and parallel to the floor (don't let your left hip go higher than your right). Keep the lower abdomen engaged to take out the compression (the arch) in the lower back.

3. Exhale as you place the sole of your left foot to the left calf muscle. Make sure the toes of your left foot are pointing to the floor.

4. On the next exhale, grab onto the left ankle with your left hand and slide the left foot up to the inside of your left thigh, keeping the toes of the left foot pointing to the floor. Avoid putting pressure on your right knee. Make sure to keep the left knee out to the side as you open the inside of your left hip.

5. Inhale as you reach both arms up over your head, fingertips pointing up to the sky. Keep them straight and shoulder-width apart. Make sure to lengthen your neck and keep your shoulder blades down your back.

6. Exhale and bring your gaze to your thumbs (Pose #1). You can experiment with rolling your head all the way back, feeling the stretch in the front of your neck (Pose #2).

7. If your shoulders are open, the neck is long, and your breathing is not constricted, you can bring your palms together on the exhale and look at your thumbs (Pose #3). With your palms pressed together, you can also experiment with rolling your head all the way back, feeling the stretch in the front of your neck (Pose #4).

8. Hold the pose for at least 30, and up to 90, seconds in order to receive the full benefits of the stretch. Exhale as you release the pose, come back to Mountain Pose (*Tadasana*), and repeat on the other side.

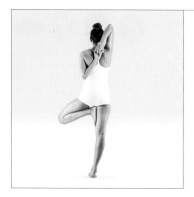

Hand Position of Cow Face Pose in Tree Pose

Hasta Gomukhasana in Vrikshasana

(HUH-stuh go-muk-AHS-uh-nuh in vrik-SHAHS-uh-nuh)

Modification: Gomukhasana arms

Pose Type: standing one-legged balance

Drishti Point: Nasagrai or Nasagre (nose)

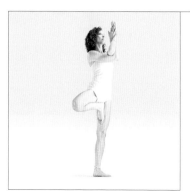

Hand Position of the Pose Dedicated to Garuda in Tree Pose

Hasta Garudasana in Vrikshasana

(HUH-stuh GUH-ru-duh-AHS-uh-nuh in vrik-SHAHS-uh-nuh)

Pose Type: standing one-legged balance

Drishti Point: Angushtamadhye or Angushta Ma Dyai (thumbs)

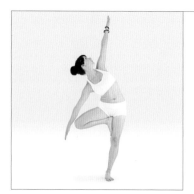

Sideways Tree Pose

Parshva Vrikshasana

(PAHRSH-vuh vrik-SHAHS-uh-nuh)

Modification: side bend toward the bent knee

Pose Type: standing one-legged balance, side bend

Drishti Point: Hastagrai or Hastagre (hands)

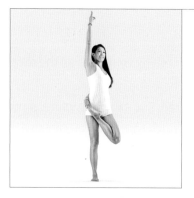

Upward One Hand Half Bound Lotus Tree Pose

Urdhva Eka Hasta Ardha Baddha Padma Vrikshasana

(OORD-vuh EY-kuh HUH-stuh UHR-duh BUH-duh PUHD-muh vrik-SHAHS-uh-nuh)

Pose Type: standing one-legged balance, binding

Drishti Point: Nasagrai or Nasagre (nose)

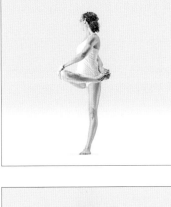

Revolved Half Bound Lotus Tree Pose

Parivritta Ardha Baddha Padma Vrikshasana
(puh-ri-VRIT-tuh UHR-duh BUH-duh PUHD-muh vrik-SHAHS-uh-nuh)
Pose Type: standing one-legged balance, twist, binding
Drishti Point: Parshva Drishti (to the right), Parshva Drishti (to the left)

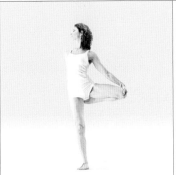

Hand to Foot Hand to Knee Tree Pose

Hasta Pada Hasta Janu Vrikshasana
(HUH-stuh PUH-duh HUH-stuh JAH-nu vrik-SHAHS-uh-nuh)
Modification: grabbing onto the foot and the knee, knee to the outside
Pose Type: standing one-legged balance
Drishti Point: Parshva Drishti (to the right), Parshva Drishti (to the left)

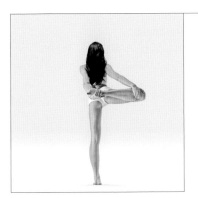

Hand to Foot Hand to Knee Tree Pose

Hasta Pada Hasta Janu Vrikshasana
(HUH-stuh PUH-duh HUH-stuh JAH-nu vrik-SHAHS-uh-nuh)
Modification: backbend, grabbing onto the foot and the knee, knee to the outside, looking straight ahead
Pose Type: standing one-legged balance, backbend
Drishti Point: Nasagrai or Nasagre (nose)

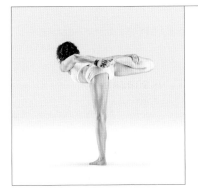

Hand to Foot Hand to Knee Toppling Tree Pose

Hasta Pada Hasta Janu Patan Vrikshasana
(HUH-stuh PUH-duh HUH-stuh JAH-nu PUH-tuhn vrik-SHAHS-uh-nuh)
Modification: grabbing onto the foot and the shin, knee to the outside
Pose Type: standing one-legged balance, forward bend
Drishti Point: Nasagrai or Nasagre (nose)

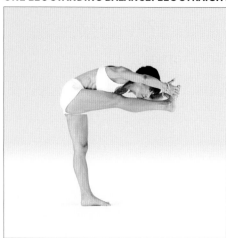

Both Hands to Foot Pose

Dwi Hasta Padasana

(dwi-huh-stuh puh-DAHS-uh-nuh)

Also Known As: Raised Up Leg and Back Stretch Pose (Utthita Eka Pada Paschimottanasana), Standing Head to Knee Pose (Dandayamana-Janushirasana)

Modification: chin to the shin

Pose Type: standing one-legged balance, forward bend

Drishti Point: Bhrumadhye or Ajna Chakra (third eye, between the eyebrows), Padayoragrai or Padayoragre (toes/feet)

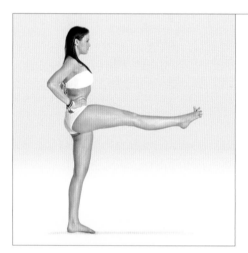

Extended One Foot Pose

Utthita Ekapadasana

(UT-ti-tuh EY-kuh-puh-DAHS-uh-nuh)

Also Known As: Extended Hand to Big Toe Pose D (Utthita Hasta Padangushtasana D; found in Ashtanga Yoga System)

Modification: hands on the hips

Pose Type: standing one-legged balance

Drishti Point: Padayoragrai or Padayoragre (toes/feet)

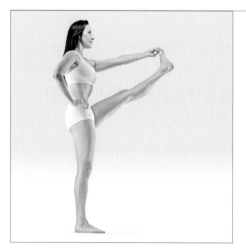

Extended Hand to Big Toe Pose 1

Utthita Hasta Padangushtasana 1

(UT-ti-tuh HUH-stuh puhd-ahng-goosh-TAHS-uh-nuh)

Also Known As: Extended Hand to Big Toe Pose A (Utthita Hasta Padangushtasana A)

Modification: lifted leg in front of the body

Pose Type: standing one-legged balance

Drishti Point: Padayoragrai or Padayoragre (toes/feet)

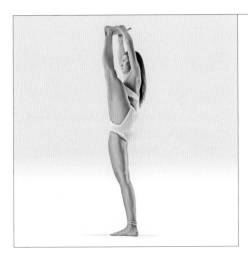

Extended Pose Dedicated to Trivikrama—Conqueror of the Three Worlds (Vishnu)

Utthita Trivikramasana

(UT-ti-tuh tri-vi-kruh-MAHS-uh-nuh)

Also Known As: Extended Hand to Foot Stretch Pose (Utthita Hastha Pada Uttanasana)
Modification: knee away from the shoulder
Pose Type: standing one-legged balance
Drishti Point: Nasagrai or Nasagre (nose)

ONE LEG STANDING BALANCE: LEG STRAIGHT TO THE SIDE

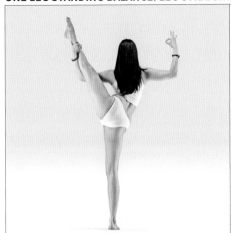

Pose Dedicated to Trivikrama—Conqueror of the Three Worlds (Vishnu)

Trivikramasana

(tri-vi-kruh-MAHS-uh-nuh)

Also Known As: Leg to the Side Pose Dedicated to Trivikrama—Conqueror of the Three Worlds (Vishnu) (Parshva Pada Trivikramasana)
Modification: arm wrapping around the leg on the same side
Pose Type: standing one-legged balance
Drishti Point: Nasagrai or Nasagre (nose)

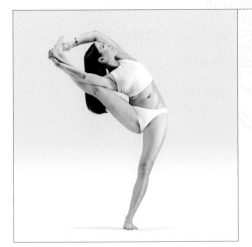

Rising Standing Sundial Pose
Utthita Stiti Surya Yantrasana

(UT-ti-tuh STI-ti SOOR-yuh yuhn-TRAHS-uh-nuh)

Also Known As: Utthita Nindra Surya Yantrasana
Modification: side bend
Pose Type: standing one-legged balance, side bend, twist
Drishti Point: Urdhva or Antara Drishti (up to the sky)

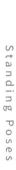

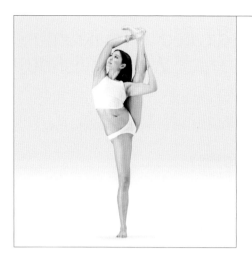

Pose Dedicated to Trivikrama—Conqueror of the Three Worlds (Vishnu)

Trivikramasana

(tri-vi-kruh-MAHS-uh-nuh)

Also Known As: Leg to the Side Pose Dedicated to Trivikrama—Conqueror of the Three Worlds (Vishnu) (Parshva Pada Trivikramasana)

Modification: both hands grabbing onto the leg, shoulder to the back of the knee, looking to the side

Pose Type: standing one-legged balance, twist

Drishti Point: Urdhva or Antara Drishti (up to the sky)

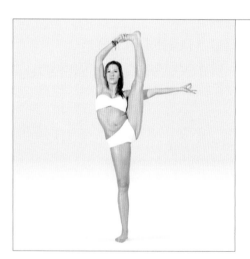

Pose Dedicated to Trivikrama—Conqueror of the Three Worlds (Vishnu)

Trivikramasana

(tri-vi-kruh-MAHS-uh-nuh)

Also Known As: Leg to the Side Pose Dedicated to Trivikrama—Conqueror of the Three Worlds (Vishnu) (Parshva Pada Trivikramasana)

Modification: one hand grabbing onto the opposite foot, shoulder to the front of the knee, other arm straight out to the side, looking straight ahead

Pose Type: standing one-legged balance

Drishti Point: Nasagrai or Nasagre (nose)

ONE LEG STANDING BALANCE: LEG STRAIGHT TO THE SIDE—BINDING & TWISTS

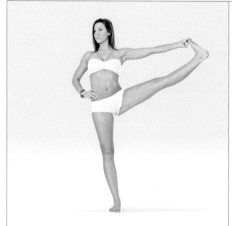

Extended Hand to Big Toe Pose 2

Utthita Hasta Padangushtasana 2

(UT-ti-tuh HUH-stuh puhd-ahng-goosh-TAHS-uh-nuh)

Also Known As: Extended Hand to Big Toe Pose B (Utthita Hasta Padangushtasana B), Standing Leg Going to the Side Pose Prep. (Utthita Parshvasahita Prep.)

Pose Type: standing one-legged balance

Drishti Point: Parshva Drishti (to the right), Parshva Drishti (to the left)

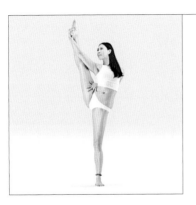

Half Bound Pose Dedicated to Trivikrama —Conqueror of the Three Worlds (Vishnu)

Ardha Baddha Trivikramasana *(UHR-duh BUH-duh tri-vi-kruh-MAHS-uh-nuh)*

Also Known As: Leg to the Side Half Bound Pose Dedicated to Trivikrama—Conqueror of the Three Worlds (Vishnu) (Parshva Pada Ardha Baddha Trivikramasana)

Modification: one arm wrapping around the leg on the same side, other arm behind the back, hand to the inside of the thigh

Pose Type: standing one-legged balance, binding

Drishti Point: Padayoragrai or Padayoragre (toes/feet)

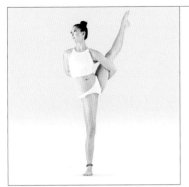

Bird of Paradise Pose

Svarga Dvijasana

(SVUHR-guh dwij-AHS-uh-nuh)

Pose Type: standing one-legged balance, binding

Drishti Point: Parshva Drishti (to the right), Parshva Drishti (to the left)

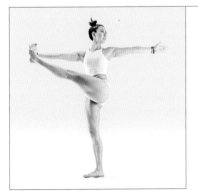

Revolved Extended Hand to Foot Pose

Parivritta Utthita Pada Hastasana

(puh-ri-VRIT-tuh UT-ti-tuh PUH-duh huh-STAHS-uh-nuh)

Also Known As: Revolved Hand to Big Toe Pose (Parivritta Hasta Padangushtasana)

Pose Type: standing one-legged balance, twist

Drishti Point: Angushtamadhye or Angushta Ma Dyai (thumbs)

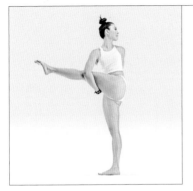

Revolved Bird of Paradise Pose

Parivritta Svarga Dvijasana

(puh-ri-VRIT-tuh SVUHR-guh dwij-AHS-uh-nuh)

Also Known As: Raised and Revolved Bound Leg Pose (Utthita Parivritta Baddha Padasana)

Pose Type: standing one-legged balance, twist, binding

Drishti Point: Parshva Drishti (to the right), Parshva Drishti (to the left)

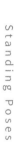

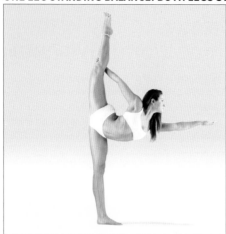

Lord of the Dance Pose

Natarajasana

(NAH-tuh-rahj-AHS-uh-nuh)

Modification: under-head grip with one hand on the same side; both legs straight

Pose Type: standing one-legged balance, backbend

Drishti Point: Hastagrai or Hastagre (hands)

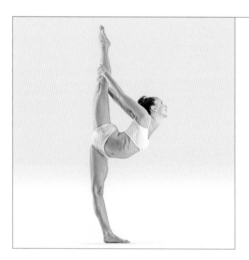

Pose Dedicated to Yogi Yogananda

Yoganandasana

(yo-gah-nuhn-DAHS-uh-nuh)

Also Known As: Pose Dedicated to Vishnu Devananda (Vishnu Devanandasana)

Modification: both legs straight, grabbing onto the back leg with an under-head grip

Pose Type: standing one-legged balance, backbend

Drishti Point: Bhrumadhye or Ajna Chakra (third eye, between the eyebrows)

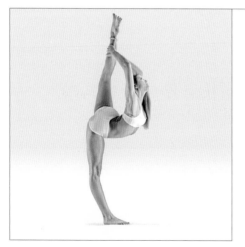

Yogi Sivananda's Pose

Sivanandasana

(shiv-ah-nuhn-DAHS-uh-nuh)

Modification: grabbing onto the shin

Pose Type: standing one-legged balance, backbend

Drishti Point: Bhrumadhye or Ajna Chakra (third eye, between the eyebrows)

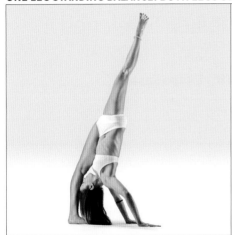

Pose Dedicated to Sage Sundaranandar

Sundaranandarasana

(sun-duh-RAH-nuhn-duh-RAHS-uh-nuh)

Modification: palms to the floor, forehead to the shin
Pose Type: standing, forward bend
Drishti Point: Nasagrai or Nasagre (nose)

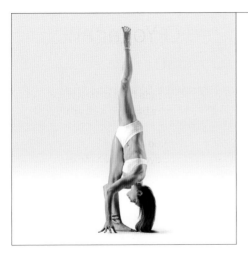

One Leg Stretched Upward Pose

Urdhva Prasarita Ekapadasana

(OORD-vuh pruh-SAH-ri-tuh ey-kuh-puhd-AHS-uh-nuh)

Modification: one hand grabbing onto the ankle on the same side, palm of the other hand to the floor, head away from the shin
Pose Type: standing one-legged balance, forward bend
Drishti Point: Padayoragrai or Padayoragre (toes/feet) or Nasagrai or Nasagre (nose)

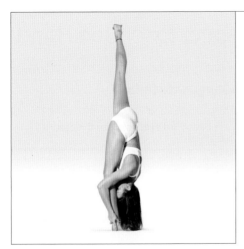

One Leg Stretched Upward Pose

Urdhva Prasarita Ekapadasana

(OORD-vuh pruh-SAH-ri-tuh ey-kuh-puhd-AHS-uh-nuh)

Modification: both hands grabbing onto the ankle, forehead to the shin
Pose Type: standing one-legged balance, forward bend
Drishti Point: Nasagrai or Nasagre (nose) if chin touches the shin

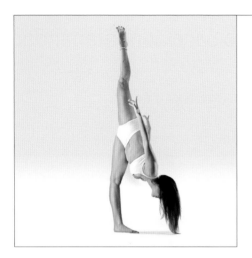

Unsupported One Leg Stretched Upward Pose

Niralamba Urdhva Prasarita Ekapadasana

(nir-AH-luhm-buh OORD-vuh pruh-SAH-ri-tuh ey-kuh-puhd-AHS-uh-nuh)

Modification: arms straight along the sides of the torso, fingertips to the sky
Pose Type: standing one-legged balance, forward bend
Drishti Point: Nasagrai or Nasagre (nose), Padayoragrai or Padayoragre (toes/feet), Bhrumadhye or Ajna Chakra (third eye, between the eyebrows)

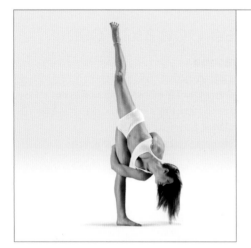

Bound Unsupported One Leg Stretched Upward Pose

Baddha Niralamba Urdhva Prasarita Ekapadasana

(BUH-duh nir-AH-luhm-buh OORD-vuh pruh-SAH-ri-tuh ey-kuh-puhd-AHS-uh-nuh-uh-nuh)

Pose Type: standing one-legged balance, forward bend, binding
Drishti Point: Nasagrai or Nasagre (nose), Padayoragrai or Padayoragre (toes/feet), Bhrumadhye or Ajna Chakra (third eye, between the eyebrows)

ONE LEG STANDING BALANCE: LEG STRAIGHT TO THE SIDE—HALF FORWARD BEND

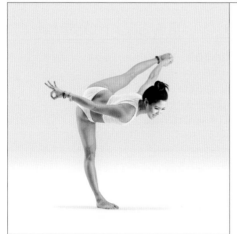

Bowing with Respect Extended Hand to Big Toe Pose 2

Nantum Utthita Hasta Padangushtasana 2

(NUHN-tum UT-ti-tuh HUH-stuh puhd-ahng-goosh-TAHS-uh-nuh)

Modification: forward bend, grabbing onto the big toe of the lifted leg; other arm extended to the side parallel to the floor
Pose Type: standing one-legged balance, forward bend
Drishti Point: Nasagrai or Nasagre (nose)

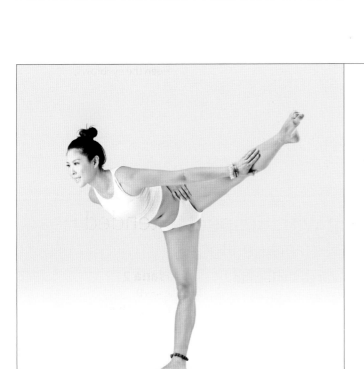

Bowing with Respect Both Hands Extended to Big Toes Pose 2

Nantum Utthita Dwi Hasta Padangushtasana 2

(NUHN-tum UT-ti-tuh DWI-huh-stuh
puhd-ahng-goosh-TAHS-uh-nuh-uh-nuh)

Modification: forward bend, grabbing onto the big toes with both hands, leg lifted higher than the hip
Pose Type: standing one-legged balance, forward bend
Drishti Point: Nasagrai or Nasagre (nose)

Bowing with Respect Half Bound Hand to Leg Pose

Nantum Ardha Baddha Hasta Padasana

(NUHN-tum UHR-duh BUH-duh HUH-stuh puhd-AHS-uh-nuh)
Modification: half forward bend
Pose Type: standing one-legged balance, forward bend, binding
Drishti Point: Bhrumadhye or Ajna Chakra (third eye, between the eyebrows)

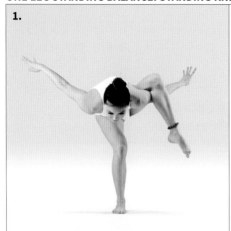

Bowing with Respect
Bird of Paradise Pose Prep.

Nantum Svarga Dvijasana Prep.

(NUHN-tum SVUHR-guh dwij-AHS-uh-nuh)

Modification: 1. standing leg bent; other knee to the back of the shoulder, leg bent

2. standing leg bent; other knee to the back of the shoulder, leg straight

Pose Type: standing one-legged balance, forward bend

Drishti Point: Nasagrai or Nasagre (nose)

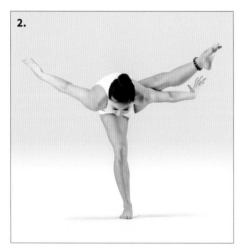

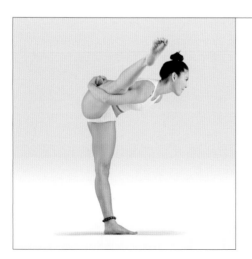

Bowing with Respect
Bird of Paradise Pose

Nantum Svarga Dvijasana

(NUHN-tum SVUHR-guh dwij-AHS-uh-nuh)

Modification: half forward bend

Pose Type: standing one-legged balance, forward bend, binding

Drishti Point: Nasagrai or Nasagre (nose)

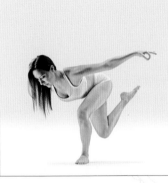

Benu Bird Pose 2

Benvasana 2

(ben-VAHS-uh-nuh)

Modification: both knees bent, chest toward the quadriceps, arms open to the sides
Pose Type: standing one-legged balance, forward bend
Drishti Point: Nasagrai or Nasagre (nose)

ONE LEG STANDING BALANCE: ONE LEG STRAIGHT TO THE BACK, HANDS TO THE FLOOR

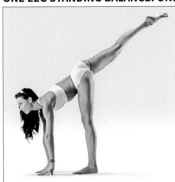

Half One Leg Stretched Upward Pose

Ardha Urdhva Prasarita Ekapadasana

(UHR-duh OORD-vuh pruh-SAH-ri-tuh ey-kuh-puh-DAHS-uh-nuh)

Also Known As: One Leg Stretched Upwards Pose Prep. (Urdhva Prasarita Ekapadasana Prep.), Warrior 3 Prep. (Virabhadrasana 3 Prep.)
Modification: fingertips to the floor
Pose Type: standing, forward bend
Drishti Point: Bhrumadhye or Ajna Chakra (third eye, between the eyebrows)

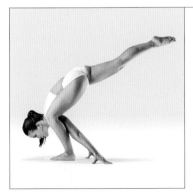

One Leg Stretched Upward Pose Prep.

Urdhva Prasarita Ekapadasana Prep.

(OORD-vuh pruh-SAH-ri-tuh ey-kuh-puh-DAHS-uh-nuh)

Modification: standing leg bent, shoulder to the back of the knee, arms extended to the back
Pose Type: standing, forward bend
Drishti Point: Bhrumadhye or Ajna Chakra (third eye, between the eyebrows)

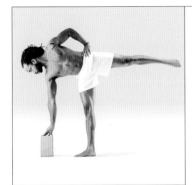

Half Moon Pose Prep.

Ardha Chandrasana Prep.

(UHR-duh chuhn-DRAHS-uh-nuh)

Modification: with yoga block prop, hand on the hip
Pose Type: standing one-legged balance, forward bend
Drishti Point: Hastagrai or Hastagre (hands)

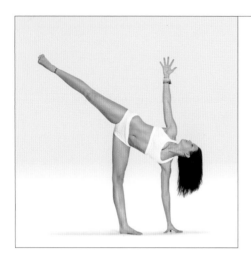

Half Moon Pose

Ardha Chandrasana

(UHR-duh chuhn-DRAHS-uh-nuh)

Pose Type: standing one-legged balance, forward bend
Drishti Point: Angushtamadhye or Angushta Ma Dyai (thumbs)

ONE LEG STANDING BALANCE: ONE LEG STRAIGHT TO THE BACK—HANDS OFF THE FLOOR

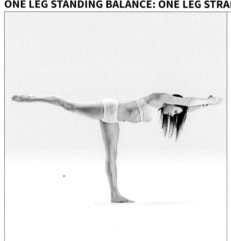

Warrior 3

Virabhadrasana 3

(VEER-uh buh-DRAHS-uh-nuh)

Also Known As: Bird Pose A (Dikasana A)
Pose Type: standing one-legged balance, forward bend
Drishti Point: Nasagrai or Nasagre (nose)

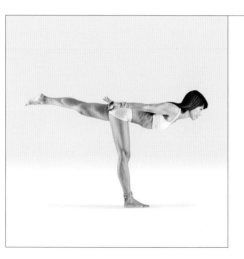

Warrior 3

Virabhadrasana 3

(VEER-uh buh-DRAHS-uh-nuh)

Also Known As: Bird Pose B (Dikasana B)
Modification: arms extended to the back and parallel to the floor
Pose Type: standing one-legged balance, forward bend
Drishti Point: Nasagrai or Nasagre (nose)

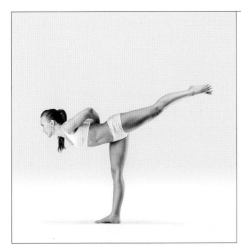

Reverse Prayer Warrior 3

Viparita Namaskar Virabhadrasana 3
(vi-puh-REE-tuh nuh-muhs-KAHR VEER-uh buh-DRAHS-uh-nuh)
Also Known As: Back of the Body Prayer Warrior 3 (Paschima Namaskara Virabhadrasana 3)
Pose Type: standing one-legged balance, forward bend
Drishti Point: Nasagrai or Nasagre (nose)

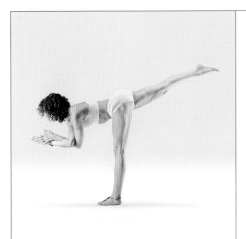

Hand Position of the Pose Dedicated to Garuda in Warrior 3

Hasta Garudasana in Virabhadrasana 3
(HUH-stuh guh-ru-DAHS-uh-nuh in VEER-uh-buh-DRAHS-uh-nuh)
Pose Type: standing one-legged balance, forward bend
Drishti Point: Angushtamadhye or Angushta Ma Dyai (thumbs)

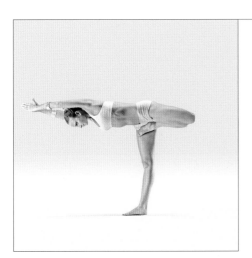

Half Lotus Warrior 3

Ardha Padma Virabhadrasana 3
(UHR-duh PUHD-muh VEER-uh-buh-DRAHS-uh-nuh-uh-nuh)
Pose Type: standing one-legged balance, forward bend
Drishti Point: Nasagrai or Nasagre (nose)

1.

Half Moon Pose
with Hands in Prayer

Ardha Chandrasana Namaskar

(UHR-duh chuhn-DRAHS-uh-nuh nuh-muhs-KAHR)
Pose Type: standing one-legged balance, forward bend
Drishti Point: 1. Nasagrai or Nasagre (nose), Bhrumad-hye or Ajna Chakra (third eye, between the eyebrows)
2. Urdhva or Antara Drishti (up to the sky)

Modification:
1. looking down
2. looking up to the sky

ardha = half
chandra = moon
namaskar = greeting with hands in
Anjali Mudra (hands in prayer)

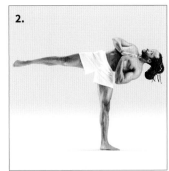

2.

How to Perform the Pose:

1. Begin by doing Extended Triangle Pose (*Utthita Trikonasana*) with the left foot in front and your left hand to the floor outside the left foot (either on the fingertips or with the palm flat on the floor). Engage your *mula bandha*, *uddhiyana bandha*, and *ujjayi* breathing.

2. Exhale as you slide your left palm out to the front while bending your left knee. Experiment with the distance to find your balance.

3. Inhale and lift your right foot off the floor until your right leg is parallel to the floor. Keep it straight and reaching away from your head. Straighten your standing left leg.

4. Exhale and rotate your chest to the side so that your shoulders stack one on top of the other.

5. On your next exhale, lift your left arm up off the floor and bring your hands into prayer at the center of your chest.

6. You can either find a gazing point on the floor that is not moving to help keep your balance (Pose #1) or challenge yourself by looking up to the sky (Pose #2).

7. Hold the pose for at least 30, and up to 90, seconds in order to receive the full benefits of the stretch. Exhale, lower your right foot to the floor, coming back into Extended Triangle Pose (*Utthita Trikonasana*), and repeat on the other side.

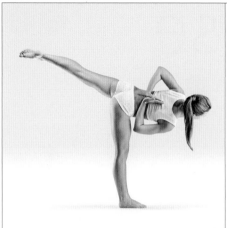

Reverse Prayer Half Moon Pose

Viparita Namaskar Ardha Chandrasana

(vi-puh-REE-tuh nuh-muhs-KAHR UHR-duh chuhn-DRAHS-uh-nuh)

Also Known As: Back of the Body Prayer Half Moon Pose (Paschima Namaskara Ardha Chandrasana)

Pose Type: standing one-legged balance, forward bend

Drishti Point: Nasagrai or Nasagre (nose)

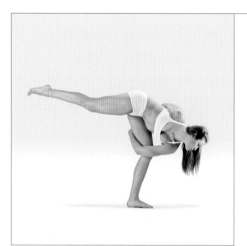

Bound Half Moon Pose

Baddha Ardha Chandrasana

(BUH-duh UHR-duh chuhn-DRAHS-uh-nuh)

Pose Type: standing one-legged balance, forward bend, binding

Drishti Point: Nasagrai or Nasagre (nose) or Padayoragrai or Padayoragre (toes/feet)

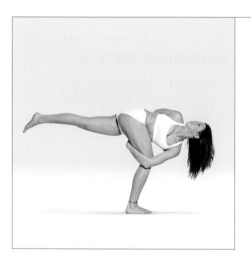

Revolved Bound Half Moon Pose

Parivritta Baddha Ardha Chandrasana

(vi-puh-REE-tuh BUH-duh UHR-duh chuhn-DRAHS-uh-nuh)

Modification: looking up to the sky

Pose Type: standing one-legged balance, forward bend, twist, binding

Drishti Point: Urdhva or Antara Drishti (up to the sky)

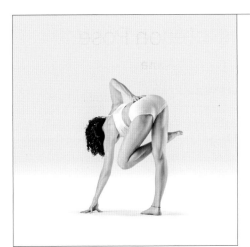

Half Firelog Pose in Half Moon Pose Prep.

Ardha Agnistambhasana in Ardha Chandrasana Prep.

(UHR-duh uhg-ni-stuhm-BAHS-uh-nuh in UHR-duh chuhn-DRAHS-uh-nuh)

Modification: foot on top of the knee, palm to the lower back

Pose Type: standing one-legged balance, forward bend

Drishti Point: Hastagrai or Hastagre (hands)

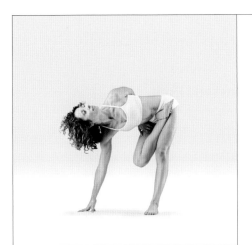

Half Bound Lotus Half Moon Pose Prep.

Ardha Baddha Padma Ardha Chandrasana Prep.

(UHR-duh BUH-duh PUHD-muh UHR-duh chuhn-DRAHS-uh-nuh)

Modification: arm behind the back, binding to the inside of the thigh of the leg in Half Lotus

Pose Type: standing one-legged balance, forward bend, twist, binding

Drishti Point: Urdhva or Antara Drishti (up to the sky)

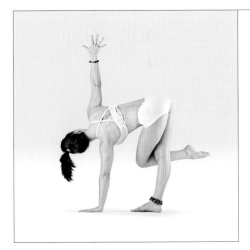

Leg Position of Half Cow Face Pose in Half Moon Pose Prep.

Pada Ardha Gomukhasana in Ardha Chandrasana Prep.

(PUH-duh UHR-duh go-muk-AHS-uh-nuh in UHR-duh chuhn-DRAHS-uh-nuh)

Also Known As: One-Legged Cow Face Pose in Half Moon Pose Prep. (Eka Pada Gomukhasana in Ardha Chandrasana Prep.)

Pose Type: standing one-legged balance, forward bend, twist

Drishti Point: Hastagrai or Hastagre (hands)

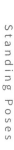

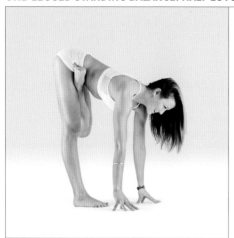

Half Bound Lotus Intense Stretch Pose Prep.

Ardha Baddha Padmottanasana Prep.

(UHR-duh BUH-duh puhd-mo-tahn-AHS-uh-nuh)

Also Known As: Half Bound Lotus Half Forward Bend Prep., Half Lotus Half Intense Stretch Pose (Ardha Padma Ardha Uttanasana), Half Lotus Half Forward Bend

Modification: half forward bend, fingertips of both hands to the floor

Pose Type: standing, forward bend

Drishti Point: Bhrumadhye or Ajna Chakra (third eye, between the eyebrows), Nasagrai or Nasagre (nose)

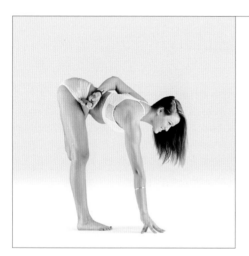

Half Bound Lotus Intense Stretch Pose Prep.

Ardha Baddha Padmottanasana Prep.

(UHR-duh BUH-duh puhd-mo-tahn-AHS-uh-nuh)

Also Known As: Half Bound Lotus Half Forward Bend

Modification: half forward bend

Pose Type: standing one-legged balance, forward bend, binding

Drishti Point: Bhrumadhye or Ajna Chakra (third eye, between the eyebrows), Nasagrai or Nasagre (nose)

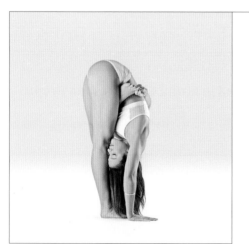

Half Bound Lotus Intense Stretch Pose

Ardha Baddha Padmottanasana

(UHR-duh BUH-duh puhd-mo-tahn-AHS-uh-nuh)

Also Known As: Half Bound Lotus Full Forward Bend

Pose Type: standing one-legged balance, forward bend, binding

Drishti Point: Nasagrai or Nasagre (nose)

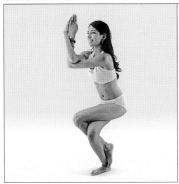

Pose Dedicated to Garuda

Garudasana

(guh-ru-DAHS-uh-nuh)

Also Known As: Eagle Pose
Modification: hands intertwined in front, low stance
Pose Type: standing one-legged balance
Drishti Point: Angushtamadhye or Angushta Ma Dyai (thumbs)

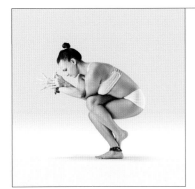

Reverse Heart Chakra Seal in Leg Position of the Pose Dedicated to Garuda

Viparita Anahata Chakra Mudra in Pada Garudasana

(vi-puh-REE-tuh un-AH-huh-tuh chuh-kruh MU-druh in PUH-duh guh-ru-DAHS-uh-nuh)

Also Known As: Reverse Heart Chakra Seal in Leg Position of the Eagle Pose
Pose Type: standing one-legged balance
Drishti Point: Nasagrai or Nasagre (nose)

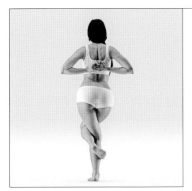

Pose Dedicated to Garuda

Garudasana

(guh-ru-DAHS-uh-nuh)

Also Known As: Eagle Pose
Modification: elbows to the knees
Pose Type: standing one-legged balance, forward bend
Drishti Point: Angushtamadhye or Angushta Ma Dyai (thumbs)

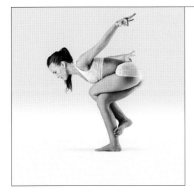

Leg Position of the Pose Dedicated to Garuda

Pada Garudasana

(PUH-duh guh-ru-DAHS-uh-nuh)

Also Known As: Leg Position of the Eagle Pose
Modification: arms straight out to the sides behind the back
Pose Type: standing one-legged balance, forward bend
Drishti Point: Nasagrai or Nasagre (nose)

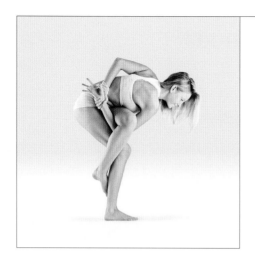

Revolved Bound Leg Position of the Pose Dedicated to Garuda

Parivritta Baddha Pada Garudasana

(puh-ri-VRIT-tuh BUH-duh PUH-duh guh-ru-DAHS-uh-nuh)

Also Known As: Revolved Bound Leg Position of the Eagle Pose

Pose Type: standing one-legged balance, forward bend, binding, twist

Drishti Point: Nasagrai or Nasagre (nose)

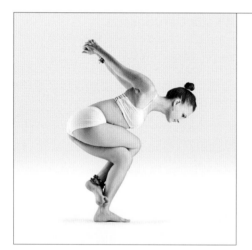

Hands Bound Leg Position of the Pose Dedicated to Garuda

Baddha Hasta Pada Garudasana

(BUH-duh HUH-stuh PUH-duh guh-ru-DAHS-uh-nuh)

Also Known As: Hands Bound Leg Position of the Eagle Pose

Pose Type: standing one-legged balance, forward bend

Drishti Point: Nasagrai or Nasagre (nose)

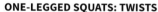

ONE-LEGGED SQUATS: TWISTS

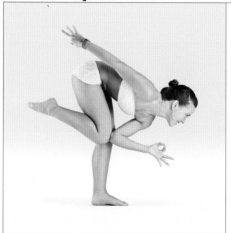

Revolved Half Standing Wind Relieving Intense Stretch Pose

Parivritta Ardha Stiti Vayu Muktyuttonasana

(puh-ri-VRIT-tuh UHR-duh STI-ti VAH-yu muk-tew-to-NAHS-uh-nuh)

Also Known As: Parivritta Ardha Nindra Vayu Muktyuttonasana; Revolved Standing Wind Relieving Half Forward Bend

Modification: knees together; elbow to the opposite knee, other arm extended to the back

Pose Type: standing one-legged balance, forward bend

Drishti Point: Bhrumadhye or Ajna Chakra (third eye, between the eyebrows), Nasagrai or Nasagre (nose)

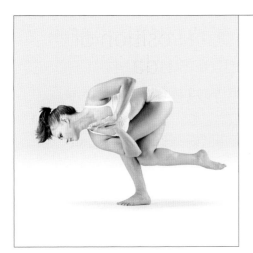

Revolved Half Standing Wind Relieving Intense Stretch Pose with Hands in Prayer

Parivritta Ardha Stiti Vayu Muktyuttonasana Namaskar

(puh-ri-VRIT-tuh UHR-duh STI-ti VAH-yu muk-tew-to-NAHS-uh-nuh nuh-muhs-KAHR)

Also Known As: Parivritta Ardha Nindra Vayu Muktyuttonasana Namaskar; Revolved Standing Wind Relieving Half Forward Bend with Hands in Prayer

Modification: back leg crossed under the front leg

Pose Type: standing one-legged balance, forward bend, twist

Drishti Point: Nasagrai or Nasagre (nose)

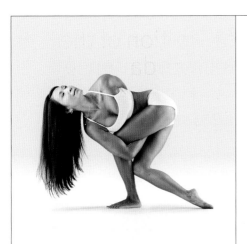

Bound Revolved Half Standing Wind Relieving Intense Stretch Pose

Baddha Parivritta Ardha Stiti Vayu Muktyuttonasana

(BUH-duh puh-ri-VRIT-tuh UHR-duh STI-ti VAH-yu muk-tew-to-NAHS-uh-nuh)

Also Known As: Baddha Parivritta Ardha Nindra Vayu Muktyuttonasana; Bound Revolved Standing Wind Relieving Half Forward Bend

Pose Type: standing one-legged balance, forward bend, twist, binding

Drishti Point: Urdhva or Antara Drishti (up to the sky)

ONE-LEGGED SQUATS: KNEES IN LINE—HEEL TO THE SITTING BONES— GRABBING ONTO THE ANKLE

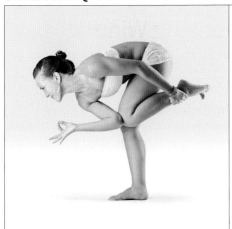

Revolved One Hand to Foot Half Standing Wind Relieving Intense Stretch Pose

Parivritta Eka Hasta Pada Ardha Stiti Vayu Muktyuttonasana

(puh-ri-VRIT-tuh EY-kuh HUH-stuh PUH-duh UHR-duh STI-ti VAH-yu muk-tew-to-NAHS-uh-nuh)

Also Known As: Parivritta Eka Hasta Pada Ardha Nindra Vayu Muktyuttonasana; Revolved One Hand to Foot Standing Wind Relieving Half Forward Bend

Modification: knees together; elbow to the opposite knee, other hand grabbing onto the ankle

Pose Type: standing one-legged balance, forward bend

Drishti Point: Bhrumadhye or Ajna Chakra (third eye, between the eyebrows), Nasagrai or Nasagre (nose)

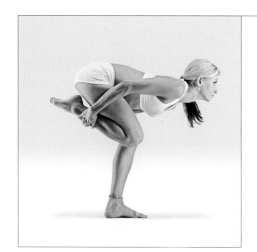

Both Hands to Foot Half Standing Wind Relieving Intense Stretch Pose

Dwi Hasta Pada Ardha Stiti Vayu Muktyuttonasana

(DWI-huh-stuh PUH-duh UHR-duh STI-ti VAH-yu muk-to-NAHS-uh-nuh)

Also Known As: Dwi Hasta Pada Ardha Nindra Vayu Muktyuttonasana

Pose Type: standing one-legged balance, forward bend

Drishti Point: Bhrumadhye or Ajna Chakra (third eye, between the eyebrows)

ONE-LEGGED SQUATS: KNEES IN LINE—HEEL TO THE SITTING BONE—HEEL OF THE STANDING LEG UP

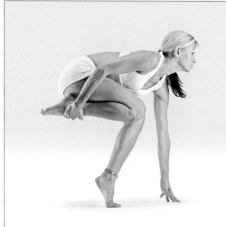

One Hand to Foot Tip Toe Half Standing Wind Relieving Intense Stretch Pose

Eka Hasta Pada Prapada Ardha Stiti Vayu Muktyuttonasana

(EY-kuh HUH-stuh PUH-duh PRUH-puh-duh UHR-duh STI-ti VAH-yu muk-to-NAHS-uh-nuh)

Also Known As: Eka Hasta Pada Prapada Ardha Nindra Vayu Muktyuttonasana

Pose Type: standing one-legged balance, forward bend

Drishti Point: Bhrumadhye or Ajna Chakra (third eye, between the eyebrows)

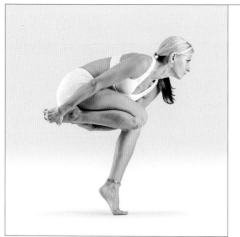

Both Hands to Foot Tip Toe Half Standing Wind Relieving Intense Stretch Pose

Dwi Hasta Pada Prapada Ardha Stiti Vayu Muktyuttonasana

(DWI-huh-stuh PUH-duh PRUH-puh-duh UHR-duh STI-ti VAH-yu muk-to-NAHS-uh-nuh)

Also Known As: Dwi Hasta Pada Prapada Ardha Nindra Vayu Muktyuttonasana

Pose Type: standing one-legged balance, forward bend

Drishti Point: Bhrumadhye or Ajna Chakra (third eye, between the eyebrows)

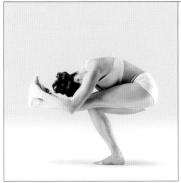

One-Legged Pose Dedicated to Yogi Shankara

Eka Pada Shankarasana

(EY-kuh PUH-duh shunk-uhr-AHS-uh-nuh)

Modification: forehead to the shin
Pose Type: standing one-legged balance, forward bend
Drishti Point: Nasagrai or Nasagre (nose)

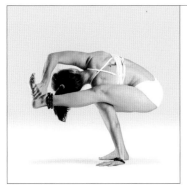

Revolved One-Legged Pose Dedicated to Yogi Shankara

Parivritta Eka Pada Shankarasana

(puh-ri-VRIT-tuh EY-kuh PUH-duh shunk-uhr-AHS-uh-nuh)

Modification: twisting to the inside of the leg
Pose Type: standing one-legged balance, forward bend, twist, side bend
Drishti Point: Urdhva or Antara Drishti (up to the sky)

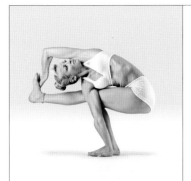

Revolved One-Legged Pose Dedicated to Yogi Shankara

Parivritta Eka Pada Shankarasana

(puh-ri-VRIT-tuh EY-kuh PUH-duh shunk-uhr-AHS-uh-nuh)

Modification: twisting to the outside of the leg
Pose Type: standing one-legged balance, forward bend, twist, side bend
Drishti Point: Urdhva or Antara Drishti (up to the sky)

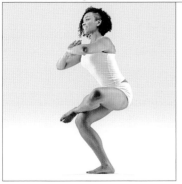

One-Legged Fierce Pose 1

Eka Pada Utkatasana 1

(EY-kuh PUH-duh ut-kuh-TAHS-uh-nuh)

Also Known As: One-Legged Prayer Fierce Pose (Eka Pada Namaskar Utkatasana)
Modification: hands in Anjali Mudra (Hands in Prayer)
Pose Type: standing one-legged balance
Drishti Point: Bhrumadhye or Ajna Chakra (third eye, between the eyebrows), Nasagrai or Nasagre (nose)

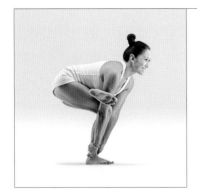

One-Legged Fierce Pose 2

Eka Pada Utkatasana 2

(EY-kuh PUH-duh ut-kuh-TAHS-uh-nuh)

Also Known As: Both Hands to Ankle One-Legged Fierce Pose (Dwi Hasta Kulpa Eka Pada Utkatasana)

Modification: both hands to the ankle

Pose Type: standing one-legged balance, forward bend

Drishti Point: Bhrumadhye or Ajna Chakra (third eye, between the eyebrows), Nasagrai or Nasagre (nose)

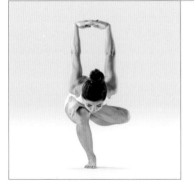

One-Legged Fierce Pose 3

Eka Pada Utkatasana 3

(EY-kuh PUH-duh ut-kuh-TAHS-uh-nuh)

Also Known As: Arms Spread One-Legged Fierce Pose (Prasarita Hasta Eka Pada Utkatasana)

Modification: arms straight out to the sides, forward bend

Pose Type: standing one-legged balance, forward bend

Drishti Point: Bhrumadhye or Ajna Chakra (third eye, between the eyebrows), Nasagrai or Nasagre (nose)

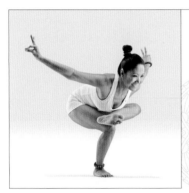

One-Legged Fierce Pose 4

Eka Pada Utkatasana 4

(EY-kuh PUH-duh ut-kuh-TAHS-uh-nuh)

Also Known As: Hands Bound One-Legged Fierce Pose (Baddha Hasta Eka Pada Utkatasana)

Modification: hands bound behind the back, forward bend

Pose Type: standing one-legged balance, forward bend

Drishti Point: Bhrumadhye or Ajna Chakra (third eye, between the eyebrows), Nasagrai or Nasagre (nose)

ONE-LEGGED SQUATS: HALF LOTUS

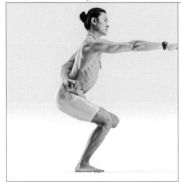

Half Bound Lotus Fierce Pose

Ardha Baddha Padma Utkatasana

(UHR-duh BUH-duh PUHD-muh ut-kuh-TAHS-uh-nuh)

Modification: hips low

Pose Type: standing one-legged balance, binding

Drishti Point: Hastagrai or Hastagre (hands)

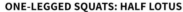

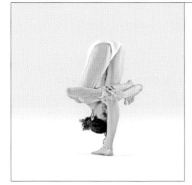

Baby Cradle Pose in Intense Stretch Pose

Hindolasana in Uttanasana

(hin-do-LAHS-uh-nuh in ut-tahn-AHS-uh-nuh)

Also Known As: Baby Cradle Pose in Full Forward Bend

Modification: foot behind the knee of the standing leg

Pose Type: standing one-legged balance, forward bend

Drishti Point: Nasagrai or Nasagre (nose)

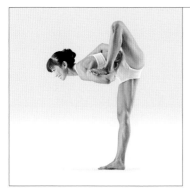

Standing Bound Yogic Staff Pose

Stiti Baddha Yoganandasana

(STI-ti BUH-duh yo-gah-nuhn-DAHS-uh-nuh)

Also Known As: Nindra Baddha Yoganandasana

Pose Type: standing one-legged balance, forward bend

Drishti Point: Nasagrai or Nasagre (nose)

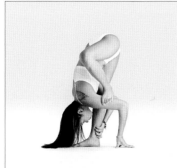

Yogic Staff Intense Stretch Pose

Yogadananda Uttanasana

(yo-gah-nuhn-duh ut-tahn-AHS-uh-nuh)

Also Known As: Yogic Staff Full Forward Bend

Pose Type: standing one-legged balance, forward bend

Drishti Point: Padayoragrai or Padayoragre (toes/feet), Nasagrai or Nasagre (nose)

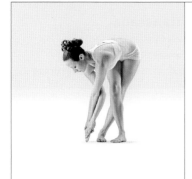

Hand Position of the Pose Dedicated to Garuda in Sideways Half Intense Stretch Pose

Hasta Garudasana in Parshva Ardha Uttanasana

(HUH-stuh guh-ru-DAHS-uh-nuh in PAHRSH-vuh UHR-duh ut-tahn-AHS-uh-nuh)

Also Known As: Hand Position of the Pose Dedicated to Garuda in Sideways Legs Crossed Half Forward Bend

Modification: legs crossed

Pose Type: standing, forward bend, twist

Drishti Point: Hastagrai or Hastagre (hands)

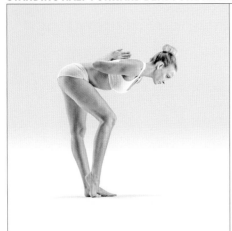

Reverse Prayer Uneven Legs Half Intense Stretch Pose

Viparita Namaskar Vishama Pada Ardha Uttanasana

(vi-puh-REE-tuh nuh-muhs-KAHR VISH-uh-muh PUH-duh UHR-duh ut-tahn-AHS-uh-nuh)

Also Known As: Back of the Body Prayer Uneven Legs Half Intense Stretch Pose (Paschima Namaskara Vishama Pada Ardha Uttanasana), Reverse Prayer Uneven Legs Half Forward Bend

Pose Type: standing, forward bend

Drishti Point: Nasagrai or Nasagre (nose)

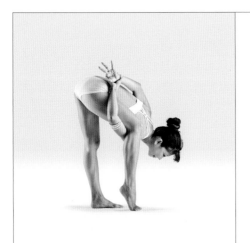

Bound Uneven Legs Half Intense Stretch Pose

Baddha Vishama Pada Ardha Uttanasana

(BUH-duh VISH-uh-muh PUH-duh UHR-duh ut-tahn-AHS-uh-nuh)

Also Known As: Bound Uneven Legs Half Forward Bend

Pose Type: standing, forward bend, binding

Drishti Point: Padayoragrai or Padayoragre (toes/feet)

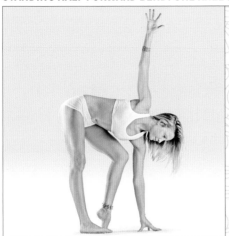

Revolved Uneven Legs Half Intense Stretch Pose

Parivritta Vishama Pada Ardha Uttanasana

(puh-ri-VRIT-tuh VISH-uh-muh PUH-duh UHR-duh ut-tahn-AHS-uh-nuh)

Also Known As: Revolved Uneven Legs Half Forward Bend

Modification: one hand to the floor, other hand up to the sky; looking down

Pose Type: standing, forward bend, twist

Drishti Point: Hastagrai or Hastagre (hands)

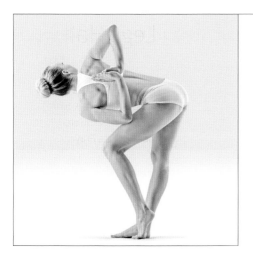

Reverse Prayer Revolved Uneven Legs Half Intense Stretch Pose

Viparita Namaskar Parivritta Vishama Pada Ardha Uttanasana

(vi-puh-REE-tuh nuh-muhs-KAHR puh-ri-VRIT-tuh VISH-uh-muh PUH-duh UHR-duh ut-tahn-AHS-uh-nuh)

Also Known As: Back of the Body Prayer Revolved Uneven Legs Half Intense Stretch Pose (Paschima Namaskara Ardha Parivritta Uttanasana), Reverse Prayer Revolved Uneven Legs Half Forward Bend

Pose Type: standing, forward bend, twist

Drishti Point: Urdhva or Antara Drishti (up to the sky)

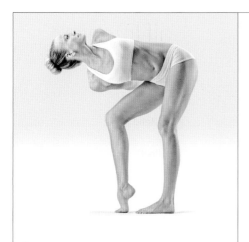

Hands Bound Revolved Uneven Legs Half Intense Stretch Pose

Baddha Hasta Parivritta Vishama Pada Ardha Uttanasana

(BUH-duh HUH-stuh puh-ri-VRIT-tuh VISH-uh-muh PUH-duh UHR-duh ut-tahn-AHS-uh-nuh)

Also Known As: Hands Bound Revolved Uneven Legs Half Forward Bend

Pose Type: standing, forward bend, twist

Drishti Point: Urdhva or Antara Drishti (up to the sky)

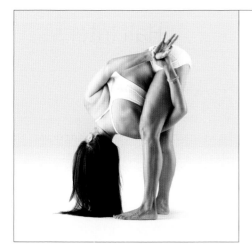

Bound Revolved Half Intense Stretch Pose

Baddha Parivritta Ardha Uttanasana

(BUH-duh puh-ri-VRIT-tuh UHR-duh ut-tahn-AHS-uh-nuh)

Also Known As: Bound Revolved Half Forward Bend

Pose Type: standing, forward bend, twist, binding

Drishti Point: Urdhva or Antara Drishti (up to the sky)

Standing Poses

85

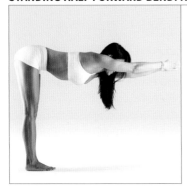

Arms Extended Half Intense Stretch Pose

Utthita Hasta Ardha Uttanasana
(UT-ti-tuh HUH-stuh UHR-duh ut-tahn-AHS-uh-nuh)
Also Known As: Arms Extended Half Forward Bend
Modification: palms pressed together
Pose Type: standing, forward bend
Drishti Point: Angushtamadhye or Angushta Ma Dyai (thumbs), Nasagrai or Nasagre (nose)

STANDING HALF FORWARD BEND: HANDS ON THE FLOOR

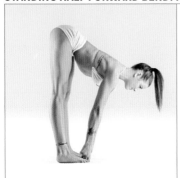

Half Foot Big Toe Pose

Ardha Padangushtasana
(UHR-duh puhd-ahng-goosh-TAHS-uh-nuh)
Pose Type: standing, forward bend
Drishti Point: Nasagrai or Nasagre (nose)

Sideways Half Intense Stretch Pose

Parshva Ardha Uttanasana
(PAHRSH-vuh UHR-duh ut-tahn-AHS-uh-nuh)
Also Known As: Sideways Half Forward Bend
Modification: fingers interlocked, palms to the floor on the outside edge of the foot
Pose Type: standing, forward bend, side bend, twist
Drishti Point: Hastagrai or Hastagre (hands)

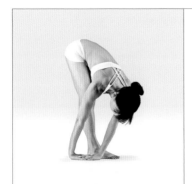

STANDING HALF FORWARD BEND: HANDS ON THE FLOOR—HEELS UP

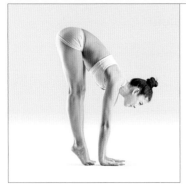

Tip Toe Half Intense Stretch Pose

Prapada Ardha Uttanasana
(PRUH-puh-duh UHR-duh ut-tahn-AHS-uh-nuh)
Also Known As: Tip Toe Half Forward Bend and Downward Facing Tree Pose Prep. (Adho Mukha Vrikshasana Prep.)
Pose Type: standing, forward bend
Drishti Point: Angushtamadhye or Angushta Ma Dyai (thumbs)

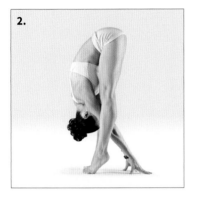

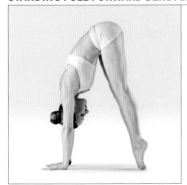

Tip Toe Intense Stretch Pose

Prapada Uttanasana
(PRUH-puh-duh ut-tahn-AHS-uh-nuh)

Also Known As: Tip Toe Full Forward Bend

Modification: arms straight and pointing to the back, both arms on the inside of the legs

1. head up

2. forehead toward the shins

Pose Type: standing, forward bend

Drishti Point: 1. Bhrumadhye or Ajna Chakra (third eye, between the eyebrows)

2. Nasagrai or Nasagre (nose)

STANDING FULL FORWARD BEND: BALLET TOES

Intense Ankle Stretch Intense Stretch Pose 1

Uttana Kulpa Uttanasana 1
(ut-TAHN-uh KUL-puh ut-tahn-AHS-uh-nuh)

Also Known As: Intense Ankle Stretch Forward Bend

Modification: legs together

Pose Type: standing, forward bend

Drishti Point: Nasagrai or Nasagre (nose)

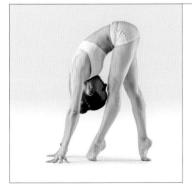

Intense Ankle Stretch Intense Stretch Pose 2

Uttana Kulpa Uttanasana 2
(ut-TAHN-uh KUL-puh ut-tahn-AHS-uh-nuh)

Also Known As: Intense Ankle Stretch Forward Bend

Modification: scissor legs

Pose Type: standing, forward bend

Drishti Point: Nasagrai or Nasagre (nose)

Standing Poses

87

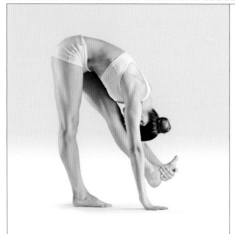

Extended One Hand to Foot Intense Stretch Pose 1

Utthita Eka Hasta Pada Uttanasana 1

(UT-ti-tuh EY-kuh HUH-stuh PUH-duh ut-tahn-AHS-uh-nuh)

Also Known As: Extended One Hand to Foot Full Forward Bend 1

Modification: hand grabbing the foot on the same side

Pose Type: standing one-legged balance, forward bend

Drishti Point: Nasagrai or Nasagre (nose)

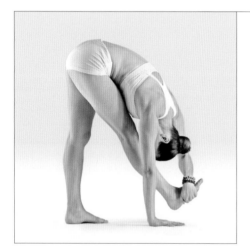

Extended One Hand to Foot Intense Stretch Pose 2

Utthita Eka Hasta Pada Uttanasana 2

(UT-ti-tuh EY-kuh HUH-stuh PUH-duh ut-tahn-AHS-uh-nuh)

Also Known As: Extended One Hand to Foot Full Forward Bend 2

Modification: hand grabbing the foot on the opposite side

Pose Type: standing one-legged balance, forward bend

Drishti Point: Nasagrai or Nasagre (nose)

STANDING FULL FORWARD BEND: HANDS TO THE FLOOR & HANDS TO THE BACK OF THE LEGS

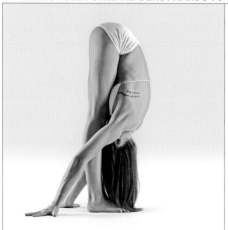

Intense Stretch Pose

Uttanasana

(ut-tahn-AHS-uh-nuh)

Also Known As: Full Forward Bend

Modification: palms to the floor, fingers pointing to the back

Pose Type: standing, forward bend

Drishti Point: Nasagrai or Nasagre (nose)

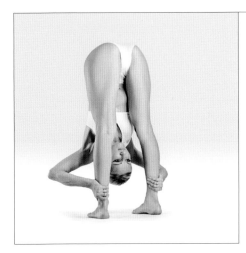

Intense Stretch Pose

Uttanasana

(ut-tahn-AHS-uh-nuh)

Also Known As: Full Forward Bend and Standing Turtle Pose (Nindra Kurmasana)
Modification: feet hip width apart, grabbing onto the calves, elbows bent
Pose Type: standing, forward bend
Drishti Point: Nasagrai or Nasagre (nose)

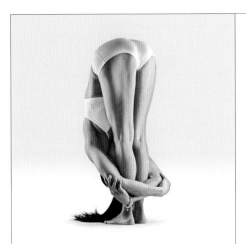

Intense Stretch Pose

Uttanasana

(ut-tahn-AHS-uh-nuh)

Also Known As: Full Forward Bend and Locked Elbows Standing Intense Stretch Pose (Baddha Padahastasana)
Modification: grabbing onto triceps behind the calves
Pose Type: standing, forward bend
Drishti Point: Nasagrai or Nasagre (nose)

STANDING FULL FORWARD BEND: GRABBING ONTO THE FEET

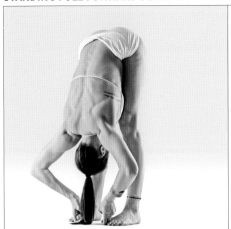

Foot Big Toe Pose

Padangushtasana

(puh-ahng-goosh-TAHS-uh-nuh)

Pose Type: standing, forward bend
Drishti Point: Nasagrai or Nasagre (nose)

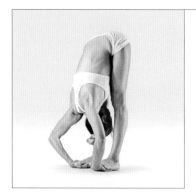

Hand Under Foot Pose

Pada Hastasana

(PUH-duh huh-STAHS-uh-nuh)

Pose Type: standing, forward bend

Drishti Point: Nasagrai or Nasagre (nose)

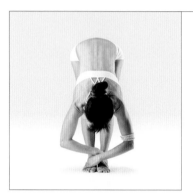

Intense Stretch Pose

Uttanasana *(ut-tahn-AHS-uh-nuh)*

Also Known As: Full Forward Bend

Modification: arms crossed, grabbing onto the outside edges of the feet, half forward bend

Pose Type: standing, forward bend

Drishti Point: Padayoragrai or Padayoragre (toes/feet) or Nasagrai or Nasagre (nose)

1.

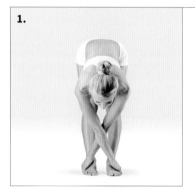

2.

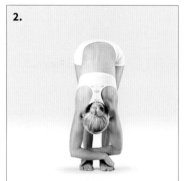

Forward Bend

Uttanasana

(ut-tahn-AHS-uh-nuh)

Also Known As: Full Forward Bend and Hands to Feet Pose Modification (Pada Hastasana)

Modification: feet hip width apart, arms crossed, grabbing onto the outside edges of the feet, elbows moving toward the feet

1. half forward bend

2. full forward bend

Pose Type: standing, forward bend

Drishti Point: 1. Padayoragrai or Padayoragre (toes/feet)

2. Nasagrai or Nasagre (nose)

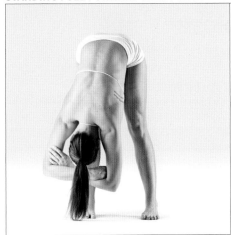

Intense Stretch Pose

Uttanasana

(ut-tahn-AHS-uh-nuh)

Also Known As: Full Forward Bend

Modification: grabbing onto the triceps, swaying from side to side

Pose Type: standing, forward bend, side bend

Drishti Point: Nasagrai or Nasagre (nose)

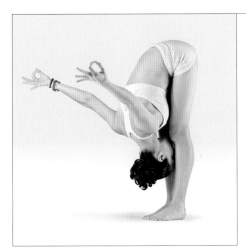

Intense Stretch Pose

Uttanasana

(ut-tahn-AHS-uh-nuh)

Also Known As: Full Forward Bend and Unsupported Forward Stretch Pose (Niralamba Uttanasana)

Modification: arms straight out to the sides behind the back, forehead to the shins

Pose Type: standing, forward bend

Drishti Point: Nasagrai or Nasagre (nose)

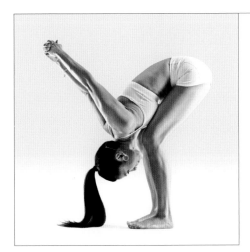

Hands Bound Forward Bend Modification

Baddha Hasta Uttanasana

(BUH-duh HUH-stuh ut-tahn-AHS-uh-nuh)

Also Known As: Hands Bound Full Forward Bend and Unsupported Forward Stretch Pose (Niralamba Uttanasana)

Modification: knees bent, chest to the quadriceps

Pose Type: standing, forward bend

Drishti Point: Nasagrai or Nasagre (nose)

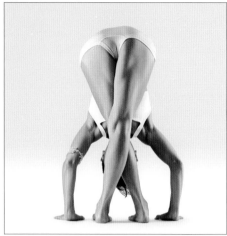

Intense Stretch Pose

Uttanasana

(ut-tahn-AHS-uh-nuh)

Also Known As: Legs Crossed Full Forward Bend

Modification: legs crossed, forehead to the shins, hands to the floor in line with the feet, elbows bent

Pose Type: standing, forward bend

Drishti Point: Nasagrai or Nasagre (nose)

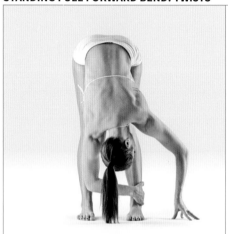

Sideways Intense Stretch

Parshva Uttanasana

(PAHRSH-vuh ut-tahn-AHS-uh-nuh)

Also Known As: Sideways Full Forward Bend

Modification: one hand grabbing onto the opposite ankle, fingertips of the other hand to the floor

Pose Type: standing, forward bend, twist

Drishti Point: Parshva Drishti (to the right), Parshva Drishti (to the left)

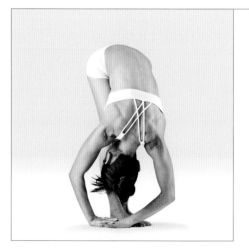

Sideways Intense Stretch

Parshva Uttanasana

(PAHRSH-vuhut-tahn-AHS-uh-nuh)

Also Known As: Sideways Full Forward Bend and Sideward Forward Stretch (Parshva Bhaga Uttanasana)

Modification: fingers interlocked, palms to the floor on the outside edge of the foot

Pose Type: standing, forward bend, twist

Drishti Point: Nasagrai or Nasagre (nose)

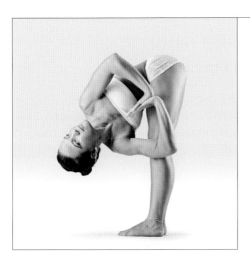

Revolved Intense Stretch Prayer Pose

Parivritta Uttana Anjalyiasana

(puh-ri-VRIT-uh ut-TAHN-uh uhn-juhl-YAHS-uh-nuh)

Also Known As: Revolved Full Forward Bend Prayer Pose
Pose Type: standing, forward bend, twist
Drishti Point: Urdhva or Antara Drishti (up to the sky)

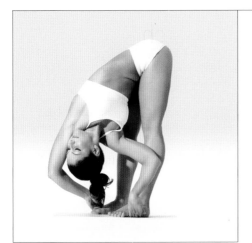

Revolved Intense Stretch

Parivritta Uttanasana

(puh-ri-VRIT-tuh ut-tahn-AHS-uh-nuh)

Also Known As: Revolved Full Forward Bend
Modification: grabbing the outside edge of the feet, feet hip width apart
Pose Type: standing, forward bend, twist
Drishti Point: Urdhva or Antara Drishti (up to the sky)

STANDING FULL FORWARD BEND: TWISTS—FEET SLIGHTLY WIDER THAN HIPS

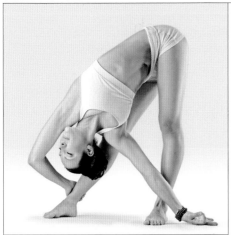

Revolved Intense Stretch

Parivritta Uttanasana

(puh-ri-VRIT-tuh ut-tahn-AHS-uh-nuh)

Also Known As: Revolved Full Forward Bend
Modification: feet wide; one hand grabbing onto the ankle, back of the other hand to the floor in front of the opposite foot
Pose Type: standing, forward bend, twist
Drishti Point: Urdhva or Antara Drishti (up to the sky)

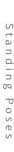

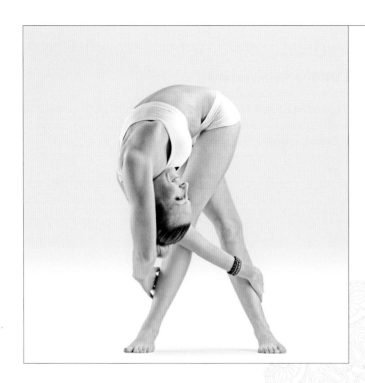

Revolved Intense Stretch

Parivritta Uttanasana

(puh-ri-VRIT-tuh ut-tahn-AHS-uh-nuh)

Also Known As: Revolved Legs Crossed Full Forward Bend
Modification: feet wide, legs crossed, feet flat on the floor
Pose Type: standing, forward bend, twist
Drishti Point: Urdhva or Antara Drishti (up to the sky)

STANDING FULL FORWARDS BEND: BINDING

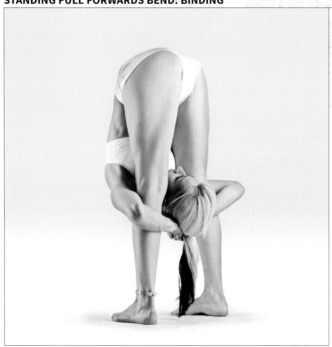

Firefly Pose 2 A

Tittibhasana 2 A

(ti-ti-BAHS-uh-nuh)

Also Known As: Intense Stretch Pose Stork Modification (Uttanasana), Standing Bound Arms Head Between Knees Pose (Utthita Baddha Hasta Janu Shirshasana)
Modification: arms wrapped around the legs, fingers interlocked behind the head
Pose Type: standing, forward bend, binding
Drishti Point: Nasagrai or Nasagre (nose)

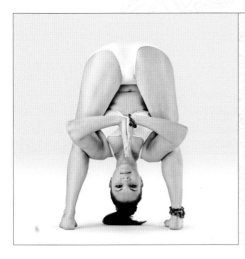

Firefly Pose 2 B

Tittibhasana 2 B

(ti-ti-BAHS-uh-nuh)

Also Known As: Inverted Firefly Prayer Pose (Viparita Tittibha Anjali Asana)
Modification: hands in Anjali Mudra (Hands in Prayer)
Pose Type: standing, forward bend
Drishti Point: Nasagrai or Nasagre (nose)

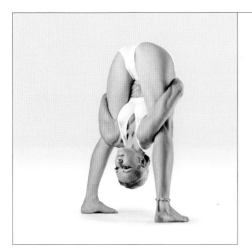

Complete Firefly Pose 2

Paripurna Tittibhasana 2

(puh-ri-POOR-nuh ti-ti-BAHS-uh-nuh)

Also Known As: Firefly Pose B (Tittibhasana B), Inverted Firefly Pose (Viparita Tittibhasana), Standing Firefly Pose Modification (Utthita Tittibhasana), Bound Firefly Pose, Standing Tortoise Pose (Nindra Kurmasana)
Modification: hands bound
Pose Type: standing, forward bend, binding
Drishti Point: Nasagrai or Nasagre (nose)

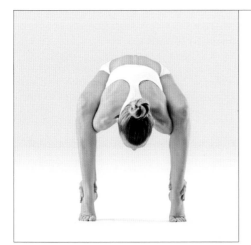

Firefly Pose 3 A Prep.

Tittibhasana 3 A Prep.

(ti-ti-BAHS-uh-nuh)

Modification: hands on the ankles, heels up
Pose Type: standing, forward bend
Drishti Point: Nasagrai or Nasagre (nose)

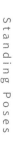

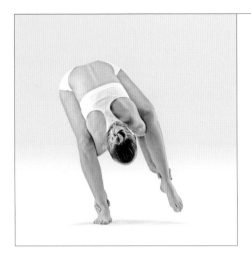

Firefly Pose 3 A

Tittibhasana 3 A

(ti-ti-BAHS-uh-nuh)

Also Known As: Firefly Pose C Prep. (Tittibhasana C Prep.)
Modification: hands on the ankles, one foot lifted
Pose Type: standing one-legged balance, forward bend
Drishti Point: Nasagrai or Nasagre (nose)

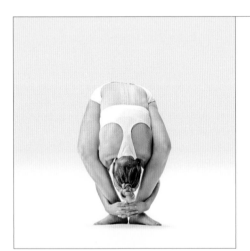

Firefly Pose 4 A

Tittibhasana 4 A

(ti-ti-BAHS-uh-nuh)

Also Known As: Firefly Pose D (Tittibhasana D), Standing Firefly Pose (Utthita Tittibhasana)
Modification: fingers interlocked in front of the ankles
Pose Type: standing, forward bend, binding
Drishti Point: Nasagrai or Nasagre (nose)

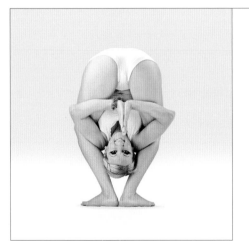

Firefly Pose 4 B

Tittibhasana 4 B

(ti-ti-BAHS-uh-nuh)

Also Known As: Inverted Both Legs Prayer Pose (Viparita DwiPada Anjaliasana)
Modification: hands in Anjali Mudra (Hands in Prayer)
Pose Type: standing, forward bend
Drishti Point: Bhrumadhye or Ajna Chakra (third eye, between the eyebrows)

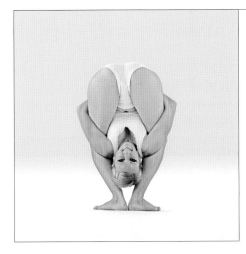

Complete Firefly Pose 4

Paripurna Tittibhasana 4

(puh-ri-POOR-nuh ti-ti-BAHS-uh-nuh)

Also Known As: Inverted Bound Legs Pose (Viparita DwiPada Baddhasana)
Modification: hands bound
Pose Type: standing, forward bend, binding
Drishti Point: Bhrumadhye or Ajna Chakra (third eye, between the eyebrows)

LEGS WIDE: STRAIGHT SPINE, TWISTS & BACKBEND

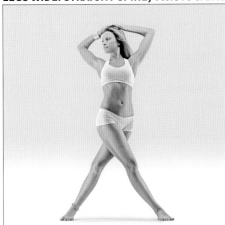

Book Stand Pose

Grantadara

(gruhn-tah-DAH-ruh)

Also Known As: Chikkyasana
Modification: hands to the head, palms facing up, looking to the side
Pose Type: standing, twist
Drishti Point: Parshva Drishti (to the right), Parshva Drishti (to the left)

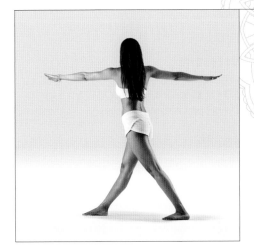

Revolved Feet Spread Mountain Pose

Parivritta Prasarita Pada Tadasana

(puh-ri-VRIT-tuh pruh-SAH-ri-tuh PUH-duh tuh-DAHS-uh-nuh)

Modification: arms straight out to the sides
Pose Type: standing, twist
Drishti Point: Parshva Drishti (to the right), Parshva Drishti (to the left)

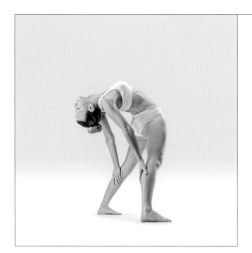

Feet Spread Mountain Pose in Hero Succession Series

Prasarita Pada Tadasana in Vira Parampara

(pruh-SAH-ri-tuh PUH-duh tuh-DAHS-uh-nuh in VEER-uh puh-ruhm-puh-RAH)

Modification: backbend, hands on the calf muscles
Pose Type: standing, backbend
Drishti Point: Bhrumadhye or Ajna Chakra (third eye, between the eyebrows)

LEGS WIDE: ARMS UP OVER THE HEAD

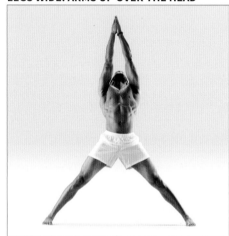

Easy Feet Spread Upward Hands Pose

Sukha Prasarita Pada Urdhva Hastasana

(SUK-kuh pruh-SAH-ri-tuh PUH-duh OORD-vuh huh-STAHS-uh-nuh)

Also Known As: Part of Hero Succession Series (Vira Parampara)
Modification: palms together, looking up
Pose Type: standing, mild backbend
Drishti Point: Angushtamadhye or Angushta Ma Dyai (thumbs)

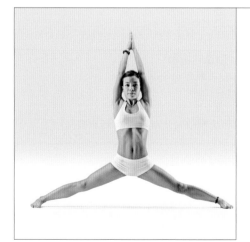

Feet Spread Upward Hands Pose

Prasarita Pada Urdhva Hastasana

(pruh-SAH-ri-tuh PUH-duh OORD-vuh huh-STAHS-uh-nuh)

Also Known As: Equal Angle Pose (Sama Konasana)
Modification: legs open extremely wide; palms together, looking straight ahead
Pose Type: standing
Drishti Point: Nasagrai or Nasagre (nose)

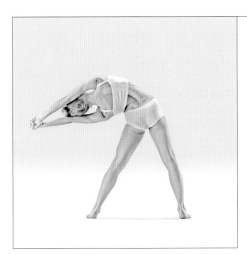

Angle Pose

Konasana

(ko-NAHS-uh-nuh)

Also Known As: Triangle Pose (Konasana)
Modification: fingers interlocked, palms together; side bend
Pose Type: standing, side bend
Drishti Point: Urdhva or Antara Drishti (up to the sky), Nasagrai or Nasagre (nose)

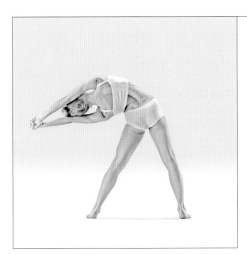

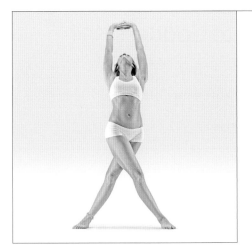

Book Stand Pose with Upward Bound Hands

Grantadara Urdhva Baddha Hastasana

(gruhn-tah-DAH-ruh OORD-vuh BUH-duh HUH-STAHS-uh-nuh)

Also Known As: Chikkiasana Urdhva Baddha Hastasana
Modification: fingers interlocked, palms facing up, looking up
Pose Type: standing
Drishti Point: Angushtamadhye or Angushta Ma Dyai (thumbs)

KALI SQUAT: HEELS DOWN—ARMS UP OVER THE HEAD

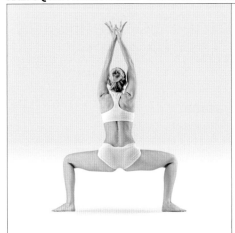

Lotus Hand Seal in Upward Hands Pose Dedicated to Goddess Kali

Padma Mudra Urdhva Hasta Kalyasana

(PUHD-muh MU-druh OORD-vuh HUH-stuh kahl-YAHS-uh-nuh)

Modification: heels down; arms extended to the sky, fingertips open
Pose Type: standing
Drishti Point: Nasagrai or Nasagre (nose)

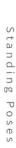

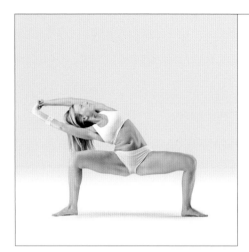

Sideways Hands Bound Pose Dedicated to Goddess Kali

Parshva Baddha Hasta Kalyasana

(PAHRSH-vuh BUH-duh HUH-stuh kahl-YAHS-uh-nuh)

Modification: side bend, fingers interlocked
Pose Type: standing, side bend
Drishti Point: Urdhva or Antara Drishti (up to the sky)

KALI SQUAT: HEELS DOWN—ARMS AT HEAD HEIGHT

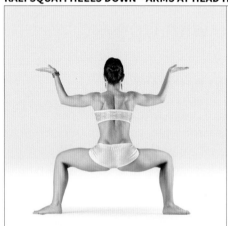

Pose Dedicated to Goddess Kali

Kalyasana

(kahl-YAHS-uh-nuh)

Modification: elbows bent, palms facing the sky, heels down
Pose Type: standing
Drishti Point: Nasagrai or Nasagre (nose)

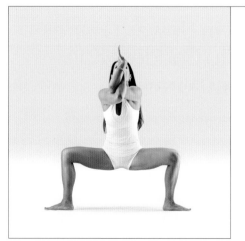

Hand Position of the Pose Dedicated to Garuda in Pose Dedicated to Goddess Kali

Hasta Garudasana in Kalyasana

(HUH-stuh guh-ru-DAHS-uh-nuh in kahl-YAHS-uh-nuh)

Pose Type: standing
Drishti Point: Angushtamadhye or Angushta Ma Dyai (thumbs)

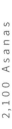

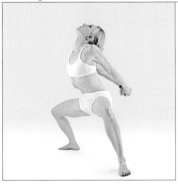

Hands Bound Pose Dedicated to Goddess Kali

Baddha Hasta Kalyasana

(BUH-duh HUH-stuh kahl-YAHS-uh-nuh)

Modification: head rolling back, heels down
Pose Type: standing, backbend
Drishti Point: Bhrumadhye or Ajna Chakra (third eye, between the eyebrows)

Bound Pose Dedicated to Goddess Kali

Baddha Kalyasana

(BUH-duh kahl-YAHS-uh-nuh)

Pose Type: standing, binding
Drishti Point: Nasagrai or Nasagre (nose)

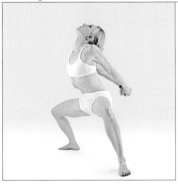

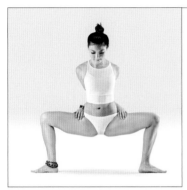

Pose Dedicated to Goddess Kali

Kalyasana

(kahl-YAHS-uh-nuh)

Modification: one hand to the forehead, arm to the knee on the same side
Pose Type: standing
Drishti Point: Parshva Drishti (to the right), Parshva Drishti (to the left)

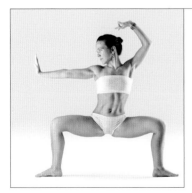

Pose Dedicated to Goddess Kali

Kalyasana

(kahl-YAHS-uh-nuh)

Modification: one arm straight and parallel to the floor, other arm bent, palm facing up
Pose Type: standing
Drishti Point: Hastagrai or Hastagre (hands)

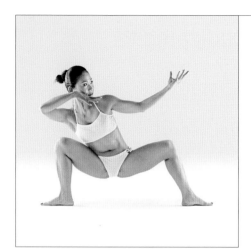

Sideways Pose Dedicated to Goddess Kali

Parshva Kalyasana

(PAHRSH-vuh kahl-YAHS-uh-nuh)

Modification: leaning to one side, one arm out to the side—elbow slightly bent, palm facing up, other hand to the face—palm down

Pose Type: standing, side bend

Drishti Point: Hastagrai or Hastagre (hands)

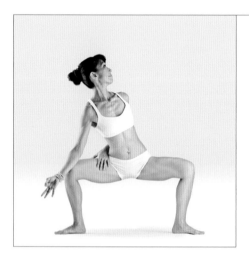

Sideways Half Bound Pose Dedicated to Goddess Kali

Parshva Ardha Baddha Kalyasana

(PAHRSH-vuh UHR-duh BUH-duh kahl-YAHS-uh-nuh)

Modification: forearm to the knee on the same side

Pose Type: standing, side bend, binding

Drishti Point: Urdhva or Antara Drishti (up to the sky)

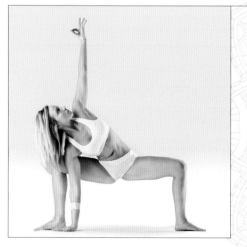

Sideways Pose Dedicated to Goddess Kali

Parshva Kalyasana

(PAHRSH-vuh kahl-YAHS-uh-nuh)

Modification: one hand to the floor, other arm up to the sky

Pose Type: standing, side bend

Drishti Point: Hastagrai or Hastagre (hands)

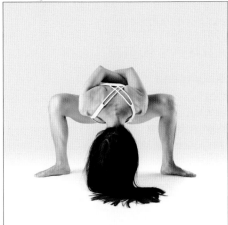

Bound Pose Dedicated to Goddess Kali

Baddha Kalyasana

(BUH-duh kahl-YAHS-uh-nuh)
Modification: forward bend
Pose Type: standing, forward bend, binding
Drishti Point: Nasagrai or Nasagre (nose)

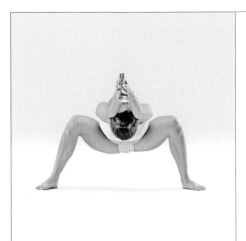

Pose Dedicated to Goddess Kali

Kalyasana

(kahl-YAHS-uh-nuh)
Modification: forward bend, arms straight and parallel to the floor, palms together
Pose Type: standing, forward bend
Drishti Point: Nasagrai or Nasagre (nose)

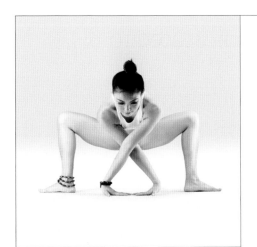

Pose Dedicated to Goddess Kali

Kalyasana

(kahl-YAHS-uh-nuh)
Modification: forward bend, arms crossed, hands to the floor
Pose Type: standing, forward bend
Drishti Point: Nasagrai or Nasagre (nose)

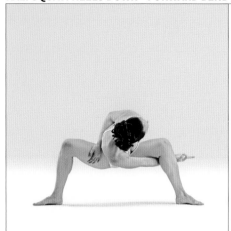

Revolved Half Bound Pose Dedicated to Goddess Kali

Parivritta Ardha Baddha Kalyasana

(puh-ri-VRIT-tuh UHR-duh BUH-duh kahl-YAHS-uh-nuh)

Modification: arm under the opposite leg
Pose Type: standing, forward bend, twist, binding
Drishti Point: Urdhva or Antara Drishti (up to the sky)

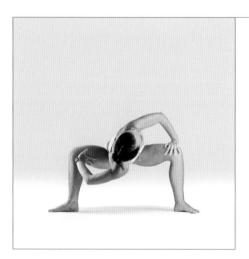

Revolved Pose Dedicated to Goddess Kali

Parivritta Kalyasana

(puh-ri-VRIT-tuh kahl-YAHS-uh-nuh)

Modification: hands to the knees
Pose Type: standing, forward bend, twist
Drishti Point: Urdhva or Antara Drishti (up to the sky)

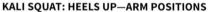

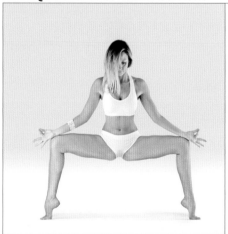

Tip Toe Pose Dedicated to Goddess Kali

Prapada Kalyasana

(PRUH-puh-duh kahl-YAHS-uh-nuh)

Modification: head down, elbows bent, back of the hands on the knees
Pose Type: standing
Drishti Point: Nasagrai or Nasagre (nose)

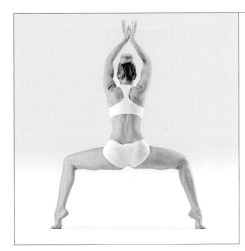

Lotus Hand Seal in Upward Hands Tip Toe Pose Dedicated to Goddess Kali

Padma Mudra in Urdhva Hasta Prapada Kalyasana

(PUHD-muh MU-druh in OORD-vuh HUH-stuh PRUH-puh-duh kahl-YAHS-uh-nuh)

Pose Type: standing
Drishti Point: Nasagrai or Nasagre (nose)

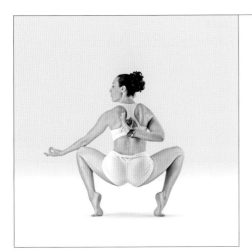

Tip Toe Pose Dedicated to Goddess Kali

Prapada Kalyasana

(PRUH-puh-duh kahl-YAHS-uh-nuh)

Modification: one hand behind the back in reverse prayer, one elbow on the knee
Pose Type: standing
Drishti Point: Hastagrai or Hastagre (hands)

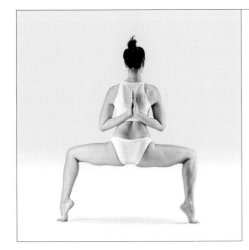

Reverse Prayer Tip Toe Pose Dedicated to Goddess Kali

Viparita Namaskar Prapada Kalyasana

(vi-puh-REE-tuh nuh-muhs-KAHR PRUH-puh-duh kahl-YAHS-uh-nuh)

Also Known As: Back of the Body Prayer Tip Toe Pose Dedicated to Goddess Kali
(Paschima Namaskar Prapada Kalyasana)
Pose Type: standing
Drishti Point: Nasagrai or Nasagre (nose)

KALI SQUAT: HEELS UP—SIDE BENDS

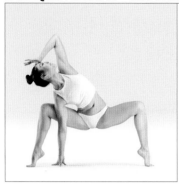

Sideways Tip Toe Pose Dedicated to Goddess Kali

Parshva Prapada Kalyasana
(PAHRSH-vuh PRUH-puh-duh kahl-YAHS-uh-nuh)

Modification: one palm to the forehead, fingertips of the other hand to the floor
Pose Type: standing, side bend
Drishti Point: Urdhva or Antara Drishti (up to the sky)

KALI SQUAT: ONE HEEL UP, ONE HEEL DOWN

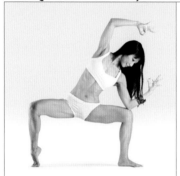

Sideways Uneven Tip Toe Pose Dedicated to Goddess Kali

Parshva Vishama Prapada Kalyasana
(PAHRSH-vuh VISH-uh-muh PRUH-puh-duh kahl-YAHS-uh-nuh)

Modification: side bend
Pose Type: standing, side bend
Dristhi Point: Padhayoragrai or Padayoragre (toes/feet)

KALI SQUAT: HEELS UP—FORWARD BENDS

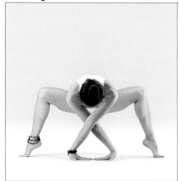

Tip Toe Pose Dedicated to Goddess Kali

Prapada Kalyasana
(PRUH-puh-duh kahl-YAHS-uh-nuh)

Modification: forward bend, arms crossed, hands to the floor, fingertips pointing toward each other
Pose Type: standing, forward bend
Drishti Point: Hastagrai or Hastagre (hands)

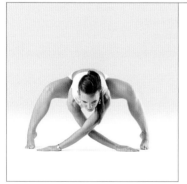

Tip Toe Pose Dedicated to Goddess Kali

Prapada Kalyasana
(PRUH-puh-duh kahl-YAHS-uh-nuh)

Modification: forward bend, arms crossed, hands to the floor, fingertips pointing away from each other
Pose Type: standing, forward bend
Drishti Point: Nasagrai or Nasagre (nose)

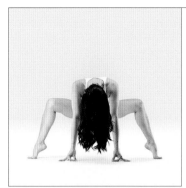

Tip Toe Pose Dedicated to Goddess Kali

Prapada Kalyasana

(PRUH-puh-duh kahl-YAHS-uh-nuh)

Modification: forward bend, hands to the floor, fingertips to the floor facing away from each other
Pose Type: standing, forward bend
Drishti Point: Hastagrai or Hastagre (hands)

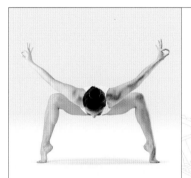

Tip Toe Pose Dedicated to Goddess Kali

Prapada Kalyasana

(PRUH-puh-duh kahl-YAHS-uh-nuh)

Modification: forward bend, arms open wide
Pose Type: standing, forward bend
Drishti Point: Nasagrai or Nasagre (nose)

KALI SQUAT: HEELS DOWN—BINDING

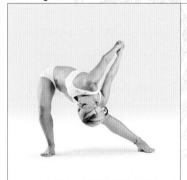

Extended Side Revolved Hands Bound Half Pose Dedicated to Goddess Kali

Utthita Parshva Parivritta Baddha Hasta Ardha Kalyasana

(UT-ti-tuh PAHRSH-vuh puh-ri-VRIT-tuh BUH-duh HUH-stuh UHR-duh kahl-YAHS-uh-nuh)
Pose Type: standing, forward bend, twist
Drishti Point: Urdhva or Antara Drishti (up to the sky)

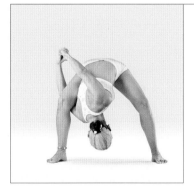

Hands Bound Pose Dedicated to Goddess Kali

Baddha Hasta Kalyasana

(BUH-duh HUH-stuh kahl-YAHS-uh-nuh)

Modification: hands bound under the leg, heels down
Pose Type: standing, forward bend, binding
Drishti Point: Nasagrai or Nasagre (nose)

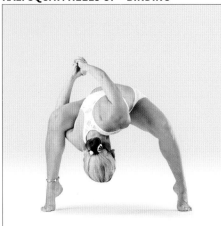

Tip Toe Hands Bound Pose Dedicated to Goddess Kali

Prapada Baddha Hasta Kalyasana

(PRUH-puh-duh kahl-YAHS-uh-nuh)

Modification: hands bound under the leg

Pose Type: standing, forward bend, binding

Drishti Point: Nasagrai or Nasagre (nose)

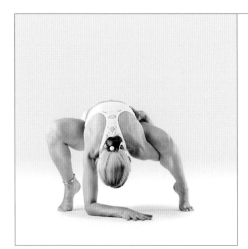

Tip Toe Half Bound Pose Dedicated to Goddess Kali

Prapada Ardha Baddha Kalyasana

(PRUH-puh-duh UHR-duh BUH-duh kahl-YAHS-uh-nuh)

Modification: one arm bound under the leg, palm to the rib cage, other forearm to the floor

Pose Type: standing, forward bend, binding

Drishti Point: Nasagrai or Nasagre (nose), Angushtamadhye or Angushta Ma Dyai (thumbs)

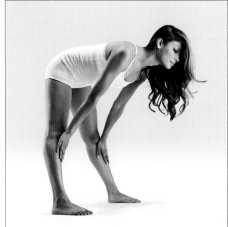

Half Feet Spread Out Intense Stretch Pose

Ardha Prasarita Padottanasana

(UHR-duh pruh-SAH-ri-tuh puhd-o-tahn-AHS-uh-nuh)

Also Known As: Feet Spread Out Half Forward Bend

Modification: legs straight, hands on the shins

Pose Type: standing, forward bend

Drishti Point: Nasagrai or Nasagre (nose)

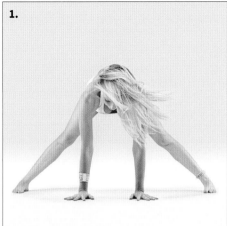

1.

Half Feet Spread Out Intense Stretch Pose

Ardha Prasarita Padottanasana

(UHR-duh pruh-SAH-ri-tuh puhd-o-tahn-AHS-uh-nuh)

Also Known As: Feet Spread Out Half Forward Bend

Modification: 1. toes pointing straight ahead, palms flat on the floor

2. toes pointing slightly outward, back of the hands to the floor, fingertips pointing toward each other

Pose Type: standing, forward bend

Drishti Point: Hastagrai or Hastagre (hands)

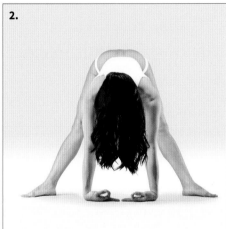

2.

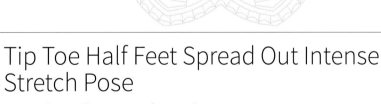

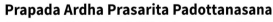

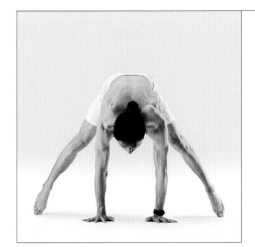

Tip Toe Half Feet Spread Out Intense Stretch Pose

Prapada Ardha Prasarita Padottanasana

(PRUH-puh-duh UHR-duh pruh-SAH-ri-tuh puhd-o-tahn-AHS-uh-nuh)

Also Known As: Tip Toe Feet Spread Out Half Forward Bend

Modification: toes pointing straight ahead, heels up, palms flat on the floor

Pose Type: standing, forward bend

Drishti Point: Hastagrai or Hastagre (hands)

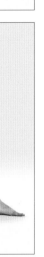

Standing Poses

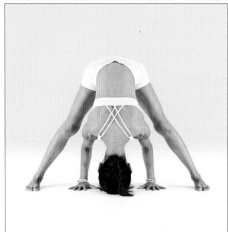

Feet Spread Out Intense Stretch Pose 1

Prasarita Padottanasana 1

(pruh-SAH-ri-tuh puhd-o-tahn-AHS-uh-nuh)

Also Known As: Feet Spread Out Intense Stretch Pose A (Prasarita Padottanasana A), Feet Spread Out Full Forward Bend A

Modification: palms to the floor, elbows bent at 90 degrees

Pose Type: standing, forward bend

Drishti Point: Nasagrai or Nasagre (nose)

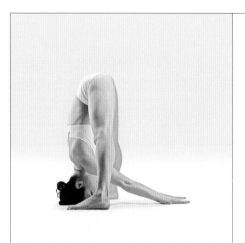

Feet Spread Out Intense Stretch Pose 1

Prasarita Padottanasana 1

(pruh-SAH-ri-tuh puhd-o-tahn-AHS-uh-nuh)

Also Known As: Feet Spread Out Intense Stretch Pose A (Prasarita Padottanasana A), Feet Spread Out Full Forward Bend A

Modification: arms straight, palms to the floor, fingertips pointing away from the head

Pose Type: standing, forward bend

Drishti Point: Hastagrai or Hastagre (hands)

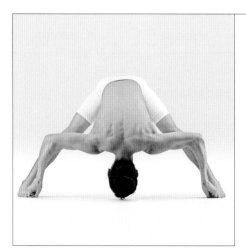

Feet Spread Out Intense Stretch Pose 4

Prasarita Padottanasana 4

(pruh-SAH-ri-tuh puhd-o-tahn-AHS-uh-nuh)

Also Known As: Feet Spread Out Intense Stretch Pose D (Prasarita Padottanasana D), Hands to Big Toes Feet Spread Out Full Forward Bend (Hasta Padangushta Prasarita Padottanasana)

Pose Type: standing, forward bend

Drishti Point: Nasagrai or Nasagre (nose)

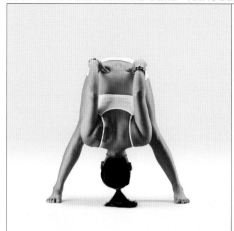

Feet Spread Out Intense Stretch Pose 2

Prasarita Padottanasana 2

(pruh-SAH-ri-tuh puhd-o-tahn-AHS-uh-nuh)

Also Known As: Feet Spread Out Intense Stretch Pose B (Prasarita Padottanasana B), Feet Spread Out Full Forward Bend

Pose Type: standing, forward bend

Drishti Point: Nasagrai or Nasagre (nose)

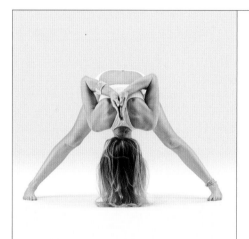

Feet Spread Out Intense Stretch Pose 5

Prasarita Padottanasana 5

(pruh-SAH-ri-tuh puhd-o-tahn-AHS-uh-nuh)

Also Known As: Reverse Prayer Feet Spread Out Full Forward Bend (Viparita Namaskar Prasarita Padottanasana)

Pose Type: standing, forward bend

Drishti Point: Nasagrai or Nasagre (nose)

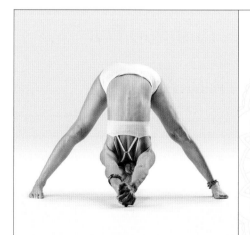

Feet Spread Out Intense Stretch Pose 3

Prasarita Padottanasana 3

(pruh-SAH-ri-tuh puhd-o-tahn-AHS-uh-nuh)

Also Known As: Feet Spread Out Intense Stretch Pose C (Prasarita Padottanasana C), Feet Spread Out Full Forward Bend, Hands Bound Wide Legs Forward Fold (Baddha Hasta Prasarita Padottanasana)

Pose Type: standing, forward bend

Drishti Point: Nasagrai or Nasagre (nose)

Standing Poses

111

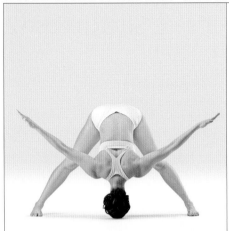

Feet Spread Out Intense Stretch Pose 6

Prasarita Padottanasana 6

(pruh-SAH-ri-tuh puhd-o-tahn-AHS-uh-nuh)

Also Known As: Feet Spread Out Full Forward Bend 6
Pose Type: standing, forward bend
Drishti Point: Nasagrai or Nasagre (nose)

Feet Spread Out Intense Stretch Pose 7

Prasarita Padottanasana 7

(pruh-SAH-ri-tuh puhd-o-tahn-AHS-uh-nuh)

Also Known As: Feet Spread Out Full Forward Bend 7
Pose Type: standing, forward bend
Drishti Point: Nasagrai or Nasagre (nose)

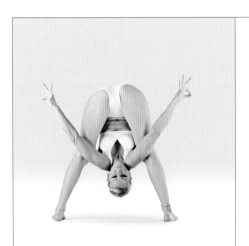

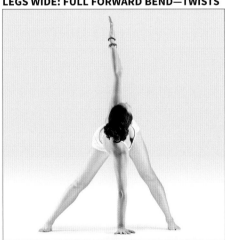

Revolved Half Feet Spread Out Intense Stretch Pose

Parivritta Ardha Prasarita Padottanasana

(puh-ri-VRIT-tuh UHR-duh pruh-SAH-ri-tuh puhd-o-tahn-AHS-uh-nuh)

Also Known As: Revolved Feet Spread Out Half Forward Bend
Modification: palm to the floor
Pose Type: standing, forward bend, twist
Drishti Point: Angushtamadhye or Angushta Ma Dyai (thumbs)

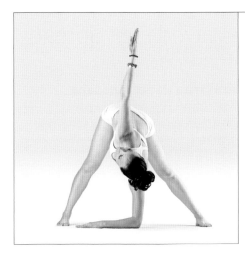

Revolved Half Feet Spread Out Intense Stretch Pose

Parivritta Ardha Prasarita Padottanasana

(puh-ri-VRIT-tuh UHR-duh pruh-SAH-ri-tuh puhd-o-tahn-AHS-uh-nuh)

Also Known As: Revolved Feet Spread Out Half Forward Bend
Modification: forearm to the floor
Pose Type: standing, forward bend, twist
Drishti Point: Angushtamadhye or Angushta Ma Dyai (thumbs)

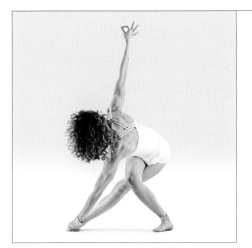

Revolved Paying Homage Feet Spread Out Intense Stretch Pose

Parivritta Namasya Prasarita Padottanasana

(puh-ri-VRIT-tuh nuh-MUHS-ya pruh-SAH-ri-tuh puhd-o-tahn-AHS-uh-nuh)

Also Known As: Revolved Paying Homage Feet Spread Out Forward Bend
Modification: legs crossed, hand to the back foot, other arm extended to the sky
Pose Type: standing, forward bend, twist
Drishti Point: Hastagrai or Hastagre (hands)

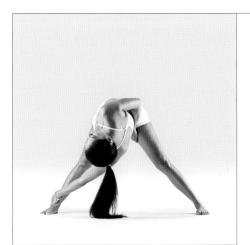

Bound Revolved Feet Spread Out Intense Stretch Pose

Baddha Parivritta Prasarita Padottanasana

(BUH-duh puh-ri-VRIT-tuh pruh-SAH-ri-tuh puhd-o-tahn-AHS-uh-nuh)

Also Known As: Bound Revolved Feet Spread Out Full Forward Bend
Modification: arm straight, looking up
Pose Type: standing, forward bend, twist, binding
Drishti Point: Urdhva or Antara Drishti (up to the sky)

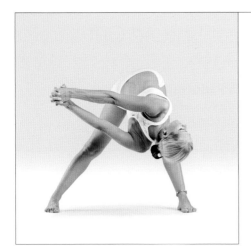

Hands Bound Revolved Feet Spread Out Intense Stretch Pose

Baddha Hasta Parivritta Prasarita Padottanasana
(BUH-duh HUH-stuh puh-ri-VRIT-tuh pruh-SAH-ri-tuh puhd-o-tahn-AHS-uh-nuh)
Also Known As: Hands Bound Revolved Feet Spread Out Full Forward Bend
Pose Type: standing, forward bend, twist
Drishti Point: Urdhva or Antara Drishti (up to the sky)

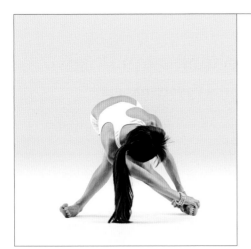

Revolved Paying Homage Feet Spread Out Intense Stretch Pose

Parivritta Namasya Prasarita Padottanasana
(puh-ri-VRIT-tuh nuh-MUHS-ya pruh-SAH-ri-tuh puhd-o-tahn-AHS-uh-nuh)
Modification: outside edges of the feet to the floor, legs crossed, forward bend, both hands on the back foot
Pose Type: standing, forward bend, twist
Drishti Point: Urdhva or Antara Drishti (up to the sky)

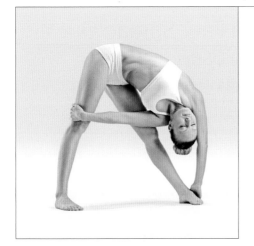

Revolved Feet Spread Out Intense Stretch Pose

Parivritta Prasarita Padottanasana
(puh-ri-VRIT-tuh pruh-SAH-ri-tuh puhd-o-tahn-AHS-uh-nuh)
Also Known As: Revolved Feet Spread Out Full Forward Bend
Modification: grabbing onto the knee and the foot
Pose Type: standing, forward bend, side bend, twist
Drishti Point: Urdhva or Antara Drishti (up to the sky)

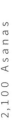

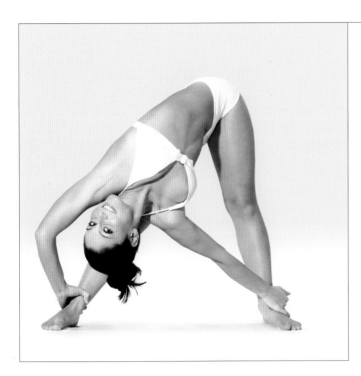

Revolved Feet Spread Out Intense Stretch Pose

Parivritta Prasarita Padottanasana

(puh-ri-VRIT-tuh pruh-SAH-ri-tuh puhd-o-tahn-AHS-uh-nuh)

Also Known As: Revolved Feet Spread Out Full Forward Bend

Modification: grabbing onto the ankles

Pose Type: standing, forward bend, side bend, twist

Drishti Point: Urdhva or Antara Drishti (up to the sky)

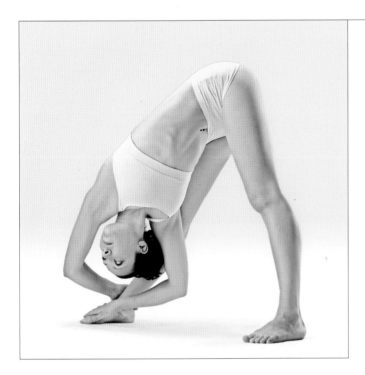

Revolved to the Side Feet Spread Out Intense Stretch Pose

Parivritta Parshva Prasarita Padottanasana

(puh-ri-VRIT-tuh PAHRSH-vuh pruh-SAH-ri-tuh puhd-o-tahn-AHS-uh-nuh)

Also Known As: Revolved to the Side Feet Spread Out Full Forward Bend)

Modification: grabbing onto the foot with both hands

Pose Type: standing, forward bend, twist

Drishti Point: Urdhva or Antara Drishti (up to the sky)

1.

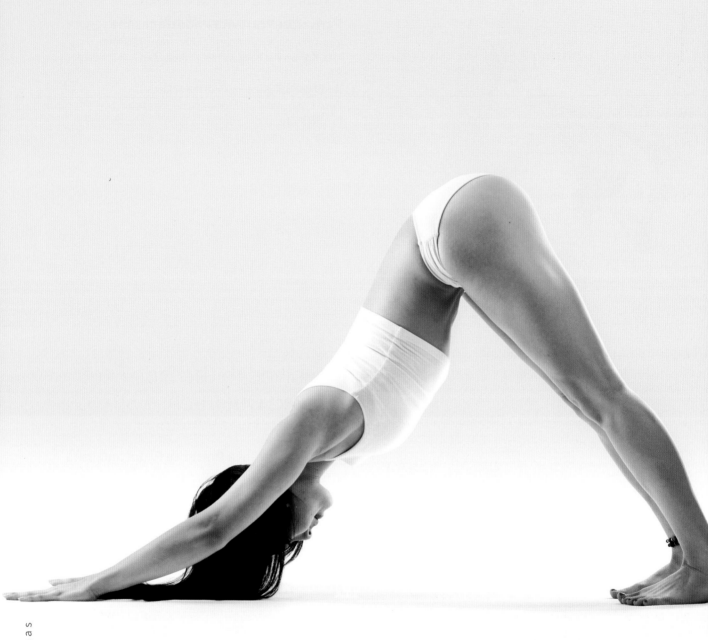

Downward Facing Dog Pose

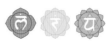

Adho Mukha Shvanasana

(uh-DO MUK-uh shwa-NAHS-uh-nuh)

Pose Type: standing, forward bend

Drishti Point: Nasagrai or Nasagre (nose)

Modification:

1. head off the floor
2. forehead to the floor

adho = downward
mukha = face
shvana = dog

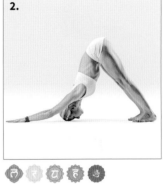

2.

How to Perform the Pose:

1. Start by lying on your stomach with your whole body flat on the floor. Place your palms on the floor at the bottom of your ribs with fingertips facing forward and elbows tucked in. Engage your *mula bandha*, *uddhiyana bandha*, and *ujjayi* breathing.

2. Exhale as you engage your core and lift your torso off the floor, and straighten your arms, coming into a distinct upside-down V shape with your sitting bones up to the sky. Your feet should be in line with your sitting bones and your hands should be shoulder width apart.

3. Try to keep your legs as straight as possible while pressing the heels to the floor. You should feel a deep stretch in the back of your thighs (the hamstrings) and your calf muscles.

4. Inhale as you lengthen your spine, keeping your neck long and your shoulder blades down your back. Try not to round your lower back, keeping it long. Exhale as you press through your chest, moving it toward your thighs. You should feel a deep stretch in the back of your shoulders.

5. You can either keep your head off the floor (Pose #1) or bring your forehead to the floor (Pose #2) if your shoulders are open.

6. Hold the pose for at least 30, and up to 90, seconds in order to receive the full benefits of the stretch.

7. To come out of the pose, inhale as you rock into Plank Pose, and exhale as you bend your elbows into Four Limbed Staff Pose (*Chaturanga Dandasana*) and lower all the way down to the floor into the starting position.

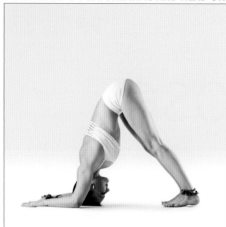

Downward Facing Pose Dedicated to Makara on the Head

Adho Mukha Shirsha Makarasana

(uh-DO MUK-uh SHEER-shuh muh-kuh-RAHS-uh-nuh)

Pose Type: forward bend, inversion, core

Drishti Point: Bhrumadhye or Ajna Chakra (third eye, between the eyebrows)

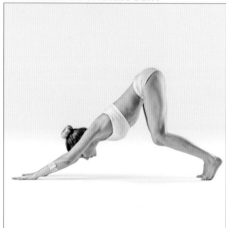

Downward Facing Dog Pose

Adho Mukha Shvanasana

(uh-DO MUK-uh shwa-NAHS-uh-nuh)

Modification: knees bent, heels up

Pose Type: standing, forward bend

Drishti Point: Nasagrai or Nasagre (nose)

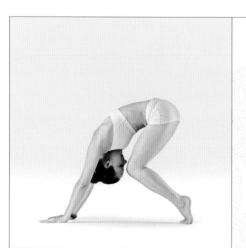

Downward Facing Dog Pose

Adho Mukha Shvanasana

(uh-DO MUK-uh shwa-NAHS-uh-nuh)

Modification: knees bent, heels up, spine in Cat Tilt, forehead toward the knees

Pose Type: standing, forward bend

Drishti Point: Nasagrai or Nasagre (nose)

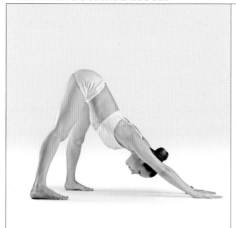

Feet Spread Downward Facing Dog Pose

Prasarita Pada Adho Mukha Shvanasana

(pruh-SAH-ri-tuh PUH-duh uh-DO MUK-uh shwa-NAHS-uh-nuh)

Modification: heels down, palms down

Pose Type: standing, forward bend

Drishti Point: Nasagrai or Nasagre (nose)

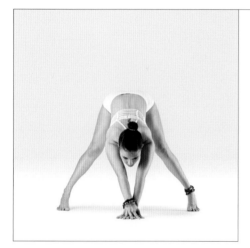

Tip Toe Feet Spread Downward Facing Dog Pose

Prapada Prasarita Pada Adho Mukha Shvanasana

(PRUH-puh-duh pruh-SAH-ri-tuh PUH-duh uh-DO MUK-uh shwa-NAHS-uh-nuh)

Modification: one palm on top of the other, fingertips to the floor, head above the arms

Pose Type: standing, forward bend

Drishti Point: Hastagrai or Hastagre (hands), Nasagrai or Nasagre (nose)

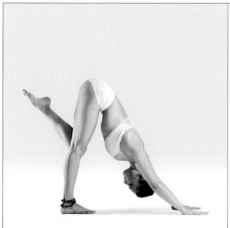

One-Legged Downward Facing Dog Pose

Eka Pada Adho Mukha Shvanasana

(EY-kuh PUH-duh uh-DO MUK-uh shwa-NAHS-uh-nuh)

Modification: back leg bent, knees together

Pose Type: standing, forward bend

Drishti Point: Padayoragrai or Padayoragre (toes/feet)

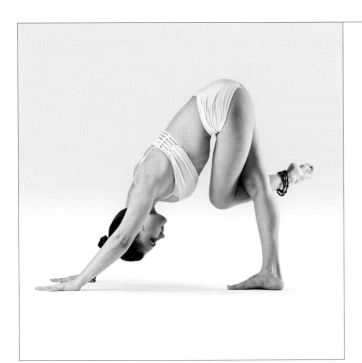

Leg Position of the Half Cow Face Pose in Downward Facing Dog Pose

Pada Ardha Gomukhasana in Adho Mukha Shvanasana

(PUH-duh URH-duh go-muk-AHS-uh-nuh in uh-DO MUK-uh shwa-NAHS-uh-nuh)

Also Known As: Leg Position of the One-Legged Cow Face Pose in Downward Facing Dog Pose (Eka Pada Gomukhasana in Adho Mukha Shvanasana)

Pose Type: standing, forward bend

Drishti Point: Padayoragrai or Padayoragre (toes/feet)

DOWNWARD DOG: ONE-ARMED

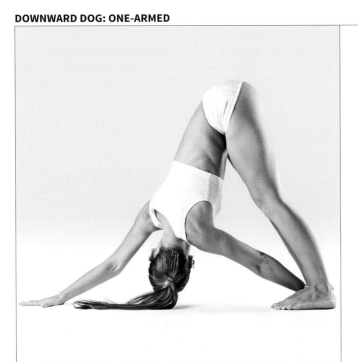

Revolved Downward Facing Dog Pose

Parivritta Adho Mukha Shvanasana

(puh-ri-VRIT-tuh uh-DO MUK-uh shwa-NAHS-uh-nuh)

Pose Type: standing, forward bend, twist

Drishti Point: Urdhva or Antara Drishti (up to the sky)

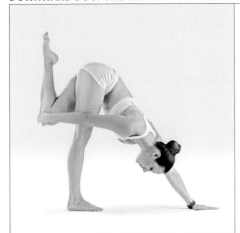

Hand to Knee One-Legged Downward Facing Dog Pose

Hasta Janu Eka Pada Adho Mukha Shvanasana

(HUH-stuh JAH-nu EY-kuh PUH-duh uh-DO MUK-uh shwa-NAHS-uh-nuh)

Modification: hand grabbing onto the opposite knee

Pose Type: standing one-legged balance, forward bend

Drishti Point: Padayoragrai or Padayoragre (toes/feet)

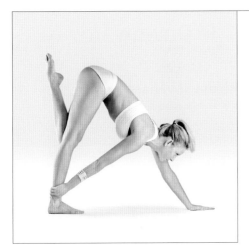

Hand to Ankle One-Legged Downward Facing Dog Pose 1

Hasta Kulpa Eka Pada Adho Mukha Shvanasana 1

(HUH-stuh KUL-puh EY-kuh PUH-duh uh-DO MUK-uh shwa-NAHS-uh-nuh)

Modification: grabbing onto the ankle on the same side; back leg bent, knees together

Pose Type: standing one-legged balance, forward bend

Drishti Point: Angushtamadhye or Angushta Ma Dyai (thumbs)

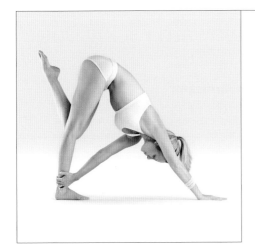

Hand to Ankle One-Legged Downward Facing Dog Pose 2

Hasta Kulpa Eka Pada Adho Mukha Shvanasana 2

(HUH-stuh KUL-puh EY-kuh PUH-duh uh-DO MUK-uh shwa-NAHS-uh-nuh)

Modification: grabbing onto the ankle on the opposite side; back leg bent, knees together

Pose Type: standing one-legged balance, forward bend

Drishti Point: Angushtamadhye or Angushta Ma Dyai (thumbs)

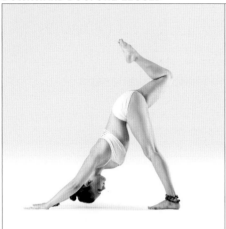

One-Legged Downward Facing Dog Pose

Eka Pada Adho Mukha Shvanasana

(EY-kuh PUH-duh uh-DO MUK-uh shwa-NAHS-uh-nuh)

Modification: knee bent
Pose Type: standing, forward bend
Drishti Point: Nasagrai or Nasagre (nose)

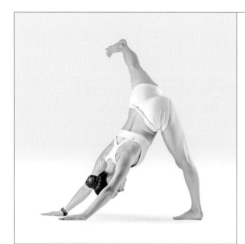

One Leg to the Side Downward Facing Dog Pose

Parshva Eka Pada Adho Mukha Shvanasana

(PAHRSH-vuh EY-kuh PUH-duh uh-DO MUK-uh shwa-NAHS-uh-nuh)

Pose Type: standing, forward bend
Drishti Point: Nasagrai or Nasagre (nose)

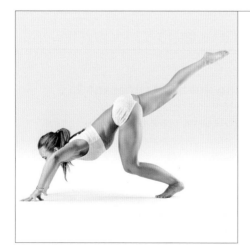

One-Legged Downward Facing Dog Pose

Eka Pada Adho Mukha Shvanasana

(EY-kuh PUH-duh uh-DO MUK-uh shwa-NAHS-uh-nuh)

Also Known As: One-Legged Downward Facing Dog Shoulder Press
Modification: bottom knee bent; elbows bent, fingertips to the floor
Pose Type: standing, forward bend
Drishti Point: Angushtamadhye or Angushta Ma Dyai (thumbs)

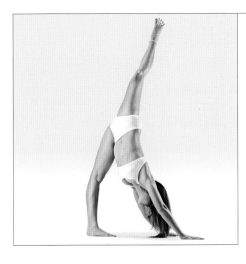

One-Legged Downward Facing Dog Pose

Eka Pada Adho Mukha Shvanasana
(EY-kuh PUH-duh uh-DO MUK-uh shwa-NAHS-uh-nuh)
Also Known As: One Leg Raised Up Downward Facing Dog Pose (Utthita Eka Pada Adho Mukha Shvanasana)
Modification: back leg straight and extended up to the sky
Pose Type: standing, forward bend
Drishti Point: Angushtamadhye or Angushta Ma Dyai (thumbs)

DOWNWARD DOG: TWISTS

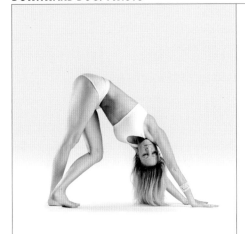

Uneven Legs Revolved Downward Facing Dog Pose 1

Vishama Pada Parivritta Adho Mukha Shvanasana 1
(VISH-uh-muh PUH-duh puh-ri-VRIT-tuh uh-DO MUK-uh shwa-NAHS-uh-nuh)
Modification: one knee bent, foot crossed over
Pose Type: standing, forward bend, twist
Drishti Point: Urdhva or Antara Drishti (up to the sky)

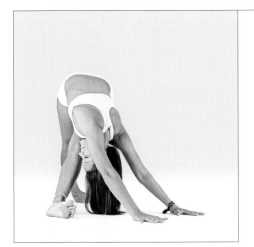

Uneven Legs Revolved Downward Facing Dog Pose 2

Vishama Pada Parivritta Adho Mukha Shvanasana 2
(VISH-uh-muh PUH-duh puh-ri-VRIT-tuh uh-DO MUK-uh shwa-NAHS-uh-nuh)
Modification: both legs straight, one leg crossed over
Pose Type: standing, forward bend, twist
Drishti Point: Parshva Drishti (to the right), Parshva Drishti (to the left)

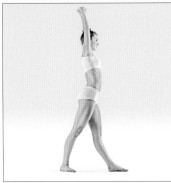

Upward Bound Hands Pose in Hero Succession Series

Urdhva Baddha Hastasana in Vira Parampara

(OORD-vuh BUH-duh huh-STAHS-uh-nuh in VEER-uh puh-ruhm-puh-RAH)

Modification: arms up to the sky, fingers interlocked, spine straight
Pose Type: standing
Drishti Point: Nasagrai or Nasagre (nose)

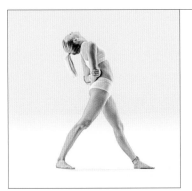

Hands Bound Pose in Hero Succession Series

Baddha Hastasana in Vira Parampara

(BUH-duh huh-STAHS-uh-nuh in VEER-uh puh-ruhm-puh-RAH)

Modification: grabbing onto the triceps behind the back
Pose Type: standing, backbend
Drishti Point: Bhrumadhye or Ajna Chakra (third eye, between the eyebrows)

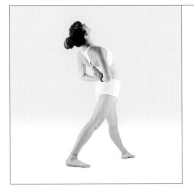

Reverse Prayer Pose in Hero Succession Series

Viparita Namaskarasana in Vira Parampara

(vi-puh-REET-tuh nuh-muhs-kahr-AHS-uh-nuh in VEER-uh puh-ruhm-puh-RAH)

Also Known As: Back of the Body Prayer in Hero Succession Series (Paschima Namaskara in Vira Parampara)
Pose Type: standing, backbend
Drishti Point: Bhrumadhye or Ajna Chakra (third eye, between the eyebrows)

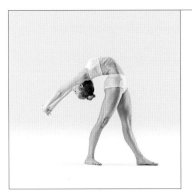

Upward Bound Hands Pose in Hero Succession Series

Urdhva Baddha Hastasana in Vira Parampara

(OORD-vuh BUH-duh huh-STAHS-uh-nuh in VEER-uh puh-ruhm-puh-RAH)

Modification: deep backbend
Pose Type: standing, backbend
Drishti Point: Bhrumadhye or Ajna Chakra (third eye, between the eyebrows), Angusthamadhye or Angustha Ma Dyai (thumbs)

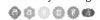

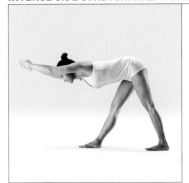

Intense Side Stretch Pose Prep.

Parshvottanasana Prep.

(pahrsh-vo-tahn-AHS-uh-nuh)

Modification: arms straight out in front, palms pressed together
Pose Type: standing, forward bend
Drishti Point: Nasagrai or Nasagre (nose)

Intense Side Stretch Pose Prep.

Parshvottanasana Prep.

(pahrsh-vo-tahn-AHS-uh-nuh)

Modification: one hand to the lower back, one arm extended out in front and parallel to the floor
Pose Type: standing, forward bend
Drishti Point: Bhrumadhye or Ajna Chakra (third eye, between the eyebrows), Hastagrai or Hastagre (hands)

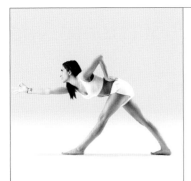

Intense Side Stretch Pose Prep.

Parshvottanasana Prep.

(pahrsh-vo-tahn-AHS-uh-nuh)

Modification: grabbing onto the triceps behind the back
Pose Type: standing, forward bend
Drishti Point: Padayoragrai or Padayoragre (toes/feet)

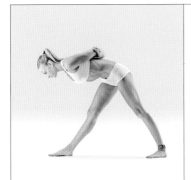

Intense Side Stretch Pose Prep.

Parshvottanasana Prep.

(pahrsh-vo-tahn-AHS-uh-nuh)

Modification: arms open to the sides
Pose Type: standing, forward bend
Drishti Point: Nasagrai or Nasagre (nose)

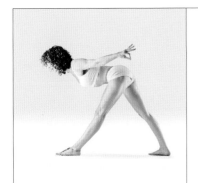

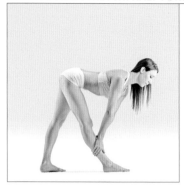

Intense Side Stretch Pose Prep.

Parshvottanasana Prep.

(pahrsh-vo-tahn-AHS-uh-nuh)

Modification: both hands on the shin on the front leg

Pose Type: standing, forward bend

Drishti Point: Padhayoragrai or Padayoragre (toes/feet)

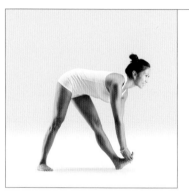

Extended Both Hands to Foot Intense Side Stretch Pose

Utthita Dwi Hasta Pada Parshvottanasana

(UT-ti-tuh DWI-huh-stuh PUH-duh pahrsh-vo-tahn-AHS-uh-nuh)

Modification: toes of the front foot flexed in and lifted off the floor

Pose Type: standing, forward bend

Drishti Point: Nasagrai or Nasagre (nose), Bhrumadhye or Ajna Chakra (third eye, between the eyebrows)

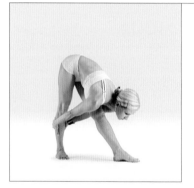

Intense Side Stretch Pose

Parshvottanasana

(pahrsh-vo-tahn-AHS-uh-nuh)

Modification: both hands grabbing onto the calf of the back leg

Pose Type: standing, forward bend

Drishti Point: Padayoragrai or Padayoragre (toes/feet)

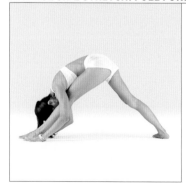

Intense Side Stretch Pose Prep.

Parshvottanasana Prep.

(pahrsh-vo-tahn-AHS-uh-nuh)

Modification: palms to the floor on either side of the front foot

Pose Type: standing, forward bend

Drishti Point: Nasagrai or Nasagre (nose)

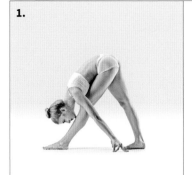

1.

Intense Side Stretch Pose Prep.

Parshvottanasana Prep.

(pahrsh-vo-tahn-AHS-uh-nuh)
Also Known As: Hero Succession Series (Vira Parampara)
Modification: arms reaching to the back, fingertips to the floor
1. chin to the shin
2. forehead to the shin
Pose Type: standing, forward bend
Drishti Point: Padayoragrai or Padayoragre (toes/feet), Nasagrai or Nasagre (nose)

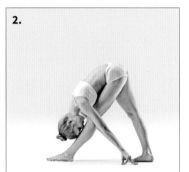

2.

INTENSE SIDE STRETCH: FULL FORWARD BEND—HANDS IN PRAYER, HANDS IN REVERSE PRAYER AND BEHIND

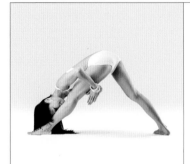

Intense Side Stretch Pose Prep.

Parshvottanasana Prep.

(pahrsh-vo-tahn-AHS-uh-nuh)
Modification: hands in Anjali Mudra (Hands in Prayer), arms wrapped around the front leg
Pose Type: standing, forward bend
Drishti Point: Nasagrai or Nasagre (nose)

Revolved Intense Side Stretch Pose

Parivritta Parshvottanasana

(puh-ri-VRIT-tuh pahrsh-vo-tahn-AHS-uh-nuh)
Modification: hands in Anjali Mudra (Hands in Prayer), arms wrapped around the front leg, twist
Pose Type: standing, forward bend, twist
Drishti Point: Urdhva or Antara Drishti (up to the sky)

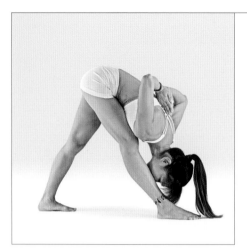

Intense Side Stretch Pose

Parshvottanasana
(pahrsh-vo-tahn-AHS-uh-nuh)

Also Known As: Reverse Prayer Intense Side Stretch Pose (Viparita Namaskar Parsvottanasana), Back of the Body Prayer Intense Side Stretch Pose (Paschima Namaskara Parshvottanasana)

Pose Type: standing, forward bend

Drishti Point: Nasagrai or Nasagre (nose)

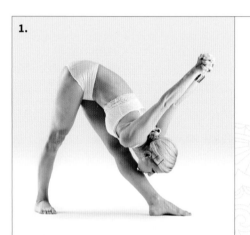

1.

Hands Bound Intense Side Stretch Pose

Baddha Hasta Parshvottanasana
(BUH-duh HUH-stuh pahrsh-vo-tahn-AHS-uh-nuh)

Modification: both legs straight

Pose Type: standing, forward bend

Drishti Point: Padayoragrai or Padayoragre (toes/feet), Nasagrai or Nasagre (nose)

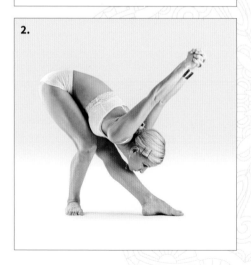

2.

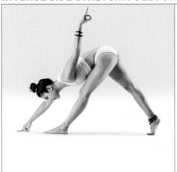

Uneven Legs Tip Toe Intense Side Stretch Pose

Vishama Pada Prapada Parshvottanasana

(VISH-uh-muh PUH-duh PRUH-puh-duh pahrsh-vo-tahn-AHS-uh-nuh)

Modification: 1. one arm stretched out to the back and up to the sky; other arm stretched out to the front, fingertips to the floor
2. both arms stretched out in front, fingertips to the floor
Pose Type: standing, forward bend
Drishti Point: Padayoragrai or Padayoragre (toes/feet)

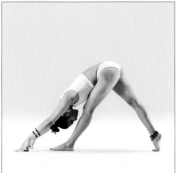

Intense Side Stretch Pose Prep.

Parshvottanasana Prep.

(pahrsh-vo-tahn-AHS-uh-nuh)

Modification: opposite arm wrapped around the front calf, chin to the shin
Pose Type: standing, forward bend
Drishti Point: Padayoragrai or Padayoragre (toes/feet)

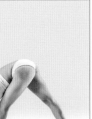

TRIANGLE POSE

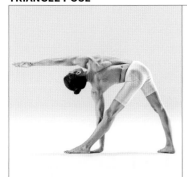

Extended Side Triangle Pose

Utthita Parshva Trikonasana

(UT-ti-tuh PAHRSH-vuh tri-ko-NAHS-uh-nuh)

Modification: top arm parallel to the floor
Pose Type: standing, forward bend, side bend
Drishti Point: Hastagrai or Hastagre (hands)

1.

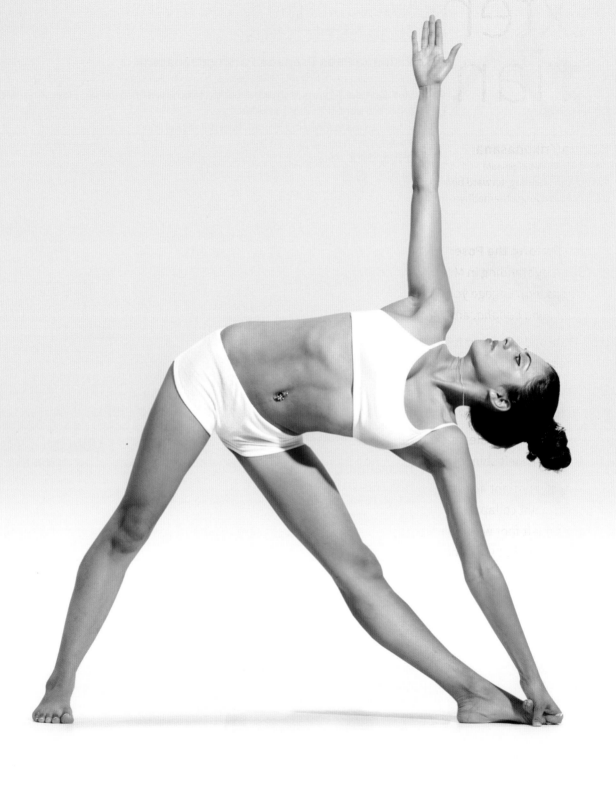

Extended Triangle Pose

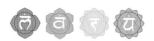

Utthita Trikonasana

(UT-ti-tuh tri-ko-NAHS-uh-nuh)

Pose Type: standing, forward bend, side bend

Drishti Point: Angusthamadhye or Angustha Ma Dyai (thumbs)

How to Perform the Pose:

1. Begin by standing in Mountain Pose (*Tadasana*). Engage your *mula bandha*, *uddhiyana bandha*, and *ujjayi* breathing.

2. Inhale and step your feet about elbow distance apart with toes facing forward and feet parallel to each other. Expand your chest and hold your arms straight out to the sides, parallel to the floor.

3. Keep your legs strong and straight by engaging your quadriceps and pulling the kneecaps up. Turn your left foot 90 degrees to the left. Turn your right foot as close to 45 degrees to the left as possible.

4. On your next exhale, reach over to the left as far as you can with good form and drop your left hand toward the left shin (or left foot or to the floor either on the inside or the outside of the left foot).

5. Reach your right arm up to the sky and look at your right thumb (the *drishti* point). Make sure that your chest is not collapsing down toward the floor by lengthening both arms, grabbing onto the big toe of your left foot with pointer finger and middle finger and thumb locked on top, and leaning back far enough so that your shoulders are stacked one on top of the other.

6. Hold the pose for at least 30, and up to 90, seconds in order to receive the full benefits of the stretch. Exhale as you release the pose. Inhale as you press strongly into both feet to come up.

7. Exhale, come back to Mountain Pose (*Tadasana*) and repeat on the other side.

Modification:
1. front view
2. back view

utittha = extended
tri = three
kona = angle

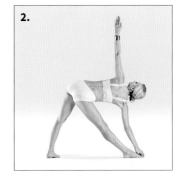

2.

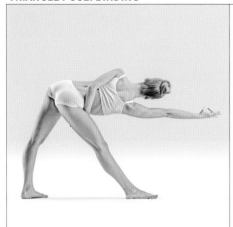

Half Bound Extended Triangle Pose

Ardha Baddha Utthita Trikonasana
(UHR-duh BUH-duh UT-ti-tuh tri-ko-NAHS-uh-nuh)
Pose Type: standing, forward bend, side bend, binding
Drishti Point: Nasagrai or Nasagre (nose)

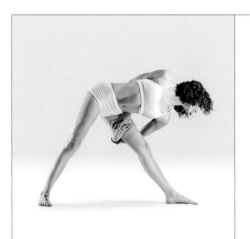

Bound Extended Triangle Pose

Baddha Utthita Trikonasana
(BUH-duh UT-ti-tuh tri-ko-NAHS-uh-nuh)
Modification: fingers interlocked on the inside of the thigh
Pose Type: standing, forward bend, side bend, binding
Drishti Point: Padayoragrai or Padayoragre (toes/feet)

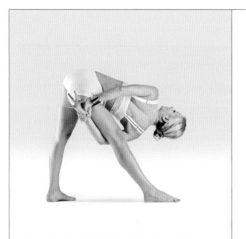

Bound Extended Triangle Pose

Baddha Utthita Trikonasana
(BUH-duh UT-ti-tuh tri-ko-NAHS-uh-nuh)
Pose Type: standing, forward bend, side bend, binding, twist
Drishti Point: Urdhva or Antara Drishti (up to the sky)

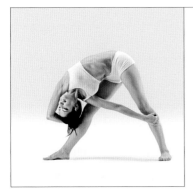

Revolved Sideways Extended Triangle Pose

Parivritta Parshva Utthita Trikonasana
(puh-ri-VRIT-tuh PAHRSH-vuh UT-ti-tuh tri-ko-NAHS-uh-nuh)
Modification: grabbing onto both shins
Pose Type: standing, forward bend, side bend, twist
Drishti Point: Urdhva or Antara Drishti (up to the sky)

TRIANGLE POSE: REVOLVED & BINDING

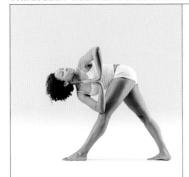

Revolved Triangle Pose

Parivritta Trikonasana
(puh-ri-VRIT-tuh tri-ko-NAHS-uh-nuh)
Also Known As: Revolved Intense Side Stretch Pose (Parivritta Parshvottanasana)
Modification: hands in Anjali Mudra (Hands in Prayer)
Pose Type: standing, forward bend, twist
Drishti Point: Urdhva or Antara Drishti (up to the sky)

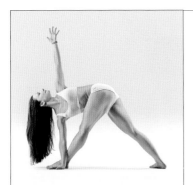

Revolved Triangle Pose

Parivritta Trikonasana
(puh-ri-VRIT-tuh tri-ko-NAHS-uh-nuh)
Pose Type: standing, forward bend, twist
Drishti Point: Angushtamadhye or Angushta Ma Dyai (thumbs)

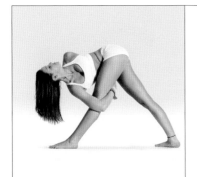

Revolved Bound Triangle Pose

Parivritta Baddha Trikonasana
(puh-ri-VRIT-tuh BUH-duh tri-ko-NAHS-uh-nuh)
Also Known As: Bound Leg Twisted Angle Pose (Baddha Pada Parivritta Konasana)
Pose Type: standing, forward bend, twist, binding
Drishti Point: Urdhva or Antara Drishti (up to the sky)

1.

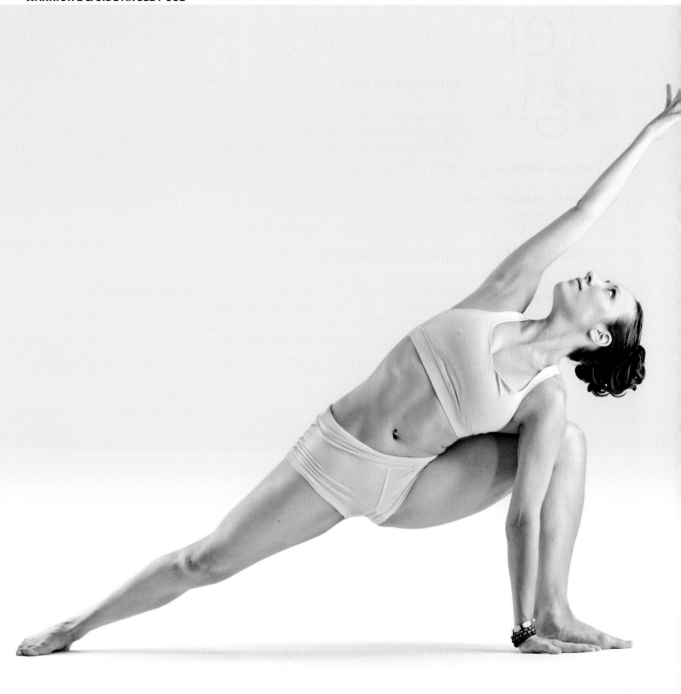

Extended Side Angle Pose

Utthita Parshva Konasana
(UT-ti-tuh pahrsh-vuh-ko-NAHS-uh-nuh)
Pose Type: standing, side bend
Drishti Point: Hastagrai or Hastagrahe (hands)

Modification:
1. arm to the inside of the thigh
2. elbow on the thigh
3. arm to the outside of the thigh

utthita = extended, rising, risen
parsva = side
kona = angle

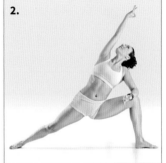
2.

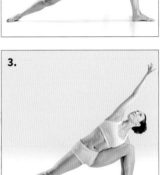
3.

How to Perform the Pose:

1. Begin by standing in Mountain Pose (*Tadasana*). Engage your *mula bandha*, *uddhiyana bandha*, and *ujjayi* breathing.

2. Inhale and step your feet about wrist-distance apart with toes facing forward and feet parallel to each other. Expand your chest and hold your arms straight out to the sides parallel to the floor.

3. Keep your legs strong and straight by engaging your quadriceps and pulling the kneecaps up. Turn your left foot 90 degrees to the left. Turn your right foot 45 degrees to the left as much as possible.

4. Exhale and bend your left knee until your left thigh is parallel to the floor, coming into Warrior 2 Pose (Virabhadrasana 2).

5. On the exhale, bend to the left and drop your left elbow to the left thigh. Reach your right arm over your head and rotate your chest to the side until your right shoulder is on top of your left shoulder.

6. You can experiment with bringing your left palm to the floor on the inside of your left thigh or the outside of your thigh.

7. Hold the pose for at least 30, and up to 90, seconds in order to receive the full benefits of the stretch. Exhale as you release the pose. Inhale as you press strongly into both feet to come up.

8. Exhale, come back to Mountain Pose (*Tadasana*) and repeat on the right side.

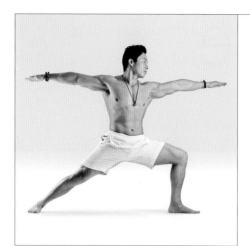

Warrior 2

Virabhadrasana 2

(veer-uh-buh-DRAHS-uh-nuh)

Also Known As: Half Side Angle Pose (Ardha Parshva Konasana)
Pose Type: standing
Drishti Point: Hastagrai or Hastagre (hands)

SIDE ANGLE POSE

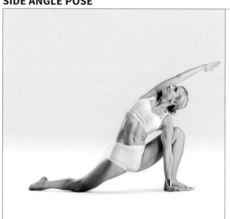

Extended Side Angle Pose Prep.

Utthita Parshva Konasana Prep.

(UT-ti-tuh pahrsh-vuh-ko-NAHS-uh-nuh)

Modification: back knee on the floor, palm to the floor on the inside of the front leg
Pose Type: standing, side bend
Drishti Point: Urdhva or Antara Drishti (up to the sky)

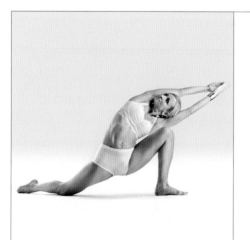

Both Arms Extended Side Angle Pose Prep.

Dwi Hasta Utthita Parshva Konasana Prep.

(DWI-huh-stuh UT-ti-tuh pahrsh-vuh-ko-NAHS-uh-nuh)

Modification: back knee on the floor
Pose Type: standing, side bend
Drishti Point: Urdhva or Antara Drishti (up to the sky)

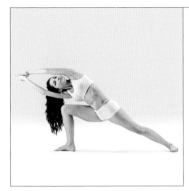

Both Arms Extended Side Angle Pose

Dwi Hasta Utthita Parshva Konasana
(DWI-huh-stuh UT-ti-tuh pahrsh-vuh-ko-NAHS-uh-nuh)
Modification: back knee off the floor
Pose Type: standing, side bend
Drishti Point: Urdhva or Antara Drishti (up to the sky)

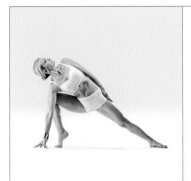

Tip Toe Extended Side Angle Pose Prep.

Prapada Utthita Parshva Konasana Prep.
(PRUH-puh-duh UT-ti-tuh pahrsh-vuh-ko-NAHS-uh-nuh)
Modification: front heel lifted, fingertips to the floor on the inside of the leg, other arm resting on the side of the torso
Pose Type: standing, side bend
Drishti Point: Urdhva or Antara Drishti (up to the sky)

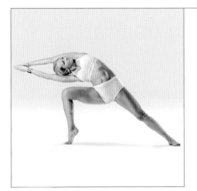

Tip Toe Both Arms Extended Side Angle Pose

Prapada Dwi Hasta Utthita Parshva Konasana
(PRUH-puh-duh DWI-huh-stuh UT-ti-tuh pahrsh-vuh-ko-NAHS-uh-nuh)
Modification: back knee off the floor
Pose Type: standing, side bend
Drishti Point: Urdhva or Antara Drishti (up to the sky)

SIDE ANGLE POSE: BINDING

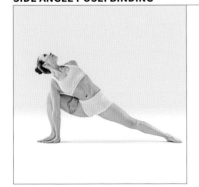

Half Bound Extended Side Angle Pose

Ardha Baddha Utthita Parshva Konasana
(UHR-duh BUH-duh UT-ti-tuh pahrsh-vuh-ko-NAHS-uh-nuh)
Modification: hand to the floor on the inside of the front leg
Pose Type: standing, side bend, binding
Drishti Point: Urdhva or Antara Drishti (up to the sky)

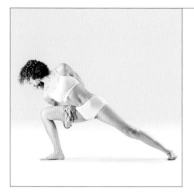

Bound Extended Side Angle Pose

Baddha Utthita Parshva Konasana

(BUH-duh UT-ti-tuh pahrsh-vuh-ko-NAHS-uh-nuh)

Modification: fingers interlocked on the inside of the front thigh

Pose Type: standing, side bend, binding

Drishti Point: Padayoragrai or Padayoragre (toes/feet)

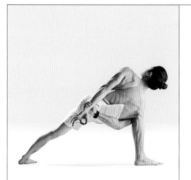

Bound Extended Side Angle Pose

Baddha Utthita Parshva Konasana

(BUH-duh UT-ti-tuh pahrsh-vuh-ko-NAHS-uh-nuh)

Also Known As: Bound Arms Side Angle Pose (Baddha Hasta Parshva Konasana)

Pose Type: standing, side bend, binding, twist

Drishti Point: Urdhva or Antara Drishti (up to the sky)

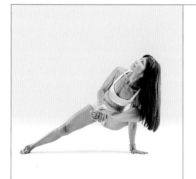

Pose Dedicated to Vishvamitra Prep.

Vishvamitrasana Prep.

(VISH-vah-mi-TRAHS-uh-nuh)

Modification: knee bent wrapped around the tricep, grabbing onto the foot

Pose Type: standing, arm balance

Drishti Point: Urdhva or Antara Drishti (up to the sky)

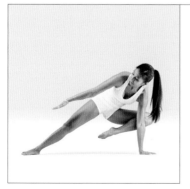

Pose Dedicated to Vishvamitra Prep.

Vishvamitrasana Prep.

(vish-vah-mi-TRAHS-uh-nuh)

Modification: knee bent, shin to the tricep

Pose Type: standing, arm balance

Drishti Point: Hastagrai or Hastagre (hands), Padayoragrai or Padayoragre (toes/feet)

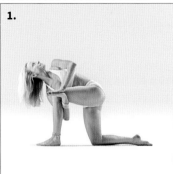

Revolved Side Angle Pose Prep.

Parivritta Parshva Konasana Prep.

(puh-ri-VRIT-tuh pahrsh-vuh-ko-NAHS-uh-nuh)

Modification: one arm under the leg, hands in Anjali Mudra (Hands in Prayer),

1. back knee on the floor, looking up to the sky
2. back knee off the floor, looking down

Pose Type: standing, twist

Drishti Point: 1. Urdhva or Antara Drishti (up to the sky)

2. Padayoragrai or Padayoragre (toes/feet)

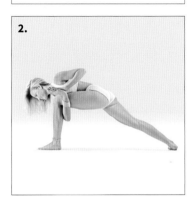

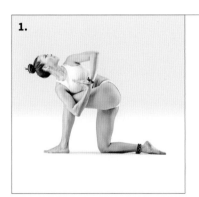

Revolved Side Angle Pose Prep.

Parivritta Parshva Konasana Prep.

(puh-ri-VRIT-tuh pahrsh-vuh-ko-NAHS-uh-nuh)

Modification: hands in Anjali Mudra (Hands in Prayer)

1. back knee on the floor, looking up to the sky
2. back knee off the floor, looking up to the sky

Pose Type: standing, twist

Drishti Point: Urdhva or Antara Drishti (up to the sky)

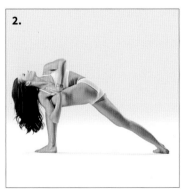

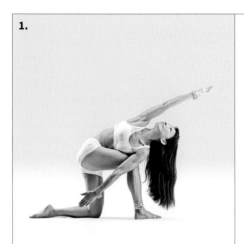

1.

Both Hands Free Revolved Side Angle Pose

Dwi Mukta Hasta Parivritta Parshva Konasana

(DWI muk-tuh HUH-stuh puh-ri-VRIT-tuh pahrsh-vuh-ko-NAHS-uh-nuh)

Modification: bottom hand off the floor, fingertips pointing in opposite directions

1. back knee on the floor
2. back knee off the floor

Pose Type: standing, twist, side bend

Drishti Point: Hastagrai or Hastagre (hands)

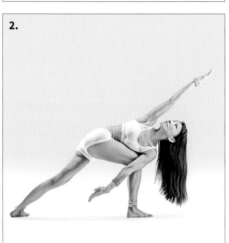

2.

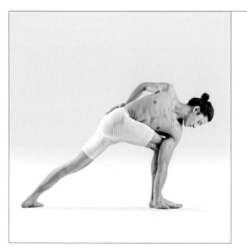

Revolved Side Angle Pose Prep.

Parivritta Parshva Konasana Prep.

(puh-ri-VRIT-tuh pahrsh-vuh-ko-NAHS-uh-nuh)

Modification: palm to the floor, other palm to lower back

Pose Type: standing, twist, side bend

Drishti Point: Hastagrai or Hastagre (hands) or Padhayoragrai or Padayoragre (toes/feet)

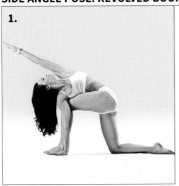

Revolved Side Angle Pose

Parivritta Parshva Konasana

(puh-ri-VRIT-tuh pahrsh-vuh-ko-NAHS-uh-nuh)

Modification: 1. palm to the floor, back knee on the floor

2. palm to the floor, back knee off the floor

Pose Type: standing, twist, side bend

Drishti Point: Hastagrai or Hastagre (hands)

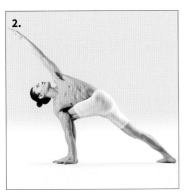

Bound Revolved Side Angle Pose

Baddha Parivritta Parshva Konasana

(BUH-duh puh-ri-VRIT-tuh pahrsh-vuh-ko-NAHS-uh-nuh)

Also Known As: Hands Bound Revolved Side Angle Pose Prep. (Baddha Hasta Parivritta Parshva Konasana Prep.)

Modification: 1. back knee on the floor

2. back knee off the floor

Pose Type: standing, twist, binding

Drishti Point: Urdhva or Antara Drishti (up to the sky)

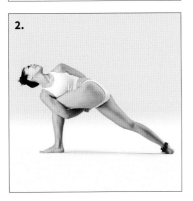

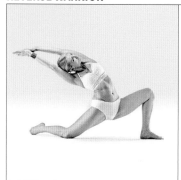

Both Arms Extended Reverse Warrior Pose Prep.

Dwi Hasta Utthita Viparita Virabhadrasana Prep.

(DWI-huh-stuh UT-ti-tuh vi-puh-REE-tuh vee-ruh-buh-DRAHS-uh-nuh)

Modification: back knee on the floor, arms straight, palms together
Pose Type: standing, backbend, side bend
Drishti Point: Urdhva or Antara Drishti (up to the sky)

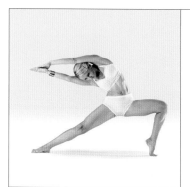

Tip Toe Both Arms Extended Reverse Warrior Pose

Prapada Dwi Hasta Utthita Viparita Virabhadrasana

(PRUH-puh-duh DWI-huh-stuh UT-ti-tuh vi-puh-REE-tuh vee-ruh-buh-DRAHS-uh-nuh)

Modification: arms straight, palms together
Pose Type: standing, backbend, side bend
Drishti Point: Bhrumadhye (third eye, between the eyebrows) or Hastagrai or Hastagre (hands)

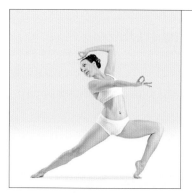

Revolved Sideways Tip Toe Reverse Warrior Pose

Parivritta Parshva Prapada Viparita Virabhadrasana

(puh-ri-VRIT-tuh PAHRSH-vuh PRUH-puh-duh vi-puh-REE-tuh vee-ruh-buh-DRAHS-uh-nuh)

Modification: front heel up, one arm in front and parallel to the floor; other elbow bent, palm facing up, hand to the crown of the head
Pose Type: standing, backbend, twist, side bend
Drishti Point: Parshva Drishti (to the right), Parshva Drishti (to the left)

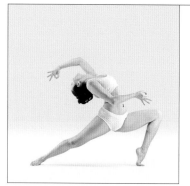

Tip Toe Reverse Warrior Pose

Prapada Viparita Virabhadrasana

(PRUH-puh-duh vi-puh-REE-tuh vee-ruh-buh-DRAHS-uh-nuh)

Modification: front heel up, both elbows bent, one arm up over the head, other arm in front of the torso
Pose Type: standing, backbend
Drishti Point: Hastagrai or Hastagre (hands)

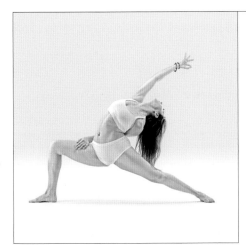

Half Bound Reverse Warrior Pose

Ardha Baddha Viparita Virabhadrasana

(UHR-duh BUH-duh vi-puh-REE-tuh vee-ruh-buh-DRAHS-uh-nuh)

Pose Type: standing, backbend, binding

Drishti Point: Hastagrai or Hastagre (hands)

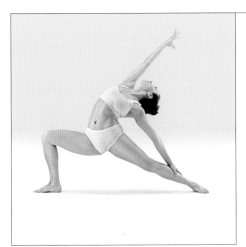

Reverse Warrior Pose

Viparita Virabhadrasana

(vi-puh-REE-tuh vee-ruh-buh-DRAHS-uh-nuh)

Also Known As: Reverse Warrior Pose 2 (Viparita Virabhadrasana 2)

Modification: hand to the calf of the back leg; low lunge, low stance

Pose Type: standing, backbend

Drishti Point: Hastagrai or Hastagre (hands)

WARRIOR 1

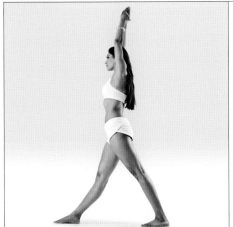

Warrior 1 Prep.

Virabhadrasana 1 Prep.

(vee-ruh-buh-DRAHS-uh-nuh)

Modification: both legs straight, palms pressed together

Pose Type: standing

Drishti Point: Nasagrai or Nasagre (nose)

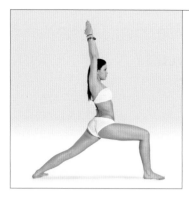

Warrior 1

Virabhadrasana 1
(vee-ruh-buh-DRAHS-uh-nuh)
Also Known As: Raised Arms Warrior Pose (Urdhva Hasta Veerasana), Hero Succession Series (Vira Parampara)
Pose Type: standing
Drishti Point: Nasagrai or Nasagre (nose)

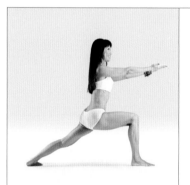

Warrior 1

Virabhadrasana 1
(vee-ruh-buh-DRAHS-uh-nuh)
Modification: arms out in front and parallel to the floor, palms facing the sky
Pose Type: standing
Drishti Point: Hastagrai or Hastagre (hands)

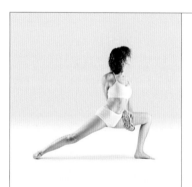

Bound Warrior 1

Baddha Virabhadrasana 1
(BUH-duh vee-ruh-buh-DRAHS-uh-nuh)
Modification: fingers interlocked on the inside of the front thigh
Pose Type: standing, binding
Drishti Point: Nasagrai or Nasagre (nose)

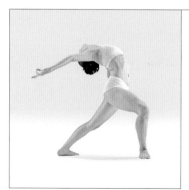

Warrior 1

Virabhadrasana 1
(vee-ruh-buh-DRAHS-uh-nuh)
Modification: arms up over the head and open to the sides; front leg, toes rotated out; deep backbend
Pose Type: standing, backbend
Drishti Point: Bhrumadhye or Ajna Chakra (third eye, between the eyebrows)

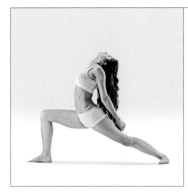

Open Heart Chakra Hands Bound Warrior

Anahata Chakra Baddha Hasta Virabhadrasana

(uh-NAH-huh-tuh CHUHK-ruh BUH-duh HUH-suh vee-ruh-buh-DRAHS-uh-nuh)

Pose Type: standing, backbend

Drishti Point: Bhrumadhye or Ajna Chakra (third eye, between the eyebrows)

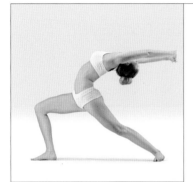

Raised Bound Hands in Warrior 1

Urdhva Baddha Hastasana in Virabhadrasana 1

(OORD-vuh BUH-duh huh-STAHS-uh-nuh in vee-ruh-buh-DRAHS-uh-nuh)

Modification: fingers interlocked deep backbend

Pose Type: standing, backbend

Drishti Point: Hastagrai or Hastagre (hands)

WARRIOR 1: FORWARD BEND—TO THE SIDE

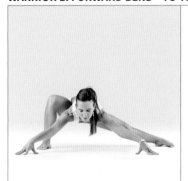

Spread Out Hands Side Angle Pose

Prasarita Hasta Parshva Konasana

(pruh-SAH-ri-tuh HUH-stuh pahrsh-vuh-ko-NAHS-uh-nuh)

Also Known As: Down Dog Lunge Pose

Pose Type: standing, forward bend

Drishti Point: Nasagrai or Nasagre (nose)

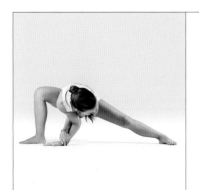

Hand Position of the Pose Dedicated to Garuda in Side Angle Pose

Hasta Garudasana in Parshva Konasana

(HUH-stuh guh-ru-DAHS-uh-nuh in pahrsh-vuh-ko-NAHS-uh-nuh)

Pose Type: standing, forward bend

Drishti Point: Padayoragrai or Padayoragre (toes/feet)

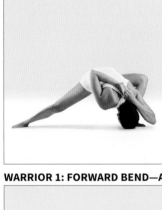

Hand Position of Cow Face Pose in Side Angle Pose

Hasta Gomukhasana in Parshva Konasana
(HUH-stuh go-muk-AHS-uh-nuh in pahrsh-vuh-ko-NAHS-uh-nuh)
Pose Type: standing, forward bend
Drishti Point: Nasagrai or Nasagre (nose)

WARRIOR 1: FORWARD BEND—ARMS BEHIND

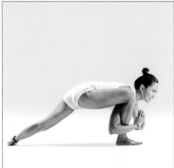

Bowing Warrior with Hands in Prayer

Nama Virabhadrasana Namaskar
(NUH-muh vee-ruh-buh-DRAHS-uh-nuh nuh-muhs-KAHR)
Pose Type: standing, forward bend
Drishti Point: Nasagrai or Nasagre (nose)

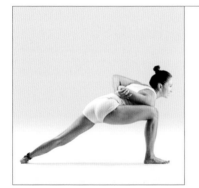

Bowing Hands Bound Warrior

Nama Baddha Hasta Virabhadrasana
(NUH-muh BUH-duh HUH-stuh vee-ruh-buh-DRAHS-uh-nuh)
Modification: grabbing onto the triceps behind the back
Pose Type: standing, forward bend
Drishti Point: Nasagrai or Nasagre (nose)

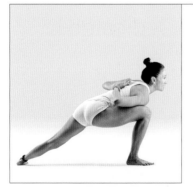

Bowing Reverse Prayer Warrior

Nama Viparita Namaskar Virabhadrasana
(NUH-muh vi-puh-REE-tuh nuh-muhs-KAHR vee-ruh-buh-DRAHS-uh-nuh)
Also Known As: Bowing Back of the Body Prayer Warrior (Nama Paschima Namaskara Virabhadrasana)
Pose Type: standing, forward bend
Drishti Point: Nasagrai or Nasagre (nose)

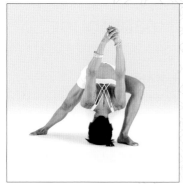

Bowing Hands Bound Warrior Pose

Nama Baddha Hasta Virabhadrasana

(NUH-muh BUH-duh HUH-stuh vee-ruh-buh-DRAHS-uh-nuh)

Also Known As: Warrior Veerastambana Pose (Veerastambanasana), Bound Hands Side Angle Pose (Baddha Hasta Parshva Konasana)

Pose Type: standing, forward bend

Drishti Point: Nasagrai or Nasagre (nose)

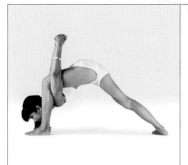

Bowing Hands Bound Warrior Pose

Nama Baddha Hasta Virabhadrasana

(NUH-muh BUH-duh HUH-stuh vee-ruh-buh-DRAHS-uh-nuh)

Also Known As: Bound Hands Side Angle Pose (Baddha Hasta Parshva Konasana)

Modification: arms bound around the front leg

Pose Type: standing, forward bend, binding

Drishti Point: Padhayoragrai or Padayoragre (toes/feet)

SIDE ANGLE POSE: HEAD BEHIND LEG

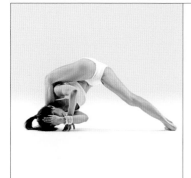

One Foot Behind the Head Side Angle Pose

Eka Pada Shirsha Parshva Konasana

(EY-kuh PUH-duh SHEER-shuh pahrsh-vuh-ko-NAHS-uh-nuh)

Modification: arms crossed in front of the chest

Pose Type: standing, forward bend

Drishti Point: Nasagrai or Nasagre (nose)

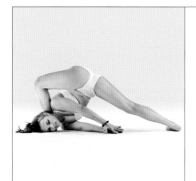

One Foot Behind the Head Side Angle Pose

Eka Pada Shirsha Parshva Konasana

(EY-kuh PUH-duh SHEER-shuh pahrsh-vuh-ko-NAHS-uh-nuh)

Modification: palms together, arms straight on the floor

Pose Type: standing, forward bend

Drishti Point: Nasagrai or Nasagre (nose)

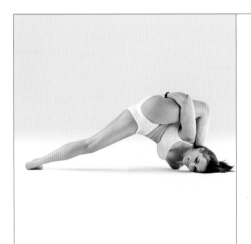

One Foot Behind the Head Bound Side Angle Pose

Eka Pada Shirsha Baddha Parshva Konasana

(EY-kuh PUH-duh SHEER-shuh BUH-duh pahrsh-vuh-ko-NAHS-uh-nuh)

Pose Type: standing, forward bend, binding

Drishti Point: Nasagrai or Nasagre (nose)

LUNGE: BACK KNEE ON THE FLOOR

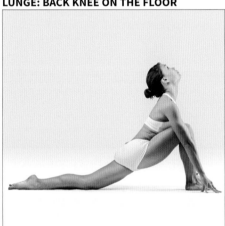

Equestrian Riding Horse Lunge Pose

Ashva Sanchalanasana

(UHSH-vuh suhn-chuh-luh-NAHS-uh-nuh)

Modification: back knee on the floor, hands to the floor on either side of the front foot, looking up to the sky

Pose Type: standing, forward bend

Drishti Point: Nasagrai or Nasagre (nose), Bhrumadhye or Ajna Chakra (third eye, between the eyebrows)

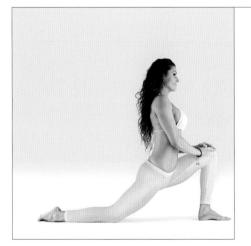

Equestrian Riding Horse Lunge Pose Prep.

Ashva Sanchalanasana Prep.

(UHSH-vuh suhn-chuh-luh-NAHS-uh-nuh)

Also Known As: Son of Anjani (Lord Hanuman) Lunge Pose Prep. (Anjaneyasana Prep.)

Modification: back knee on the floor, both hands on the front knee

Pose Type: standing

Drishti Point: Nasagrai or Nasagre (nose)

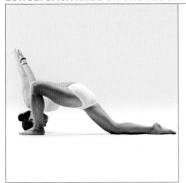

Hands Bound Extended Lizard Tail Lunge Pose

Baddha Hasta Uttana Pristhasana

(BUH-duh HUH-stuh ut-TAHN-uh prish-TAHS-uh-nuh)

Also Known As: Bowing Warrior Pose Prep. (Nama Virabhadrasana Prep.)

Modification: back knee on the floor, forehead to the floor

Pose Type: standing, forward bend

Drishti Point: Nasagrai or Nasagre (nose)

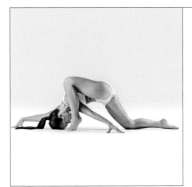

Tip Toe Extended Lizard Tail Lunge Pose

Prapada Uttana Pristhasana

(PRUH-puh-duh ut-TAHN-uh prish-TAHS-uh-nuh)

Modification: back knee on the floor, shoulder to the back of the knee, one arm straight out in front, other arm straight to the back, forehead to the floor

Pose Type: standing, forward bend

Drishti Point: Nasagrai or Nasagre (nose)

1.

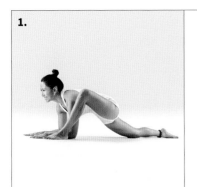

Extended Lizard Tail Lunge Pose

Uttana Pristhasana

(ut-TAHN-uh prish-TAHS-uh-nuh)

Modification: back knee on the floor

1. forearms to the floor on the inside of the foot
2. forearms to the floor on either side of the foot

Pose Type: standing , forward bend

Drishti Point: Nasagrai or Nasagre (nose)

2.

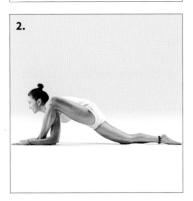

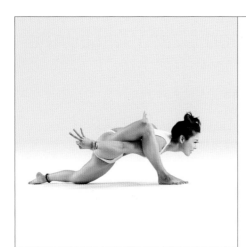

Unsupported Extended Lizard Tail Lunge Pose

Niralamba Uttana Pristhasana

(nir-AH-luhm-buh ut-TAHN-uh prish-TAHS-uh-nuh)

Also Known As: God Favour Seeking Sacrifice Ritual Pose (Yajnasana), Christ's Cross Pose

Modification: arms straight out to the sides

Pose Type: standing, forward bend

Drishti Point: Nasagrai or Nasagre (nose)

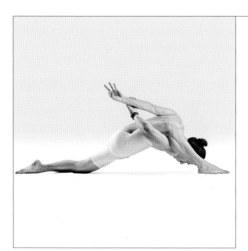

Bound Extended Lizard Tail Lunge Pose

Baddha Uttana Pristhasana

(BUH-duh ut-TAHN-uh prish-TAHS-uh-nuh)

Also Known As: Bound God Favor Seeking Sacrifice Ritual Pose (Baddha Yajnasana), Bound Christ's Cross Pose)

Modification: back knee on the floor

Pose Type: standing, forward bend, binding

Drishti Point: Nasagrai or Nasagre (nose)

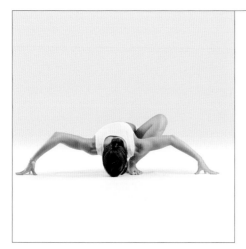

Hands Spread Out Extended Lizard Tail Lunge Pose

Prasarita Hasta Uttana Pristhasana

(pruh-SAH-ri-tuh HUH-stuh ut-TAHN-uh prish-TAHS-uh-nuh)

Also Known As: God Favour Seeking Sacrifice Ritual Pose (Yajnasana), Christ's Cross Pose

Modification: back knee on the floor, shin to the tricep

Pose Type: standing, forward bend

Drishti Point: Nasagrai or Nasagre (nose)

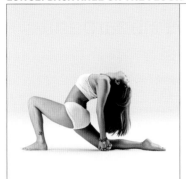

Bound Hands Son of Anjani (Lord Hanuman) Lunge Pose

Baddha Hasta Anjaneyasana *(BUH-duh HUH-stuh uhn-juh-ney-AHS-uh-nuh)*
Also Known As: Open Heart Chakra Hands Bound Equestrian Riding Horse Pose (Anahata Chakra Baddha Hasta Ashva Sanchalanasana)
Modification: back knee on the floor, backbend, hands to the floor on the inside of the back knee
Pose Type: standing, forward bend
Drishti Point: Bhrumadhye or Ajna Chakra (third eye, between the eyebrows)

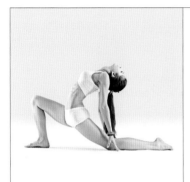

Son of Anjani (Lord Hanuman) Lunge Pose

Anjaneyasana *(uhn-juh-ney-AHS-uh-nuh)*
Also Known As: Open Heart Chakra Equestrian Riding Horse Pose (Anahata Chakra Ashva Sanchalanasana)
Modification: back knee on the floor, backbend, fingertips to the floor on either side of the back knee
Pose Type: standing, backbend
Drishti Point: Bhrumadhye or Ajna Chakra (third eye, between the eyebrows)

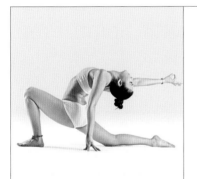

One Hand Son of Anjani (Lord Hanuman) Lunge Pose

Eka Hasta Anjaneyasana *(EY-kuh HUH-stuh uhn-juh-ney-AHS-uh-nuh)*
Also Known As: Equestrian Riding Horse Pose (Ashva Sanchalanasana)
Modification: back knee on the floor, one arm extended up over the head, other hand to the floor
Pose Type: standing, backbend
Drishti Point: Bhrumadhye or Ajna Chakra (third eye, between the eyebrows)

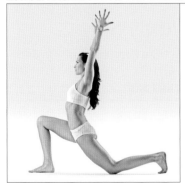

Son of Anjani (Lord Hanuman) Lunge Pose

Anjaneyasana *(uhn-juh-ney-AHS-uh-nuh)*
Also Known As: Crescent Lunge Pose
Modification: front heel on the floor, back knee down, back toes curled in; arms shoulder width apart, fingertips up to the sky
Pose Type: standing, mild backbend
Drishti Point: Bhrumadhye or Ajna Chakra (third eye, between the eyebrows), Nasagrai or Nasagre (nose)

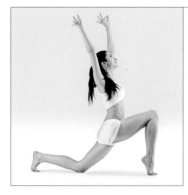

Tip Toe Son of Anjani (Lord Hanuman) Lunge Pose

Prapada Anjaneyasana *(PRUH-puh-duh uhn-juh-ney-AHS-uh-nuh)*
Also Known As: Tip Toe Crescent Lunge Pose
Modification: front heel off the floor, back knee down, back toes curled in; arms shoulder width apart, fingertips up to the sky
Pose Type: standing, mild backbend
Drishti Point: Bhrumadhye or Ajna Chakra (third eye, between the eyebrows), Nasagrai or Nasagre (nose)

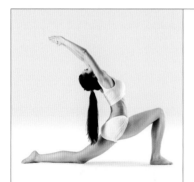

Son of Anjani (Lord Hanuman) Lunge Pose

Anjaneyasana *(uhn-juh-ney-AHS-uh-nuh)*
Also Known As: Monkey Pose (Kapyasana), Crescent Lunge Pose
Modification: arms up over the head, back knee on the floor, palms pressed together
Pose Type: standing, mild backbend
Drishti Point: Bhrumadhye or Ajna Chakra (third eye, between the eyebrows), Angusthamadhye or Angustha Ma Dyai (thumbs)

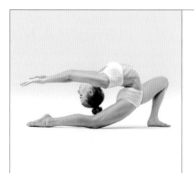

Standing Pose of the Heavenly Spirits Prep.

Stiti Valakhilyasana Prep. *(STI-ti VAH-luh-kil-YAHS-uh-nuh)*
Also Known As: Nindra Valakhilyasana; Son of Anjani (Lord Hanuman) Lunge Pose (Anjaneyasana), Crescent Lunge Pose)
Modification: back knee on the floor, arms up over the head, palms open to the sky, arms parallel to the floor
Pose Type: standing, backbend
Drishti Point: Bhrumadhye or Ajna Chakra (third eye, between the eyebrows)

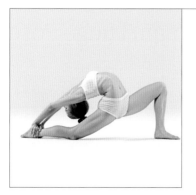

Standing Pose of the Heavenly Spirits

Stiti Valakhilyasana *(STI-ti VAH-luh-kil-YAHS-uh-nuh)*
Also Known As: Nindra Valakhilyasana
Modification: back knee to the floor, grabbing the back heel with overhead grip
Pose Type: standing, backbend
Drishti Point: Bhrumadhye or Ajna Chakra (third eye, between the eyebrows)

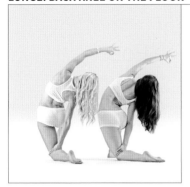

Sideways Son of Anjani (Lord Hanuman) Lunge Pose

Parshva Anjaneyasana
(PAHRSH-vuh uhn-juh-ney-AHS-uh-nuh)

Modification: back knee on the floor; one hand to the inside of the opposite knee, other arm up over the head

Pose Type: standing, side bend, backbend

Drishti Point: Angushtamadhye or Angushta Ma Dyai (thumbs)

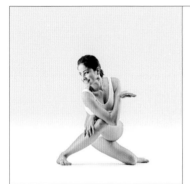

Revolved Paying Homage Lunge Pose

Parivritta Namasyasana
(puh-ri-VRIT-tuh nuh-muh-SYAHS-uh-nuh)

Also Known As: Curtsey Lunge

Modification: front leg crossed over to the side, opposite elbow over the front knee, back knee on the floor

Pose Type: standing, twist

Drishti Point: Parshva Drishti (to the right), Parshva Drishti (to the left)

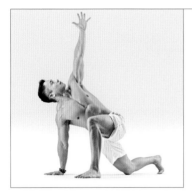

Revolved Son of Anjani (Lord Hanuman) Lunge Pose

Parivritta Anjaneyasana
(puh-ri-VRIT-tuh uhn-juh-ney-AHS-uh-nuh)

Modification: back knee on the floor, toes curled in; one hand to the floor, other arm up in the sky; twisting to the inside of the front knee

Pose Type: standing, twist

Drishti Point: Angushtamadhye or Angushta Ma Dyai (thumbs)

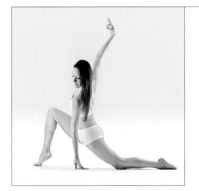

Tip Toe Sideways Son of Anjani (Lord Hanuman) Lunge Pose

Prapada Parshva Anjaneyasana
(PRUH-puh-duh PAHRSH-vuh uhn-juh-ney-AHS-uh-nuh)

Modification: back knee on the floor, toes pointed to the back, one hand to the floor, other arm up in the sky, twisting to the outside of the front knee

Pose Type: standing, twist

Drishti Point: Padayoragrai or Padayoragre (toes/feet)

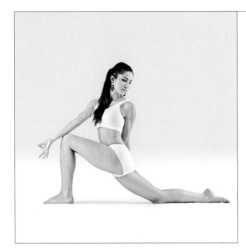

Revolved Son of Anjani (Lord Hanuman) Lunge Pose

Parivritta Anjaneyasana

(puh-ri-VRIT-tuh uhn-juh-ney-AHS-uh-nuh)

Also Known As: Revolved Monkey Pose (Parivritta Anjaneyasana)
Modification: back knee on the floor
Pose Type: standing, twist
Drishti Point: Padhayoragrai or Padayoragre (toes/feet)

LUNGE: BACK KNEE ON THE FLOOR UNDER THE HIP SOCKET

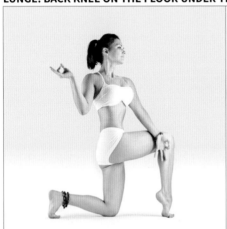

Tip Toe Revolved Son of Anjani (Lord Hanuman) Lunge Pose

Prapada Parivritta Anjaneyasana

(PRUH-puh-duh puh-ri-VRIT-tuh uhn-juh-ney-AHS-uh-nuh)

Pose Type: standing, twist
Drishti Point: Nasagrai or Nasagre (nose)

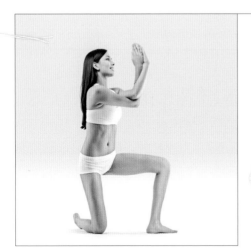

Horse Pose Prep.

Vatayanasana Prep.

(vah-tah-yuh-NAHS-uh-nuh)

Modification: back knee and foot on the floor
Pose Type: standing
Drishti Point: Angushtamadhye or Angushta Ma Dyai (thumbs)

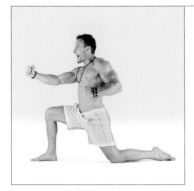

Fighting Warrior Pose 1

Yudhasana 1

(yu-DAHS-uh-nuh)
Pose Type: standing
Drishti Point: Hastagrai or Hastagre (hands)

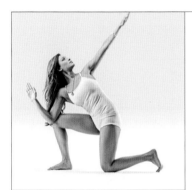

Fighting Warrior Pose 2

Yudhasana 2

(yu-DAHS-uh-nuh)
Modification: back knee on the floor
Pose Type: standing
Drishti Point: Hastagrai or Hastagre (hands)

LUNGE: BACK KNEE ON THE FLOOR UNDER THE HIP SOCKET—FORWARD BEND

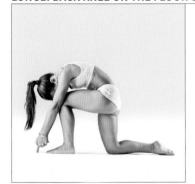

Half Equestrian Riding Horse Lunge Pose

Ardha Ashva Sanchalanasana

(UHR-duh UHSH-vuh suhn-chuh-luh-NAHS-uh-nuh)
Modification: spine in Cat Tilt, back knee down, toes pointing away from the head
Pose Type: standing, forward bend
Drishti Point: Nasagrai or Nasagre (nose)

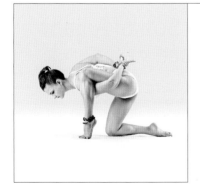

Tip Toe Bound Son of Anjani (Lord Hanuman) Lunge Pose

Prapada Baddha Anjaneyasana

(PRUH-puh-duh BUH-duh uhn-juh-ney-AHS-uh-nuh)
Modification: front leg bound, back knee on the floor, toes pointing away from the head
Pose Type: standing, forward bend, binding
Drishti Point: Nasagrai or Nasagre (nose)

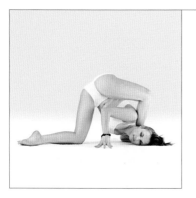

One Foot Behind the Head Extended Lizard Tail Lunge Pose

Eka Pada Shirsha Uttana Pristhasana

(EY-kuh PUH-duh SHEER-shuh ut-TAHN-uh prish-TAHS-uh-nuh)

Modification: back knee under the hip, toes pointing away from the head
Pose Type: standing, forward bend
Drishti Point: Nasagrai or Nasagre (nose)

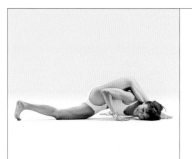

One Foot Behind the Head Extended Lizard Tail Lunge Pose

Eka Pada Shirsha Uttana Pristhasana

(EY-kuh PUH-duh SHEER-shuh ut-TAHN-uh prish-TAHS-uh-nuh)

Modification: legs working toward full vertical splits, toes of the back leg curled in
Pose Type: standing, forward bend
Drishti Point: Nasagrai or Nasagre (nose)

LUNGE: BACK KNEE ON THE FLOOR UNDER THE HIP SOCKET—BACKBEND

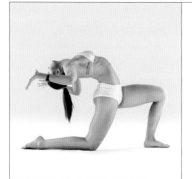

Son of Anjani (Lord Hanuman) Lunge Pose

Anjaneyasana

(uhn-juh-ney-AHS-uh-nuh)

Modification: deep backbend; chest open, arms to the side, elbows bent; back knee on the floor, toes pointing away from the head
Pose Type: standing, backbend
Drishti Point: Bhrumadhye or Ajna Chakra (third eye, between the eyebrows)

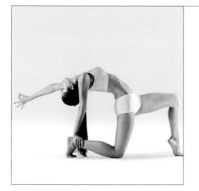

Tip Toe One Hand to Foot Son of Anjani (Lord Hanuman) Lunge Pose

Prapada Eka Hasta Pada Anjaneyasana

(PRUH-puh-duh EY-kuh HUH-stuh PUH-duh uhn-juh-ney-AHS-uh-nuh)

Modification: deep backbend; hand to the ankle on the same side
Pose Type: standing, backbend
Drishti Point: Bhrumadhye or Ajna Chakra (third eye, between the eyebrows)

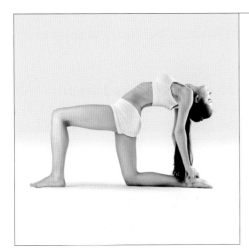

Both Hands to Foot Son of Anjani (Lord Hanuman) Lunge Pose

Dwi Hasta Pada Anjaneyasana

(DWI-huh-stuh PUH-duh uhn-juh-ney-AHS-uh-nuh)

Modification: backbend
Pose Type: standing, backbend
Drishti Point: Bhrumadhye or Ajna Chakra (third eye, between the eyebrows)

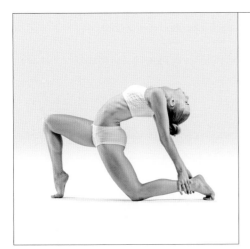

Tip Toe Both Hands to Foot Son of Anjani (Lord Hanuman) Lunge Pose

Prapada Dwi Hasta Pada Anjaneyasana

(PRUH-puh-duh DWI-huh-stuh PUH-duh uhn-juh-ney-AHS-uh-nuh)

Modification: deep backbend, back knee on the floor, back toes curled in
Pose Type: standing, backbend
Drishti Point: Bhrumadhye or Ajna Chakra (third eye, between the eyebrows)

LUNGE: BACK KNEE ON THE FLOOR—FOOT OFF THE FLOOR

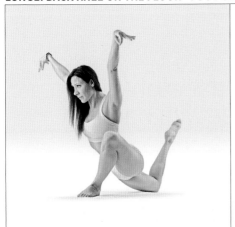

One-Legged King Pigeon Pose 2 Prep.

Eka Pada Raja Kapotasana 2 Prep.

(EY-kuh PUH-duh RAH-juh kuh-po-TAHS-uh-nuh)

Modification: arms open wide and raised
Pose Type: standing, forward bend
Drishti Point: Nasagrai or Nasagre (nose)

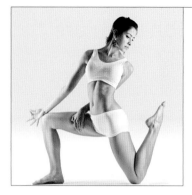

Half Bound Revolved One-Legged King Pigeon Pose 2 Prep.

Ardha Baddha Parivritta Eka Pada Raja Kapotasana 2 Prep.

(UHR-duh BUH-duh puh-ri-VRIT-tuh EY-kuh PUH-duh RAH-juh kuh-po-TAHS-uh-nuh)

Pose Type: standing, twist, binding

Drishti Point: Padayoragrai or Padayoragre (toes/feet)

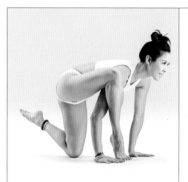

Tip Toe Extended Lizard Tail Lunge Pose Prep.

Prapada Uttana Pristhasana Prep.

(PRUH-puh-duh ut-TAHN-uh prish-TAHS-uh-nuh)

Modification: arms straight to semi-straight, back foot lifted off the floor

Pose Type: standing, forward bend

Drishti Point: Nasagrai or Nasagre (nose), Bhrumadhye or Ajna Chakra (third eye, between the eyebrows)

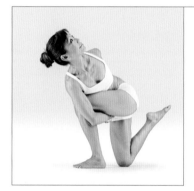

Bound Revolved Side Angle Pose Prep.

Baddha Parivritta Parshva Konasana Prep.

(BUH-duh puh-ri-VRIT-tuh pahrsh-vuh-ko-NAHS-uh-nuh)

Also Known As: Bound Revolved Son of Anjani (Lord Hanuman) Lunge Pose Prep. (Anjaneyasana Prep.)

Modification: back knee bent, heel toward the sitting bone

Pose Type: standing, forward bend, twist, binding

Drishti Point: Urdhva or Antara Drishti (up to the sky)

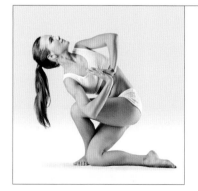

Foot to Knee Revolved Son of Anjani (Lord Hanuman) Lunge Pose with Hands in Prayer

Janu Pada Parivritta Anjaneyasana Namaskar

(JAH-nu PUH-duh puh-ri-VRIT-tuh uhn-juh-ney-AHS-uh-nuh nuh-muhs-KAHR)

Pose Type: standing, forward bend, twist

Drishti Point: Urdhva or Antara Drishti (up to the sky)

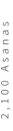

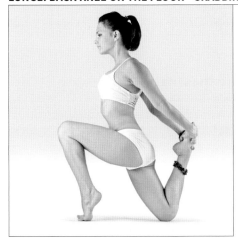

Tip Toe One-Legged King Pigeon Pose 2 Prep.

Prapada Eka Pada Raja Kapotasana 2 Prep.

(PRUH-puh-duh EY-kuh PUH-duh RAH-juh kuh-po-TAHS-uh-nuh)

Modification: both hands grabbing onto the back foot with under-head grip

Pose Type: standing, mild backbend

Drishti Point: Nasagrai or Nasagre (nose)

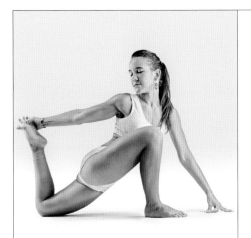

Revolved One-Legged King Pigeon Pose 2 Prep.

Parivritta Eka Pada Raja Kapotasana 2 Prep.

(puh-ri-VRIT-tuh EY-kuh PUH-duh RAH-juh kuh-po-TAHS-uh-nuh)

Modification: grabbing onto the back foot with the opposite hand using an under-head grip, twisting toward the front knee

Pose Type: standing, twist

Drishti Point: Padayoragrai or Padayoragre (toes/feet)

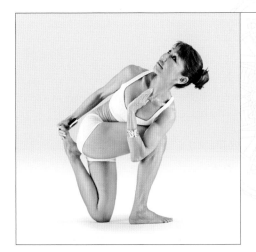

One Hand in Prayer Revolved One-Legged King Pigeon Pose 2 Prep.

Eka Hasta Namaskar Parivritta Eka Pada Raja Kapotasana 2 Prep.

(EY-kuh HUH-stuh nuh-muhs-KAHR puh-ri-VRIT-tuh EY-kuh PUH-duh RAH-juh kuh-po-TAHS-uh-nuh)

Modification: opposite hand to the back foot, other hand to the heart

Pose Type: standing, forward bend, twist

Drishti Point: Urdhva or Antara Drishti (up to the sky)

Standing Poses

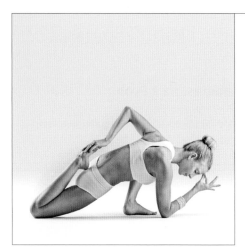

One Hand to Foot Extended Lizard Tail Lunge Pose

Eka Hasta Pada Uttana Pristhasana

(EY-kuh HUH-stuh PUH-duh ut-TAHN-uh prish-TAHS-uh-nuh)

Modification: forward bend, elbow to the floor, grabbing onto the back foot with opposite hand, heel to the glutes
Pose Type: standing, forward bend
Drishti Point: Nasagrai or Nasagre (nose)

LUNGE: BACK KNEE ON THE FLOOR—FOOT TO THE HIP SOCKET

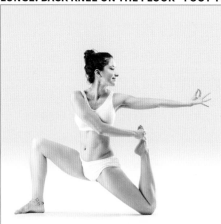

Spear Pose Prep.

Kuntasana Prep.

(kun-TAHS-uh-nuh)

Modification: grabbing onto the foot with one hand, arm crossed over in front, other arm parallel to the floor, foot away from the hip
Pose Type: standing, twist
Drishti Point: Hastagrai or Hastagre (hands)

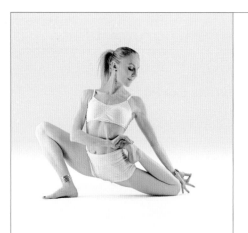

Spear Pose

Kuntasana

(kun-TAHS-uh-nuh)

Modification: grabbing onto the foot with one hand, arm crossed over in front, other hand to the knee, foot close to the hip
Pose Type: standing, twist
Drishti Point: Hastagrai or Hastagre (hands)

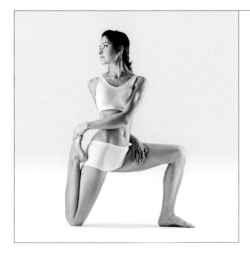

Both Hands Bound Revolved Spear Pose Prep.

Dwi Hasta Baddha Parivritta Kuntasana Prep.

(dwi HUH-stuh BUH-duh puh-ri-VRIT-tuh kun-TAHS-uh-nuh)
Pose Type: standing, twist, binding
Drishti Point: Parshva Drishti (to the right), Parshva Drishti (to the left)

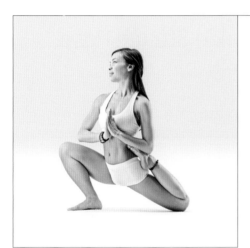

Spear Pose with Hands in Prayer

Kuntasana Namaskar

(kun-TAHS-uh-nuh nuh-muhs-KAHR)
Pose Type: standing
Drishti Point: Nasagrai or Nasagre (nose)

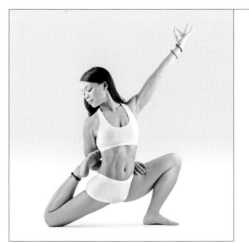

Half Bound Revolved Spear Pose Prep.

Ardha Baddha Parivritta Kuntasana Prep.

(UHR-duh-BUH-duh puh-ri-VRIT-tuh kun-TAHS-uh-nuh)
Modification: foot to the inside of the elbow
Pose Type: standing, twist, binding
Drishti Point: Padayoragrai or Padayoragre (toes/feet)

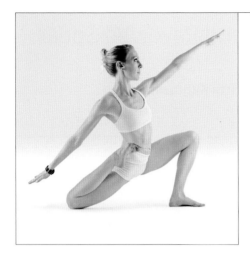

Spear Pose

Kuntasana

(kun-TAHS-uh-nuh)

Pose Type: standing

Drishti Point: Hastagrai or Hastagre (hands)

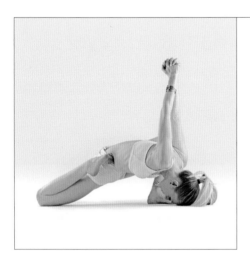

Hands Bound Ankle Stretch Pose

Baddha Hasta Kulpasana

(BUH-duh HUH-stuh kul-PAHS-uh-nuh)

Pose Type: standing, forward bend

Drishti Point: Nasagrai or Nasagre (nose)

LUNGE: BACK KNEE ON THE FLOOR—HEAD BEHIND THE FRONT LEG, GRABBING ONTO THE BACK FOOT

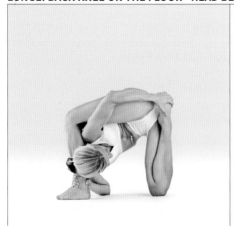

One Foot Behind the Head Extended Lizard Tail Lunge Pose

Eka Pada Shirsha Uttana Pristhasana

(EY-kuh PUH-duh SHEER-shuh ut-TAHN-uh prish-TAHS-uh-nuh)

Modification: grabbing onto the foot with the opposite hand, back knee under the hips

Pose Type: standing, forward bend

Drishti Point: Nasagrai or Nasagre (nose)

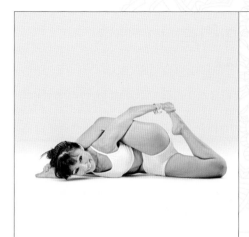

One Foot Behind the Head Extended Lizard Tail Lunge Pose

Eka Pada Shirsha Uttana Pristhasana

(EY-kuh PUH-duh SHEER-shuh ut-TAHN-uh prish-TAHS-uh-nuh)

Modification: grabbing onto the foot with the opposite hand, chest and quadriceps on the floor

Pose Type: standing, forward bend

Drishti Point: Nasagrai or Nasagre (nose)

LUNGE: BACK KNEE ON FLOOR—ONE-LEGGED KING PIGEON 2

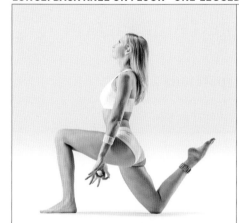

One-Legged King Pigeon Pose 2 Prep.

Eka Pada Raja Kapotasana 2 Prep.

(EY-kuh PUH-duh RAH-juh kuh-po-TAHS-uh-nuh)

Modification: back knee bent toward the glutes, front heel down; arms on the sides, spine straight

Pose Type: standing

Drishti Point: Bhrumadhye or Ajna Chakra (third eye, between the eyebrows)

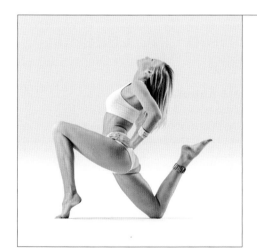

Tip Toe One-Legged King Pigeon Pose 2 Prep.

Prapada Eka Pada Raja Kapotasana 2 Prep.

(PRUH-puh-duh EY-kuh PUH-duh RAH-juh kuh-po-TAHS-uh-nuh)

Modification: back knee bent toward the glutes, heel of the top foot up; hands on the hips, backbend

Pose Type: standing, backbend

Drishti Point: Bhrumadhye or Ajna Chakra (third eye, between the eyebrows)

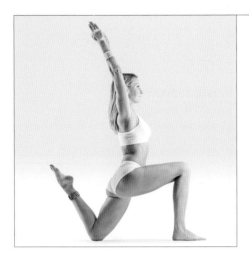

One-Legged King Pigeon Pose 2

Eka Pada Raja Kapotasana 2

(EY-kuh PUH-duh RAH-juh kuh-po-TAHS-uh-nuh)

Modification: prep.—arms up over the head, back knee bent toward the glutes

Pose Type: standing, mild backbend

Drishti Point: Nasagrai or Nasagre (nose)

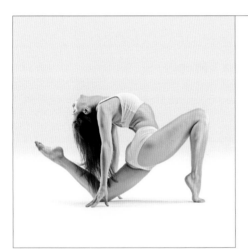

Tip Toe One-Legged King Pigeon Pose 2 Prep.

Prapada Eka Pada Raja Kapotasana 2 Prep.

(PRUH-puh-duh EY-kuh PUH-duh RAH-juh kuh-po-TAHS-uh-nuh)

Modification: fingertips to the floor, front heel lifted

Pose Type: standing, backbend

Drishti Point: Bhrumadhye or Ajna Chakra (third eye, between the eyebrows)

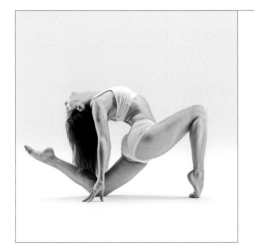

Intense Ankle Stretch One-Legged King Pigeon Pose 2

Uttana Kulpa Eka Pada Raja Kapotasana 2

(ut-TAH-nuh kul-puh EY-kuh PUH-duh RAH-juh kuh-po-TAHS-uh-nuh)

Modification: prep.—fingertips to the floor, front toes curled under

Pose Type: standing, backbend

Drishti Point: Bhrumadhye or Ajna Chakra (third eye, between the eyebrows)

1.

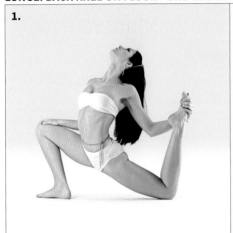

One-Legged King Pigeon Pose 2 Prep.

Eka Pada Raja Kapotasana 2 Prep.

(EY-kuh PUH-duh RAH-juh kuh-po-TAHS-uh-nuh)

Modification: 1. grabbing onto the foot on the same side

2. grabbing onto the foot with the hand on the same side, foot toward the hip

3. grabbing onto the foot with the opposite hand, foot twisted toward the opposite glute

Pose Type: standing, backbend

Drishti Point: Bhrumadhye or Ajna Chakra (third eye, between the eyebrows)

2.

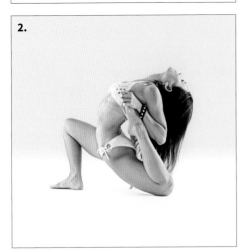

3.

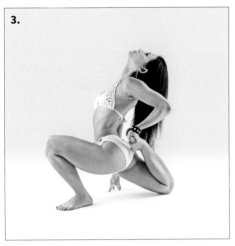

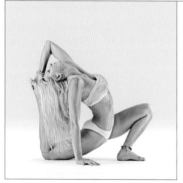

Revolved One-Legged King Pigeon Pose 2

Parivritta Eka Pada Raja Kapotasana 2

(puh-ree-VRIT-tuh EY-kuh PUH-duh RAH-juh kuh-po-TAHS-uh-nuh)

Pose Type: standing, forward bend, twist

Drishti Point: Parsva Drishti (to the right), Parsva Drishti (to the left)

Mermaid Pose 2

Naginyasana 2

(nuh-gin-YAHS-uh-nuh)

Pose Type: standing, backbend

Drishti Point: Bhrumadhye or Ajna Chakra (third eye, between the eyebrows)

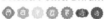

LUNGE: BACK KNEE ON FLOOR—ONE-LEGGED KING PIGEON 2—OVERHEAD GRIP

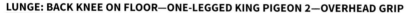

One-Legged King Pigeon Pose 2

Eka Pada Raja Kapotasana 2

(EY-kuh PUH-duh RAH-juh kuh-po-TAHS-uh-nuh)

Modification: grabbing onto the foot with the opposite hand, palm of the other hand to the floor on the side

1. foot to the head

2. heel to the forehead

Pose Type: standing, backbend

Drishti Point: Bhrumadhye or Ajna Chakra (third eye, between the eyebrows)

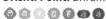

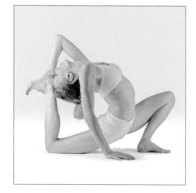

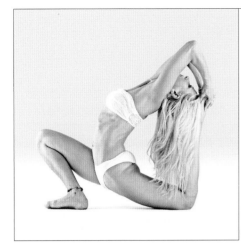

One-Legged King Pigeon Pose 2

Eka Pada Raja Kapotasana 2

(EY-kuh PUH-duh RAH-juh kuh-po-TAHS-uh-nuh)

Modification: both hands grabbing onto the foot

1. foot to the head
2. heel to the forehead

Pose Type: standing, backbend

Drishti Point: Bhrumadhye or Ajna Chakra (third eye, between the eyebrows)

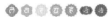

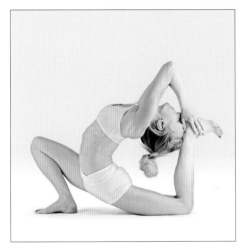

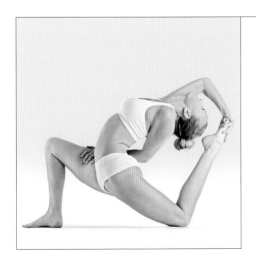

Half Bound One-Legged King Pigeon Pose 2

Ardha Baddha Eka Pada Raja Kapotasana 2

(UHR-duh BUH-duh EY-kuh PUH-duh RAH-juh kuh-po-TAHS-uh-nuh)

Pose Type: standing, backbend, binding

Drishti Point: Bhrumadhye or Ajna Chakra (third eye, between the eyebrows)

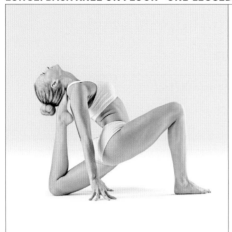

Necklace Pose Prep.

Graivasana Prep.

(gr-eye-VAHS-uh-nuh)

Also Known As: Chain Pose (Gaivasana)

Modification: back foot to the back of the head, hands to the floor

Pose Type: standing, backbend

Drishti Point: Bhrumadhye or Ajna Chakra (third eye, between the eyebrows)

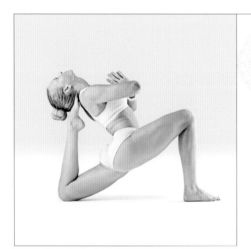

Necklace Pose Prep.

Graivasana Prep.

(gr-eye-VAHS-uh-nuh)

Also Known As: Chain Pose (Gaivasana)

Modification: back foot to the back of the head, hands in Anjali Mudra (Hands in Prayer)

Pose Type: standing, backbend

Drishti Point: Bhrumadhye or Ajna Chakra (third eye, between the eyebrows)

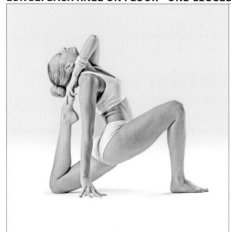

Bound Hand to Foot Supported One-Legged King Pigeon Pose 2

Baddha Hasta Pada Salamba Eka Pada Raja Kapotasana 2

(BUH-duh HUH-stuh PUH-duh SAH-luhm-buh EY-kuh PUH-duh RAH-juh kuh-po-TAHS-uh-nuh)

Modification: arm crossed in front of the neck, other hand to the floor

Pose Type: standing, backbend

Drishti Point: Bhrumadhye or Ajna Chakra (third eye, between the eyebrows)

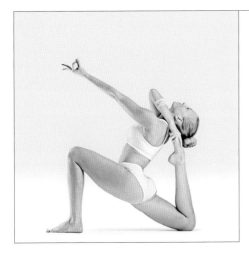

Bound Hand to Foot Unsupported One-Legged King Pigeon Pose 2

Baddha Hasta Pada Niralamba Eka Pada Raja Kapotasana 2

(BUH-duh HUH-stuh PUH-duh nir-AH-luhm-buh EY-kuh PUH-duh RAH-juh kuh-po-TAHS-uh-nuh)

Modification: arm crossed in front of the neck, other arm straight out in front

Pose Type: standing, backbend

Drishti Point: Bhrumadhye or Ajna Chakra (third eye, between the eyebrows)

LUNGE: FRONT LEG STRAIGHT—BACKBEND

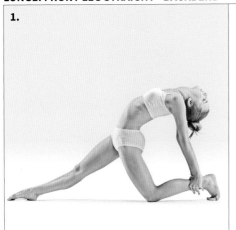

1.

Both Hands to Foot Son of Anjani (Lord Hanuman) Lunge Pose

Dwi Hasta Pada Anjaneyasana

(DWI-huh-stuh PUH-duh uhn-juh-ney-AHS-uh-nuh)

Modification: front leg straight
1. back knee on the floor
2. back knee off the floor

Pose Type: standing, backbend

Drishti Point: Bhrumadhye or Ajna Chakra (third eye, between the eyebrows)

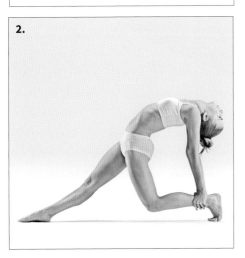

2.

1.

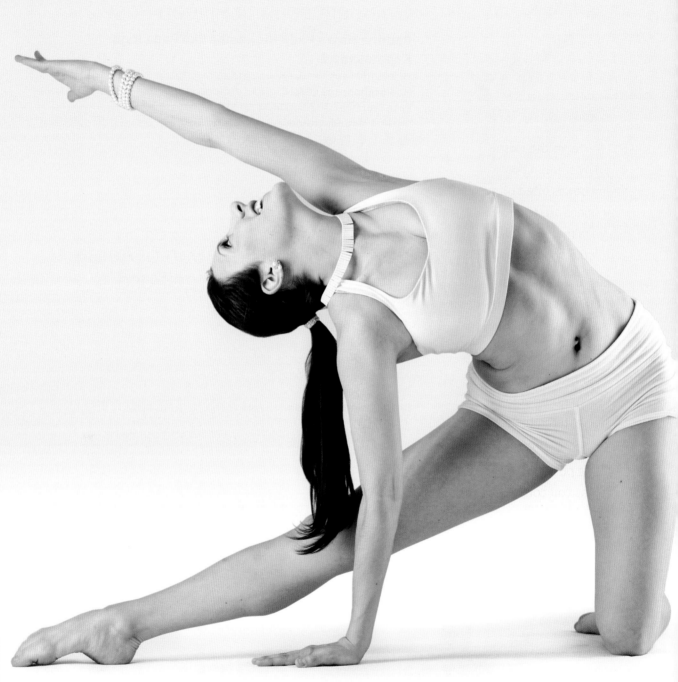

Gate Pose

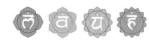

Parighasana

(puh-ri-GAHS-uh-nuh)
Pose Type: standing, side bend
Drishti Point: Hastagrai or Hastagrahe (hands)

How to Perform the Pose:

1. Begin by standing on your knees with sitting bones lifted off the feet. (Make sure your knees are comfortable by rolling up the yoga mat a couple of times.) Engage your *mula bandha*, *uddhiyana bandha*, and *ujjayi* breathing.

Modification: bending to the opposite side of the bent knee on the floor
1. palm to the floor, toes of the straight leg pointing to the side
2. hand on the shin, toes of the straight leg pointing straight ahead

parigha = iron bar used for locking a gate

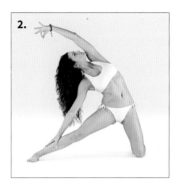

2. Exhale and extend your right leg straight out to the side with the right foot on the floor. You can either point the toes to the right (Pose #1) or point your toes straight ahead, lifting the arch and pressing the outside edge of the right foot to the floor (Pose #2).

3. Inhale as you expand your chest and hold your arms straight out to the sides, parallel to the floor.

4. On your next exhale, side bend to the right and bring your right hand onto your right shin (Pose #2), while extending your left arm over your head to the right with the palm facing down. Make sure your chest is rotated to face forward and not collapsing toward the floor. Look toward your right hand. You can also experiment with dropping your right palm to the floor on the inside of your right leg (Pose #1).

5. Hold the pose for at least 30, and up to 90, seconds in order to receive the full benefits of the stretch. Inhale as you come up and bring your right knee back to the floor by your left knee. Repeat on the other side.

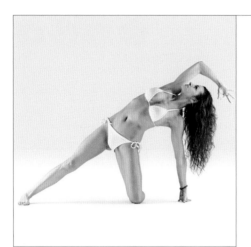

Gate Pose

Parighasana
(puh-ri-GAHS-uh-nuh)
Modification: bending to the side of the bent knee on the floor, hand to the floor on the outside of the bent leg, toes of the straight leg pointing straight ahead
Pose Type: standing, side bend
Drishti Point: Urdhva or Antara Drishti (up to the sky)

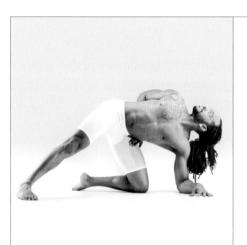

Half Bound Gate Pose

Ardha Baddha Parighasana
(UHR-duh BUH-duh puh-ri-GAHS-uh-nuh)
Modification: bending to the side of the bent knee on the floor, forearm to the floor on the side of the bent leg, toes of the straight leg pointing straight ahead
Pose Type: standing, side bend, binding
Drishti Point: Urdhva or Antara Drishti (up to the sky)

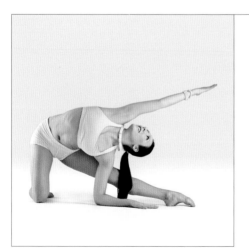

Gate Pose

Parighasana
(puh-ri-GAHS-uh-nuh)
Modification: bending to the opposite side of the bent knee on the floor, fore-arm to the floor, toes of the straight leg pointing to the side
Pose Type: standing, forward bend, side bend
Drishti Point: Hastagrai or Hastagre (hands)

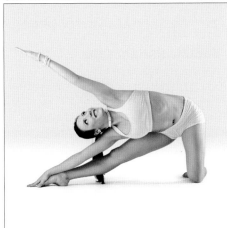

Gate Pose

Parighasana

(puh-ri-GAHS-uh-nuh)

Modification: bending to the opposite side of the bent knee on the floor, palm to the top of the foot of the straight leg, toes of the straight leg pointing to the side

Pose Type: standing, forward bend, side bend

Drishti Point: Hastagrai or Hastagre (hands)

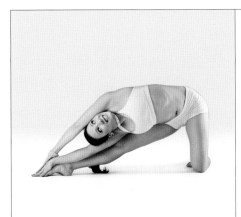

Gate Pose

Parighasana

(puh-ri-GAHS-uh-nuh)

Modification: bending to the opposite side of the bent knee on the floor, both hands to the top of the foot of the straight leg, toes of the straight leg pointing to the side

Pose Type: standing, forward bend, side bend

Drishti Point: Urdhva or Antara Drishti (up to the sky)

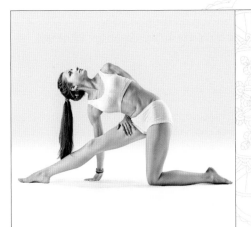

Revolved Half Bound Gate Pose
Parivritta Ardha Baddha Parighasana

(puh-ri-VRIT-tuh UHR-duh BUH-duh puh-ri-GAHS-uh-nuh)

Modification: hand to the floor on the outside of the straight leg, rotating the chest to the sky, toes of the straight leg pointing to the side

Pose Type: standing, side bend, binding

Drishti Point: Urdhva or Antara Drishti (up to the sky)

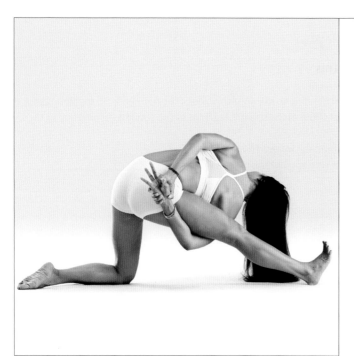

Revolved Bound Gate Pose

Parivritta Baddha Parighasana

(puh-ri-VRIT-tuh BUH-duh puh-ri-GAHS-uh-nuh)

Modification: toes of the straight leg flexed in, toes of the bent leg pointing away from the head

Pose Type: standing, forward bend, side bend, binding

Drishti Point: Urdhva or Antara Drishti (up to the sky)

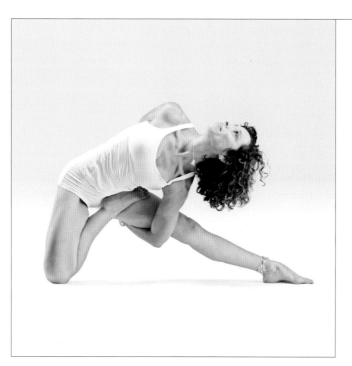

Revolved Bound Half Lotus Gate Pose

Parivritta Baddha Ardha Padma Parighasana

(puh-ri-VRIT-tuh BUH-duh UHR-duh PUHD-muh puh-ri-GAHS-uh-nuh)

Modification: toes of the straight leg pointing to the side

Pose Type: standing, side bend, binding

Drishti Point: Urdhva or Antara Drishti (up to the sky)

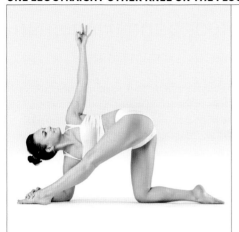

Revolved Gate Pose

Parivritta Parighasana

(puh-ri-VRIT-tuh puh-ri-GAHS-uh-nuh)

Modification: forearm to the floor, hand grabbing onto the opposite foot, other arm straight up to the sky, toes of the straight leg pointed to the side, toes of the bent leg pointing away from the head

Pose Type: standing, forward bend, twist

Drishti Point: Hastagrai or Hastagre (hands)

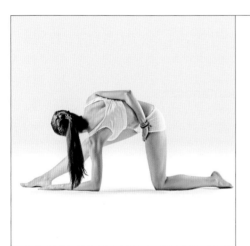

Revolved Half Bound Gate Pose

Parivritta Ardha Baddha Parighasana

(puh-ri-VRIT-tuh UHR-duh BUH-duh puh-ri-GAHS-uh-nuh)

Modification: forearm to the floor, twisting toward the straight leg, toes of the straight leg pointing to the side

Pose Type: standing, forward bend, twist, binding

Drishti Point: Urdhva or Antara Drishti (up to the sky)

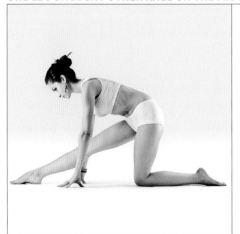

Half Pose Dedicated to Lord Hanuman

Ardha Hanumanasana

(UHR-duh huh-nu-mahn-AHS-uh-nuh)

Also Known As: Pose Dedicated to Lord Hanuman Prep. (Hanumanasana Prep.)

Modification: back toes pointed away from the head, fingertips to the floor on the outsides of the straight leg

Pose Type: standing, forward bend

Drishti Point: Padayoragrai or Padayoragre (toes/feet)

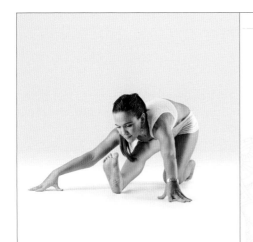

Half Pose Dedicated to Lord Hanuman

Ardha Hanumanasana
(UHR-duh huh-nu-mahn-AHS-uh-nuh)

Also Known As: Pose Dedicated to Lord Hanuman Prep. (Hanumanasana Prep.)
Modification: back toes curled in, toes of the straight leg flexed in, arms extended to the front, fingertips to the floor
Pose Type: standing, forward bend
Drishti Point: Padayoragrai or Padayoragre (toes/feet)

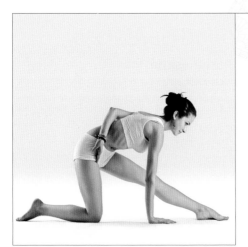

Half Bound Half Pose Dedicated to Lord Hanuman

Ardha Baddha Ardha Hanumanasana
(UHR-duh BUH-duh UHR-duh huh-nu-mahn-AHS-uh-nuh)

Also Known As: Pose Dedicated to Lord Hanuman Prep. (Hanumanasana Prep.)
Modification: toes of the bent leg pointed away from the head
Pose Type: standing, forward bend, binding
Drishti Point: Padayoragrai or Padayoragre (toes/feet)

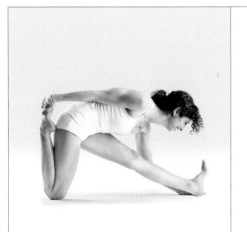

Half Pose Dedicated to Lord Hanuman

Ardha Hanumanasana
(UHR-duh huh-nu-mahn-AHS-uh-nuh)

Also Known As: Pose Dedicated to Lord Hanuman Prep. (Hanumanasana Prep.)
Modification: toes of the straight leg flexed in; hand grabbing onto the back foot on the same side, heel to the sitting bone
Pose Type: standing, forward bend
Drishti Point: Padayoragrai or Padayoragre (toes/feet)

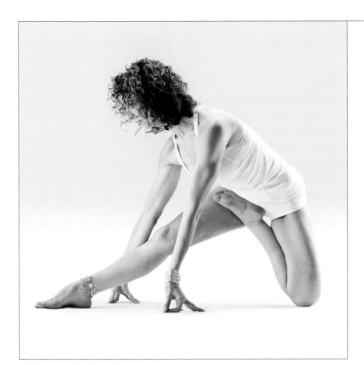

Half Lotus Half Pose Dedicated to Lord Hanuman

Ardha Padma Ardha Hanumanasana

(UHR-duh PUHD-muh UHR-duh huh-nu-mahn-AHS-uh-nuh)

Also Known As: Pose Dedicated to Lord Hanuman Prep. (Hanumanasana Prep.)

Modification: fingertips of both hands on the sides of the straight leg

Pose Type: standing, forward bend

Drishti Point: Padayoragrai or Padayoragre (toes/feet)

HORSE POSE: FORWARD BEND, BINDING & TWIST

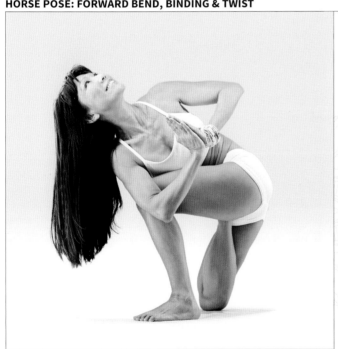

Revolved Leg Position of Horse Pose with Hands in Prayer

Parivritta Pada Vatayanasana Namaskar

(puh-ri-VRIT-tuh PUH-duh vah-tah-yuh-NAHS-uh-nuh nuh-muhs-KAHR)

Pose Type: standing, twist

Drishti Point: Urdhva or Antara Drishti (up to the sky)

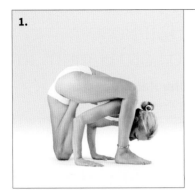

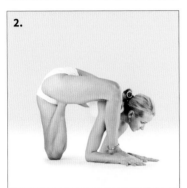

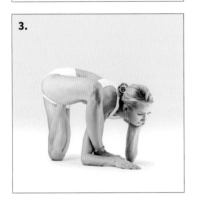

Half Lotus Extended Lizard Tail Lunge Pose

Ardha Padma Uttana Pristhasana

(UHR-duh PUHD-muh ut-TAHN-uh prish-TAHS-uh-nuh)

Modification: 1. palms to the floor, elbows bent 90 degrees

2. forearms to the floor

3. one forearm to the floor; other elbow to the floor, hand to the face

Pose Type: standing, forward bend

Drishti Point: 1 & 3. Nasagrai or Nasagre (nose)

2. Padhayoragrai or Padayoragre (toes/feet) and Angusthamadhye or Angushta Ma Dyai (thumbs)

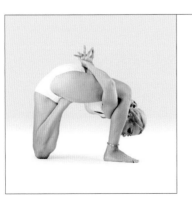

Bound Half Lotus Extended Lizard Tail Lunge Pose

Baddha Ardha Padma Uttana Pristhasana

(BUH-duh UHR-duh PUHD-muh ut-TAHN-uh prish-TAHS-uh-nuh)

Pose Type: standing, forward bend, binding

Drishti Point: Padayoragrai or Padayoragre (toes/feet)

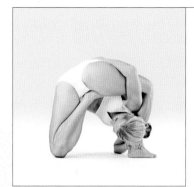

One Foot Behind the Head Bound Half Lotus Extended Lizard Tail Lunge Pose

Eka Pada Shirsha Baddha Ardha Padma Uttan Pristhasana

(EY-kuh PUH-duh SHEER-shuh BUH-duh UHR-duh PUHD-muh ut-TAHN-uh prish-TAHS-uh-nuh)

Pose Type: standing, forward bend, binding

Drishti Point: Urdhva or Antara Drishti (up to the sky)

HORSE POSE: SPINE STRAIGHT

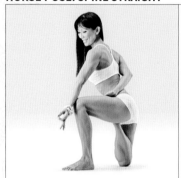

Half Bound Revolved Leg Position of Horse Pose

Ardha Baddha Parivritta Pada Vatayanasana

(UHR-duh BUH-duh puh-ri-VRIT-tuh PUH-duh vah-tah-yuh-NAHS-uh-nuh)

Modification: wrist to the knee of the front leg

Pose Type: standing, binding

Drishti Point: Hastagrai or Hastagre (hands)

1.

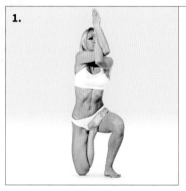

Horse Pose

Vatayanasana

(vah-tah-yuh-NAHS-uh-nuh)

Also Known As: Sea Horse Pose

Modification: 1. Front View

2. Side View

Pose Type: standing

Drishti Point: Angushtamadhye or Angushta Ma Dyai (thumbs)

2.

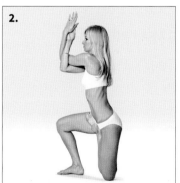

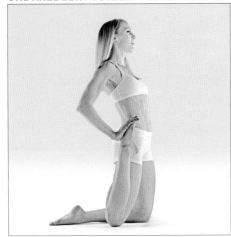

One-Legged Frog Pose in Camel Pose

Eka Pada Bhekasana in Ushtrasana

(EY-kuh PUH-duh bey-KAHS-uh-nuh in oosh-TRAHS-uh-nuh)

Modification: spine straight

Pose Type: standing (on the knees)

Drishti Point: Bhrumadhye or Ajna Chakra (third eye, between the eyebrows)

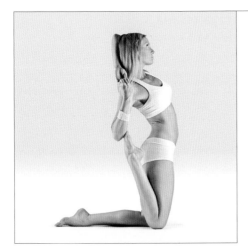

Mermaid Arm Position in Half Camel Pose

Hasta Naginyasana in Ardha Ushtrasana

(HUH-stuh nuh-gin-YAHS-uh-nuh in UHR-duh oosh-TRAHS-uhna)

Modification: spine straight

Pose Type: standing (on the knees), mild backbend, binding

Drishti Point: Bhrumadhye or Ajna Chakra (third eye, between the eyebrows)

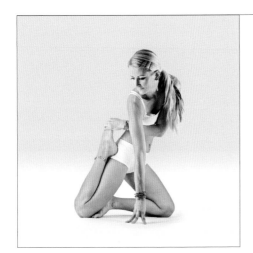

Revolved One-Legged Frog Pose in One-Legged King Pigeon 1 Version B

Parivritta Eka Pada Bhekasana in Eka Pada Raja Kapotasana 1 B

(puh-ri-VRIT-tuh EY-kuh PUH-duh bey-KAHS-uh-nuh in EY-kuh PUH-duh RAH-juh kuh-po-TAHS-uh-nuh)

Modification: fingertips to the floor in front

Pose Type: standing (on the knees), twist, binding

Drishti Point: Padhayoragrai or Padayoragre (toes/feet)

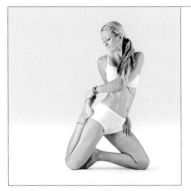

Half Bound Revolved One-Legged Frog Pose in One-Legged King Pigeon 1 Version B

Ardha Baddha Parivritta Eka Pada Bhekasana in Eka Pada Raja Kapotasana 1 B

(UHR-duh BUH-duh puh-ri-VRIT-tuh EY-kuh PUH-duh bey-KAHS-uh-nuh in EY-kuh PUH-duh RAH-juh kuh-po-TAHS-uh-nuh)

Pose Type: standing (on the knees), twist, binding
Drishti Point: Padayoragrai or Padayoragre (toes/feet)

COW FACE POSE AND GARUDA ON THE KNEES

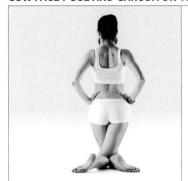

Leg Position of Cow Face Pose on the Knees

Janu Pada Gomukhasana

(JAH-nu PUH-duh go-moo-KAHS-uh-nuh)

Modification: hands on the hips
Pose Type: standing (on the knees)
Drishti Point: Nasagrai or Nasagre (nose)

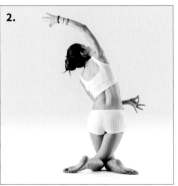
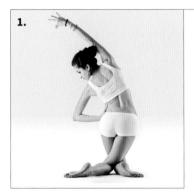

Leg Position of Cow Face Pose on the Knees

Janu Pada Gomukhasana

(JAH-nu PUH-duh go-moo-KAHS-uh-nuh)

Modification: 1. one hand on the hip, other arm straight over the head, side bend
2. one arm crossed in front of the body, other arm over the head, elbow bent, side bend
Pose Type: 1. standing (on the knees)
2. standing (on the knees), side bend
Drishti Point: Padayoragrai or Padayoragre (toes/feet), Hastagrai or Hastagre (hands)

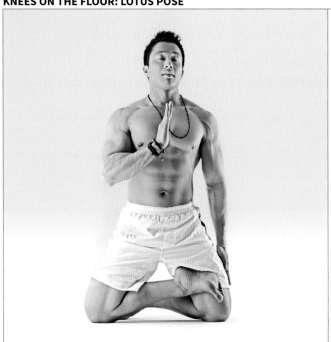

Half Pose Dedicated to Sage Goraksha

Ardha Gorakshasana

(UHR-duh go-rak-SHAHS-uh-nuh)

Modification: spine straight, one hand to the heart, other hand to the side of the thigh

Pose Type: standing (on the knees), balance

Drishti Point: Nasagrai or Nasagre (nose), Hastagrai or Hastagre (hands)

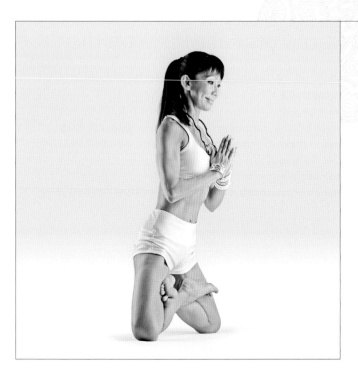

Pose Dedicated to Sage Goraksha

Gorakshasana

(go-ruhk-SHAHS-uh-nuh)

Also Known As: Yogic Seat Pose A (Yogapithasana A)

Modification: hands in Anjali Mudra (Hands in Prayer)

Pose Type: standing (on the knees), balance

Drishti Point: Nasagrai or Nasagre (nose), Hastagrai or Hastagre (hands)

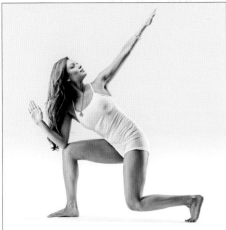

Fighting Warrior Pose 2

Yudhasana 2

(yu-DAHS-uh-nuh)

Modification: back knee off the floor

Pose Type: standing

Drishti Point: Hastagrai or Hastagre (hands)

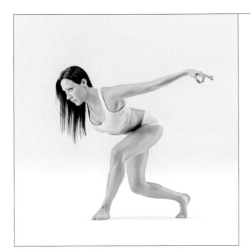

Son of Anjani (Lord Hanuman) Lunge Pose

Anjaneyasana

(uhn-juh-ney-AHS-uh-nuh)

Modification: arms open wide, forward bend, back knee bent and off the floor

Pose Type: standing, forward bend

Drishti Point: Nasagrai or Nasagre (nose)

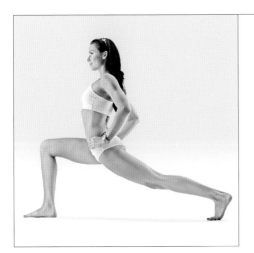

Son of Anjani (Lord Hanuman) Lunge Pose

Anjaneyasana

(uhn-juh-ney-AHS-uh-nuh)

Also Known As: Warrior 1 Modification (Virabhadrasana 1 Modification)

Modification: hands on the hips, back knee off the floor

Pose Type: standing

Drishti Point: Nasagrai or Nasagre (nose)

Standing Poses

183

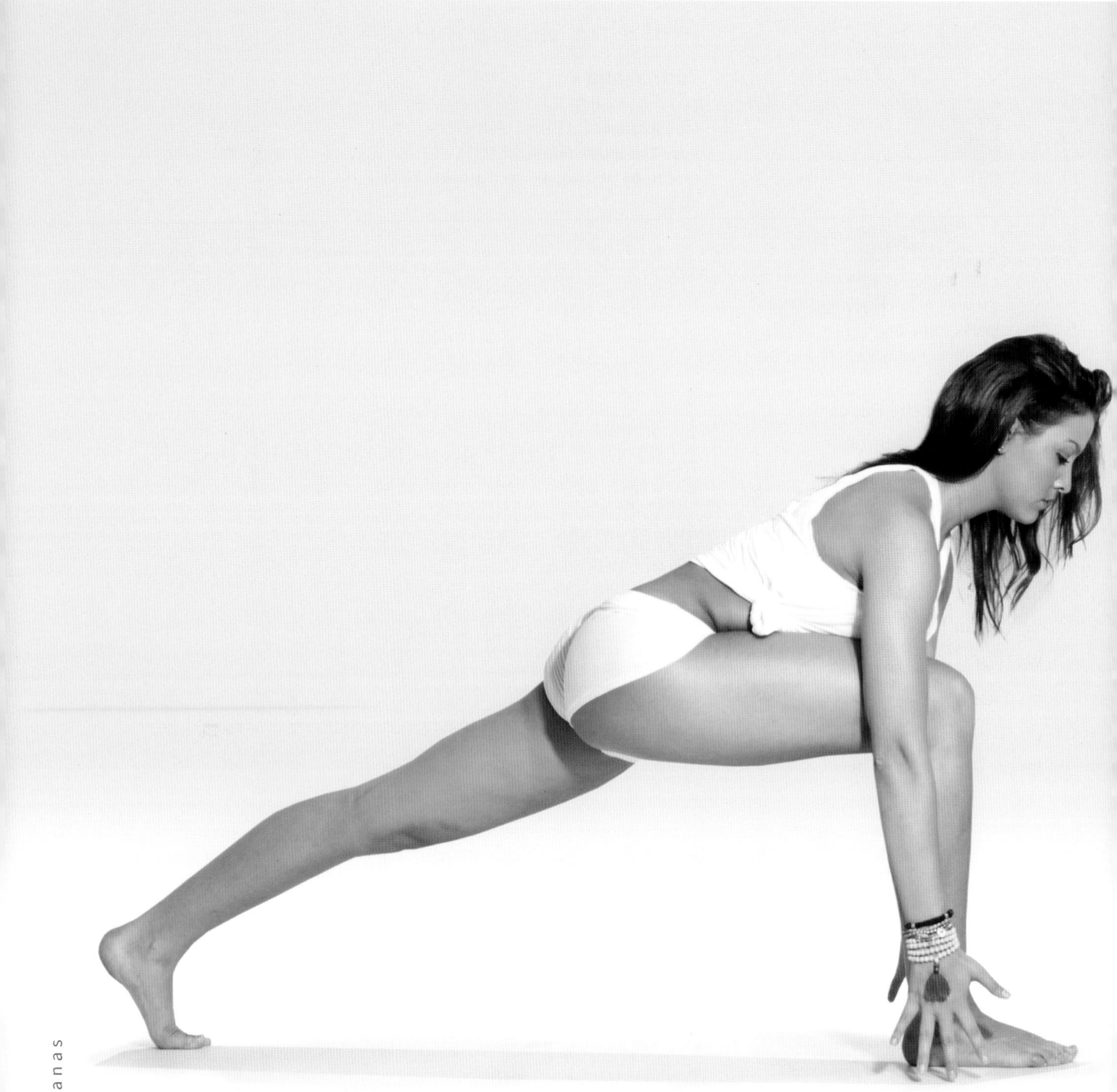

Equestrian Riding Horse Pose

Ashva Sanchalanasana
(UHSH-vuh suhn-chuh-luh-NAHS-un-nuh)
Pose Type: standing, forward bend
Drishti Point: Bhrumadhye or Ajna Chakra (third eye, between the eyebrows) or Padhayoragrai or Padayoragre (toes/feet)

Modification: back knee off the floor, fingertips off the floor on either side of the front foot

ashva sanchala = horse, riding posture

How to Perform the Pose:

1. Begin in Intense Stretch Pose (*Uttanasana*), also known as Full Forward Bend Pose. Engage your *mula bandha*, *uddhiyana bandha*, and *ujjayi* breathing.

2. Inhale and bend your knees enough for your fingertips to touch the floor on the sides of the feet.

3. Exhale as you step your left foot to the back, keeping your toes curled in, your left knee off the floor and keep your left leg strong and straight. Make sure your right knee is on top of your right ankle to prevent wear and tear on your knee joint.

4. Rest your torso on your right thigh. Inhale as you lengthen your spine, stretching your body in two opposing directions: crown of the head moving to the front and the heel of the right foot pushing to the back. You can look at the toes of the right foot.

5. Hold the pose for at least 30, and up to 90, seconds in order to receive the full benefits of the stretch.

6. Exhale as you step your left foot to the front in line with your right foot, and repeat on the other side.

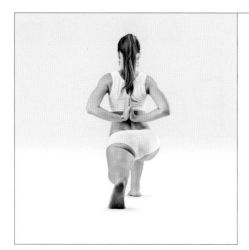

Reverse Prayer Son of Anjani (Lord Hanuman) Lunge Pose

Viparita Namaskar Anjaneyasana

(vi-puh-REE-tuh nuh-muhs-KAHR uhn-juh-ney-AHS-uh-nuh)

Also Known As: Back of the Body Prayer Son of Anjani (Lord Hanuman) Lunge Pose (Paschima Namaskara Anjaneyasana)
Modification: back knee off the floor
Pose Type: standing
Drishti Point: Nasagrai or Nasagre (nose)

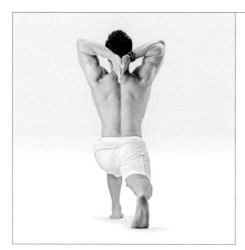

Son of Anjani (Lord Hanuman) Lunge Pose

Anjaneyasana

(uhn-juh-ney-AHS-uh-nuh)

Modification: palms together, thumbs to upper back, back knee off the floor
Pose Type: standing
Drishti Point: Nasagrai or Nasagre (nose)

LUNGE: BACK KNEE OFF THE FLOOR, BACK LEG STRAIGHT—BACKBENDS

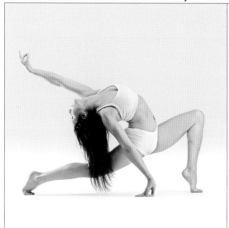

Tip Toe One Hand Son of Anjani (Lord Hanuman) Lunge Pose

Prapada Eka Hasta Anjaneyasana

(PRUH-puh-duh EY-kuh HUH-stuh uhn-juh-ney-AHS-uh-nuh)

Modification: deep backbend, one arm up over the head; fingertips of the other hand to the floor, back knee off the floor
Pose Type: standing, backbend
Drishti Point: Bhrumadhye or Ajna Chakra (third eye, between the eyebrows)

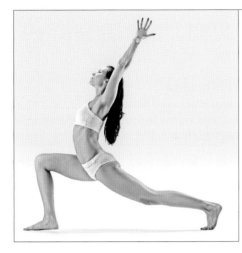

Son of Anjani (Lord Hanuman) Lunge Pose

Anjaneyasana
(uhn-juh-ney-AHS-uh-nuh)
Also Known As: Warrior 1 Modification (Virabhadrasana 1 Modification), Crescent Lunge Pose
Modification: hands up over the head and shoulder width apart, back knee off the floor
Pose Type: standing, mild backbend
Drishti Point: Bhrumadhye or Ajna Chakra (third eye, between the eyebrows)

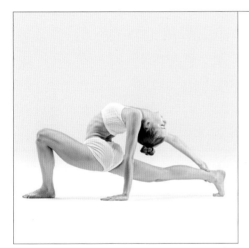

One Hand Rising Standing Pose of the Heavenly Spirits

Eka Hasta Utthita Stiti Valakhilyasana
(EY-kuh HUH-stuh UT-ti-tuh STI-ti vah-luh-khil-YAHS-uh-nuh)
Also Known As: Eka Hasta Utthita Nindra Valakhilyasana; Son of Anjani (Lord Hanuman) Lunge Pose (Anjaneyasana)
Modification: grabbing the back ankle overhead on the same side, other hand to the floor, back knee off the floor
Pose Type: standing, backbend
Drishti Point: Bhrumadhye or Ajna Chakra (third eye, between the eyebrows)

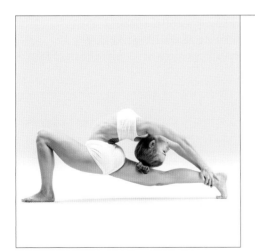

Rising Standing Pose of the Heavenly Spirits

Utthita Stiti Valakhilyasana
(UT-ti-tuh STI-ti vah-luh-khil-YAHS-uh-nuh)
Also Known As: Utthita Nindra Valakhilyasana; Son of Anjani (Lord Hanuman) Lunge Pose (Anjaneyasana)
Modification: grabbing the back ankle overhead with both hands, back knee off the floor
Pose Type: standing, backbend
Drishti Point: Bhrumadhye or Ajna Chakra (third eye, between the eyebrows)

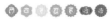

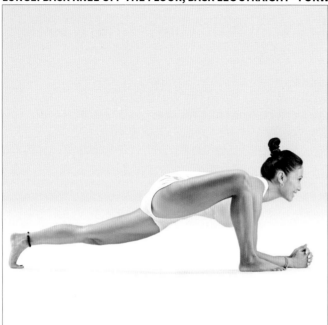

Extended Lizard Tail Lunge Pose

Uttana Pristhasana

(ut-TAH-nuh prish-TAHS-uh-nuh)

Modification: elbows to the floor on the inside of the front leg, back knee off the floor
Pose Type: standing, forward bend
Drishti Point: Nasagrai or Nasagre (nose)

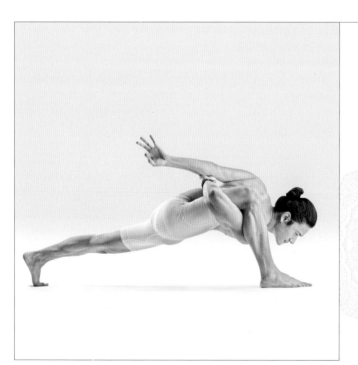

Pose Dedicated to Sage Punnakeesar Lunge

Punnakeesarasana

(pu-nuh-kee-suh-RAHS-uh-nuh)

Also Known As: Bound God Favor Seeking Sacrifice Ritual Pose (Baddha Yajnasana), Bound Christ's Cross Pose
Modification: back knee off the floor
Pose Type: standing, forward bend, binding
Drishti Point: Padhayoragrai or Padayoragre (toes/feet)

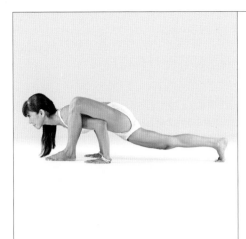

Extended Lizard Tail Lunge Pose

Uttana Pristhasana

(ut-TAH-nuh prish-TAHS-uh-nuh)

Modification: elbows bent at 90 degrees, palms to the floor, back knee off the floor

Pose Type: standing, forward bend

Drishti Point: Nasagrai or Nasagre (nose), Bhrumadhye or Ajna Chakra (third eye, between the eyebrows)

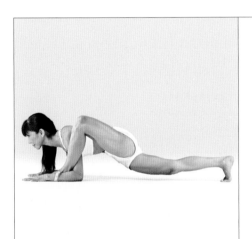

Extended Lizard Tail Lunge Pose

Uttana Pristhasana

(ut-TAH-nuh prish-TAHS-uh-nuh)

Modification: forearms to the floor on either side of the front foot, back knee off the floor

Pose Type: standing, forward bend

Drishti Point: Nasagrai or Nasagre (nose), Bhrumadhye or Ajna Chakra (third eye, between the eyebrows)

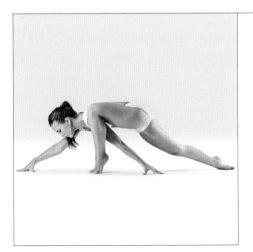

Tip Toe Extended Lizard Tail Lunge Pose

Prapada Uttana Pristhasana

(PRUH-puh-duh ut-TAH-nuh prish-TAHS-uh-nuh)

Modification: arms straight and reaching in the opposite directions, heel of the front leg up, top of the back foot to the floor, back knee off the floor

Pose Type: standing, forward bend

Drishti Point: Nasagrai or Nasagre (nose)

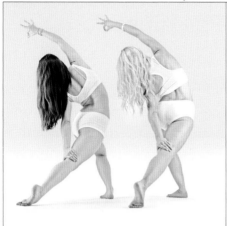

Sideways Son of Anjani (Lord Hanuman) Lunge Pose

Parshva Anjaneyasana

(PAHRSH-vuh uhn-juh-ney-AHS-uh-nuh)

Modification: top of the back foot on the floor, back knee off the floor

Pose Type: standing, side bend, backbend

Drishti Point: Hastagrai or Hastagre (hands)

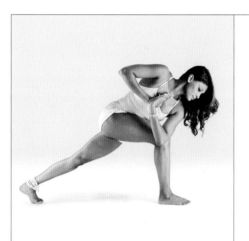

Revolved Son of Anjani (Lord Hanuman) Lunge Pose with Hands in Prayer

Parivritta Anjaneyasana Namaskar

(puh-ri-VRIT-tuh uhn-juh-ney-AHS-uh-nuh nuh-muhs-KAHR)

Modification: elbow over knee, back knee off the floor

Pose Type: standing, twist

Drishti Point: Padayoragrai or Padayoragre (toes/feet)

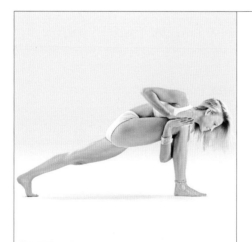

Revolved Son of Anjani (Lord Hanuman) Lunge Pose with Hands in Prayer

Parivritta Anjaneyasana Namaskar

(puh-ri-VRIT-tuh uhn-juh-ney-AHS-uh-nuh nuh-muhs-KAHR)

Modification: arm under the knee, back knee off the floor

Pose Type: standing, twist

Drishti Point: Padayoragrai or Padayoragre (toes/feet)

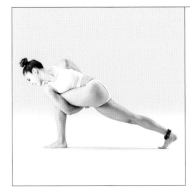

Bound Revolved Son of Anjani (Lord Hanuman) Lunge Pose

Baddha Parivritta Anjaneyasana

(BUH-duh puh-ri-VRIT-tuh uhn-juh-ney-AHS-uh-nuh)
Modification: back knee off the floor
Pose Type: standing, twist, binding
Drishti Point: Padhayoragrai or Padayoragre (toes/feet)

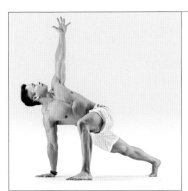

Revolved Son of Anjani (Lord Hanuman) Lunge Pose

Parivritta Anjaneyasana

(puh-ri-VRIT-tuh uhn-juh-ney-AHS-uh-nuh)
Modification: one hand to the floor, other arm up in the sky, twisting to the inside of the front knee, back knee off the floor
Pose Type: standing, twist
Drishti Point: Angushtamadhye or Angushta Ma Dyai (thumbs)

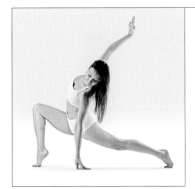

Tip Toe Sideways Son of Anjani (Lord Hanuman) Lunge Pose

Prapada Parshva Anjaneyasana

(PRUH-puh-duh PAHRSH-vuh uhn-juh-ney-AHS-uh-nuh)
Modification: one hand to the floor, other arm up in the sky, twisting to the outside of the front knee, back knee off the floor
Pose Type: standing, twist
Drishti Point: Hastagrai or Hastagre (hands)

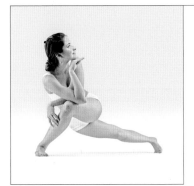

Revolved Paying Homage Lunge Pose

Parivritta Namasyasana

(puh-ri-VRIT-tuh nuh-muhs-YAHS-uh-muh)
Also Known As: Curtsey Lunge
Modification: front leg crossed over to the side, opposite elbow over the front knee, back knee off the floor
Pose Type: standing, twist
Drishti Point: Parshva Drishti (to the right), Parshva Drishti (to the left)

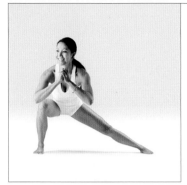

Extended Leg to the Side Squat Pose

Utthita Parshva Pada Upaveshasana

(UT-ti-tuh PAHRSH-vuh PUH-duh u-puh-vey-SHAHS-uh-nuh)

Also Known As: Plyo Side Lunge

Modification: high stance, fingers interlocked in front of the chest

Pose Type: standing

Drishti Point: Nasagrai or Nasagre (nose)

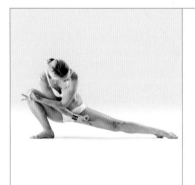

Tip Toe Extended Leg to the Side Squat Pose

Prapada Utthita Parshva Pada Upaveshasana

(PRUH-puh-duh UT-ti-tuh PAHRSH-vuh PUH-duh u-puh-vey-SHAHS-uh-nuh)

Modification: high stance; arms straight out to the sides, toes of the straight leg flexed in

Pose Type: standing

Drishti Point: Hastagrai or Hastagre (hands)

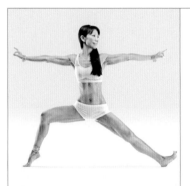

Extended Leg to the Side Squat Pose

Utthita Parshva Pada Upaveshasana

(UT-ti-tuh PAHRSH-vuh PUH-duh u-puh-vey-SHAHS-uh-nuh)

Modification: arms crossed in front of the chest, forward bend

Pose Type: standing, forward bend

Drishti Point: Padayoragrai or Padayoragre (toes/feet)

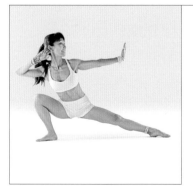

Extended Leg to the Side Squat Pose

Utthita Parshva Pada Upaveshasana

(UT-ti-tuh PAHRSH-vuh PUH-duh u-puh-vey-SHAHS-uh-nuh)

Modification: leaning toward the bent leg, one arm straight to the side, fingertips flexed in; other elbow to the side, fingertips to the back of the head

Pose Type: standing, side bend

Drishti Point: Hastagrai or Hastagre (hands)

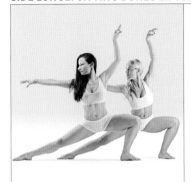

Extended Leg to the Side Squat Pose

Utthita Parshva Pada Upaveshasana

(UT-ti-tuh PAHRSH-vuh PUH-duh u-puh-vey-SHAHS-uh-nuh)

Modification: side bend toward the straight leg, one arm parallel to the floor, other arm extended to the sky

Pose Type: standing

Drishti Point: Hastagrai or Hastagre (hands)

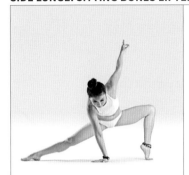

Tip Toe Extended Leg to the Side Squat Pose

Prapada Utthita Parshva Pada Upaveshasana

(PRUH-puh-duh UT-ti-tuh PAHRSH-vuh PUH-duh u-puh-vey-SHAHS-uh-nuh)

Modification: one palm to the floor

Pose Type: standing, forward bend

Drishti Point: Hastagrai or Hastagre (hands)

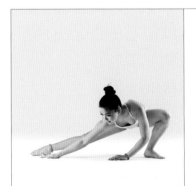

Extended Leg to the Side Squat Pose

Utthita Parshva Pada Upaveshasana

(UT-ti-tuh PAHRSH-vuh PUH-duh u-puh-vey-SHAHS-uh-nuh)

Modification: both hands to the floor, side bending toward the straight leg

Pose Type: standing, forward bend, side bend

Drishti Point: Hastagrai or Hastagre (hands)

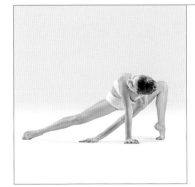

Intense Ankle Stretch Extended Leg to the Side Squat Pose

Uttana Kulpa Utthita Parshva Pada Upaveshasana

(ut-TAH-nuh kul-puh UT-ti-tuh PAHRSH-vuh PUH-duh u-puh-vey-SHAHS-uh-nuh)

Modification: both palms to the floor, arms crossed

Pose Type: standing, forward bend, twist

Drishti Point: Urdhva or Antara Drishti (up to the sky)

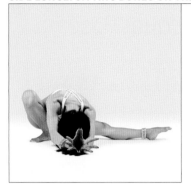

Lotus Hand Seal Extended Leg to the Side Squat Pose

Padma Mudra Utthita Parshva Pada Upaveshasana

(PUHD-muh MU-druh UT-ti-tuh PAHRSH-vuh PUH-duh u-puh-vey-SHAHS-uh-nuh)

Modification: forward bend, forehead to the floor, arms extended in front

Pose Type: standing, forward bend

Drishti Point: Nasagrai or Nasagre (nose)

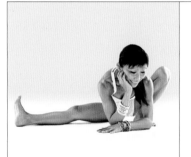

Uneven Arms Extended Leg to the Side Squat Pose

Vishama Hasta Utthita Parshva Pada Upaveshasana

(VISH-uh-muh HUH-stuh UT-ti-tuh PAHRSH-vuh PUH-duh u-puh-vey-SHAHS-uh-nuh)

Modification: forward bend, one forearm to the floor, other hand to the face

Pose Type: standing, seated, forward bend

Drishti Point: Nasagrai or Nasagre (nose)

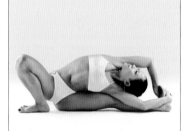

Revolved Extended Leg to the Side Squat Pose 1

Parivritta Utthita Parshva Pada Upaveshasana 1

(puh-ri-VRIT-tuh UT-ti-tuh PAHRSH-vuh PUH-duh u-puh-vey-SHAHS-uh-nuh)

Modification: both hands to the foot of the straight leg

Pose Type: standing, seated, forward bend, side bend, twist

Drishti Point: Urdhva or Antara Drishti (up to the sky)

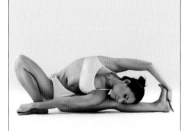

Revolved Extended Leg to the Side Squat Pose 2

Parivritta Utthita Parshva Pada Upaveshasana 2

(puh-ri-VRIT-tuh UT-ti-tuh PAHRSH-vuh PUH-duh u-puh-vey-SHAHS-uh-nuh)

Modification: grabbing onto both feet

Pose Type: standing, seated, forward bend, side bend, twist

Drishti Point: Hastagrai or Hastagre (hands), Padayoragrai or Padayoragre (toes/feet)

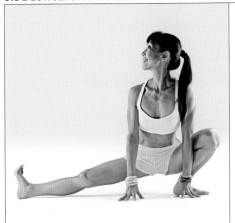

Extended Leg to the Side Squat Pose

Utthita Parshva Pada Upaveshasana

(UT-ti-tuh PAHRSH-vuh PUH-duh u-puh-vey-SHAHS-uh-nuh)

Modification: fingertips to the floor, toes of the straight leg flexed in

Pose Type: standing, forward bend

Drishti Point: Parshva Drishti (to the right), Parshva Drishti (to the left)

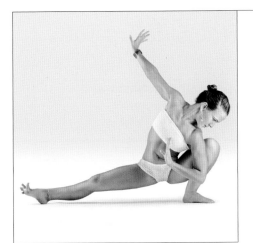

Knee to Shoulder Extended Leg to the Side Squat Pose

Janu Bhuja Utthita Parshva Pada Upaveshasana

(JAH-nu BHU-juh UT-ti-tuh PAHRSH-vuh PUH-duh u-puh-vey-SHAHS-uh-nuh)

Modification: toes of the straight leg pointed

Pose Type: standing, forward bend, side bend

Drishti Point: Padayoragrai or Padayoragre (toes/feet)

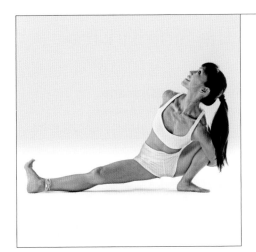

Bound Extended Leg to the Side Squat Pose

Baddha Utthita Parshva Pada Upaveshasana

(BUH-duh UT-ti-tuh PAHRSH-vuh PUH-duh u-puh-vey-SHAHS-uh-nuh)

Modification: binding around the shin of the bent leg, toes of the straight leg flexed in

Pose Type: standing, side bend, binding

Drishti Point: Urdhva or Antara Drishti (up to the sky)

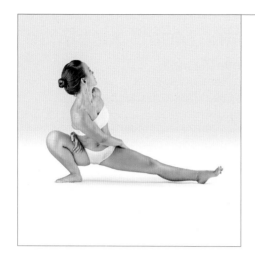

Revolved Half Bound Extended Leg to the Side Squat Pose

Parivritta Ardha Baddha Utthita Parshva Pada Upaveshasana

(puh-ri-VRIT-tuh UHR-duh BUH-duh UT-ti-tuh PAHRSH-vuh PUH-duh u-puh-vey-SHAHS-uh-nuh)

Modification: toes of the straight leg pointed
Pose Type: standing, side bend, binding
Drishti Point: Urdhva or Antara Drishti (up to the sky)

SIDE LUNGE: SITTING BONE TO THE HEEL—ARMS HIGHER THAN HEAD LEVEL

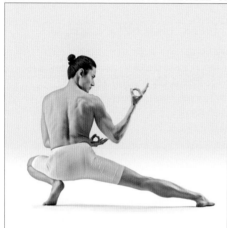

Extended Leg to the Side Tip Toe Squat Pose

Utthita Parshva Pada Prapada Upaveshasana

(UT-ti-tuh PAHRSH-vuh PUH-duh PRUH-puh-duh u-puh-vey-SHAHS-uh-nuh)

Modification: toes of the straight leg to the floor
Pose Type: standing, forward bend
Drishti Point: Hastagrai or Hastagre (hands)

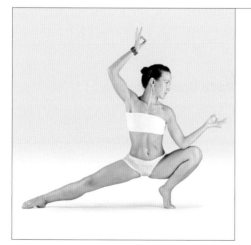

Extended Leg to the Side Tip Toe Squat Pose

Utthita Parshva Pada Prapada Upaveshasana

(UT-ti-tuh PAHRSH-vuh PUH-duh PRUH-puh-duh u-puh-vey-SHAHS-uh-nuh)

Modification: elbow to the knee of the bent leg, toes of the straight leg to the floor
Pose Type: standing, forward bend
Drishti Point: Hastagrai or Hastagre (hands)

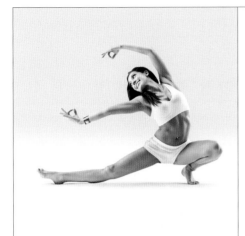

Extended Leg to the Side Tip Toe Squat Pose

Utthita Parshva Pada Prapada Upaveshasana

(UT-ti-tuh PAHRSH-vuh PUH-duh PRUH-puh-duh u-puh-vey-SHAHS-uh-nuh)

Modification: side bend toward the straight leg, one arm parallel to the floor, other arm extended to the sky, toes of the straight leg pointed
Pose Type: standing, side bend
Drishti Point: Hastagrai or Hastagre (hands)

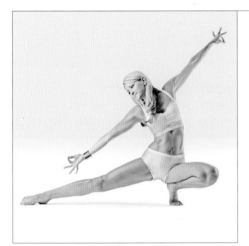

Extended Leg to the Side Tip Toe Squat Pose

Utthita Parshva Pada Prapada Upaveshasana

(UT-ti-tuh PAHRSH-vuh PUH-duh PRUH-puh-duh u-puh-vey-SHAHS-uh-nuh)

Modification: side bend toward the straight leg, arms extended to the side and straight, toes of the straight leg to the floor
Pose Type: standing, side bend
Drishti Point: Hastagrai or Hastagre (hands), Padayoragrai or Padayoragre (toes/feet)

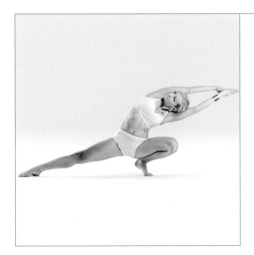

Both Arms Extended Leg to the Side Tip Toe Squat Pose

Dwi Hasta Utthita Parshva Pada Prapada Upaveshasana

(DWI-huh-stuh UT-ti-tuh PAHRSH-vuh PUH-duh PRUH-puh-duh u-puh-vey-SHAHS-uh-nuh)

Modification: side bend toward the bent leg, toes of the straight leg to the floor
Pose Type: standing, side bend
Drishti Point: Urdhva or Antara Drishti (up to the sky)

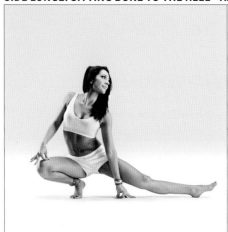

Extended Leg to the Side Tip Toe Squat Pose

Utthita Parshva Pada Prapada Upaveshasana

(UT-ti-tuh PAHRSH-vuh PUH-duh PRUH-puh-duh u-puh-vey-SHAHS-uh-nuh)

Modification: one hand on the knee, other hand to the floor, toes of the straight leg pointed

Pose Type: standing, forward bend

Drishti Point: Parshva Drishti (to the right), Parshva Drishti (to the left)

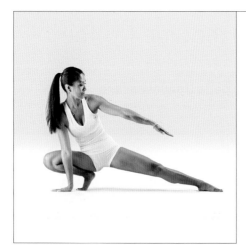

Extended Leg to the Side Tip Toe Squat Pose

Utthita Parshva Pada Prapada Upaveshasana

(UT-ti-tuh PAHRSH-vuh PUH-duh PRUH-puh-duh u-puh-vey-SHAHS-uh-nuh)

Modification: one palm to the floor, other arm straight and parallel to the straight leg, toes of the straight leg to the floor

Pose Type: standing

Drishti Point: Padayoragrai or Padayoragre (toes/feet), Hastagrai or Hastagre (hands)

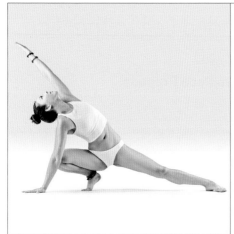

Extended Leg to the Side Tip Toe Squat Pose

Utthita Parshva Pada Prapada Upaveshasana

(UT-ti-tuh PAHRSH-vuh PUH-duh PRUH-puh-duh u-puh-vey-SHAHS-uh-nuh)

Modification: side bending toward the bent knee, one hand to the floor, other arm extended up over the head, toes of the straight leg to the floor

Pose Type: standing, side bend

Drishti Point: Hastagrai or Hastagre (hands)

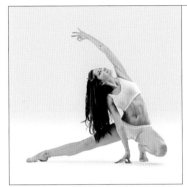

Extended Leg to the Side Tip Toe Squat Pose

Utthita Parshva Pada Prapada Upaveshasana

(UT-ti-tuh PAHRSH-vuh PUH-duh PRUH-puh-duh u-puh-vey-SHAHS-uh-nuh)

Modification: side bending toward the straight leg, one hand to the floor, other arm extended up over the head, toes of the straight leg to the floor

Pose Type: standing, side bend

Drishti Point: Hastagrai or Hastagre (hands)

SIDE LUNGE: SITTING BONE TO THE HEEL—TWISTS & BINDING

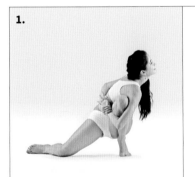

Revolved Extended Leg to the Side Tip Toe Squat Pose with Hands in Prayer

Parivritta Utthita Parshva Pada Prapada Upaveshasana Namaskar

(puh-ri-VRIT-tuh UT-ti-tuh PAHRSH-vuh PUH-duh PRUH-puh-duh u-puh-vey-SHAHS-uh-nuh nuh-muhs-KAHR)

Modification: toes of the straight leg to the floor

Pose Type: standing, forward bend, twist

Drishti Point: Urdhva or Antara Drishti (up to the sky)

1.

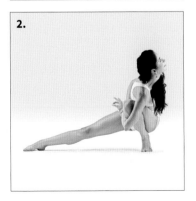

Revolved Bound Extended Leg to the Side Tip Toe Squat Pose

Parivritta Baddha Utthita Parshva Pada Prapada Upaveshasana

(puh-ri-VRIT-tuh BUH-duh UT-ti-tuh PAHRSH-vuh PUH-duh PRUH-puh-duh u-puh-vey-SHAHS-uh-nuh)

Modification: toes of the straight leg to the floor

1. knee on the floor

2. knee off the floor

Pose Type: standing, twist, binding

Drishti Point: Nasagrai or Nasagre (nose), Bhrumadhye or Ajna Chakra (third eye, between the eyebrows)

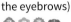

2.

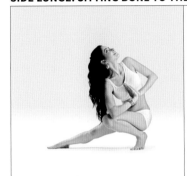

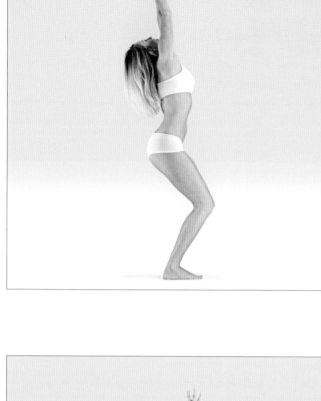

Fierce Pose

Utkatasana
(OOT-kuh-TAHS-uh-nuh)
Also Known As: Chair Pose
Modification: palms pressed together, high squat
Pose Type: standing, mild backbend
Drishti Point: Angushtamadhye or Angushta Ma Dyai (thumbs)

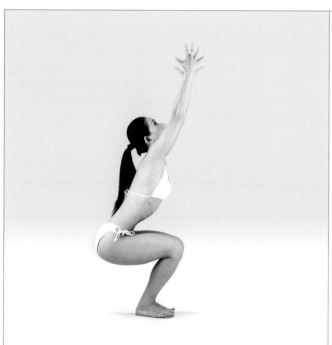

Fierce Pose

Utkatasana
(OOT-kuh-TAHS-uh-nuh)
Also Known As: Chair Pose
Modification: hands shoulder width apart, low squat
Pose Type: standing
Drishti Point: Angushtamadhye or Angushta Ma Dyai (thumbs)

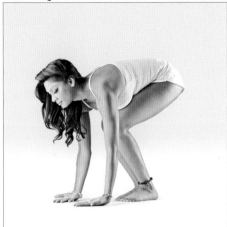

Wagtail Bird Pose Prep.

Khanjanasana Prep.

(kuhn-juh-NAHS-uh-nuh)

Modification: hands to the floor, palms facing up, feet together
Pose Type: standing, forward bend
Drishti Point: Nasagrai or Nasagre (nose), Bhrumadhye/Ajna Chakra (third eye, between the eyebrows)

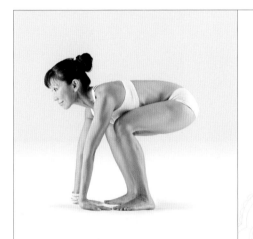

Intense Wrist Stretch Fierce Pose

Uttana Manibandha Utkatasana

(ut-TAH-nuh muh-ni-BUHN-duh OOT-kuh-TAHS-uh-nuh)

Also Known As: Intense Wrist Stretch Chair Pose
Modification: palms to the floor, fingertips facing the toes
Pose Type: standing, forward bend
Drishti Point: Nasagrai or Nasagre (nose)

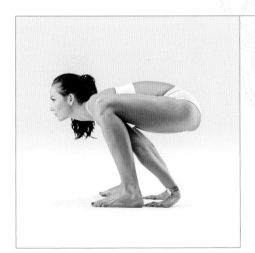

Wagtail Bird Pose

Khanjanasana

(kuhn-juh-NAHS-uh-nuh)

Also Known As: Shoulder Pressure Pose Prep. (Bhujapidasana Prep.)
Modification: shoulders to the back of the knees, fingertips to the heel
Pose Type: standing, forward bend
Drishti Point: Bhrumadhye/Ajna Chakra (third eye, between the eyebrows)

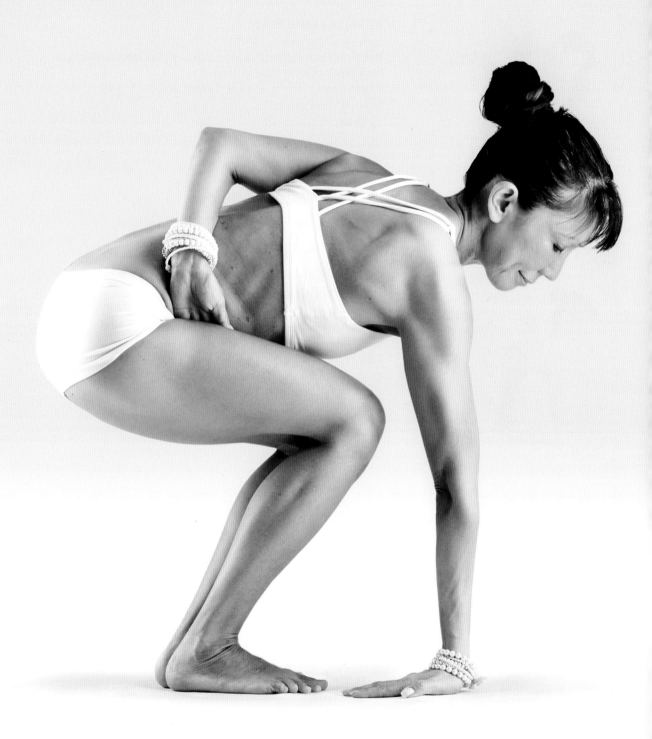

Intense Wrist Stretch Half Bound
Fierce Pose

Uttana Manibandha Ardha Baddha Utkatasana

(ut-TAH-nuh muh-ni-BUHN-duh UHR-duh OOT-kuh-TAHS-uh-nuh)

Also Known As: Intense Wrist Stretch Half Bound Chair Pose

Pose Type: standing, forward bend, binding

Drishti Point: Hastagrai or Hastagrahe (hands)

Modification: hand to the floor, fingertips pointing toward the toes

ut = intense
tan = to stretch, to extend
manibandha = wrist
ardha = half
baddha = bound
utkata = fierce

How to Perform the Pose:

1. Begin by standing in Mountain Pose (*Tadasana*). Engage your *mula bandha*, *uddhiyana bandha*, and *ujjayi* breathing.

2. Exhale, bend your knees until your thighs are parallel to the floor, and drop both your hands to the floor. Rest your torso on top of your thighs.

3. Inhale as you externally rotate your right arm to point the fingertips of your right hand toward your feet.

4. On your next inhale, bring your left arm behind your back and your left hand to the inside of your right thigh. Try to seal the gap between your ribcage and your elbow.

5. Hold the pose for at least 30, and up to 90, seconds in order to receive the full benefits of the stretch.

6. Exhale as you release your left arm and bring your left hand to the floor. Repeat on the right side.

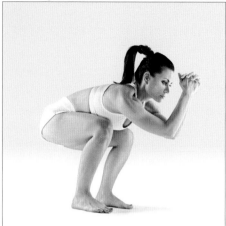

Elephant Old Form

Gaja Vadivu

(GUH-juh vah-dee-vuh)

Pose Type: standing, forward bend

Drishti Point: Angushtamadhye or Angushta Ma Dyai (thumbs)

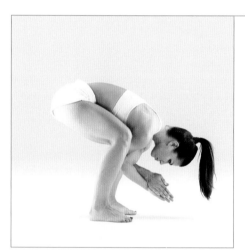

Hand Position of the Pose Dedicated to Garuda in Half Intense Stretch Pose

Hasta Garudasana in Ardha Uttanasana

(HUH-stuh guh-ru-DAHS-uh-nuh in UHR-duh ut-tahn-AHS-uh-nuh)

Also Known As: Hand Position of the Pose Dedicated to Garuda in Half Forward Bend

Modification: knees bent, feet hip width apart

Pose Type: standing, forward bend

Drishti Point: Angushtamadhye or Angushta Ma Dyai (thumbs)

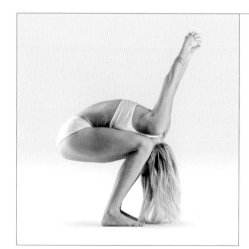

Hands Bound Ear Pressure Fierce Pose

Baddha Hasta Karnapida Utkatasana

(BUH-duh HUH-stuh kahr-nuh-PEE-duh ut-kuh-TAHS-uh-nuh)

Also Known As: Hands Bound Ear Pressure Chair Pose

Pose Type: standing, forward bend

Drishti Point: Nasagrai or Nasagre (nose)

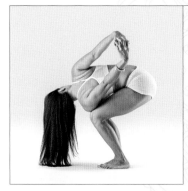

Hands Bound Revolved Fierce Pose

Baddha Hasta Parivritta Utkatasana

(Buh-duh HUH-stuh puh-ri-VRIT-tuh ut-kuh-TAHS-uh-nuh)

Also Known As: Hands Bound Revolved Chair Pose

Pose Type: standing, forward bend, twist

Drishti Point: Urdhva or Antara Drishti (up to the sky)

CHAIR SQUAT: HIGH STANCE—TWIST, ONE HAND TO THE FLOOR

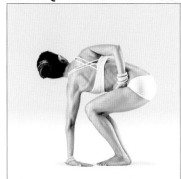

Intense Wrist Stretch Revolved Half Bound Pose Dedicated to Yogi Shankara

Uttana Manibandha Parivritta Ardha Baddha Shankarasana

(ut-TAHN-uh muh-ni-BUHN-duh puh-ri-VRIT-tuh UHR-duh BUH-duh shuhng-kuhr-AHS-uh-nuh)

Pose Type: standing, forward bend, twist, binding

Drishti Point: Urdhva or Antara Drishti (up to the sky)

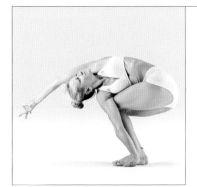

Revolved Pose Dedicated to Yogi Shankara

Parivritta Sankarasana

(puh-ri-VRIT-tuh shuhng-kuhr-AHS-uh-nuh)

Pose Type: standing, forward bend, side bend, twist

Drishti Point: Urdhva or Antara Drishti (up to the sky)

CHAIR SQUAT: HIGH STANCE—TWIST AND ELBOW OVER THE KNEE

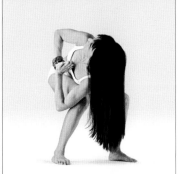

Revolved Fierce Pose

Parivritta Utkatasana

(puh-ri-VRIT-tuh ut-kuh-TAHS-uh-nuh)

Also Known As: Revolved Chair Pose

Modification: feet wide apart, hands in Anjali Mudra (Hands in Prayer)

Pose Type: standing, forward bend, twist

Drishti Point: Urdhva or Antara Drishti (up to the sky)

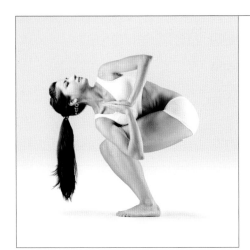

Revolved Fierce Pose

Parivritta Utkatasana

(puh-ri-VRIT-tuh ut-kuh-TAHS-uh-nuh)

Also Known As: Revolved Chair Pose
Modification: feet together, hands in Anjali Mudra (Hands in Prayer)
Pose Type: standing, forward bend, twist
Drishti Point: Urdhva or Antara Drishti (up to the sky)

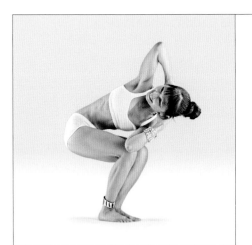

Revolved Fierce Pose

Parivritta Utkatasana

(puh-ri-VRIT-tuh ut-kuh-TAHS-uh-nuh)

Also Known As: Revolved Chair Pose
Modification: hands behind the head
Pose Type: standing, forward bend, twist
Drishti Point: Urdhva or Antara Drishti (up to the sky)

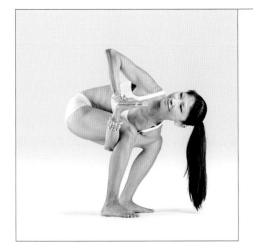

Revolved Fierce Pose

Parivritta Utkatasana

(puh-ri-VRIT-tuh ut-kuh-TAHS-uh-nuh)

Also Known As: Revolved Chair Pose
Modification: arm wrapped under the knee, hands in Anjali Mudra (Hands in Prayer)
Pose Type: standing, forward bend, twist
Drishti Point: Urdhva or Antara Drishti (up to the sky)

1.

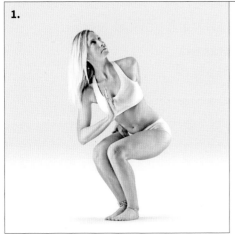

One Hand Bound Revolved Fierce Pose

Eka Hasta Baddha Parivritta Utkatasana

(EY-kuh HUH-stuh BUH-duh puh-ri-VRIT-tuh ut-kuh-TAHS-uh-nuh)

Also Known As: One Hand Bound Revolved Chair Pose

Modification: 1. one hand to the heart

2. hand grabbing onto the biceps, other elbow over the opposite knee

Pose Type: standing, forward bend, twist, binding

Drishti Point: 1. Urdhva or Antara Drishti (up to the sky)

2. Padhayoragrai or Padayoragre (toes/feet)

2.

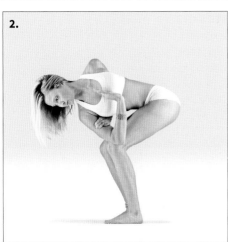

Revolved One Leg Bound Fierce Pose

Parivritta Eka Pada Baddha Utkatasana

(puh-ri-VRIT-tuh EY-kuh PUH-duh BUH-duh ut-kuh-TAHS-uh-nuh)

Also Known As: Revolved One Leg Bound Chair Pose

Pose Type: standing, forward bend, twist, binding

Drishti Point: Padayoragrai or Padayoragre (toes/feet)

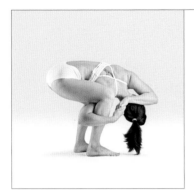

Revolved One Leg Bound Fierce Pose

Parivritta Eka Pada Baddha Utkatasana

(puh-ri-VRIT-tuh EY-kuh PUH-duh BUH-duh ut-kuh-TAHS-uh-nuh)

Also Known As: Revolved One Leg Bound Chair Pose
Modification: binding around one leg, hands bound overhead
Pose Type: standing, forward bend, twist, binding
Drishti Point: Urdhva or Antara Drishti (up to the sky)

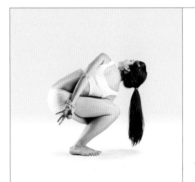

Revolved Both Legs Bound Fierce Pose

Parivritta Dwi Pada Baddha Utkatasana

(puh-ri-VRIT-tuh DWI-puh-duh BUH-duh ut-kuh-TAHS-uh-nuh)

Also Known As: Revolved Both Legs Bound Chair Pose
Pose Type: standing, forward bend, twist, binding
Drishti Point: Urdhva or Antara Drishti (up to the sky)

CHAIR SQUAT: HIGH STANCE HEELS UP—CHEST AWAY FROM QUADRICEPS

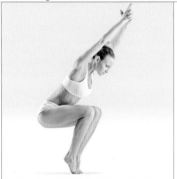

Tip Toe Fierce Pose 1

Prapada Utkatasana 1

(PRUH-puh-duh ut-kuh-TAHSuh-nuh)

Also Known As: Tip Toe Chair Pose 1
Modification: arms up over the head, fingers interlocked
Pose Type: standing, forward bend
Drishti Point: Nasagrai or Nasagre (nose)

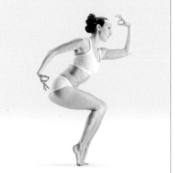

Tip Toe Fierce Pose 3

Prapada Utkatasana 3

(PRUH-puh-duh ut-kuh-TAHSuh-nuh)

Also Known As: Tip Toe Chair Pose 3
Modification: both elbows bent, one arm up in front, one arm down to the back
Pose Type: standing, forward bend
Drishti Point: Hastagrai or Hastagre (hands)

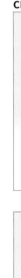

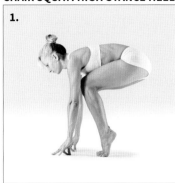

1.

Crane Pose Prep.

Bakasana Prep.

(buhk-AHS-uh-nuh)

Modification: hands to the floor in front of the feet
1. fingertips to the floor
2. palms flat to the floor, arms shoulder width apart, fingertips pointing away from the head
Pose Type: standing, forward bend
Drishti Point: Hastagrai or Hastagre (hands), Nasagrai or Nasagre (nose)

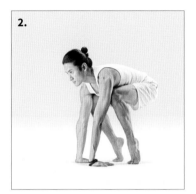

2.

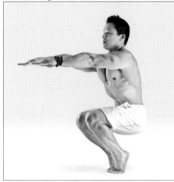

Tip Toe Fierce Pose

Prapada Utkatasana

(PRUH-puh-duh ut-kuh-TAHS-uh-nuh)

Also Known As: Awkward Pose (Utkatasana)
Modification: arms out in front and parallel to the floor, sitting bones lifted off the heels
Pose Type: standing
Drishti Point: Angushtamadhye or Angushta Ma Dyai (thumbs)

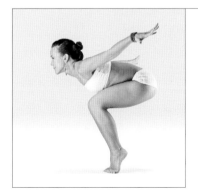

Tip Toe Fierce Pose 2

Prapada Utkatasana 2

(PRUH-puh-duh ut-kuh-TAHS-uh-nuh)

Also Known As: Tip Toe Chair Pose 2 and Tip Toe Diver's Pose
Modification: arms extended to the back, chest to the quadriceps, palms facing down
Pose Type: standing, forward bend
Drishti Point: Nasagrai or Nasagre (nose), Bhrumadhye or Ajna Chakra (third eye, between the eyebrows)

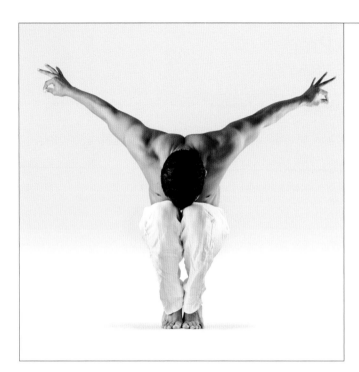

Head to Knees Tip Toe Fierce Pose 2

Janu Shirsha Prapada Utkatasana 2

(JAH-nu SHEER-shuh PRUH-puh-duh ut-kuh-TAHS-uh-nuh)

Also Known As: Head to Knees Tip Toe Chair Pose 2 and Head to Knees Tip Toe Diver's Pose

Modification: knees together, arms straight out to the sides, forehead to the knees

Pose Type: standing, forward bend

Drishti Point: Nasagrai or Nasagre (nose)

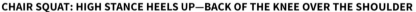

CHAIR SQUAT: HIGH STANCE HEELS UP—BACK OF THE KNEE OVER THE SHOULDER

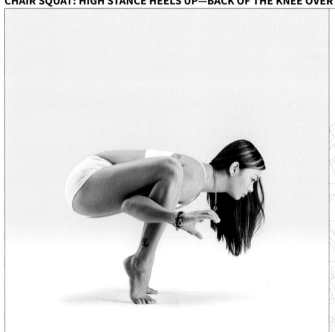

Unsupported Tip Toe Wagtail Pose 1

Niralamba Prapada Khanjanasana 1

(nir-ah-LUHM-buh PRUH-puh-duh kuhn-juh-NAHS-uh-nuh)

Modification: elbows bent, hands reaching to the front

Pose Type: standing, forward bend

Drishti Point: Nasagrai or Nasagre (nose)

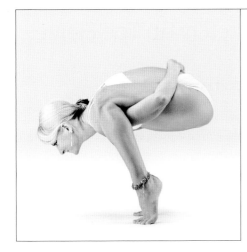

Unsupported Bound Tip Toe Wagtail Pose

Niralamba Baddha Prapada Khanjanasana
(nir-ah-LUHM-buh BUH-duh PRUH-puh-duh kuhn-juh-NAHS-uh-nuh)
Pose Type: standing, forward bend, binding
Drishti Point: Nasagrai or Nasagre (nose)

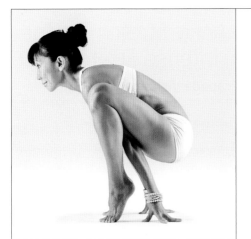

Supported Tip Toe Wagtail Pose

Salamba Prapada Khanjanasana
(sah-LUHM-buh PRUH-puh-duh kuhn-juh-NAHS-uh-nuh)
Pose Type: standing, forward bend
Drishti Point: Nasagrai or Nasagre (nose), Bhrumadhye or Ajna Chakra (third eye, between the eyebrows)

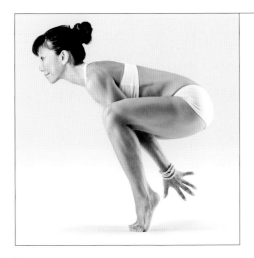

Unsupported Tip Toe Wagtail Pose 2

Niralamba Prapada Khanjanasana 2
(nirsah-LUHM-buh PRUH-puh-duh kuhn-juh-NAHS-uh-nuh)
Modification: fingertips reaching away from the head, palms pressed together, high stance
Pose Type: standing, forward bend
Drishti Point: Nasagrai or Nasagre (nose), Bhrumadhye or Ajna Chakra (third eye, between the eyebrows)

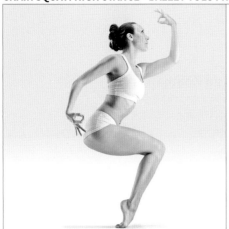

Intense Ankle Stretch Tip Toe Fierce Pose 3

Uttana Kulpa Prapada Utkatasana 3

(ut-TAH-nuh KUL-puh PRUH-puh-duh ut-kuh-TAHS-uh-nuh)

Also Known As: Intense Ankle Stretch Tip Toe Chair Pose 3

Modification: both elbows bent, one arm up in front, one arm down to the back

Pose Type: standing, balance

Drishti Point: Hastagrai or Hastagre (hands)

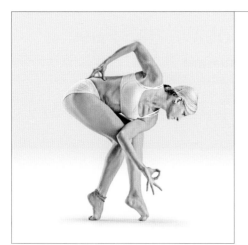

Revolved Intense Ankle Stretch Tip Toe Uneven Legs Half Intense Stretch Pose

Parivritta Uttana Kulpa Prapada Vishama Pada Ardha Uttanasana

(puh-ri-VRIT-tuh ut-TAH-nuh KUL-puh PRUH-puh-duh VISH-uh-muh PUH-duh UHR_duh ut-tahn-AHS-uh-nuh)

Also Known As: Revolved Intense Ankle Stretch Tip Toe Uneven Legs Half Forward Bend

Modification: fingertips off the floor

Pose Type: standing, balance, forward bend, twist

Drishti Point: Hastagrai or Hastagre (hands)

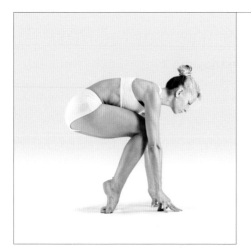

Intense Ankle Stretch Tip Toe Fierce Pose Prep.

Uttana Kulpa Prapada Utkatasana Prep.

(ut-TAH-nuh KUL-puh PRUH-puh-duh ut-kuh-TAHS-uh-nuh)

Also Known As: Intense Ankle Stretch Tip Toe Chair Pose Prep.

Modification: fingertips to the floor

Pose Type: standing, forward bend

Drishti Point: Hastagrai or Hastagre (hands)

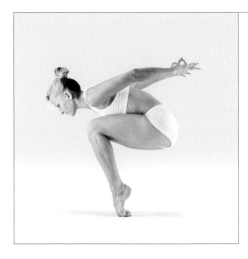

Intense Ankle Stretch Tip Toe Fierce Pose 2

Uttana Kulpa Prapada Utkatasana 2

(ut-TAH-nuh KUL-puh PRUH-puh-duh ut-kuh-TAHS-uh-nuh)

Also Known As: Intense Ankle Stretch Tip Toe Chair Pose 2 and Intense Ankle Stretch Tip Toe Diver's Pose
Modification: arms extended to the back, chest to the quadriceps
Pose Type: standing, balance, forward bend
Drishti Point: Nasagrai or Nasagre (nose)

CHAIR SQUAT: HIGH STANCE HEELS UP—ANKLES CROSSED, HANDS TO THE FLOOR

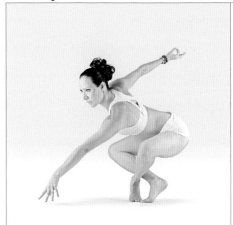

Revolved Tip Toe Pose

Parivritta Prapadasana

(puh-ri-VRIT-tuh pruh-puh-DAHS-uh-nuh)

Modification: ankles crossed, one arm to the back, other hand toward the floor in front of the feet
Pose Type: standing, forward bend, twist
Drishti Point: Hastagrai or Hastagre (hands)

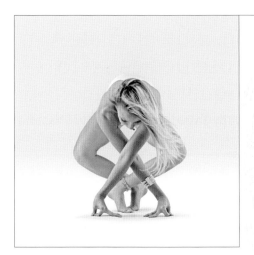

Tip Toe Pose

Prapadasana

(pruh-puh-DAHS-uh-nuh)

Modification: ankles crossed, arms crossed, fingertips to the floor in front of the feet
Pose Type: standing, forward bend
Drishti Point: Hastagrai or Hastagre (hands)

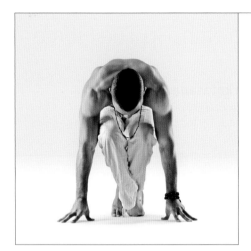

Pendant Pose Prep.

Lolasana Prep.

(lo-LAHS-uh-nuh)

Modification: ankles crossed

Pose Type: standing, forward bend

Drishti Point: Angushtamadhye or Angushta Ma Dyai (thumbs), Nasagrai or Nasagre (nose)

SQUAT: HEELS UP—LEGS CROSSED

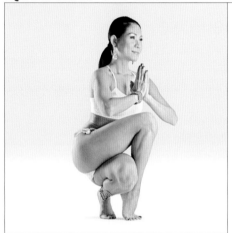

Easy Leg Position of the Pose Dedicated to Garuda in Yoga Squat with Hands in Prayer

Sukha Pada Garudasana in Upaveshasana Namaskar

(SUK-kuh PUH-duh guh-ru-DAHS-uh-nuh in u-puh-veysh-AHS-uh-nuh nuh-muhs-KAHR)

Pose Type: standing, forward bend

Drishti Point: Nasagrai or Nasagre (nose), Hastagrai or Hastagrahe (hands)

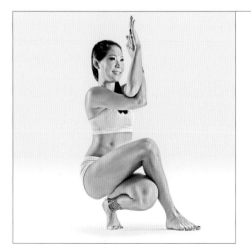

Easy Leg Position and Complete Arm Position of the Pose Dedicated to Garuda in Yoga Squat

Sukha Pada Paripurna Hasta Garudasana in Upaveshasana

(SUK-kuh PUH-duh puh-ri-POOR-nuh HUH-stuh guh-ru-DAHS-uh-nuh in u-puh-veysh-AHS-uh-nuh)

Pose Type: standing, forward bend

Drishti Point: Angushtamadhye or Angushta Ma Dyai (thumbs)

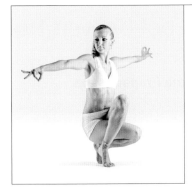

Revolved Easy Leg Position of the Pose Dedicated to Garuda in Yoga Squat

Parivritta Sukha Pada Garudasana in Upaveshasana

(puh-ri-VRIT-tuh SUK-kuh PUH-duh guh-ru-DAHS-uh-nuh in u-puh-veysh-AHS-uh-nuh)

Modification: both knees off the floor, arms open wide and straight
Pose Type: standing, forward bend, twist
Drishti Point: Hastagrai or Hastagrahe (hands)

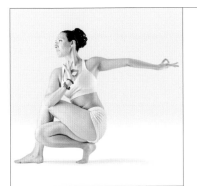

Revolved Easy Leg Position of the Pose Dedicated to Garuda in Yoga Squat

Parivritta Sukha Pada Garudasana in Upaveshasana

(puh-ri-VRIT-tuh SUK-kuh PUH-duh guh-ru-DAHS-uh-nuh in u-puh-veysh-AHS-uh-nuh)

Modification: bottom knee on the floor, arms open wide and straight
Pose Type: standing, forward bend, twist
Drishti Point: Hastagrai or Hastagrahe (hands)

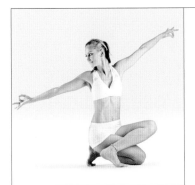

Revolved Easy Leg Position of the Pose Dedicated to Garuda in Yoga Squat

Parivritta Sukha Pada Garudasana in Upaveshasana

(puh-ri-VRIT-tuh SUK-kuh PUH-duh guh-ru-DAHS-uh-nuh in u-puh-veysh-AHS-uh-nuh)

Modification: elbow over the opposite knee, other arm straight out to the side
Pose Type: standing, forward bend, twist
Drishti Point: Parshva Drishti (to the right), Parshva Drishti (to the left)

SQUAT: HEELS UP—KNEES APART

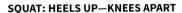

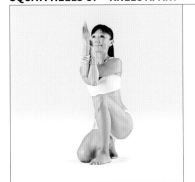

Hand Position of the Pose Dedicated to Garuda in Half Tip Toe Hero Pose

Hasta Garudasana in Ardha Prapada Virasana

(HUH-stuh guh-ru-DAHS-uh-nuh in UHR-duh PRUH-puh-duh veer-AHS-uh-nuh)

Modification: one knee on the floor, one foot to the floor on the inside of the knee
Pose Type: standing, forward bend
Drishti Point: Angushtamadhye or Angushta Ma Dyai (thumbs)

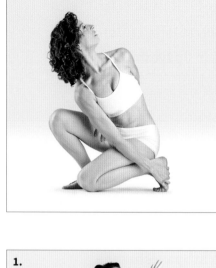

Half Bound Hand to Foot Uneven Tip Toe Pose

Ardha Baddha Hasta Pada Vishama Prapadasana

(UHR-duh BUH-duh HUH-stuh PUH-duh VISH-uh-muh pruh-puh-DAHS-uh-nuh)

Modification: one hand crossed in front, grabbing onto the heel; other hand to the inner thigh on the opposite side

Pose Type: standing, forward bend, twist, binding

Drishti Point: Urdhva or Antara Drishti (up to the sky)

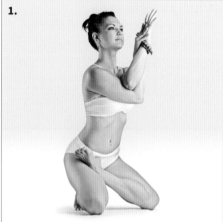

Hand Position of the Pose Dedicated to Garuda in Half Lotus Tip Toe Pose

Hasta Garudasana in Ardha Padma Prapadasana

(HUH-stuh guh-ru-DAHS-uh-nuh in UHR-duh PUHD-muh pruh-puh-DAHS-uh-nuh)

Modification: 1. Both knees on the floor

2. One knee on the floor

Pose Type: standing

Drishti Point: 1. Angusthamadhye or Angustha Ma Dyai (thumbs)

2. Nasagrai or Nasagre (nose)

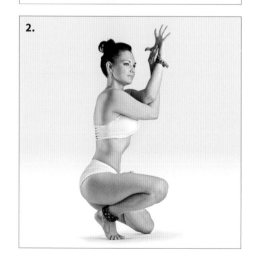

1.

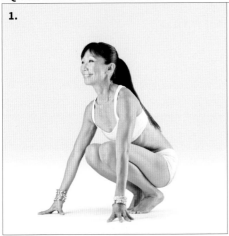

Tip Toe Pose

Prapadasana

(pruh-puh-DAHS-uh-nuh)

Also Known As: Noose Pose Prep. (Pasasana Prep.)

Modification: 1. fingertips to the floor on the outside of the knees

2. one hand to the heart, other hand to the floor

3. hands on the hips

Pose Type: standing, forward bend

Drishti Point: Nasagrai or Nasagre (nose)

2.

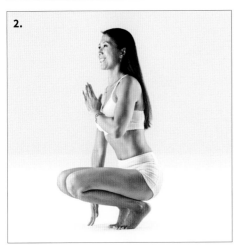

3.

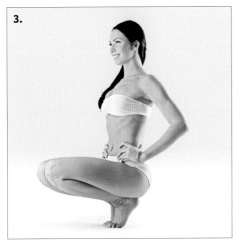

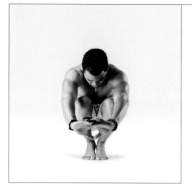

Hands Bound Tip Toe Pose

Baddha Hasta Prapadasana

(BUH-duh HUH-stuh pruh-puh-DAHS-uh-nuh)

Modification: arms straight out in front, palms facing out, chest to the quadriceps
Pose Type: standing, forward bend
Drishti Point: Angushtamadhye or Angushta Ma Dyai (thumbs)

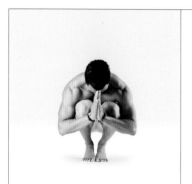

Tip Toe Pose with Hands in Prayer

Prapadasana Namaskar

(pruh-puh-DAHS-uh-nuh nuh-muhs-KAHR)

Modification: knees together, chest to the quadriceps
Pose Type: standing, forward bend
Drishti Point: Nasagrai or Nasagre (nose)

SQUAT: HEELS UP—KNEES TOGETHER—ARMS HEAD LEVEL OR ABOVE HEAD

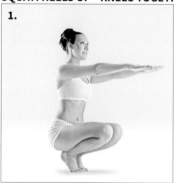

Tip Toe Pose

Prapadasana

(pruh-puh-DAHS-uh-nuh)

Also Known As: Garland Pose Prep. (Malasana Prep.), Full Squat Pose (Purna Utkatasana)
Modification: 1. arms straight out in front and parallel to the floor
2. arms up over the head, palms pressed together, elbows bent
Pose Type: standing
Drishti Point: Hastagrai or Hastagre (hands)
Drishti Point: 1. Hastagrai or Hastagrahe (hands)
2. Nasagrai or Nasagre (nose)

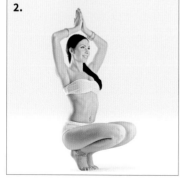

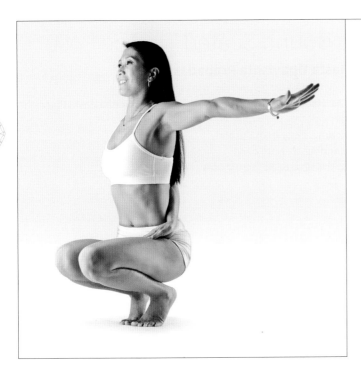

Half Bound Tip Toe Pose

Ardha Baddha Prapadasana

(UHR-duh BUH-duh pruh-puh-DAHS-uh-nuh)

Modification: one hand binding to the opposite hip behind the back, other arm straight and extended out to the side

Pose Type: standing, binding

Drishti Point: Nasagrai or Nasagre (nose)

SQUAT: HEELS UP—KNEES TOGETHER—KNEES SHOULDER LEVEL

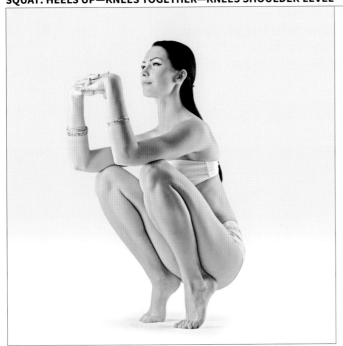

Seated Tip Toe Pose

Upavishta Prapadasana

(u-puh-VISH-tuh pruh-puh-DAHS-uh-nuh)

Also Known As: Crouching Tip Toe Pose; Upavistha Prapadasana

Modification: elbows resting on the knees, fingers interlocked in front of the face

Pose Type: standing, forward bend

Drishti Point: Angushtamadhye or Angushta Ma Dyai (thumbs)

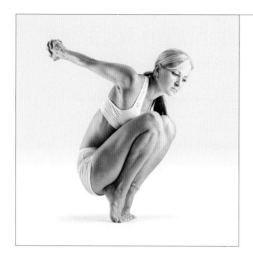

Hands Bound Seated Tip Toe Pose

Baddha Hasta Upavishta Prapadasana

(BUH-duh HUH-stuh u-puh-VISH-tuh pruh-puh-DAHS-uh-nuh)

Also Known As: Hands Bound Crouching Tip Toe Pose; Baddha Hasta Upavistha Prapadasana

Modification: arms away from the body

Pose Type: standing, forward bend

Drishti Point: Nasagrai or Nasagre (nose)

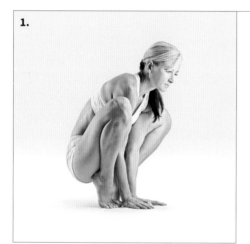

Knees to the Shoulders Seated Tip Toe Pose

Janu Bhuja Upavishta Prapadasana

(JAH-nu BHU-juh u-puh-VISH-tuh pruh-puh-DAHS-uh-nuh)

Also Known As: Knees to the Shoulders Crouching Tip Toe Pose; Janu Bhuja Upavistha Prapadasana

Modification: 1. palms together to the floor
2. palms apart and to the floor, elbows bent

Pose Type: standing, forward bend

Drishti Point: Nasagrai or Nasagre (nose)

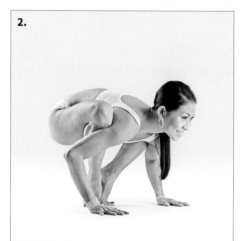

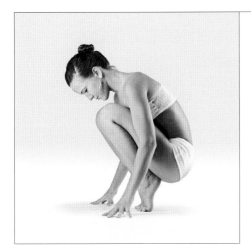

Supported Seated Tip Toe Pose

Salamba Upavishta Prapadasana

(sah-LUHM-buh u-puh-VISH-tuh pruh-puh-DAHS-uh-nuh)

Also Known As: Supported Crouching Tip Toe Pose; Salamba Upavistha Prapadasana

Modification: fingertips to the floor in front of the feet

Pose Type: standing, forward bend

Drishti Point: Nasagrai or Nasagre (nose)

1.

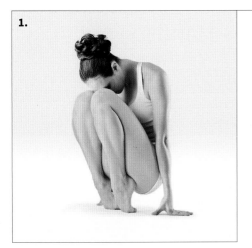

Supported/Unsupported Intense Ankle Stretch Seated Tip Toe Pose

Salamba/Niralamba Uttana Kulpa Upavishta Prapadasana

(sah-LUHM-buh-/nir-ah-LUHM-buh ut-TAHN-uh KUL-puh u-puh-VISH-tuh pruh-puh-DAHS-uh-nuh)

Also Known As: Supported/Unsupported Intense Ankle Stretch Crouching Tip Toe Pose; Salamba/Niralamba Uttana Kulpa Upavistha Prapadasana

Modification: 1. hands to the floor by the hips

2. arms wrapped around the shins, grabbing onto the triceps

Pose Type: 1. standing, forward bend

2. standing, balance, forward bend

Drishti Point: Nasagrai or Nasagre (nose)

2.

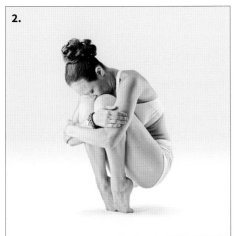

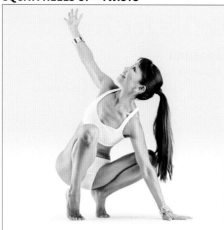

Tip Toe Easy Noose Pose Prep.

Prapada Sukha Pashasana Prep.

(PRUH-puh-duh SUK-kuh puh-SHAHS-uh-nuh)

Modification: elbow on the inside of the thigh, arms open wide
Pose Type: standing, twist
Drishti Point: Hastagrai or Hastagre (hands)

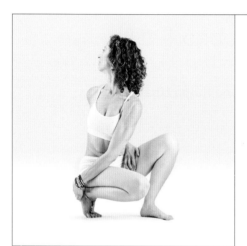

Uneven Legs One Hand to Foot Noose Pose

Vishama Pada Eka Hasta Pada Pashasana

(VISH-uh-muh PUH-duh EY-kuh HUH-stuh PUH-duh puh-SHAS-uh-nuh)

Modification: one heel up, one heel down
Pose Type: standing, twist, binding
Drishti Point: Parshva Drishti (to the right), Parshva Drishti (to the left)

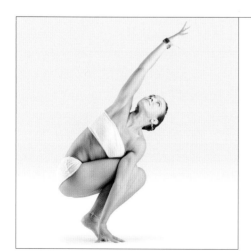

Extended Side Tip Toe Noose Pose

Utthita Parshva Prapada Pashasana

(UT-ti-tuh PAHRSH-vuh PRUH-puh-duh puh-SHAHS-uh-nuh)

Modification: one hand to the floor, other arm extended up over the head
Pose Type: standing, forward bend, twist
Drishti Point: Hastagrai or Hastagre (hands)

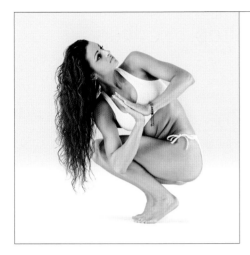

Tip Toe Noose Pose with Hands in Prayer

Prapada Pashasana Namaskar

(PRUH-puh-duh puh-SHAHS-uh-nuh nuh-muhs-KAHR)

Pose Type: standing, twist

Drishti Point: Urdhva or Antara Drishti (up to the sky)

1.

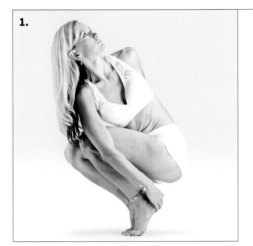

One Hand to the Foot Tip Toe Noose Pose

Eka Hasta Pada Prapada Pashasana

(EY-kuh HUH-stuh PUH-duh PRUH-puh-duh puh-SHAHS-uh-nuh)

Modification: one hand to the opposite heel, other hand binding to the opposite hip behind the back

1. right side view
2. left side view

Pose Type: standing, twist, binding

Drishti Point: Urdhva or Antara Drishti (up to the sky)

2.

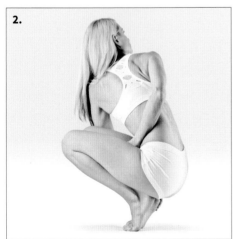

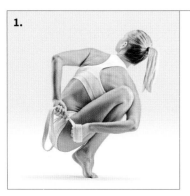

Tip Toe Noose Pose Prep.

Prapada Pashasana Prep.

(PRUH-puh-duh puh-SHAHS-uh-nuh)

Modification: 1. binding around one leg with a strap

2. binding around one leg without a strap

Pose Type: standing, twist, binding

Drishti Point: Urdhva or Antara Drishti (up to the sky)

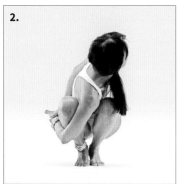

Tip Toe Noose Pose

Prapada Pashasana

(PRUH-puh-duh puh-SHAHS-uh-nuh)

Modification: binding around both legs

Pose Type: standing, forward bend, twist, binding

Drishti Point: Nasagrai or Nasagre (nose)

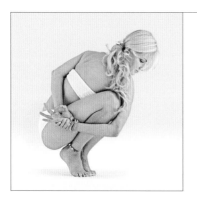

SQUAT: HEELS DOWN—ARMS BELOW HEAD

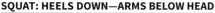

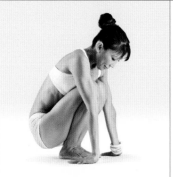

Intense Wrist Stretch Garland Pose Prep.

Uttana Manibandha Malasana Prep.

(ut-TAH-nuh muh-ni-BUHN-duh mah-LAHS-uh-nuh)

Modification: heels down, knees together, palms to the floor, fingers facing the toes, chest to the quadriceps

Pose Type: standing, forward bend

Drishti Point: Nasagrai or Nasagre (nose)

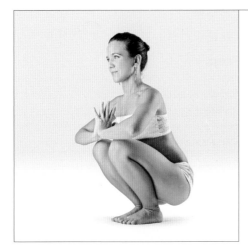

Garland Pose with Hands in Prayer Prep.

Malasana Namaskar Prep.

(mah-LAHS-uh-nuh nuh-muhs-KAHR)

Modification: heels down

Pose Type: standing, forward bend

Drishti Point: Bhrumadhye or Ajna Chakra (third eye, between the eyebrows), Nasagrai or Nasagre (nose)

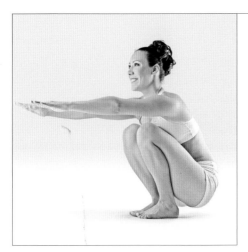

Garland Pose Prep.

Malasana Prep.

(mah-LAHS-uh-nuh)

Also Known As: Full Squat Pose (Purna Utkatasana)

Modification: knees together, heels down; arms straight out to the front, palms down

Pose Type: standing, forward bend

Drishti Point: Hastagrai or Hastagre (hands)

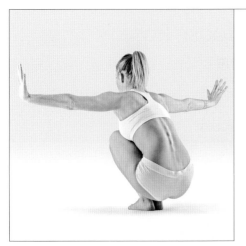

Arms Spread Out Garland Pose Prep.

Prasarita Hasta Malasana Prep.

(pruh-SAH-ri-tuh HUH-stuh mah-LAHS-uh-nuh)

Also Known As: Full Squat Pose (Purna Utkatasana), Flying Bird Pose (Khagasana)

Modification: knees together, heels down, arms straight out to the side

Pose Type: standing, forward bend

Drishti Point: Nasagrai or Nasagre (nose)

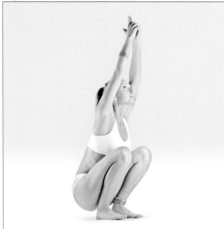

Upward Hands Garland Pose Prep.

Urdhva Hasta Malasana Prep.

(OORD-vuh HUH-stuh mah-LAHS-uh-nuh)

Also Known As: Full Squat Pose (Purna Utkatasana)
Modification: knees together, hands to the sky
Pose Type: standing, forward bend
Drishti Point: Angushtamadhye or Angushta Ma Dyai (thumbs)

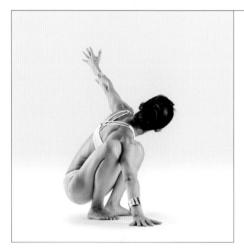

Easy Noose Pose

Sukha Pashasana

(SUK-kuh puh-SHAHS-uh-nuh)

Also Known As: Revolved Yoga Squat (Parivritta Upaveshasana)
Modification: heels down, shoulder between the knees, one palm flat on the floor, other arm straight out to the back
Pose Type: standing, forward bend, twist
Drishti Point: Hastagrai or Hastagre (hands)

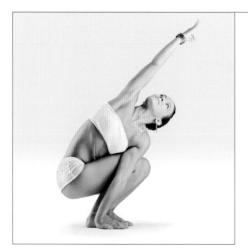

Extended Side Noose Pose

Utthita Parshva Pashasana

(UT-ti-tuh PAHRSH-vuh puh-SHAHS-uh-nuh)

Modification: heels down, one hand to the floor, other arm extended up over the head
Pose Type: standing, forward bend, twist
Drishti Point: Hastagrai or Hastagre (hands)

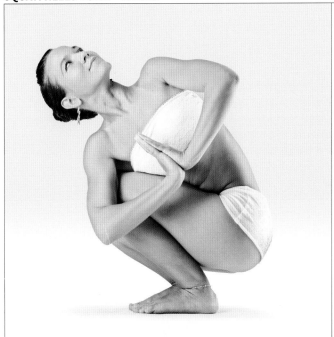

Noose Pose with Hands in Prayer

Pashasana Namaskar

(puh-SHAHS-uh-nuh nuh-muhs-KAHR)

Modification: heels down

Pose Type: standing, forward bend, twist

Drishti Point: Urdhva or Antara Drishti (up to the sky)

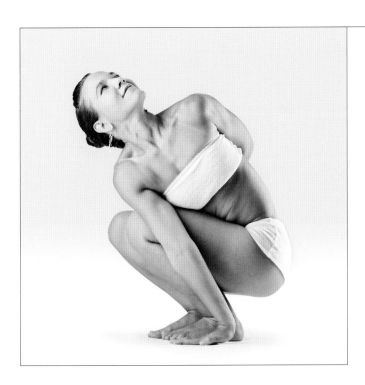

Half Bound Noose Pose

Ardha Baddha Pashasana

(UHR-duh BUH-duh puh-SHAHS-uh-nuh)

Modification: heels down

Pose Type: standing, forward bend, twist, binding

Drishti Point: Urdhva or Antara Drishti (up to the sky)

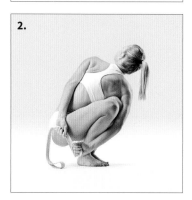

Noose Pose

Pashasana

(puh-SHAHS-uh-nuh)

Modification: heels down, binding with a strap

1. binding around one leg
2. binding around both legs

Pose Type: standing, forward bend, twist, binding

Drishti Point: Urdhva or Antara Drishti (up to the sky)

2.

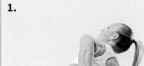

1.

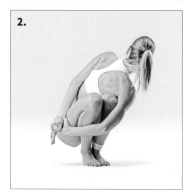

Noose Pose

Pashasana

(puh-SHAHS-uh-nuh)

Modification: heels down, binding around both legs

1. side view
2. front view

Pose Type: standing, forward bend, twist, binding

Drishti Point: Urdhva or Antara Drishti (up to the sky)

2.

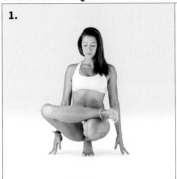

One-Legged Tip Toe Pose

Eka Pada Prapadasana

(EY-kuh PUH-duh pruh-puh-DAHS-uh-nuh)

Also Known As: Half Bound Lotus Tip Toe Pose Prep. (Ardha Baddha Padma Padangush-tasana Prep.)

Modification: 1. both hands to the floor on the sides

2. hands in Anjali Mudra (Hands in Prayer)

Pose Type: standing one-legged balance

Drishti Point: Nasagrai or Nasagre (nose)

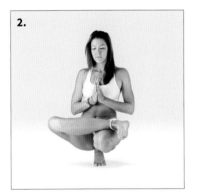

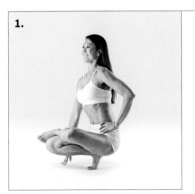

One-Legged Tip Toe Pose

Eka Pada Prapadasana

(EY-kuh PUH-duh pruh-puh-DAHS-uh-nuh)

Also Known As: Half Bound Lotus Tip Toe Pose Prep. (Ardha Baddha Padma Padangush-tasana Prep.)

Modification: 1. one hand on the hip, other hand to the floor

2. one hand on the hip, one arm up over the head

Pose Type: standing one-legged balance

Drishti Point: Nasagrai or Nasagre (nose)

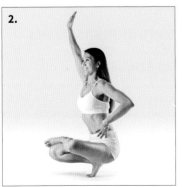

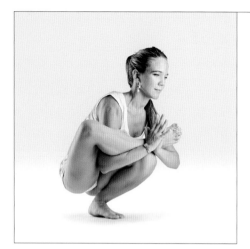

Baby Cradle Pose with Hands in Prayer in One-Legged Garland Pose

Hindolasana Namaskar in Eka Pada Malasana

(hin-do-LAHS-uh-nuh EY-kuh PUH-duh mah-LAHS-uh-nuh)

Also Known As: Baby Cradle Pose with Hands in Prayer in One-Legged Yoga Squat (Hindolasana Namaskar in Eka Pada Upavesashana)

Pose Type: standing one-legged balance, forward bend

Drishti Point: Nasagrai or Nasagre (nose)

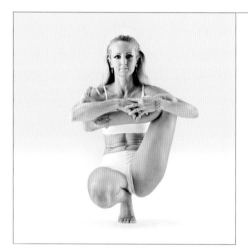

Baby Cradle Pose in One-Legged Tip Toe Pose 1

Hindolasana in Eka Pada Prapadasana 1

(hin-do-LAHS-uh-nuh in EY-kuh PUH-duh pruh-puh-DAHS-uh-nuh)

Pose Type: standing one-legged balance, forward bend

Drishti Point: Nasagrai or Nasagre (nose)

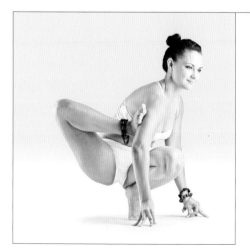

Half Yogic Staff Pose Prep. in One-Legged Tip Toe Pose

Ardha Yogadandasana Prep. in Eka Pada Prapadasana

(UHR-duh yo-guh-duhn-DAHS-uh-nuh in EY-kuh PUH-duh pruh-puh-DAHS-uh-nuh)

Pose Type: standing one-legged balance, forward bend

Drishti Point: Nasagrai or Nasagre (nose)

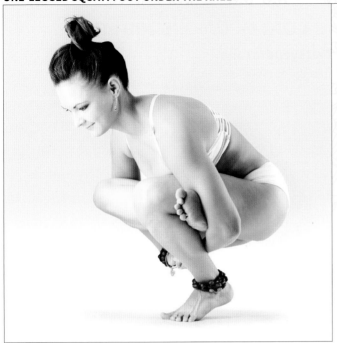

Baby Cradle Pose in One-Legged Tip Toe Pose 2

Hindolasana in Eka Pada Prapadasana 2

(hin-do-LAHS-uh-nuh in EY-kuh PUH-duh pruh-puh-DAHS-uh-nuh)

Pose Type: standing one-legged balance, forward bend

Drishti Point: Nasagrai or Nasagre (nose)

Supported Revolved One-Legged Tip Toe Pose

Salamba Parivritta Eka Pada Prapadasana

(sah-LUHM-buh puh-ri-VRIT-tuh EY-kuh PUH-duh pruh-puh-DAHS-uh-nuh)

Modification: foot under the knee

Pose Type: standing one-legged balance, forward bend, twist

Drishti Point: Padayoragrai or Padayoragre (toes/feet)

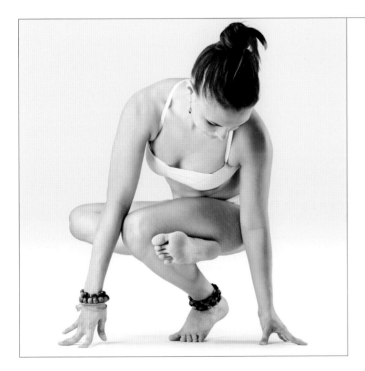

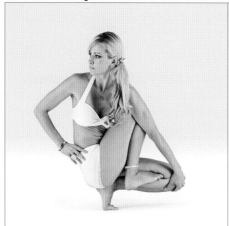

Tip Toe Lord of the Fishes Pose

Prapada Matsyendrasana

(PRUH-puh-duh muhts-y-eyn-DRAHS-uh-nuh)

Pose Type: standing one-legged balance, twist

Drishti Point: Parshva Drishti (to the right), Parshva Drishti (to the left)

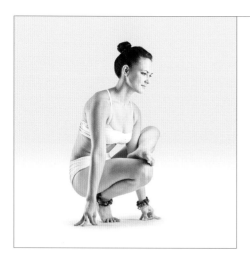

Supported One-Legged Tip Toe Pose

Salamba Eka Pada Prapadasana

(sah-LUHM-buh EY-kuh PUH-duh pruh-puh-DAHS-uh-nuh)

Modification: leg wrapped around the tricep, fingertips to the floor

Pose Type: standing one-legged balance

Drishti Point: Nasagrai or Nasagre (nose)

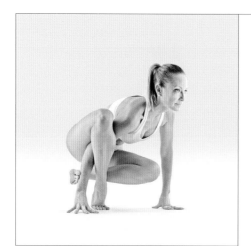

Supported One-Legged Tip Toe Pose

Salamba Eka Pada Prapadasana

(sah-LUHM-buh EY-kuh PUH-duh pruh-puh-DAHS-uh-nuh)

Modification: hands to the floor, shoulder to the back of the knee, other foot wrapped around the forearm

Pose Type: standing one-legged balance, forward bend

Drishti Point: Nasagrai or Nasagre (nose)

1.

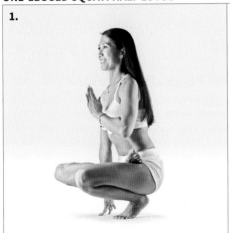

Half Bound Lotus Tip Toe Pose
Ardha Baddha Padma Prapadasana
(UHR-duh BUH-duh PUHD-muh pruh-puh-DAHS-uh-nuh)

Also Known As: Half Bound Lotus Tip Toe Pose (Ardha Baddha Padma Padan-gushtasana)

Modification: 1. fingertips to the floor, other hand to the heart

2. binding, other hand to the heart

3. binding, other arm out to the side, parallel to the floor

Pose Type: 1. standing one-legged balance

2 & 3. standing one-legged balance, binding

Drishti Point: Nasagrai or Nasagre (nose)

2.

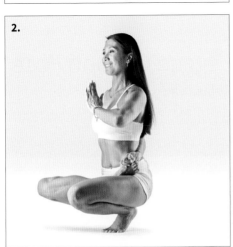

3.

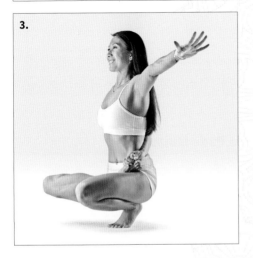

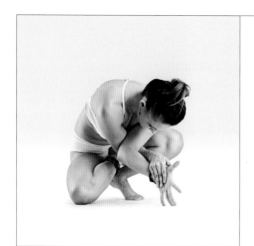

Hand Position of the Pose Dedicated to Garuda in Half Lotus Tip Toe Pose

Hasta Garudasana in Ardha Padma Prapadasana

(HUH-stuh guh-ru-DAHS-uh-nuh in UHR-duh-PUHD-muh pruh-puh-DAHS-uh-nuh)

Modification: knee on the floor, forward bend

Pose Type: standing one-legged balance, forward bend

Drishti Point: Angushtamadhye or Angushta Ma Dyai (thumbs)

ONE-LEGGED SQUAT: HALF LOTUS—HEEL DOWN

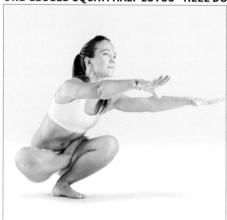

Half Lotus One-Legged Garland Pose

Ardha Padma Eka Pada Malasana

(UHR-duh PUHD-muh EY-kuh PUH-duh mah-LAHS-uh-nuh)

Also Known As: Half Lotus One-Legged Yoga Squat (Ardha Padma Eka Pada Upaveshasana)

Modification: arms parallel to the floor

Pose Type: standing one-legged balance

Drishti Point: Angushtamadhye or Angushta Ma Dyai (thumbs)

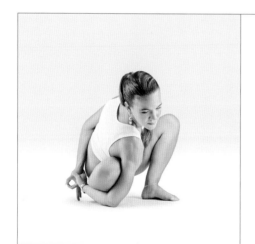

Half Lotus Bound One-Legged Garland Pose

Ardha Padma Baddha Eka Pada Malasana

(UHR-duh PUHD-muh BUH-duh EY-kuh PUH-duh mah-LAHS-uh-nuh)

Also Known As: Half Lotus Bound One-Legged Yoga Squat (Ardha Padma Baddha Eka Pada Upavesasana)

Pose Type: standing one-legged balance, forward bend, binding

Drishti Point: Nasagrai or Nasagre (nose)

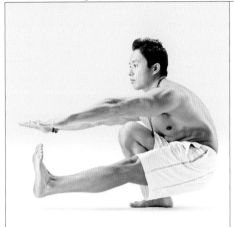

Hand to Foot Pose Squatting Prep.

Hasta Padasana Prep.

(HUH-stuh puh-DAHS-uh-nuh)

Modification: leg straight and lifted off the floor, arms parallel to the floor
Pose Type: standing one-legged balance
Drishti Point: Angushtamadhye or Angushta Ma Dyai (thumbs)

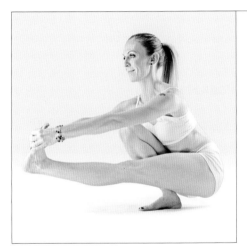

Hands to Foot Squatting Pose 1

Hasta Padasana 1

(HUH-stuh puh-DAHS-uh-nuh)

Also Known As: Pose Dedicated to Sage Marichi Modification (Marichyasana Modification)
Modification: both hands to the foot, heel down
Pose Type: standing one-legged balance
Drishti Point: Padayoragrai or Padayoragre (toes/feet)**Drishti Point:** Nasagrai or Nasagre (nose) or Padhayoragrai or Padayoragre (toes/feet)

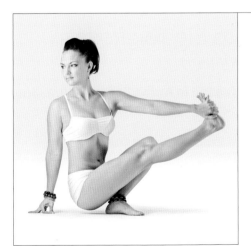

Revolved Supported Hand to Foot Pose Squatting

Parivritta Salamba Hasta Padasana

(puh-ri-VRIT-tuh SAH-luhm-buh HUH-stuh puh-DAHS-uh-nuh)

Modification: one hand to the floor
Pose Type: standing one-legged balance, twist
Drishti Point: Parshva Drishti (to the right), Parshva Drishti (to the left)

Standing Poses

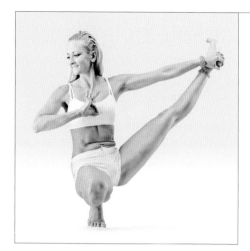

Hand to Foot to the Side Tip Toe Pose

Hasta Pada Parshva Prapadasana

(HUH-stuh PUH-duh PAHRSH-vuh pruh-puh-DAHS-uh-nuh)

Pose Type: standing one-legged balance

Drishti Point: Parshva Drishti (to the right), Parshva Drishti (to the left)

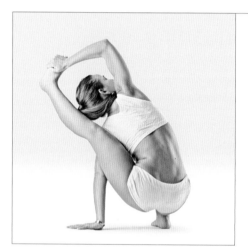

Sundial Pose in One-Legged Garland Pose

Surya Yantrasana in Eka Pada Malasana

(SOOR-yuh yuhn-TRAHS-uh-nuh in EY-kuh PUH-duh mah-LAHS-uh-nuh)

Also Known As: Sundial Pose in One-Legged Yoga Squat (Surya Yantrasana in Eka Pada Upavesasana)

Pose Type: standing one-legged balance, forward bend, twist

Drishti Point: Urdhva or Antara Drishti (up to the sky)

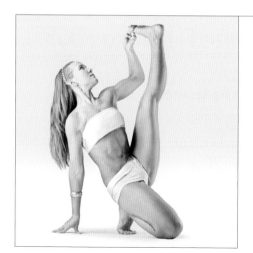

Extended Hand to Big Toe Pose in Half Tip Toe Hero Pose

Utthita Hasta Padangushtasana in Ardha Prapada Virasana

(UT-ti-tuh HUH-stuh puhd-ahng-goosh-TAHS-uh-nuh in UHR-duh PRUH-puh-duh veer-AHS-uh-nuh)

Pose Type: standing one-legged balance, forward bend

Drishti Point: Padayoragrai or Padayoragre (toes/feet)

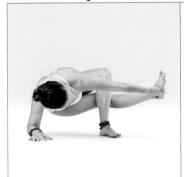

Baby Grasshopper Pose

Bala Shalabhasana

(BUH-luh shuh-luh-BAHS-uh-nuh)

Also Known As: Baby Locust Pose

Modification: chest facing the floor, forearm on the floor

Pose Type: standing one-legged balance, forward bend, twist

Drishti Point: Padayoragrai or Padayoragre (toes/feet)

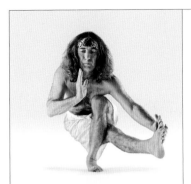

Hand to Foot Pose 2

Hasta Padasana 2

(HUH-stuh puh-DAHS-uh-nuh)

Modification: leg crossed over, one hand to the foot, other hand to the heart

Pose Type: standing one-legged balance, forward bend

Drishti Point: Padayoragrai or Padayoragre (toes/feet), Angushtamadhye or Angushta Ma Dyai (thumbs)

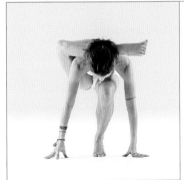

Supported One Foot Behind the Head Tip Toe Pose Prep. 1

Salamba Eka Pada Shirsha Prapadasana Prep. 1

(SAH-luhm-buh EY-kuh PUH-duh SHEER-shuh pruh-puh-DAHS-uh-nuh)

Modification: heel up, sitting bones lifted

Pose Type: standing one-legged balance, forward bend

Drishti Point: Angushtamadhye or Angushta Ma Dyai (thumbs)

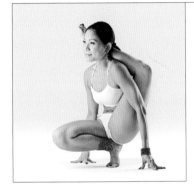

Supported One Foot Behind the Head Tip Toe Pose Prep. 2

Salamba Eka Pada Shirsha Prapadasana Prep. 2

(SAH-luhm-buh EY-kuh PUH-duh SHEER-shuh pruh-puh-DAHS-uh-nuh)

Modification: hands to the floor

Pose Type: standing one-legged balance

Drishti Point: Nasagrai or Nasagre (nose)

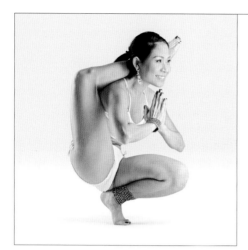

One Foot Behind the Head Tip Toe Pose

Eka Pada Shirsha Prapadasana

(EY-kuh PUH-duh SHEER-shuh pruh-puh-DAHS-uh-nuh)

Also Known As: Tip Toe Balance Foot Behind The Head Pose (Padangushta Eka Pada Shirshasana), One Foot Behind the Head Tip Toe Pose (Eka Pada Shirsha Padangushtasana)

Pose Type: standing one-legged balance

Drishti Point: Nasagrai or Nasagre (nose)

SQUAT: HEELS DOWN—KNEES WIDE

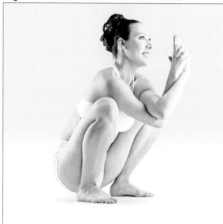

Hand Position of the Pose Dedicated to Garuda in Garland Pose

Hasta Garudasana in Malasana

(HUH-stuh guh-ru-DAHS-uh-nuh in mah-LAHS-uh-nuh)

Also Known As: Hand Position of the Pose Dedicated to Garuda in Yoga Squat (Hasta Garudasana in Upaveshasana)

Pose Type: standing, forward bend

Drishti Point: Angushtamadhye or Angushta Ma Dyai (thumbs)

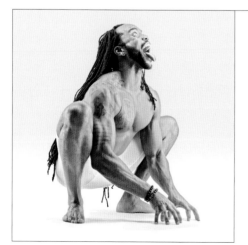

Lion Pose Dedicated to an Avatar of Lord Vishnu in Garland Pose

Narasimhasana in Malasana

(nuh-ruh-sim-HAHS-uh-nuh in mah-LAHS-uh-nuh)

Also Known As: Lion Pose in Yoga Squat (Simhasana in Upaveshasana)

Modification: heels down

Pose Type: standing, forward bend

Drishti Point: Bhrumadhye or Ajna Chakra (third eye, between the eyebrows)

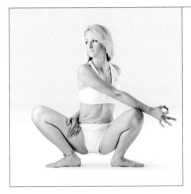

Half Bound Revolved Garland Pose

Ardha Baddha Parivritta Malasana

(UHR-duh BUH-duh puh-ri-VRIT-tuh mah-LAHS-uh-nuh)

Also Known As: Half Bound Revolved Yoga Squat (Ardha Baddha Parivritta Upaveshasana)

Modification: forearm on the knee

Pose Type: standing, twist, binding

Drishti Point: Parshva Drishti (to the right), Parshva Drishti (to the left)

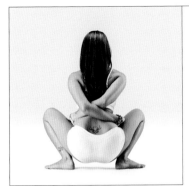

Bound Garland Pose

Baddha Malasana

(BUH-duh mah-LAHS-uh-nuh)

Also Known As: Bound Yoga Squat (Baddha Upaveshasana)

Pose Type: standing, binding

Drishti Point: Nasagrai or Nasagre (nose)

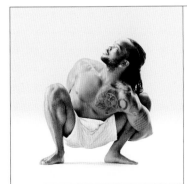

One Leg Bound Garland Pose

Eka Pada Baddha Malasana

(EY-kuh PUH-duh BUH-duh mah-LAHS-uh-nuh)

Also Known As: One Leg Bound Yoga Squat (Eka Pada Baddha Upaveshasana)

Modification: heels down, binding around one of the legs, knees open wide

Pose Type: standing, binding, forward bend

Drishti Point: Urdhva or Antara Drishti (up to the sky)

SQUAT: ONE HEEL UP, ONE HEEL DOWN—KNEES WIDE

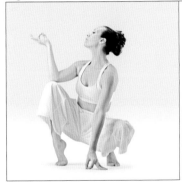

Uneven Legs Garland Pose

Vishama Pada Malasana

(VISH-uh-muh PUH-duh mah-LAHS-uh-nuh)

Also Known As: Uneven Legs Yoga Squat (Vishama Pada Upaveshasana)

Modification: one knee higher than the other; fingertips of one hand to the floor, other elbow on the knee

Pose Type: standing, forward bend

Drishti Point: Hastagrai or Hastagre (hands)

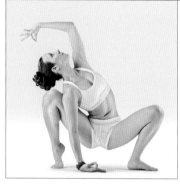

Sideways Uneven Legs Garland Pose

Parshva Vishama Pada Malasana

(PAHRSH-vuh VISH-uh-muh PUH-duh mah-LAHS-uh-nuh)

Also Known As: Sideways Uneven Legs Yoga Squat (Parshva Vishama Pada Upaveshasana)
Modification: one heel up, one heel down, one arm up over the head into a side bend, back of the other hand on the floor
Pose Type: standing, forward bend, side bend
Drishti Point: Hastagrai or Hastagre (hands)

SQUAT: HEELS DOWN—KNEES WIDE, FORWARD BENDS

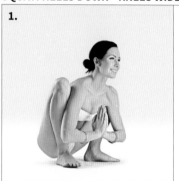

1.

Garland Pose

Malasana

(mah-LAHS-uh-nuh)

Also Known As: Yoga Squat (Upaveshasana)
Modification: 1. hands in Anjali Mudra (Hands in Prayer)
2. arms straight out in front; palms down, head up
3. arms straight out in front; palms down, head down
Pose Type: standing, forward bend
Drishti Point: Nasagrai or Nasagre (nose)

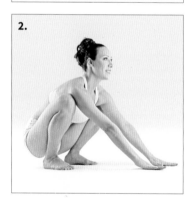

2.

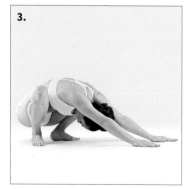

3.

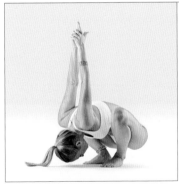

Hands Bound Garland Pose

Baddha Hasta Malasana

(BUH-duh HUH-stuh mah-LAHS-uh-nuh)

Also Known As: Hands Bound Yoga Squat (Baddha Hasta Upaveshasana)
Pose Type: standing, forward bend
Drishti Point: Nasagrai or Nasagre (nose)

SQUAT: HEELS DOWN—KNEES WIDE, FORWARD BENDS—BINDING

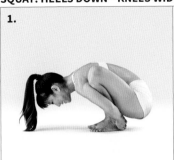

1.

Garland Pose

Malasana

(mah-LAHS-uh-nuh)

Also Known As: Tortoise Pose Squat (Kurmasana Modification)
Modification: grabbing onto heels
1. head off the floor
2. forehead to the floor
Pose Type: standing, forward bend
Drishti Point: Nasagrai or Nasagre (nose)

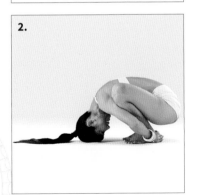

2.

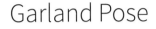

Garland Pose

Malasana

(mah-LAHS-uh-nuh)

Also Known As: Golden Belt Pose (Kanchyasana)
Modification: hands bound, heels down
Pose Type: standing, forward bend, binding
Drishti Point: Nasagrai or Nasagre (nose)

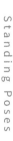

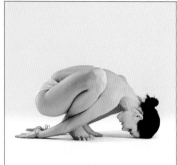

Garland Pose

Malasana

(mah-LAHS-uh-nuh)

Modification: heels up, arms stretched out to the back, palms facing up, forehead to the floor

Pose Type: standing, forward bend

Drishti Point: Nasagrai or Nasagre (nose)

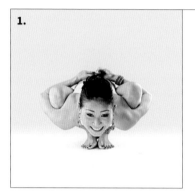

1.

Garland Pose

Malasana

(mah-LAHS-uh-nuh)

Also Known As: Golden Belt Pose (Kanchyasana)

Modification: heels up, hands bound

1. front view
2. side view

Pose Type: standing, forward bend, binding

Drishti Point: Nasagrai or Nasagre (nose)

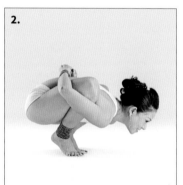

2.

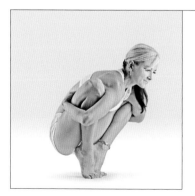

Garland Pose

Malasana

(mah-LAHS-uh-nuh)

Modification: heels up, arms binding around the shins, hands between thighs and rib cage

Pose Type: standing, forward bend, binding

Drishti Point: Nasagrai or Nasagre (nose)

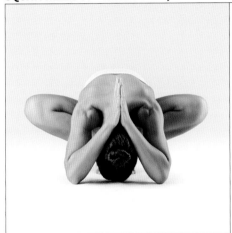

Garland Pose

Malasana

(mah-LAHS-uh-nuh)

Modification: forehead to the floor, thumbs to the upper back
Pose Type: standing, forward bend
Drishti Point: Nasagrai or Nasagre (nose)

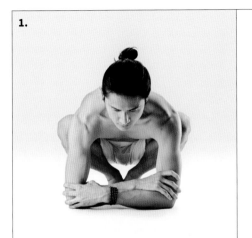

1.

Garland Pose

Malasana

(mah-LAHS-uh-nuh)

Modification: forearms to the floor
1. grabbing onto the triceps
2. forearms on the floor, palms pressed together
Pose Type: standing, forward bend
Drishti Point: 1. Nasagrai or Nasagre (nose)
2. Angusthamadhye or Angustha Ma Dyai (thumbs)

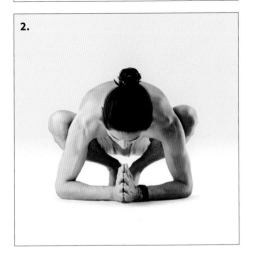

2.

4.

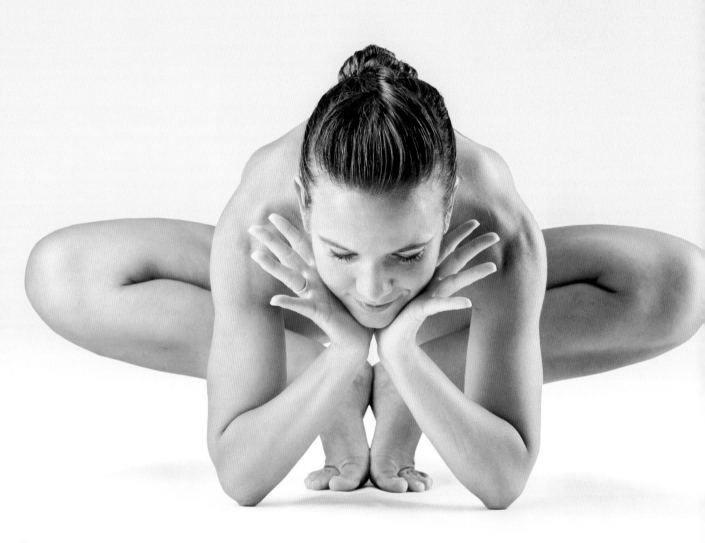

Garland Pose

Malasana

(mah-LAHS-uh-nuh)
Pose Type: standing, forward bend
Drishti Point: 1 & 2. Angusthamadhye or Angustha Ma Dyai (thumbs) 3 & 4. Nasagrai or Nasagre (nose)

How to Perform the Pose:

1. Begin by standing in Mountain Pose (*Tadasana*). Engage your *mula bandha*, *uddhiyana bandha*, and *ujjayi* breathing.

2. Exhale as you bend your knees, lift your heels, and drop your sitting bones to your heels.

3. Inhale as you open your knees out to the sides. Exhale as you drop your chest between your knees and lower your forearms to the floor. Your knees should end up on the outsides of your shoulders.

4. You can experiment with various arm positions. Start with your palms flat on the floor (Pose #1), then bring either one hand to your face (Pose #2) or both hands to your face (Pose #3) and then spread your fingers out (Pose #4).

5. Hold the pose for at least 30, and up to 90, seconds in order to receive the full benefits of the stretch.

6. To come out of the pose, inhale as you lift your chest and bring your knees together. Exhale as you press into your feet, straighten your legs, and come back to Mountain Pose (*Tadasana*).

Modification:
1. forearms and palms to the floor
2. one forearm and palm to the floor, other elbow to the floor hand to the face
3. both hands to the face, elbows on the floor
4. both hands to the face, fingers spread open in a Padma Mudra - Lotus Hand Seal elbows, on the floor

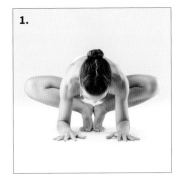

1.

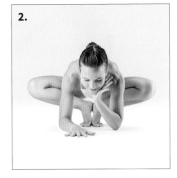

2.

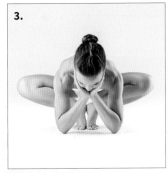

3.

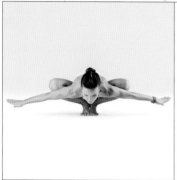

Garland Pose

Malasana

(mah-LAHS-uh-nuh)

Also Known As: Full Squat Pose (Kunthasana)
Modification: hands wide, knees on top of the triceps
Pose Type: standing, forward bend
Drishti Point: Nasagrai or Nasagre (nose)

1.

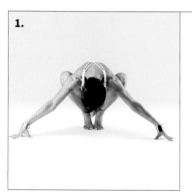

Garland Pose

Malasana

(mah-LAHS-uh-nuh)

Modification: heels up
1. knees to the armpits; hands out to the sides, fingertips to the floor
2. forehead to the floor; elbows bent at 90 degrees, fingertips to the floor
3. forehead to the floor; hands off the floor, arms out to the sides
Pose Type: standing, forward bend
Drishti Point: Nasagrai or Nasagre (nose)

2.

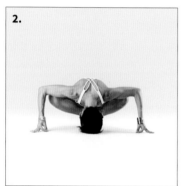

3.

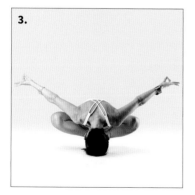

246   2,100 Asanas

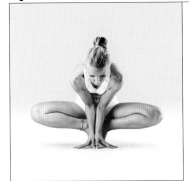

Supported Tip Toe Pose

Salamba Prapadasana

(SAH-luhm-buh pruh-puh-DAHS-uh-nuh)

Modification: knees open, elbows and wrists together, fingertips touching the floor in front of the feet

Pose Type: standing, forward bend

Drishti Point: Nasagrai or Nasagre (nose)

Intense Wrist Stretch Supported Tip Toe Pose

Uttana Manibandha Salamba Prapadasana

(ut-TAH-nuh muh-ni-BUHN-duh SAH-luhm-buh pruh-puh-DAHS-uh-nuh)

Modification: knees open wide; palms on the floor, fingertips toward the feet

Pose Type: standing, forward bend

Drishti Point: Nasagrai or Nasagre (nose)

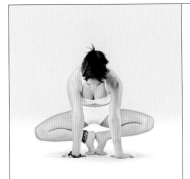

Lion Pose Dedicated to an Avatar of Lord Vishnu in Tip Toe Pose

Narasimhasana in Prapadasana

(nuh-ruh-sim-HAHS-uh-nuh in pruh-puh-DAHS-uh-nuh)

Also Known As: Lion Pose in Tip Toe Pose (Simhasana in Prapadasana)

Modification: feet wide apart

Pose Type: standing, forward bend

Drishti Point: Bhrumadhye or Ajna Chakra (third eye, between the eyebrows)

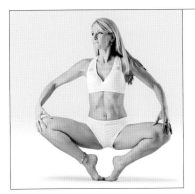

Unsupported Intense Ankle Stretch Tip Toe Pose

Niralamba Uttana Kulpa Prapadasana

(nir-AH-luhm-buh ut-TAH-nuh KUL-puh pruh-puh-DAHS-uh-nuh)

Modification: hands on the knees

Pose Type: standing, balance

Drishti Point: Nasagrai or Nasagre (nose)

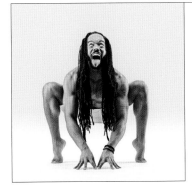

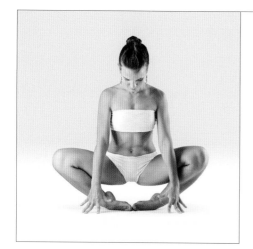

Supported Intense Ankle Stretch Tip Toe Pose

Salamba Uttana Kulpa Prapadasana

(SAH-luhm-buh ut-TAH-nuh KUL-puh pruh-puh-DAHS-uh-nuh)

Modification: fingertips to the floor
Pose Type: standing, balance
Drishti Point: Nasagrai or Nasagre (nose)

SQUAT: HEELS UP—KNEES WIDE, ARM MODIFICATIONS

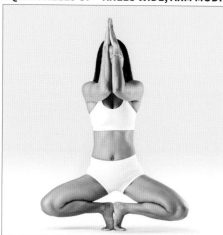

Tip Toe Pose

Prapadasana

(pruh-puh-DAHS-uh-nuh)

Modification: knees open wide; palms together, elbows together
Pose Type: standing
Drishti Point: Angushtamadhye or Angushta Ma Dyai (thumbs)

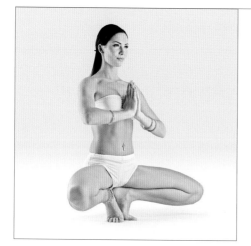

Tip Toe Pose

Prapadasana

(pruh-puh-DAHS-uh-nuh)

Modification: knees open wide, hands in Anjali Mudra (Hands in Prayer)
Pose Type: standing
Drishti Point: Nasagrai or Nasagre (nose)

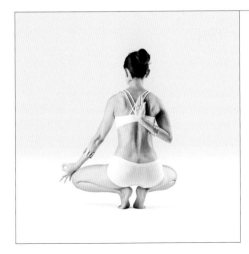

One Hand in Reverse Prayer Tip Toe Pose

Eka Hasta Viparita Namaskar Prapadasana
(EY-kuh HUH-stuh vi-puh-REE-tuh nuh-muhs-KAHR pruh-puh-DAHS-uh-nuh)
Modification: knees open wide; one hand to the knee
Pose Type: standing
Drishti Point: Nasagrai or Nasagre (nose)

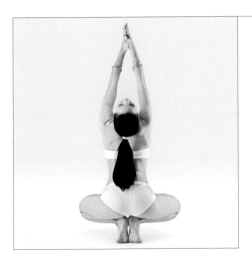

Upward Hands Tip Toe Pose

Urdhva Hasta Prapadasana
(OORD-vuh HUH-stuh pruh-puh-DAHS-uh-nuh)
Modification: knees open wide; arms extended up to the sky, head rolling back
Pose Type: standing, mild backbend
Drishti Point: Angushtamadhye or Angushta Ma Dyai (thumbs)

SQUAT: HEELS UP—KNEES WIDE, KNEES ON THE FLOOR—ARM MODIFICATIONS

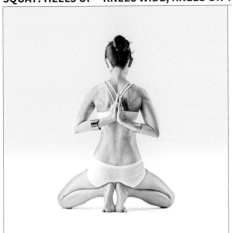

Reverse Prayer Root Lock Pose Prep.

Viparita Namaskar Mulabhandasana Prep.
(vi-puh-REE-tuh nuh-muhs-KAHR moo-luh-buhn-DAHS-uh-nuh)
Also Known As: Back of the Body Prayer Tip Toe Pose (Paschima Namaskara Prapadasana)
Modification: knees open wide; knees to the floor
Pose Type: standing
Drishti Point: Nasagrai or Nasagre (nose)

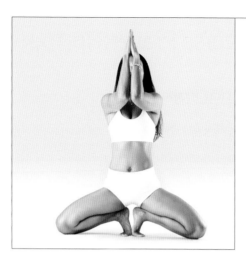

Root Lock Pose Prep.

Mulabhandasana Prep.

(moo-luh-buhn-DAHS-uh-nuh)

Also Known As: Tip Toe Pose Modification (Prapadasana Modification)
Modification: knees open wide; palms and elbows together; knees to the floor
Pose Type: standing
Drishti Point: Angushtamadhye or Angushta Ma Dyai (thumbs)

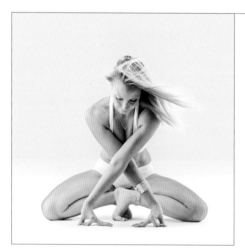

Root Lock Pose Prep.

Mulabhandasana Prep.

(moo-luh-buhn-DAHS-uh-nuh)

Also Known As: Tip Toe Pose Modification (Prapadasana Modification)
Modification: knees open wide; elbows and ankles crossed; knees to the floor, fingertips to the floor
Pose Type: standing, forward bend
Drishti Point: Hastagrai or Hastagre (hands)

ROOT LOCK POSE

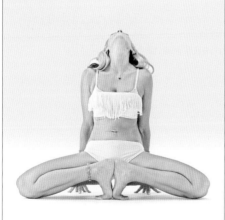

Root Lock Pose Prep.

Mulabhandasana Prep.

(moo-luh-buhn-DAHS-uh-nuh)

Also Known As: Twisted Feet Bound Angle Pose (Parivritta Pada Baddha Konasana)
Modification: fingertips to the floor behind the hips, sitting bones off the floor
Pose Type: standing, mild backbend
Drishti Point: Urdhva or Antara Drishti (up to the sky)

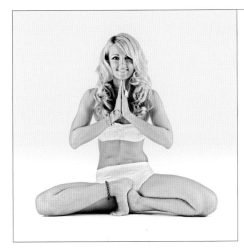

Womb Staff Pose

Yoni Dandasana

(YO-ni duhn-DAHS-uh-nuh)

Also Known As: Root Lock Pose Modification (Mulabandhasana Modification)
Pose Type: seated
Drishti Point: Nasagrai or Nasagre (nose)

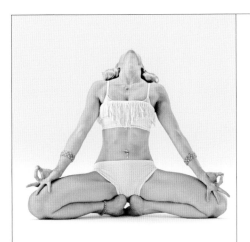

Root Lock Pose

Mulabhandasana

(moo-luh-buhn-DAHS-uh-nuh)

Also Known As: Perineal Contraction Pose (Mula Bandhasana)
Modification: palms up on the knees, head rolled back
Pose Type: seated, mild backbend
Drishti Point: Urdhva or Antara Drishti (up to the sky)

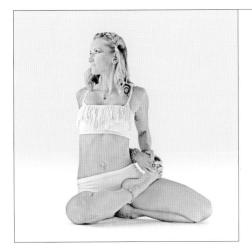

Pose Dedicated to Sage Vamadeva 1

Vamadevasana 1

(vah-muh-dey-VAHS-uh-nuh)

Modification: both hands binding to the top foot
Pose Type: seated, twist, binding
Drishti Point: Parsva Drishti (to the right), Parsva Drishti (to the left)

Seated Poses

EASY POSE: KNEES HIGH

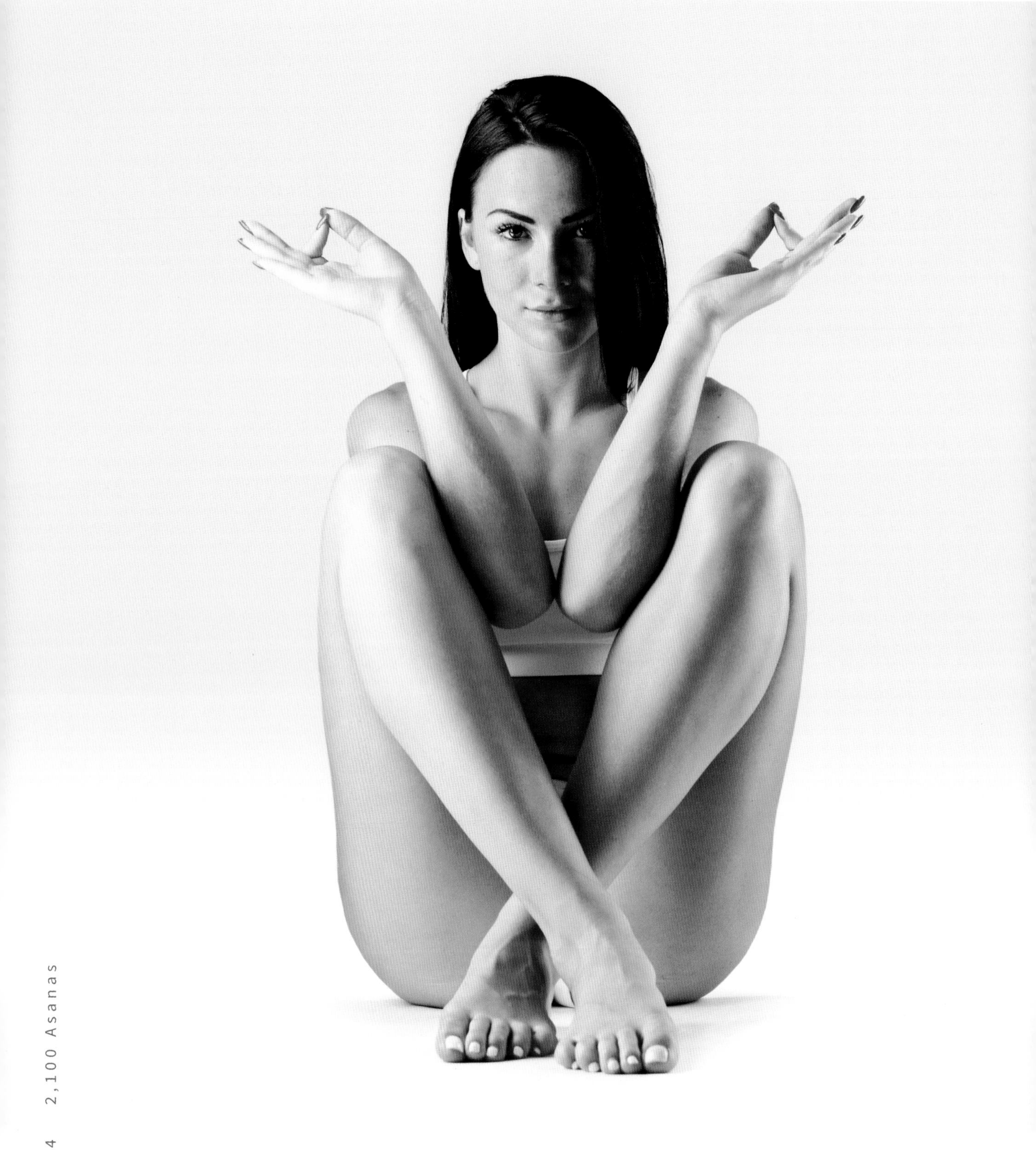

Easy Pose

Sukhasana

(suk-AHS-uh-nuh)

Pose Type: seated, forward bend

Drishti Point: Nasagrai or Nasagre (nose)

Modification: knees in line with the shoulders, elbows to the inside of the knees

sukha = easy, lightness

How to Perform the Pose:

1. Begin by sitting on the floor with both your legs straight out in front of you. Engage your *mula bandha*, *uddhiyana bandha*, and *ujjayi* breathing.

2. Exhale as you bring your feet toward you and cross them at the ankles. Keep the soles of your feet flat on the floor and your knees in line with your shoulders.

3. Inhale, stretch your arms up to the sky to lengthen your spine, and exhale as you bring your elbows together on the inside of your knees.

4. Inhale as you open your palms up to sky with your fingertips pointing to the outsides. Exhale as you bring you thumbs and pointer fingers together.

5. Hold the pose for at least 30, and up to 90, seconds in order to receive the full benefits of the stretch.

6. Exhale as you release the pose, coming back to starting position with both your legs straight out.

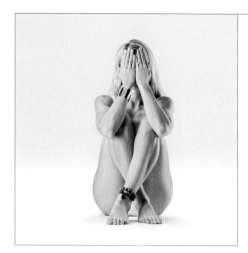

Easy Pose

Sukhasana

(suk-AHS-uh-nuh)

Modification: knees to the chest, elbows to the outside of the knees, palms covering the face

Pose Type: seated, forward bend

Drishti Point: Bhrumadhye or Ajna Chakra (third eye, between the eyebrows)

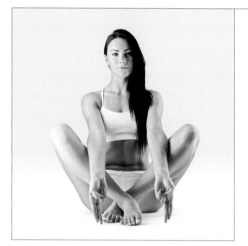

Easy Pose

Sukhasana

(suk-AHS-uh-nuh)

Modification: knees high, forearms to the shins

Pose Type: seated

Drishti Point: Nasagrai or Nasagre (nose), Bhrumadhye or Ajna Chakra (third eye, between the eyebrows)

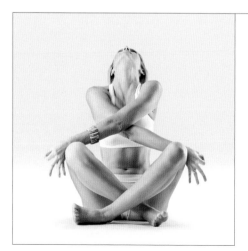

Easy Pose

Sukhasana

(suk-AHS-uh-nuh)

Modification: elbows crossed, backs of both hands to the knees

Pose Type: seated, mild backbend

Drishti Point: Bhrumadhye or Ajna Chakra (third eye, between the eyebrows)

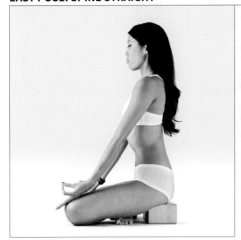

Easy Pose

Sukhasana

(suk-AHS-uh-nuh)

Modification: on the yoga block
Pose Type: seated
Drishti Point: Bhrumadhye or Ajna Chakra (third eye, between the eyebrows)

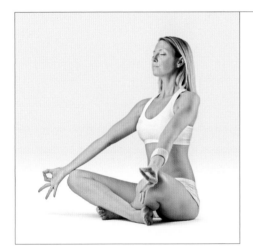

Easy Pose

Sukhasana

(suk-AHS-uh-nuh)

Pose Type: seated
Drishti Point: Bhrumadhye or Ajna Chakra (third eye, between the eyebrows)

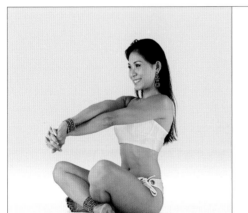

Bound Hands Easy Pose

Baddha Hasta Sukhasana

(BUH-duh HUH-stuh suk-AHS-uh-nuh)

Modification: arms in front, arms straight
Pose Type: seated
Drishti Point: Hastagrai or Hastagre (hands), Bhrumadhye or Ajna Chakra (third eye, between the eyebrows)

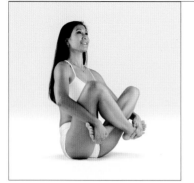

Embryo in the Womb Pose in Easy Pose

Garbha Pindasana in Sukhasana

(GUHR-buh pin-DAHS-uh-nuh in suk-AHS-uh-nuh)

Modification: grabbing onto the outside edges of the feet
Pose Type: seated, forward bend, core
Drishti Point: Bhrumadhye or Ajna Chakra (third eye, between the eyebrows)

EASY POSE: TWISTS & SIDE BENDS

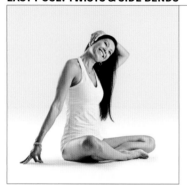

Easy Pose

Sukhasana

(suk-AHS-uh-nuh)

Modification: neck stretch
Pose Type: seated
Drishti Point: Nasagrai or Nasagre (nose)

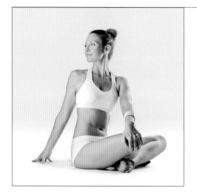

Revolved Easy Pose

Parivritta Sukhasana

(puh-ri-VRIT-tuh suk-AHS-uh-nuh)

Pose Type: seated, twist
Drishti Point: Parshva Drishti (to the right), Parshva Drishti (to the left)

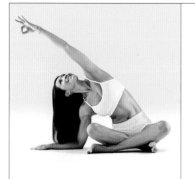

Sideways Easy Pose

Parshva Sukhasana

(PAHRSH-vuh suk-AHS-uh-nuh)

Modification: one forearm to the floor, other arm extended up over the head
Pose Type: seated, side bend
Drishti Point: Hastagrai or Hastagre (hands)

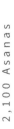

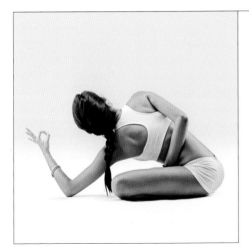

Revolved Bound Easy Pose

Parivritta Baddha Sukhasana

(puh-ri-VRIT-tuh BUH-duh suk-AHS-uh-nuh)

Modification: elbow to the floor

Pose Type: seated, forward bend, twist, binding

Drishti Point: Urdhva or Antara Drishti (up to the sky)

ACCOMPLISHED ONE POSE

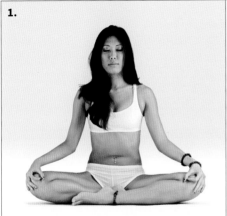

1.

Accomplished One Pose

Siddhasana

(sid-DAHS-anna)

Modification: 1. one heel in front of the other

2. one foot tucked between the hamstring and the calf

Pose Type: seated

Drishti Point: Bhrumadhye or Ajna Chakra (third eye, between the eyebrows)

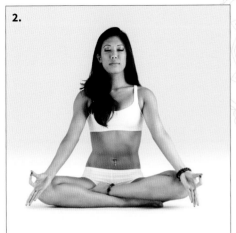

2.

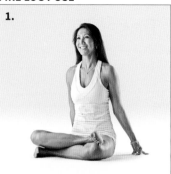

Fire Log Pose

Agnistambhasana

(uhg-ni-stuhm-BAHS-anna)

Modification: 1. spine straight, fingertips to the floor behind the hips

2. leaning forward, palms on the floor by the thighs

Pose Type: 1. seated

2. seated, forward bend

Drishti Point: Nasagrai or Nasagre (nose), Bhrumadhye or Ajna Chakra (third eye, between the eyebrows)

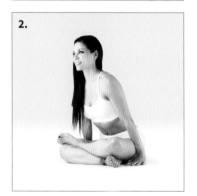

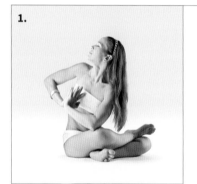

Revolved Fire Log Pose

Parivritta Agnistambhasana

(puh-ri-VRIT-tuh uhg-ni-stuhm-BAHS-uh-nuh)

Modification: hands in Anjali Mudra (Hands in Prayer)

1. elbow to the knee

2. elbow to the foot

Pose Type: seated, forward bend, twist

Drishti Point: Urdhva or Antara Drishti (up to the sky); Parshva Drishti (to the right), Parshva Drishti (to the left)

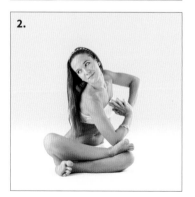

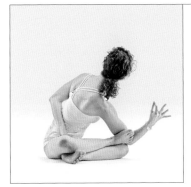

Revolved Bound Fire Log Pose

Parivritta Baddha Agnistambhasana

(puh-ri-VRIT-tuh BUH-duh uhg-ni-stuhm-BAHS-uh-nuh)

Modification: one elbow to the sole of the top foot, other arm behind the back, hand to the inside of the thigh

Pose Type: seated, forward bend, twist, binding

Drishti Point: Urdhva or Antara Drishti (up to the sky)

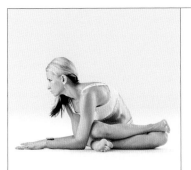

Revolved Fire Log Pose

Parivritta Agnistambhasana

(puh-ri-VRIT-tuh uhg-ni-stuhm-BAHS-uh-nuh)

Modification: forearms to the floor

Pose Type: seated, forward bend, twist

Drishti Point: Bhrumadhye or Ajna Chakra (third eye, between the eyebrows)

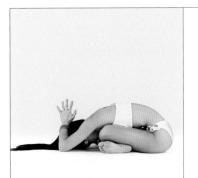

Fire Log Pose

Agnistambhasana

(uhg-ni-stuhm-BAHS-uh-nuh)

Modification: forward bend, palms together, fingers spread wide; elbows and forehead on the floor

Pose Type: seated, forward bend

Drishti Point: Nasagrai or Nasagre (nose)

HALF LOTUS POSE

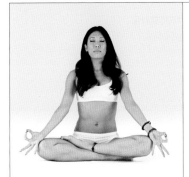

Half Lotus Pose

Ardha Padmasana

(UHR-duh puhd-MAHS-uh-nuh)

Modification: back of the hands on the knees

Pose Type: seated

Drishti Point: Nasagrai or Nasagre (nose)

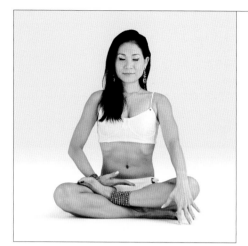

Half Lotus Pose

Ardha Padmasana

(UHR-duh puhd-MAHS-uh-nuh)

Modification: Salute to the Buddha Mudra Hand Position: one palm facing up, fingertips of the other hand to the floor
Pose Type: seated
Drishti Point: Nasagrai or Nasagre (nose)

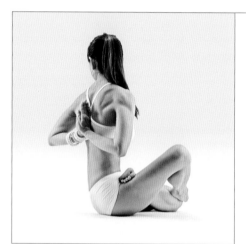

Reverse Prayer Revolved Half Lotus Pose

Viparita Namaskar Parivritta Ardha Padmasana

(vi-puh-REE-tuh nuh-muhs-KAHR puh-ri-VRIT-tuh UHR-duh puhd-MAHS-uh-nuh)

Also Known As: Back of the Body Prayer Revolved Half Lotus Pose (Paschima Namaskara Parivritta Ardha Padmasana)
Modification: top foot resting on the bottom knee
Pose Type: seated, twist
Drishti Point: Parshva Drishti (to the right), Parshva Drishti (to the left)

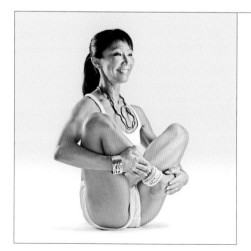

Embryo in the Womb Pose in Half Lotus Pose

Garbha Pindasana in Ardha Padmasana

(guhr-buh-pin-DAHS-uh-nuh in UHR-duh puhd-MAHS-uh-nuh)

Modification: knees lifted toward the chest
Pose Type: seated, forward bend, core
Drishti Point: Nasagrai or Nasagre (nose)

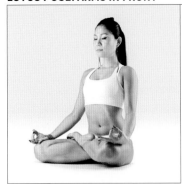

Lotus Pose

Padmasana

(puhd-MAHS-uh-nuh)

Modification: back of the hands on the knees
Pose Type: seated
Drishti Point: Nasagrai or Nasagre (nose)

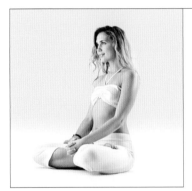

Lotus Pose

Padmasana

(puhd-MAHS-uh-nuh)

Modification: fingers interlocked, hands resting on the lap
Pose Type: seated
Drishti Point: Nasagrai or Nasagre (nose), Bhrumadhye or Ajna Chakra (third eye, between the eyebrows)

LOTUS POSE: ARMS BEHIND

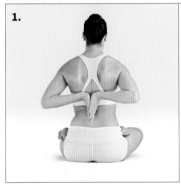

1.

Reverse Prayer Lotus Pose

Viparita Namaskar Padmasana

(vi-puh-REE-tuh nuh-muhs-KAHR puhd-MAHS-uh-nuh)

Also Known As: Back of the Body Prayer Lotus Pose (Paschima Namaskara Padmasana)
Modification: 1. fingertips pointing down
2. fingertips pointing up
Pose Type: seated
Drishti Point: Nasagrai or Nasagre (nose)

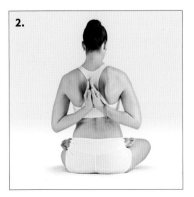

2.

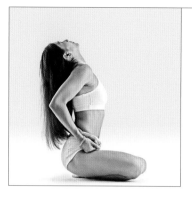

Bound Lotus Pose

Baddha Padmasana

(BUH-duh puhd-MAHS-uh-nuh)

Modification: both hands to one foot, one arm behind the back
Pose Type: seated, mild backbend, binding
Drishti Point: Bhrumadhye or Ajna Chakra (third eye, between the eyebrows)

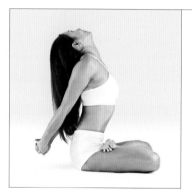

Bound Lotus Pose

Baddha Padmasana

(BUH-duh puhd-MAHS-uh-nuh)

Modification: both arms behind the back
Pose Type: seated, mild backbend, binding
Drishti Point: Bhrumadhye or Ajna Chakra (third eye, between the eyebrows)

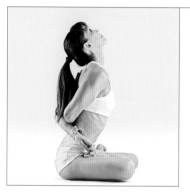

Hands Bound Lotus Pose

Baddha Hasta Padmasana

(BUH-duh HUH-stuh puhd-MAHS-uh-nuh)

Modification: backbend
Pose Type: seated, backbend
Drishti Point: Bhrumadhye or Ajna Chakra (third eye, between the eyebrows)

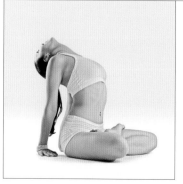

Lotus Pose

Padmasana

(puhd-MAHS-uh-nuh)

Modification: palms to the floor behind the hips; fingertips facing forward, backbend
Pose Type: seated, backbend
Drishti Point: Bhrumadhye or Ajna Chakra (third eye, between the eyebrows)

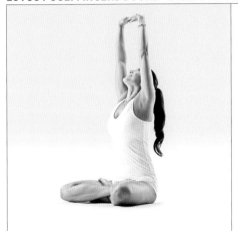

Raised Bound Hands Lotus Pose

Urdhva Baddha Hasta Padmasana

(OORD-vuh BUH-duh HUH-stuh puhd-MAHS-uh-nuh)

Also Known As: Seated Mountain Pose A (Parvatasana A)
Pose Type: seated, mild backbend
Drishti Point: Angushtamadhye (Thumbs)

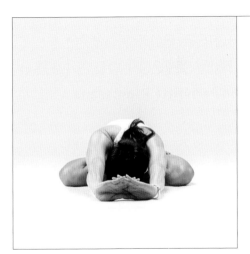

Simple Yoga Seal

Laghu Yoga Mudra

(LUH-gu YO-guh MU-druh)

Also Known As: Seated Mountain Pose B (Parvatasana B)
Pose Type: seated, forward bend
Drishti Point: Nasagrai or Nasagre (nose)

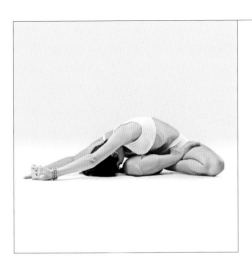

Sideways Simple Yoga Seal

Parshva Laghu Yoga Mudra

(PAHRSH-vuh LUH-gu YO-guh MU-druh)

Modification: fingers interlocked, palms facing out; arms straight to the side, forward bend
Pose Type: seated, forward bend, side bend
Drishti Point: Nasagrai or Nasagre (nose)

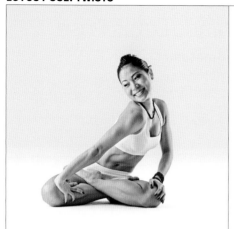

Pose Dedicated to Siddhar Vaasamuni—Easy Version

Sukha Vaasamunvasana

(SUK-uh vah-sah-moo-NYAHS-uh-nuh)

Pose Type: seated, side bend, forward bend, twist

Drishti Point: Parshva Drishti (to the right), Parshva Drishti (to the left)

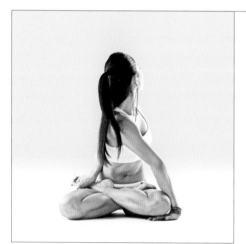

Arms of Twist Dedicated to Sage Bharadvaja 2 in Revolved Lotus Pose

Hasta Bharadvajasana 2 in Parivritta Padmasana

(HUH-stuh buh-ruhd-vuhj-AHS-uh-nuh in puh-ri-VRIT-uh puhd-MAHS-uh-nuh)

Pose Type: seated, twist, binding

Drishti Point: Parshva Drishti (to the right), Parshva Drishti (to the left)

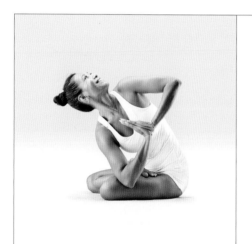

Revolved Lotus Pose

Parivritta Padmasana

(puh-ri-VRIT-uh puhd-MAHS-uh-nuh)

Modification: hands in Anjali Mudra (Hands in Prayer)

Pose Type: seated, forward bend, twist

Drishti Point: Urdhva or Antara Drishti (up to the sky)

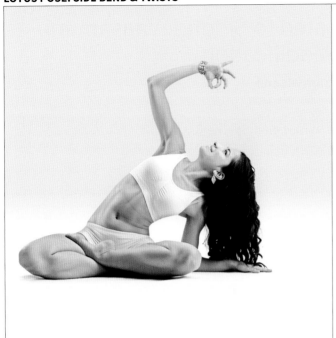

Sideways Lotus Pose

Parshva Padmasana

(PAHRSH-vuh puhd-MAHS-uh-nuh)
Modification: forearm to the floor
Pose Type: seated, side bend
Drishti Point: Hastagrai or Hastagre (hands)

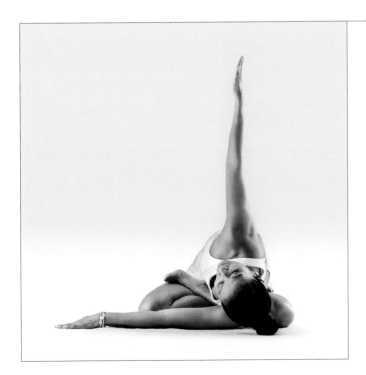

Revolved Western Intense Stretch Pose Lotus Pose

Parivritta Paschimottana Padmasana

(puh-ri-VRIT-uh puhsh-chi-mo-TAHN-nuh puhd-MAHS-uh-nuh)
Also Known As: Revolved Forward Bend Lotus Pose
Modification: shoulder to the floor, other arm extended to the sky
Pose Type: seated, forward bend, twist
Drishti Point: Angushtamadhye or Angushta Ma Dyai (thumbs)

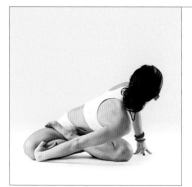

Pose Dedicated to Siddhar Vaasamuni—One Hand Modification

Eka Hasta Vaasamunvasana

(EY-kuh HUH-stuh [vah-sah-moo]-NYAHS-uh-nuh)

Pose Type: seated, forward bend, twist

Drishti Point: Urdhva or Antara Drishti (up to the sky)

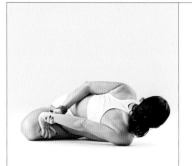

Pose Dedicated to Siddhar Vaasamuni

Vaasamunvasana

([vah-sah-moo-NYAHS-uh-nuh)

Pose Type: seated, forward bend, twist, binding

Drishti Point: Urdhva or Antara Drishti (up to the sky)

LOTUS POSE: FORWARD BEND

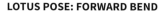

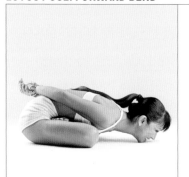

Yogic Seal Pose

Yoga Mudrasana

(YO-guh mu-DRAHS-uh-nuh)

Also Known As: Yoga Pose (Yogasana)

Modification: grabbing onto the wrist behind the back

Pose Type: seated, forward bend

Drishti Point: Nasagrai or Nasagre (nose) or Bhrumadhye or Ajna Chakra (third eye, between the eyebrows)

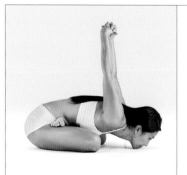

Hands Bound Lotus Pose

Baddha Hasta Padmasana

(BUH-duh HUH-stuh puhd-MAHS-uh-nuh)

Also Known As: Yoga Seal (Yoga Mudra)

Modification: chin to the floor, forward bend

Pose Type: seated, forward bend

Drishti Point: Nasagrai or Nasagre (nose) or Bhrumadhye or Ajna Chakra (third eye, between the eyebrows)

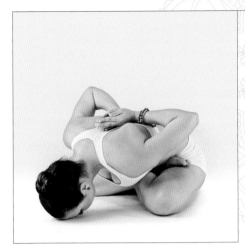

Reverse Prayer Yogic Seal Pose

Viparita Namaskar Yoga Mudrasana

(vi-puh-REE-tuh nuh-muhs-KAHR YO-guh mu-DRAHS-uh-nuh)

Also Known As: Back of the Body Prayer Yogic Seal Pose (Paschima Namaskara Yoga Mudrasana)

Modification: forehead to the floor

Pose Type: seated, forward bend

Drishti Point: Nasagrai or Nasagre (nose)

1.

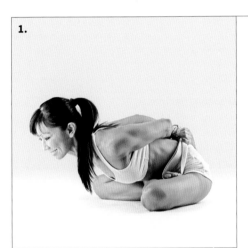

Yogic Seal Pose Prep.

Yoga Mudrasana Prep.

(YO-guh mu-DRAHS-uh-nuh)

Modification: 1. using a yoga strap

2. wrists crossed behind the back, reaching toward the feet

Pose Type: seated, forward bend, binding

Drishti Point: Bhrumadhye or Ajna Chakra (third eye, between the eyebrows)

2.

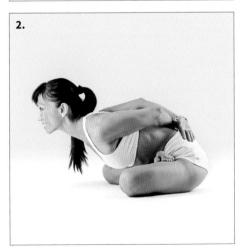

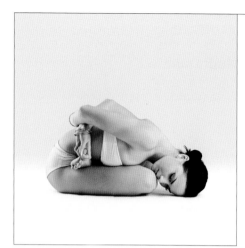

Sideways Yogic Seal Pose

Parshva Yoga Mudrasana

(PARHSH-vuh YO-guh mu-DRAHS-uh-nuh)

Also Known As: Sideways Bound Lotus Pose (Parshva Baddha Padmasana)

Modification: chin to the knee

Pose Type: seated, forward bend, binding, twist

Drishti Point: Bhrumadhye or Ajna Chakra (third eye, between the eyebrows)

1.

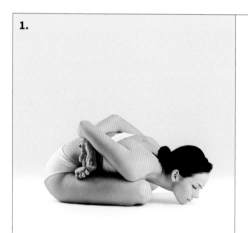

Yogic Seal Pose

Yoga Mudrasana

(YO-guh mu-DRAHS-uh-nuh)

Also Known As: Bound Lotus Pose (Baddha Padmasana)

Modification: 1. side view

2. front view

Pose Type: seated, forward bend, binding

Drishti Point: Bhrumadhye or Ajna Chakra (third eye, between the eyebrows)

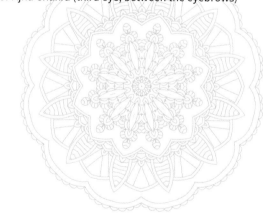

2.

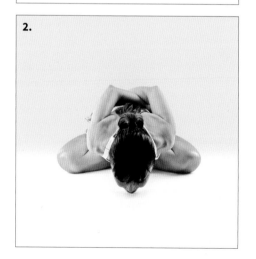

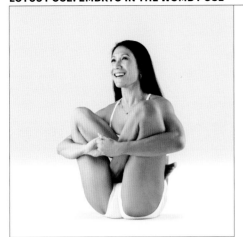

Embryo in the Womb Pose

Garbha Pindasana

(guhr-buh pin-DAHS-uh-nuh)

Modification: arms wrapped around the legs

Pose Type: seated, forward bend, core

Drishti Point: Nasagrai or Nasagre (nose), Bhrumadhye or Ajna Chakra (third eye, between the eyebrows)

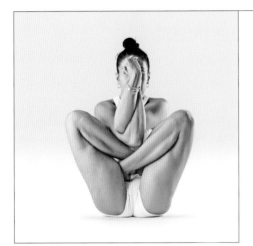

Hand Position of the Pose Dedicated to Garuda in Yoga Pose A

Hasta Garudasana in Yogasana A

(HUH-stuh guh-ru-DAHS-uh-nuh in yo-GAHS-uh-nuh)

Pose Type: seated, forward bend, core

Drishti Point: Angushtamadhye or Angustha Ma Dyai (thumbs)

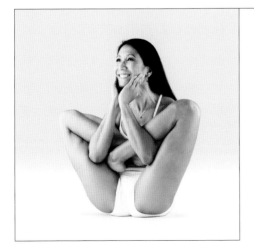

Embryo in the Womb Pose

Garbha Pindasana

(guhr-buh pin-DAHS-uh-nuh)

Pose Type: seated, forward bend, core

Drishti Point: Bhrumadhye or Ajna Chakra (third eye, between the eyebrows) or Nasagrai or Nasagre (nose)

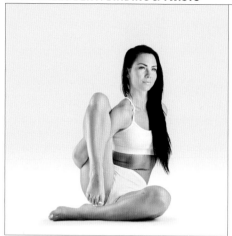

Bound Sundial Pose

Baddha Surya Yantrasana

(BUH-duh SOOR-yuh yuhn-TRAHS-uh-nuh)

Modification: both knees bent
Pose Type: seated, forward bend, binding
Drishti Point: Nasagrai or Nasagre (nose)

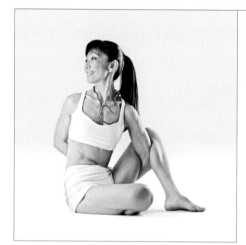

Revolved Pose Dedicated to Sage Marichi

Parivritta Marichyasana

(puh-ri-VRIT-tuh muh-ree-CHYAHS-uh-nuh)

Modification: twisting to the inside, foot to the thigh, binding under the leg
Pose Type: seated, forward bend, twist, binding
Drishti Point: Parshva Drishti (to the right), Parshva Drishti (to the left)

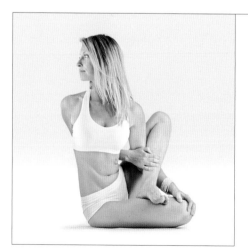

Half Lord of the Fishes Pose 3

Ardha Matsyendrasana 3

(UH-ruh muhts-yeyn-DRAHS-uh-nuh)

Modification: looking to the back
Pose Type: seated, forward bend, twist, binding
Drishti Point: Parshva Drishti (to the right), Parshva Drishti (to the left)

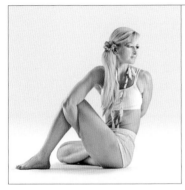

Pose Dedicated to Sage Marichi 4

Marichyasana 4

(muh-ree-CHYAHS-uh-nuh)
Modification: binding under the knee
Pose Type: seated, forward bend, twist, binding
Drishti Point: Parshva Drishti (to the right), Parshva Drishti (to the left)

BOTH KNEES BENT: BINDING & TWISTS—ARM THREADED UNDER

1.

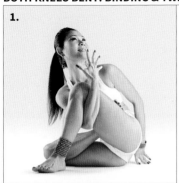

Half Pose Dedicated to Sage Agasthiyar

Ardha Agasthiyarasana

(UHR-duh uh-guhs-ti-yahr-AH-suh-nuh)
Modification: 1. one arm threaded through
2. full expression of the pose
Pose Type: 1. seated, forward bend, twist, binding
2. seated, forward bend, binding
Drishti Point: Urdhva or Antara Drishti (up to the sky), Nasagrai or Nasagre (nose), or Bhrumadhye or Ajna Chakra (third eye, between the eyebrows)

2.

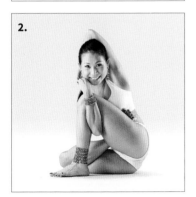

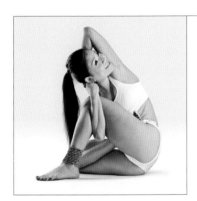

Revolved Half Pose Dedicated to Sage Agasthiyar

Parivritta Ardha Agasthiyarasana

(puh-ri-VRIT-tuh UHR-duh uh-guhs-ti-yahr-AH-suh-nuh)
Pose Type: seated, forward bend, binding, twist
Drishti Point: Urdhva or Antara Drishti (up to the sky)

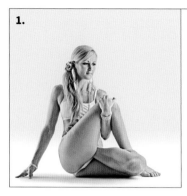

Pose Dedicated to Sage Agasthiyar

Agasthiyarasana

(uh-guhs-ti-yahr-AH-suh-nuh)

Modification: 1. prep. one arm threaded under the knee, fingertips of the other hand to the floor
2. full expression of the pose
Pose Type: seated, forward bend, binding
Drishti Point: 1. Hastagrai or Hastagre (hands)
2. Nasagrai or Nasagre (nose)

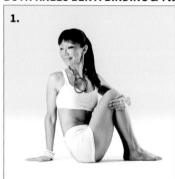

BOTH KNEES BENT: BINDING & TWISTS—KNEES TOGETHER

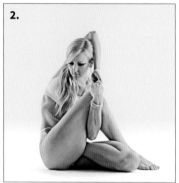

Seated Noose Pose Prep.

Upavishta Pashasana

(u-puh-VISH-tuh puh-SHAHS-uh-nuh)

Also Known As: Half Noose Pose (Ardha Pashasana), Upavistha Pashasana
Modification: 1. grabbing onto the knees
2. elbow over the opposite knee
Pose Type: seated, forward bend, twist
Drishti Point: Parshva Drishti (to the right), Parshva Drishti (to the left)

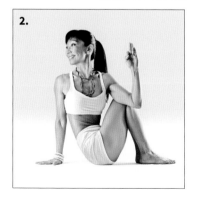

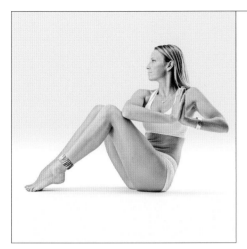

Seated Noose Pose Prep.

Upavishta Pashasana

(u-puh-VISH-tuh puh-SHAHS-uh-nuh)
Also Known As: Upavistha Pashasana
Modification: heels lifted; elbow over the opposite knee, hands in Anjali Mudra (Hands in Prayer)
Pose Type: seated, forward bend, twist, core
Drishti Point: Parshva Drishti (to the right), Parshva Drishti (to the left)

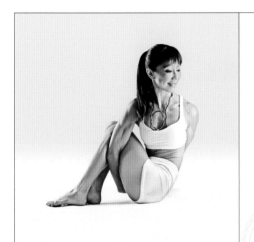

Seated Noose Pose

Upavishta Pashasana

(u-puh-VISH-tuh puh-SHAHS-uh-nuh)
Also Known As: Upavistha Pashasana
Modification: binding around both legs under the knees
Pose Type: seated, forward bend, twist, binding
Drishti Point: Parshva Drishti (to the right), Parshva Drishti (to the left)

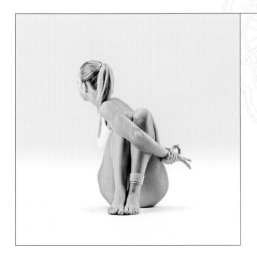

Seated Noose Pose

Upavishta Pashasana

(u-puh-VISH-tuh puh-SHAHS-uh-nuh)
Also Known As: Upavistha Pashasana
Modification: binding around both shins
Pose Type: seated, forward bend, twist, binding
Drishti Point: Parshva Drishti (to the right), Parshva Drishti (to the left)

1.

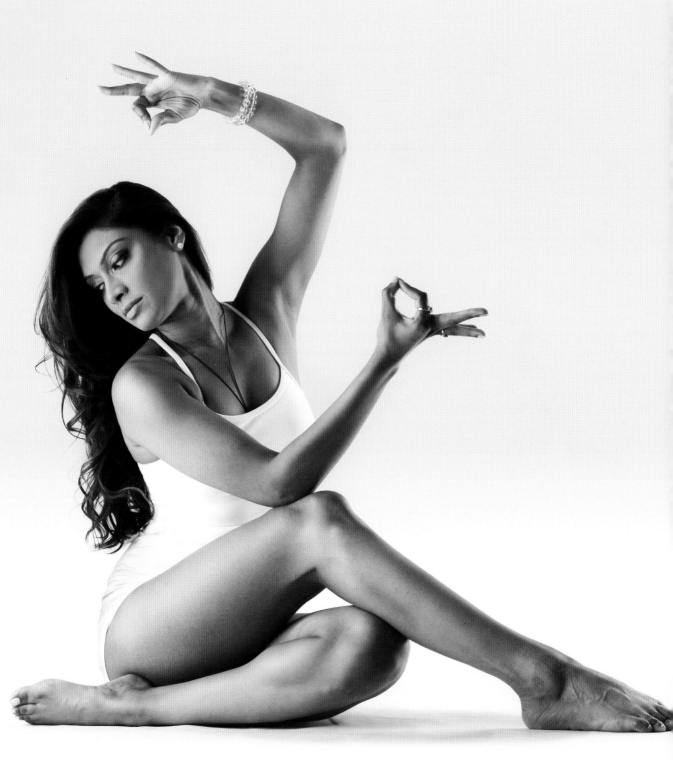

Half Lord of the Fishes Pose

Ardha Matsyendrasana

UHR-duh muhts-yeyn-DRAHS-uh-nuh

Pose Type: seated, forward bend, side bend, twist

Drishti Point: Padhayoragrai or Padayoragre (toes/feet)

How to Perform the Pose:

1. Begin by sitting on the floor with both your legs straight out in front of you. Engage your *mula bandha*, *uddhiyana bandha*, and *ujjayi* breathing.

Modification: side bend twist:
1. elbow to the knee on the same side
2. elbow to the opposite knee

ardha = half
Matsyendra = a Hindu sage and one of the first teachers of Hatha yoga, a legend, king of the fish

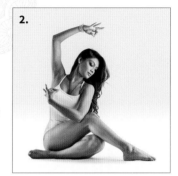

2.

2. Exhale as you bend the right knee toward your right shoulder and then bring it over your left leg so that your right foot is flat on the floor on the outside of your left shin.

3. Exhale and bend your left knee, bringing your left heel toward your right sitting bone. Keep the left knee and both your sitting bones evenly on the floor.

4. Exhale as you bring your right elbow to your right knee. Inhale as you bring your left arm up over your head and look towards your left foot (Pose #1).

5. To execute pose #2, exhale as you bring your left elbow over the right knee. Inhale as you bring your right arm up and exhale as you bend your right elbow and look over toward your right foot.

6. Hold the pose for at least 30, and up to 90, seconds in order to receive the full benefits of the stretch.

7. Inhale as you release the twist and exhale as you bring both your legs out in front of you. Repeat on the other side.

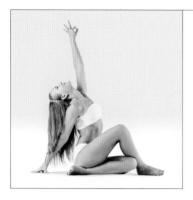

Half Lord of the Fishes Pose

Ardha Matsyendrasana

(UHR-duh muhts-yeyn-DRAHS-uh-nuh)
Modification: backbend
Pose Type: seated, backbend, forward bend
Drishti Point: Hastagrai or Hastagre (hands)

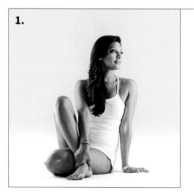

1.

Half Lord of the Fishes Pose

Ardha Matsyendrasana

(UHR-duh muhts-yeyn-DRAHS-uh-nuh)
Modification: twisting to the inside
1. grabbing onto the ankle
2. elbow over the knee
Pose Type: seated, forward bend, twist
Drishti Point: Parshva Drishti (to the right), Parshva Drishti (to the left)

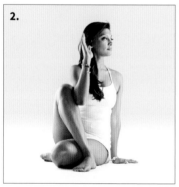

2.

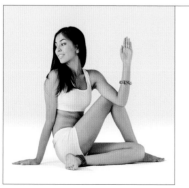

Half Lord of the Fishes Pose
Ardha Matsyendrasana

(UHR-duh muhts-yeyn-DRAHS-uh-nuh)
Modification: twisting to the outside, elbow over the knee; palm of the other hand to the floor
Pose Type: seated, forward bend, twist
Drishti Point: Parshva Drishti (to the right), Parshva Drishti (to the left)

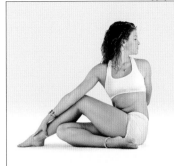

Half Lord of the Fishes Pose 1

Ardha Matsyendrasana 1

(UHR-duh muhts-yeyn-DRAHS-uh-nuh)

Modification: grabbing onto the ankle, other arm behind the back, hand to the inside of the thigh

Pose Type: seated, forward bend, twist, binding

Drishti Point: Parshva Drishti (to the right), Parshva Drishti (to the left)

BOTH KNEES BENT: BINDING FORWARD BEND & TWIST

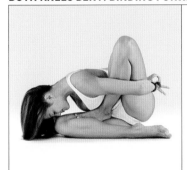

Pose Dedicated to Sage Marichi 3 Prep.

Marichyasana 3 Prep.

(muh-ree-CHYAHS-uh-nuh)

Also Known As: Pose Dedicated to Sage Marichi B (Marichyasana B)

Modification: top foot to the bottom thigh, binding around the shin, nose to the knee

Pose Type: seated, forward bend, binding

Drishti Point: Nasagrai or Nasagre (nose)

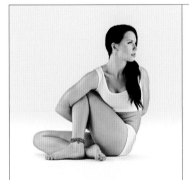

Pose Dedicated to Sage Marichi 4 Prep.

Marichyasana 4 Prep.

(muh-ree-CHYAHS-uh-nuh)

Modification: sitting in a cross-legged position, one knee dropped to the side, foot by the sitting bones; other knee bent toward the shoulder, binding around the shin on the outside of the leg

Pose Type: seated, forward bend, twist, binding

Drishti Point: Parshva Drishti (to the right), Parshva Drishti (to the left)

BOTH KNEES BENT: BINDING & TWIST

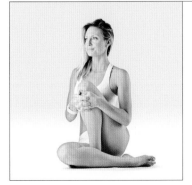

Pose Dedicated to Sage Marichi 3 Prep.

Marichyasana 3 Prep.

(muh-ree-CHYAHS-uh-nuh)

Also Known As: Pose Dedicated to Sage Marichi B (Marichyasana B)

Modification: spine straight, bottom knee wrapped around the foot, fingers interlocked on the shin

Pose Type: seated, forward bend

Drishti Point: Nasagrai or Nasagre (nose), Bhrumadhye or Ajna Chakra (third eye, between the eyebrows)

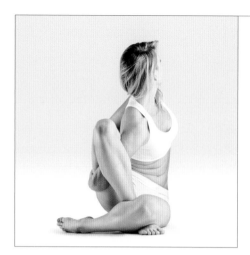

Pose Dedicated to Sage Marichi 3 Prep.

Marichyasana 3 Prep.

(muh-ree-CHYAHS-uh-nuh)

Also Known As: Pose Dedicated to Sage Marichi B Modification (Marichyasana B Modification)

Modification: bottom knee wrapped around the foot, binding under the thigh

Pose Type: seated, forward bend, twist, binding

Drishti Point: Parshva Drishti (to the right), Parshva Drishti (to the left)

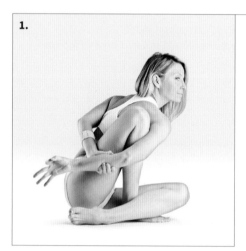

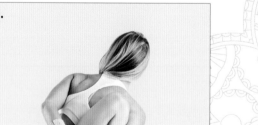

Pose Dedicated to Sage Marichi 3 Prep.

Marichyasana 3 Prep.

(muh-ree-CHYAHS-uh-nuh)

Also Known As: Pose Dedicated to Sage Marichi B Modification (Marichyasana B Modification)

Modification: knee wrapped around the foot, binding over the shin

Pose Type: 1. seated, forward bend, binding

2. seated, forward bend, twist, binding

Drishti Point: Parshva Drishti (to the right), Parshva Drishti (to the left)

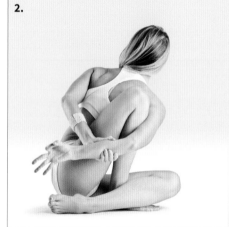

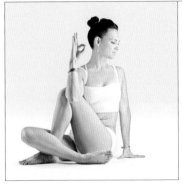

Half Lord of the Fishes Pose 1 Prep.

Ardha Matsyendrasana 1

(UHR-duh muhts-yeyn-DRAHS-uh-nuh)

Modification: foot under the knee, twisting to the outside
Pose Type: seated, forward bend, twist
Drishti Point: Parshva Drishti (to the right), Parshva Drishti (to the left)

HALF LOTUS POSE: KNEE BENT TOWARD THE CHEST

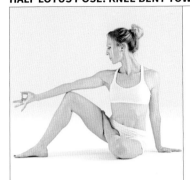

Pose Dedicated to Sage Marichi Prep.

Marichyasana Prep.

(muh-ree-CHYAHS-uh-nuh)

Modification: prep.—elbow to the knee on the same side, palm to the floor behind the hips
Pose Type: seated, forward bend
Drishti Point: Hastagrai or Hastagre (hands)

Pose Dedicated to Sage Marichi Prep.

Marichyasana Prep.

(muh-ree-CHYAHS-uh-nuh)

Modification: prep.—arms wrapping around the leg
Pose Type: seated, forward bend
Drishti Point: Nasagrai or Nasagre (nose)

HALF LOTUS POSE: BINDING & TWISTS—KNEE BENT TOWARD THE CHEST

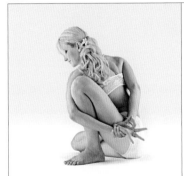

Pose Dedicated to Sage Marichi 3

Marichyasana 3

(muh-ree-CHYAHS-uh-nuh)

Also Known As: Pose Dedicated to Sage Marichi B (Marichyasana B)
Modification: sitting up straight
Pose Type: seated, forward bend, binding
Drishti Point: Nasagrai or Nasagre (nose)

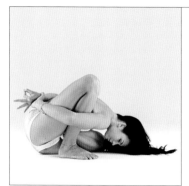

Pose Dedicated to Sage Marichi 3

Marichyasana 3

(muh-ree-CHYAHS-uh-nuh)

Also Known As: Pose Dedicated to Sage Marichi B (Marichyasana B)
Modification: full forward bend
Pose Type: seated, forward bend, binding
Drishti Point: Nasagrai or Nasagre (nose)

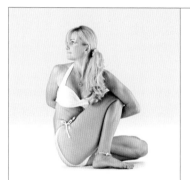

Pose Dedicated to Sage Marichi 4

Marichyasana 4

(muh-ree-CHYAHS-uh-nuh)

Also Known As: Pose Dedicated to Sage Marichi D (Marichyasana D)
Modification: sitting bones on the floor
Pose Type: seated, forward bend, twist, binding
Drishti Point: Parshva Drishti (to the right), Parshva Drishti (to the left)

LOTUS POSE: BINDING & TWISTS—KNEE BENT TOWARD THE CHEST

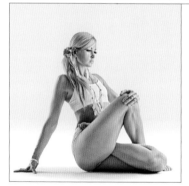

Full Lord of the Fishes Pose Prep.

Paripurna Matsyendrasana Prep.

(puh-ri-POOR-nuh muhts-yeyn-DRAHS-uh-nuh)

Modification: one palm to the floor behind the hips, grabbing onto the knee with the opposite hand
Pose Type: seated, forward bend
Drishti Point: Nasagrai or Nasagre (nose)

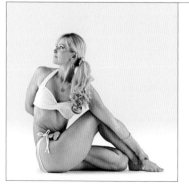

Full Lord of the Fishes Pose

Paripurna Matsyendrasana

(puh-ri-POOR-nuh muhts-yeyn-DRAHS-uh-nuh)

Also Known As: Full Lord of the Fishes Pose (Poorna Matsyendrasana)
Pose Type: seated, forward bend, twist, binding
Drishti Point: Parshva Drishti (to the right), Parshva Drishti (to the left)

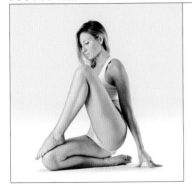

Root Lord of the Fishes Pose Prep.

Mula Matsyendrasana Prep.

(MOOL-uh muhts-yeyn-DRAHS-uh-nuh)

Modification: heel to the perineum, other foot resting on the knee, fingertips to the floor by the hips

Pose Type: seated, forward bend

Drishti Point: Padayoragrai or Padayoragre (toes/feet)

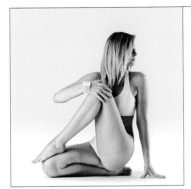

Half Root Lord of the Fishes Pose

Ardha Mula Matsyendrasana

(UHR-duh MOOL-uh muhts-yeyn-DRAHS-uh-nuh)

Modification: heel to the perineum, other foot resting on the knee, fingertips of one hand to the floor by the hips, other hand grabbing onto the opposite knee

Pose Type: seated, forward bend, twist

Drishti Point: Parshva Drishti (to the right), Parshva Drishti (to the left)

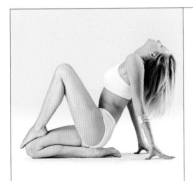

Root Lord of the Fishes Pose Prep.

Mula Matsyendrasana Prep.

(MOOL-uh muhts-yeyn-DRAHS-uh-nuh)

Modification: backbend, heel to the perineum, other foot resting on the knee, fingertips to the floor behind the hips

Pose Type: seated, backbend, forward bend

Drishti Point: Bhrumadhye or Ajna Chakra (third eye, between the eyebrows)

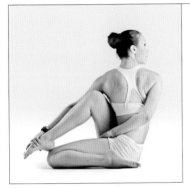

Pose Dedicated to Sage Marichi 6 Prep.

Marichyasana 6 Prep.

(muh-ree-CHYAHS-uh-nuh)

Also Known As: Pose Dedicated to Sage Marichi F (Marichyasana F)

Modification: opposite hand grabbing onto the foot, heel resting on the knee, other arm behind the back to the inside of the thigh, looking over the shoulder to the back

Pose Type: seated, forward bend, twist, binding

Drishti Point: Parshva Drishti (to the right), Parshva Drishti (to the left)

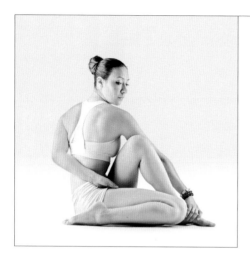

Pose Dedicated to Sage Marichi 6 Prep.

Marichyasana 6 Prep.

(muh-ree-CHYAHS-uh-nuh)

Also Known As: Pose Dedicated to Sage Marichi F (Marichyasana F)
Modification: opposite hand grabbing onto the foot, foot flat to the floor, other arm behind the back to the inside of the thigh, looking toward the foot
Pose Type: seated, forward bend, twist, binding
Drishti Point: Parshva Drishti (to the right), Parshva Drishti (to the left)

BOUND ANGLE POSE: ARMS IN FRONT

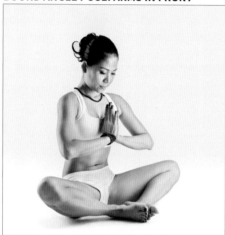

Bound Angle Pose with Hands in Prayer

Baddha Konasana Namaskar

(BUH-duh ko-NAHS-uh-nuh nuh-muhs-KAHR)

Modification: hands in Anjali Mudra (Hands in Prayer)
Pose Type: seated
Drishti Point: Nasagrai or Nasagre (nose) or Hastagrai or Hastagre (hands)

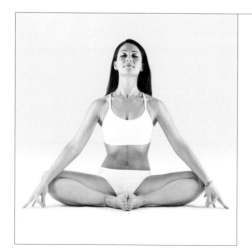

Bound Angle Pose

Baddha Konasana

(BUH-duh ko-NAHS-uh-nuh)

Modification: fingertips touching the floor
Pose Type: seated
Drishti Point: Bhrumadhye or Ajna Chakra (third eye, between the eyebrows)

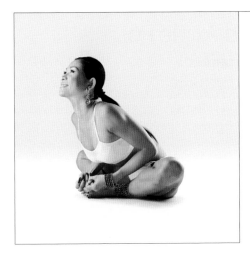

Bound Angle Pose

Baddha Konasana

(BUH-duh ko-NAHS-uh-nuh)

Modification: half forward bend, opening the soles of the feet up to the sky
Pose Type: seated, forward bend
Drishti Point: Bhrumadhye or Ajna Chakra (third eye, between the eyebrows)

BOUND ANGLE POSE: ARMS BEHIND

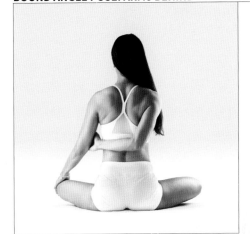

Bound Angle Pose

Baddha Konasana

(BUH-duh ko-NAHS-uh-nuh)

Modification: one hand to the knee; other hand behind, grabbing onto the bicep
Pose Type: seated, binding
Drishti Point: Nasagrai or Nasagre (nose)

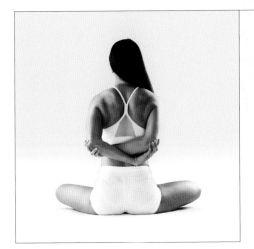

Bound Hands Bound Angle Pose

Baddha Hasta Baddha Konasana

(BUH-duh HUH-stuh BUH-duh ko-NAHS-uh-nuh)

Modification: arms behind, grabbing onto the elbows
Pose Type: seated
Drishti Point: Nasagrai or Nasagre (nose)

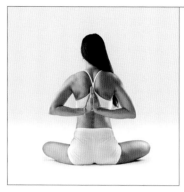

Reverse Prayer Bound Angle Pose

Viparita Namaskar Baddha Konasana

(vi-puh-REE-tuh nuh-muhs-KAHR BUH-duh ko-NAHS-uh-nuh)

Also Known As: Back of the Body Prayer Bound Angle Pose (Paschima Namaskara Baddha Konasana)

Pose Type: seated

Drishti Point: Nasagrai or Nasagre (nose)

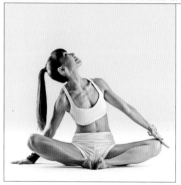

Hand Position of Cow Face Pose in Bound Angle Pose

Hasta Gomukhasana in Baddha Konasana

(HUH-stuh go-muk-AHS-uh-nuh in BUH-duh ko-NAHS-uh-nuh)

Pose Type: seated

Drishti Point: Nasagrai or Nasagre (nose)

BOUND ANGLE POSE: SIDE BEND & BINDING

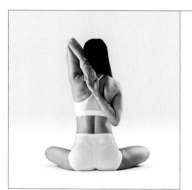

Sideways Bound Angle Pose

Parshva Baddha Konasana

(PAHRSH-vuh BUH-duh ko-NAHS-uh-nuh)

Pose Type: seated, side bend

Drishti Point: Urdhva or Antara Drishti (up to the sky)

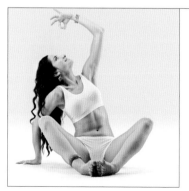

Sideways Star Pose

Parshva Tarasana

(PAHRSH-vuh tahr-AHS-uh-nuh)

Pose Type: seated, side bend

Drishti Point: Hastagrai or Hastagre (hands)

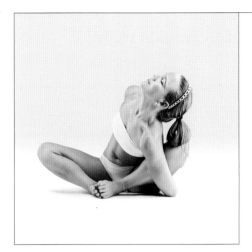

Sideways Bound Leg Bound Angle Pose

Parshva Baddha Pada Baddha Konasana

(PAHRSH-vuh BUH-duh PUH-duh BUH-duh ko-NAHS-uh-nuh)

Modification: binding around one leg, arm wrapped around the shin
Pose Type: seated, forward bend, side bend, twist, binding
Drishti Point: Urdhva or Antara Drishti (up to the sky)

BOUND ANGLE POSE: HEELS CLOSE, FEET LIFTED, SITTING BONES LIFTED AND FORWARD BEND

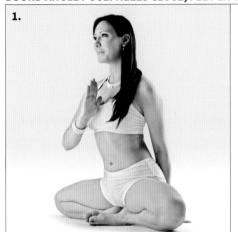

1.

Pose Dedicated to Sage Goraksha

Gorakshasana

(go-rahk-SHAHS-uh-nuh)

Modification: feet in Bound Angle Pose (Baddha Konasana), sitting on the heels
1. one hand to the centre of the chest, other hand to the floor behind the hips
2. hands in Anjali Mudra (Hands in Prayer)
Pose Type: seated, balance
Drishti Point: Nasagrai or Nasagre (nose), Bhrumadhye or Ajna Chakra (third eye, between the eyebrows)

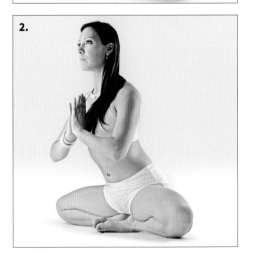

2.

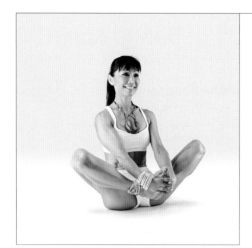

Equilibrium Bound Angle Pose 1

Tulya Baddha Konasana 1

(TUL-yuh BUH-duh ko-NAHS-uh-nuh)

Modification: feet lifted off the floor

Pose Type: seated, forward bend, core

Drishti Point: Nasagrai or Nasagre (nose), Bhrumadhye or Ajna Chakra (third eye, between the eyebrows)

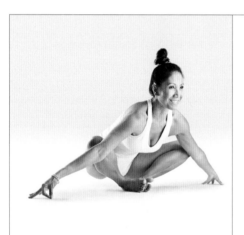

Equilibrium Bound Angle Pose 2

Tulya Baddha Konasana 2

(TUL-yuh BUH-duh ko-NAHS-uh-nuh)

Modification: sitting bones lifted off the floor

Pose Type: seated, forward bend, core

Drishti Point: Nasagrai or Nasagre (nose), Bhrumadhye or Ajna Chakra (third eye, between the eyebrows)

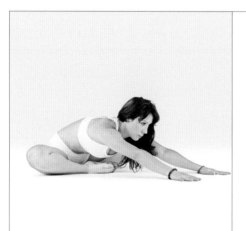

Bound Angle Pose

Baddha Konasana

(BUH-duh ko-NAHS-uh-nuh)

Modification: forward bend; arms straight to the front, palms down

Pose Type: seated, forward bend

Drishti Point: Angushtamadhye or Angushta Ma Dyai (thumbs) or Nasagrai or Nasagre (nose)

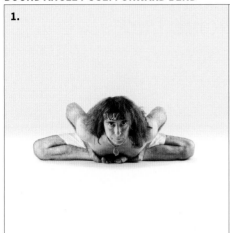

Bound Angle Pose

Baddha Konasana
(BUH-duh ko-NAHS-uh-nuh)
Modification: 1. half forward bend
2. full forward bend, chin to the floor
Pose Type: seated, forward bend
Drishti Point: Nasagrai or Nasagre (nose) or Bhrumadhye or Ajna Chakra (third eye, between the eyebrows)

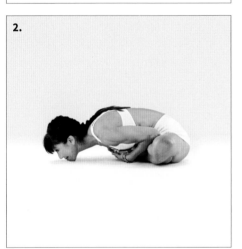

Bound Angle Pose

Baddha Konasana
(BUH-duh ko-NAHS-uh-nuh)
Modification: elbows bent and to the floor, forehead to the floor, palms together, fingers spread wide
Pose Type: seated, forward bend
Drishti Point: Bhrumadhye or Ajna Chakra (third eye, between the eyebrows) or Nasagrai or Nasagre (nose)

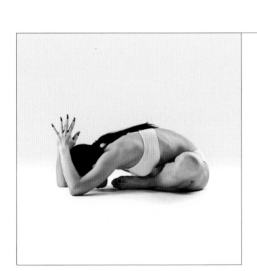

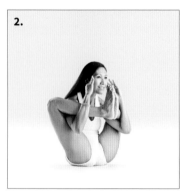

Easy Embryo in the Womb Pose

Sukha Garbha Pindasana

(SUK-uh GUHR-buh pin-DAHS-uh-nuh)

Modification: arms under the legs

1. hands to the feet
2. fingertips to the temples
3. hands to the sides; heels touching, feet to the sides

Pose Type: seated, forward bend, core

Drishti Point: Bhrumadhye or Ajna Chakra (third eye, between the eyebrows)

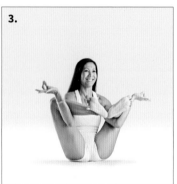

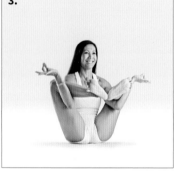

Easy Embryo in the Womb Pose

Sukha Garbha Pindasana

(SUK-uh GUHR-buh pin-DAHS-uh-nuh)

Also Known As: Yoga Pose A Prep. (Yogasana A Prep.)

Modification: shins into armpits, hands in Anjali Mudra (Hands in Prayer)

Pose Type: seated, forward bend, core

Drishti Point: Bhrumadhye or Ajna Chakra (third eye, between the eyebrows)

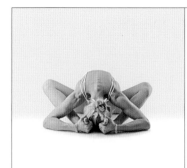

Star Pose

Tarasana

(tahr-AHS-uh-nuh)
Pose Type: seated, forward bend
Drishti Point: Nasagrai or Nasagre (nose)

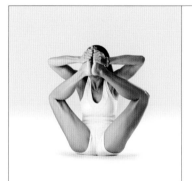

Upward Star Pose

Urdhva Tarasana

(OORD-vuh tahr-AHS-uh-nuh)
Pose Type: seated, forward bend, core
Drishti Point: Padhayoragrai or Padayoragre (toes/feet) or Nasagrai or Nasagre (nose)

LEGS IN FRONT: KNEES BENT

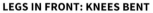

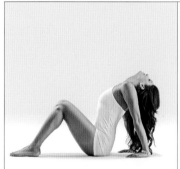

Seated Eastern Intense Stretch Pose

Upavishta Purvottanasana

(u-puh-VISH-tuh poor-vo-TAHS-uh-nuh)
Also Known As: Reverse Plank Prep.; Upavistha Purvottanasana
Pose Type: seated, backbend
Drishti Point: Bhrumadhye or Ajna Chakra (third eye, between the eyebrows)

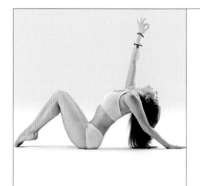

One Hand Seated Eastern Intense Stretch Pose

Eka Hasta Upavishta Purvottanasana

(EY-kuh HUH-stuh u-puh-VISH-tuh poor-vo-TAHS-uh-nuh)
Also Known As: One Hand Reverse Plank Prep.; Eka Hasta Upavistha Purvottanasana
Pose Type: seated, backbend
Drishti Point: Bhrumadhye or Ajna Chakra (third eye, between the eyebrows), Hastagrai or Hastagre (hands)

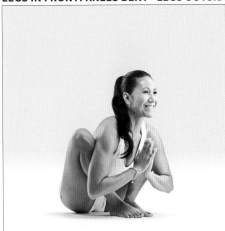

Seated Knee to Shoulder Pose

Upavishta Janu Bhujasana

(u-puh-VISH-tuh JAH-nu buj-AHS-uh-nuh)

Also Known As: Upavistha Janu Bhujasana
Modification: hands in Anjali Mudra (Hands in Prayer)
Pose Type: seated, forward bend
Drishti Point: Nasagrai or Nasagre (nose), Bhrumadhye or Ajna Chakra (third eye, between the eyebrows)

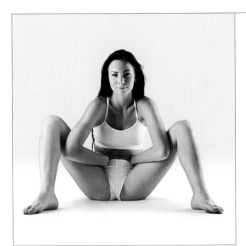

Broken Wing Pose

Avabhinna Pakshakasana

(uh-vuh-BIN-uh puhk-shuh-KAHS-uh-nuh)

Pose Type: seated, forward bend
Drishti Point: Nasagrai or Nasagre (nose), Bhrumadhye or Ajna Chakra (third eye, between the eyebrows)

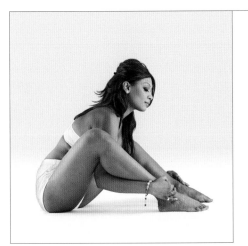

Tortoise Pose Prep.

Kurmasana Prep.

(koor-MAHS-uh-nuh)

Modification: grabbing onto the ankles
Pose Type: seated, forward bend
Drishti Point: Padhayoragrai or Padayoragre (toes/feet) or Nasagrai or Nasagre (nose)

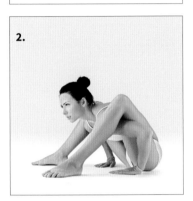

1.

Tortoise Pose Prep.

Kurmasana Prep.

(koor-MAHS-uh-nuh)
Modification: 1. arms straight
2. elbows bent
Pose Type: seated, forward bend
Drishti Point: Nasagrai or Nasagre (nose,) Bhrumadhye or Ajna Chakra (third eye, between the eyebrows)

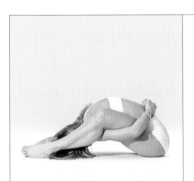

2.

Sleeping Tortoise Pose Prep.

Supta Kurmasana Prep.

(SUP-tuh koor-MAHS-uh-nuh)
Modification: feet unhooked
Pose Type: seated, forward bend, binding
Drishti Point: Bhrumadhye or Ajna Chakra (third eye, between the eyebrows)

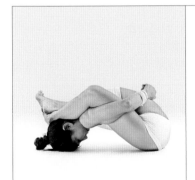

Sleeping Tortoise Pose

Supta Kurmasana

(SUP-tuh koor-MAHS-uh-nuh)
Pose Type: seated, forward bend, binding
Drishti Point: Bhrumadhye or Ajna Chakra (third eye, between the eyebrows)

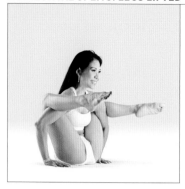

Half Upward Seated Angle Pose Prep.

Ardha Urdhva Upavistha Konasana Prep.

(UHR-duh OORD-vuh u-puh-VISH-tuh ko-NAHS-uh-nuh)

Modification: shoulders to the back of the knees, palms to the floor, knees bent
Pose Type: seated, forward bend, core
Drishti Point: Bhrumadhye or Ajna Chakra (third eye, between the eyebrows), Nasagrai or Nasagre (nose)

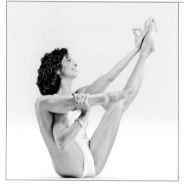

Bound Legs in Half Pose Dedicated to Sage Koormamuni

Baddha Pada Ardha Koormamunyasana

(BUH-duh PUH-duh UHR-duh koor-muh-mun-YAHS-uh-nuh)

Pose Type: seated, forward bend, core, binding
Drishti Point: Bhrumadhye or Ajna Chakra (third eye, between the eyebrows), Nasagrai or Nasagre (nose)

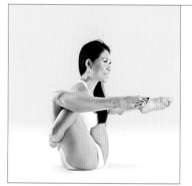

Half Upward Seated Angle Pose Prep. in One Hand to Foot Boat Pose

Ardha Urdhva Upavishta Konasana Prep. in Eka Hasta Pada Navasana

(UHR-duh OORD-vuh u-puh-VISH-tuh ko-NAHS-uh-nuh in EY-kuh HUH-stuh PUH-duh nuh-VAHS-uh-nuh)

Also Known As: Ardha Urdhva Upavistha Konasana Prep. in Eka Hasta Pada Navasana
Modification: one leg straight, back of the other knee to the shoulder
Pose Type: seated, forward bend, core
Drishti Point: Hastagrai or Hastagre (hands) or Padhayoragrai or Padayoragre (toes/feet)

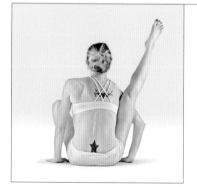

Half Upward Seated Angle Pose

Ardha Urdhva Upavishta Konasana

(UHR-duh OORD-vuh u-puh-VISH-tuh ko-NAHS-uh-nuh)

Also Known As: Ardha Urdhva Upavishta Konasana
Modification: palms to the floor, one leg straight up to the sky; other foot to the floor, knee to the chest
Pose Type: seated, forward bend
Drishti Point: Nasagrai or Nasagre (nose)

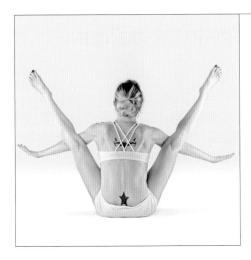

Upward Seated Angle Pose

Urdhva Upavishta Konasana

(UHR-duh OORD-vuh u-puh-VISH-tuh ko-NAHS-uh-nuh)

Also Known As: Urdhva Upavistha Konasana
Modification: arms open to the sides, triceps to the back of the knees
Pose Type: seated, forward bend, core
Drishti Point: Bhrumadhye or Ajna Chakra (third eye, between the eyebrows), Nasagrai or Nasagre (nose)

HORIZONTAL SPLITS: LEGS LIFTED & STRAIGHT

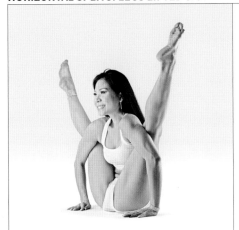

Seated Firefly Pose

Upavishta Tittibhasana

(u-puh-VISH-tuh ti-ti-BAHS-uh-nuh)

Also Known As: Upward Seated Angle Pose Prep. (Urdhva Upavishta Konasana Prep.), Pose Dedicated to Sage Koormamuni Prep. (Koormamunyasana Prep.), Upavistha Tittibhasana
Modification: palms to the floor, shoulders to the back of the knees
Pose Type: seated, forward bend, core
Drishti Point: Bhrumadhye or Ajna Chakra (third eye, between the eyebrows), Nasagrai or Nasagre (nose)

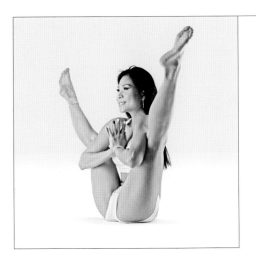

Pose Dedicated to Sage Koormamuni

Koormamunyasana

(koor-muh-mun-YAHS-uh-nuh)

Modification: hands in Anjali Mudra (Hands in Prayer)
Pose Type: seated, forward bend, core
Drishti Point: Bhrumadhye or Ajna Chakra (third eye, between the eyebrows), Nasagrai or Nasagre (nose)

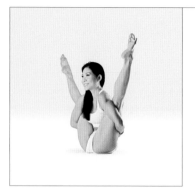

Pose Dedicated to Sage Koormamuni— Bound Legs

Baddha Pada Koormamunyasana
(BUH-duh PUH-duh koor-muh-mun-YAHS-uh-nuh)
Modification: legs straight
Pose Type: seated, forward bend, core, binding
Drishti Point: Bhrumadhye or Ajna Chakra (third eye, between the eyebrows), Nasagrai or Nasagre (nose)

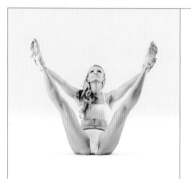

Hands to Feet Upward Seated Angle Pose

Pada Hasta Urdhva Upavishta Konasana
(PUH-duh HUH-stuh OORD-vuh u-puh-VISH-tuh ko-NAHS-uh-nuh)
Also Known As: Pada Hasta Urdhva Upavistha Konasana
Modification: grabbing onto the outside edges of the feet
Pose Type: seated, forward bend, core
Drishti Point: Bhrumadhye or Ajna Chakra (third eye, between the eyebrows), Urdhva or Antara Drishti (up to the sky)

Big Toe Upward Seated Angle Pose

Padangushta Urdhva Upavishta Konasana
(puhd-ahng-GOOSH-tuh OORD-vuh u-puh-VISH-tuh ko-NAHS-uh-nuh)
Also Known As: Padangushta Urdhva Upavistha Konasana
Modification: grabbing onto the big toes, arms parallel to the floor
Pose Type: seated, forward bend, core
Drishti Point: Bhrumadhye or Ajna Chakra (third eye, between the eyebrows) or Urdhva or Antara Drishti (up to the sky)

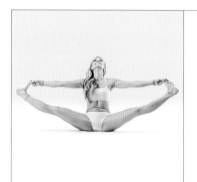

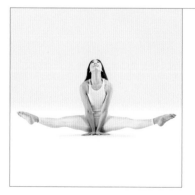

Upward Seated Angle Pose

Urdhva Upavishta Konasana
(OORD-vuh u-puh-VISH-tuh ko-NAHS-uh-nuh)
Also Known As: Urdhva Upavistha Konasana
Modification: palms to the floor, heels of the palms touching, fingertips pointing to the sides; feet lifted, toes pointed
Pose Type: seated, forward bend, core
Drishti Point: Bhrumadhye or Ajna Chakra (third eye, between the eyebrows), Urdhva or Antara Drishti (up to the sky)

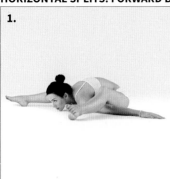

1.

Tortoise Pose

Kurmasana

(koor-MAHS-uh-nuh)

Modification: 1. knees bent

2. legs straight

Pose Type: seated, forward bend

Drishti Point: Bhrumadhye or Ajna Chakra (third eye, between the eyebrows)

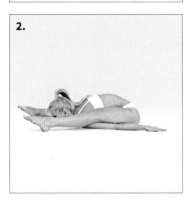

2.

Equal Angle Pose

Samakonasana

(suh-muh-ko-NAHS-uh-nuh)

Modification: forward bend, forearms to the floor

Pose Type: seated, forward bend

Drishti Point: Bhrumadhye or Ajna Chakra (third eye, between the eyebrows)

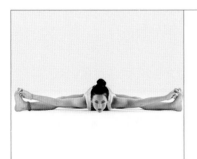

Big Toe Seated Angle Pose

Padangushta Upavishta Konasana

(puhd-ahng-GOOSH-tuh u-puh-VISH-tuh ko-NAHS-uh-nuh)

Also Known As: Padangushta Upavistha Konasana

Modification: forward bend, chin to the floor

Pose Type: seated, forward bend

Drishti Point: Bhrumadhye or Ajna Chakra (third eye, between the eyebrows)

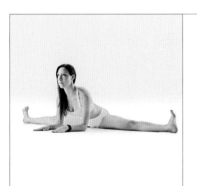

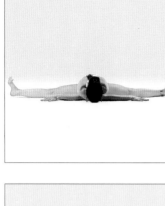

Equal Angle Pose

Samakonasana

(suh-muh-ko-NAHS-uh-nuh)

Modification: forward bend, arms crossed in front
Pose Type: seated, forward bend
Drishti Point: Bhrumadhye or Ajna Chakra (third eye, between the eyebrows), Nasagrai or Nasagre (nose)

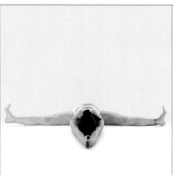

Equal Angle Pose

Samakonasana

(suh-muh-ko-NAHS-uh-nuh)

Modification: forward bend, arms extended to the front
Pose Type: seated, forward bend
Drishti Point: Nasagrai or Nasagre (nose)

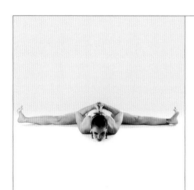

Reverse Prayer Equal Angle Pose

Viparita Namaskar Samakonasana

(vi-puh-REE-tuh nuh-muhs-KAHR suh-muh-ko-NAHS-uh-nuh)

Also Known As: Back of the Body Prayer Equal Angle Pose (Paschima Namaskara Samakonasana)
Pose Type: seated, forward bend
Drishti Point: Bhrumadhye or Ajna Chakra (third eye, between the eyebrows)

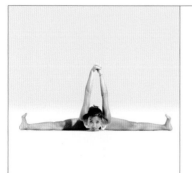

Hands Bound Equal Angle Pose

Baddha Hasta Samakonasana

(BUH-duh HUH-stuh suh-muh-ko-NAHS-uh-nuh)

Modification: forward bend
Pose Type: seated, forward bend
Drishti Point: Bhrumadhye or Ajna Chakra (third eye, between the eyebrows)

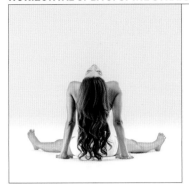

Seated Angle Pose

Upavishta Konasana
(u-puh-VISH-tuh ko-NAHS-uh-nuh)

Also Known As: Upavistha Konasana
Modification: mild version, backbend
Pose Type: seated, backbend
Drishti Point: Bhrumadhye or Ajna Chakra (third eye, between the eyebrows)

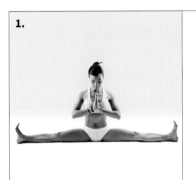

1.

Seated Angle Pose

Upavishta Konasana
(u-puh-VISH-tuh ko-NAHS-uh-nuh)

Also Known As: Upavistha Konasana
Modification: 1. hands in Anjali Mudra (Hands in Prayer), toes flexed in
2. hands in reverse prayer, toes flexed in
Pose Type: seated
Drishti Point: Nasagrai or Nasagre (nose) or Hastagrai or Hastagre (hands)

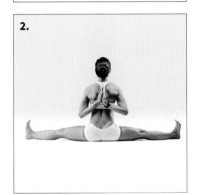

2.

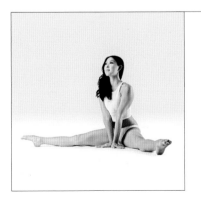

Seated Angle Pose

Upavishta Konasana
(u-puh-VISH-tuh ko-NAHS-uh-nuh)

Also Known As: Upavistha Konasana
Modification: palms to the floor in front of the hips, heels of the palms touching, fingertips pointing to the side, straight spine, toes pointed
Pose Type: seated
Drishti Point: Bhrumadhye or Ajna Chakra (third eye, between the eyebrows)

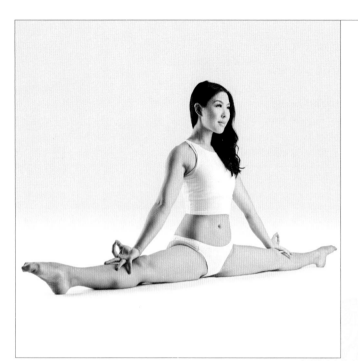

Equal Angle Pose

Samakonasana

(su-muh-ko-NAHS-uh-nuh)

Modification: hands on the knees, spine straight
Pose Type: seated
Drishti Point: Bhrumadhye or Ajna Chakra (third eye, between the eyebrows), Nasagrai or Nasagre (nose)

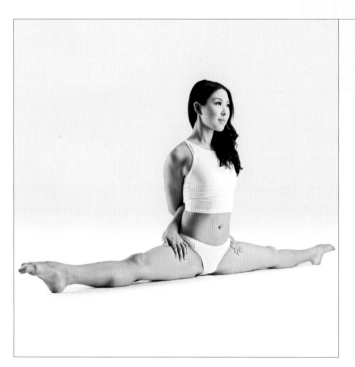

Bound Equal Angle Pose

Baddha Samakonasana

(BUH-duh su-muh-ko-NAHS-uh-nuh)

Pose Type: seated, binding
Drishti Point: Bhrumadhye or Ajna Chakra (third eye, between the eyebrows), Nasagrai or Nasagre (nose)

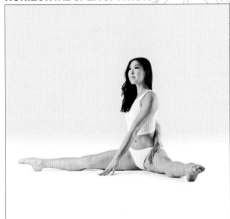

Half Bound Seated Angle Pose
Ardha Baddha Upavishta Konasana
(UHR-duh BUH-duh u-puh-VISH-tuh ko-NAHS-uh-nuh)
Also Known As: Ardha Baddha Upavistha Konasana
Modification: toes pointed, one hand binding behind the back, fingertips of the other hand to the floor in front of the hips
Pose Type: seated, binding
Drishti Point: Bhrumadhye or Ajna Chakra (third eye, between the eyebrows), Nasagrai or Nasagre (nose)

1.

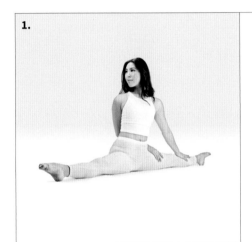

Revolved Half Bound Equal Angle Pose
Parivritta Samakonasana
(puh-ri-VRIT-tuh suh-muh-ko-NAHS-uh-nuh)
Modification: 1. toes pointed, both hands on one leg
2. toes flexed in, one hand to the leg, other hand to the floor
Pose Type: seated, twist, binding
Drishti Point: Parshva Drishti (to the right), Parshva Drishti (to the left)

2.

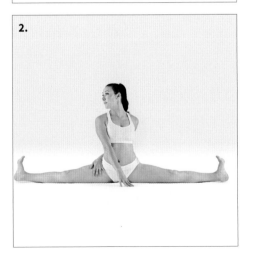

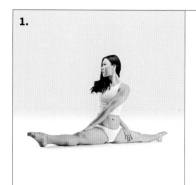

Revolved Bound Equal Angle Pose

Parivritta Baddha Samakonasana

(puh-ri-VRIT-tuh BUH-duh suh-muh-ko-NAHS-uh-nuh)

Modification: 1. toes pointed

2. toes flexed in

Pose Type: seated, twist, binding

Drishti Point: Parshva Drishti (to the right), Parshva Drishti (to the left)

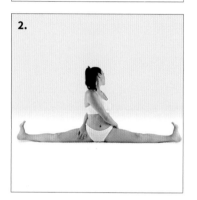

HORIZONTAL SPLITS: SIDE BENDS

Sideways Equal Angle Pose

Parshva Samakonasana

(PAHRSH-vuh suh-muh-ko-NAHS-uh-nuh)

Modification: side bend, fingertips to the back of the head; elbow to the floor

Pose Type: seated, side bend

Drishti Point: Urdhva or Antara Drishti (up to the sky)

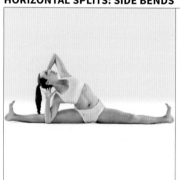

Both Hands to Foot Revolved Seated Angle Pose

Dwi Hasta Pada Parivritta Upavishta Konasana

(DWI-huh-stuh PUH-duh puh-ri-VRIT-tuh u-puh-VISH-tuh ko-NAHS-uh-nuh)

Also Known As: Dwi Hasta Pada Parivritta Upavistha Konasana

Pose Type: seated, side bend, twist

Drishti Point: Urdhva or Antara Drishti (up to the sky)

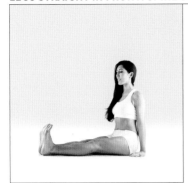

Staff Pose

Dandasana
(duhn-DAHS-uh-nuh)
Pose Type: seated
Drishti Point: Nasagrai or Nasagre (nose), Padhayoragrai or Padayoragre (toes/feet)

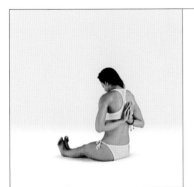

Reverse Prayer Staff Pose

Viparita Namaskar Dandasana
(vi-puh-REE-tuh nuh-muhs-KAHR duhn-DAHS-uh-nuh)
Also Known As: Back of the Body Prayer Staff Pose (Paschima Namaskara Dandasana)
Pose Type: seated
Drishti Point: Padayoragrai or Padayoragre (toes/feet), Nasagrai or Nasagre (nose)

1.

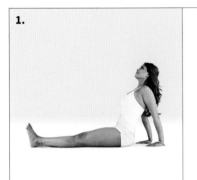

2.

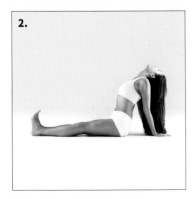

Staff Pose

Dandasana
(duhn-DAHS-uh-nuh)
Modification: 1. fingertips pointing to the heels
2. fingertips pointing away from the heels, head rolling back
Pose Type: seated, mild backbend
Drishti Point: Bhrumadhye or Ajna Chakra (third eye, between the eyebrows)

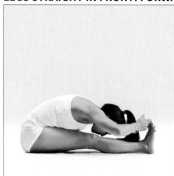

Western Intense Stretch Pose

Paschimottanasana

(puhsh-chi-mo-tahn-AHS-uh-nuh)

Also Known As: Seated Forward Bend
Modification: grabbing onto the big toes
Pose Type: seated, forward bend
Drishti Point: Padayoragrai or Padayoragre (toes/feet), Nasagrai or Nasagre (nose)

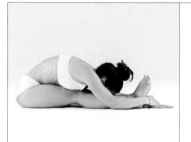

Western Intense Stretch Pose

Paschimottanasana

(puhsh-chi-mo-tahn-AHS-uh-nuh)

Also Known As: Seated Forward Bend
Modification: grabbing onto the balls of the feet
Pose Type: seated, forward bend
Drishti Point: Padayoragrai or Padayoragre (toes/feet), Nasagrai or Nasagre (nose)

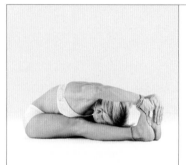

Western Intense Stretch Pose

Paschimottanasana

(puhsh-chi-mo-tahn-AHS-uh-nuh)

Also Known As: Seated Forward Bend
Modification: grabbing onto the wrist
Pose Type: seated, forward bend
Drishti Point: Padayoragrai or Padayoragre (toes/feet), Nasagrai or Nasagre (nose)

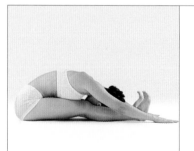

Western Intense Stretch Pose

Paschimottanasana

(puhsh-chi-mo-tahn-AHS-uh-nuh)

Also Known As: Seated Forward Bend
Modification: palms down
Pose Type: seated, forward bend
Drishti Point: Padayoragrai or Padayoragre (toes/feet), Nasagrai or Nasagre (nose)

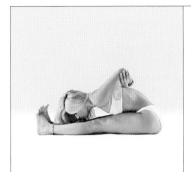

Bound Hands Western Intense Stretch Pose

Baddha Hasta Paschimottanasana

(BUH-duh HUH-stuh puhsh-chi-mo-tahn-AHS-uh-nuh)

Also Known As: Seated Forward Bend

Pose Type: seated, forward bend

Drishti Point: Padayoragrai or Padayoragre (toes/feet), Nasagrai or Nasagre (nose)

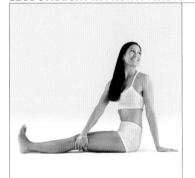

Reverse Prayer Western Intense Stretch Pose

Viparita Namaskar Paschimottanasana

(vi-puh-REE-tuh nuh-muhs-KAHR puhsh-chi-mo-tahn-AHS-uh-nuh)

Also Known As: Back of the Body Prayer Western Intense Stretch Pose (Paschima Namaskara Paschimottanasana), Reverse Prayer Forward Bend

Pose Type: seated, forward bend

Drishti Point: Padayoragrai or Padayoragre (toes/feet), Nasagrai or Nasagre (nose)

LEGS STRAIGHT IN FRONT: TWISTS

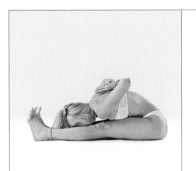

Revolved Staff Pose

Parivritta Dandasana

(puh-ri-VRIT-tuh duhn-DAHS-uh-nuh)

Pose Type: seated, twist

Drishti Point: Parshva Drishti (to the right), Parshva Drishti (to the left)

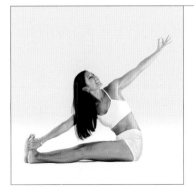

Revolved Upward One Arm Extended Hand to Foot Staff Pose

Parivritta Urdhva Eka Hasta Utthita Hasta Pada Dandasana

(puh-ri-VRIT-tuh OORD-vuh EY-kuh HUH-stuh UT-tu-tuh HUH-stuh PUH-duh duhn-DAHS-uh-nuh)

Pose Type: seated, forward bend, twist

Drishti Point: Hastagrai or Hastagre (hands)

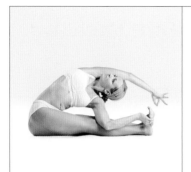

One Hand Revolved Western Intense Stretch Pose

Eka Hasta Parivritta Paschimottanasana
(EY-kuh HUH-stuh puh-ri-VRIT-tuh puhsh-chi-mo-tahn-AHS-uh-nuh)
Also Known As: One Hand Revolved Seated Forward Bend
Modification: one hand to the foot
Pose Type: seated, forward bend, side bend, twist
Drishti Point: Urdhva or Antara Drishti (up to the sky)

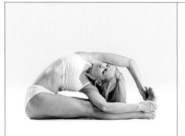

Two Hands Revolved Western Intense Stretch Pose

Dwi Hasta Parivritta Paschimottanasana
(DWI-huh-stuh puh-ri-VRIT-tuh puhsh-chi-mo-tahn-AHS-uh-nuh)
Also Known As: Two Hands Revolved Forward Bend
Pose Type: seated, forward bend, side bend, twist
Drishti Point: Urdhva or Antara Drishti (up to the sky)

LEGS STRAIGHT: ON THE SIDE & SCISSOR LEGS

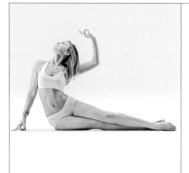

Upward Side Infinity Pose

Urdhva Parshva Anantasana
(OORD-vuh PARSH-vuh uh-nuhn-TAHS-uh-nuh)
Pose Type: seated, side bend
Drishti Point: Urdhva or Antara Drishti (up to the sky)

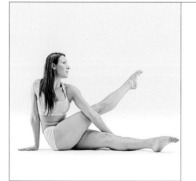

One Leg Upward Hand to Knee Revolved Staff Pose

Urdhva Eka Pada Janu Hasta Parivritta Dandasana
(OORD-vuh EY-kuh PUH-duh JAH-nu HUH-stuh puh-ri-VRIT-tuh duhn-DAHS-uh-nuh)
Pose Type: seated, forward bend, twist
Drishti Point: Padayoragrai or Padayoragre (toes/feet)

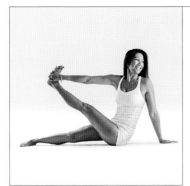

One Leg Upward Hand to Foot Revolved Staff Pose

Urdhva Eka Pada Hasta Pada Parivritta Dandasana

(OORD-vuh EY-kuh PUH-duh HUH-stuh PUH-duh puh-ri-VRIT-tuh duhn-DAHS-uh-nuh)

Pose Type: seated, forward bend, twist

Drishti Point: Parsva Drishti (to the right), Parsva Drishti (to the left)

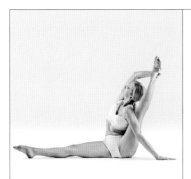

One Hand to Foot Archer's Pose

Eka Hasta Pada Akarna Dhanurasana

(EY-kuh HUH-stuh PUH-duh AH-kuhr-nuh duh-nur-AHS-uh-nuh)

Modification: both legs straight, knee behind the shoulder, other palm to the floor

Pose Type: seated, twist

Drishti Point: Urdhva or Antara Drishti (up to the sky)

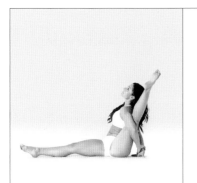

Bound Leg Archer's Pose

Baddha Pada Akarna Dhanurasana

(BUH-duh PUH-duh AH-kuhr-nuh duh-nur-AHS-uh-nuh)

Pose Type: seated, twist, binding

Drishti Point: Urdhva or Antara Drishti (up to the sky)

ONE LEG STRAIGHT, ONE LEG BENT

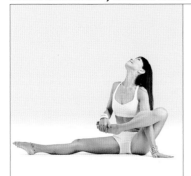

Archer's Pose Prep.

Akarna Dhanurasana Prep.

(AH-kuhr-nuh duh-nur-AHS-uh-nuh)

Modification: knee wrapping around the arm

Pose Type: seated, mild backbend

Drishti Point: Urdhva or Antara Drishti (up to the sky)

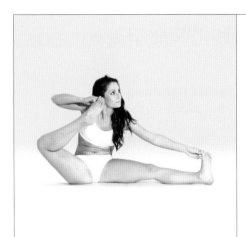

Archer's Pose

Akarna Dhanurasana

(AH-kuhr-nuh duh-nur-AHS-uh-nuh)

Modification: foot to the ear

Pose Type: seated, forward bend

Drishti Point: Bhrumadhye or Ajna Chakra (third eye, between the eyebrows)

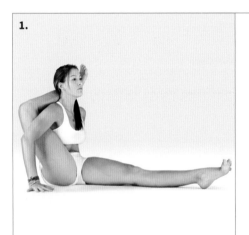

1.

Foot Behind the Head Pose

Eka Pada Shirshasana

(EY-kuh PUH-duh sheer-SHAHS-uh-nuh)

Also Known As: Foot Behind the Head Pose A (Eka Pada Shirshasana A)

Modification: leg straight

1. palms to the floor by the hips

2. hands in Anjali Mudra (Hands in Prayer)

Pose Type: seated

Drishti Point: Bhrumadhye or Ajna Chakra (third eye, between the eyebrows)

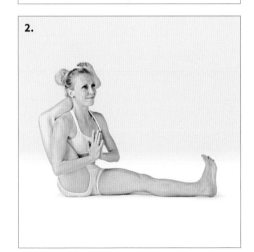

2.

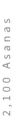

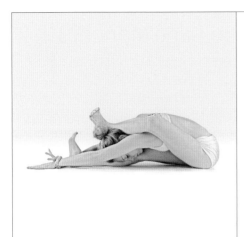

Pose Dedicated to Skanda

Skandasana

(skuhn-DAHS-uh-nuh)

Also Known As: Foot Behind the Head Pose B (Eka Pada Shirshasana B)
Pose Type: seated, forward bend
Drishti Point: Bhrumadhye or Ajna Chakra (third eye, between the eyebrows), Nasagrai or Nasagre (nose)

ONE LEG STRAIGHT, ONE LEG BENT: TWISTS

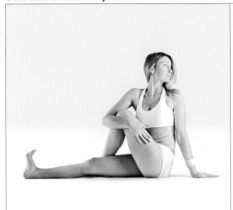

Easy Lord of the Fishes Pose Prep.

Sukha Matsyendrasana Prep.

(SUK-uh muhts-yeyn-DRAHS-uh-nuh)

Modification: one leg straight, arm wrapped around the bent knee
Pose Type: seated, forward bend, twist
Drishti Point: Parshva Drishti (to the right), Parshva Drishti (to the left)

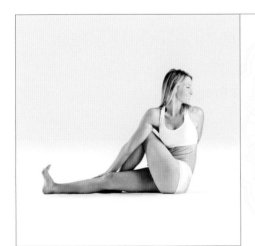

Easy Lord of the Fishes Pose

Sukha Matsyendrasana

(SUK-uh muhts-yeyn-DRAHS-uh-nuh)

Pose Type: seated, forward bend, twist, binding
Drishti Point: Parshva Drishti (to the right), Parshva Drishti (to the left)

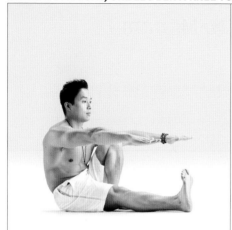

Pose Dedicated to Sage Marichi 1 & 2 Prep.

Marichyasana 1 & 2 Prep.
(muh-ree-CHYAHS-uh-nuh)
Also Known As: Pose Dedicated to Sage Marichi A & C Prep. (Marichyasana A & C Prep.)
Modification: arms parallel to the floor in front of the chest
Pose Type: seated, forward bend
Drishti Point: Hastagrai or Hastagre (hands)

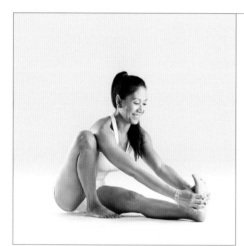

Pose Dedicated to Sage Marichi 1 & 2 Prep.

Marichyasana 1 & 2 Prep.
(muh-ree-CHYAHS-uh-nuh)
Also Known As: Pose Dedicated to Sage Marichi A & C Prep. (Marichyasana A & C Prep.)
Modification: both hands grabbing onto the foot of the straight leg
Pose Type: seated, forward bend
Drishti Point: Padhayoragrai or Padayoragre (toes/feet)

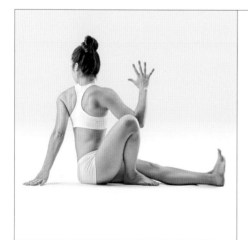

Revolved Pose Dedicated to Sage Marichi 1 Prep.

Parivritta Marichyasana 1 Prep.
(puh-ri-VRIT-tuh muh-ree-CHYAHS-uh-nuh)
Modification: twisting to the inside of the bent knee, elbow to the knee
Pose Type: seated, forward bend, twist
Drishti Point: Parshva Drishti (to the right), Parshva Drishti (to the left)

1.

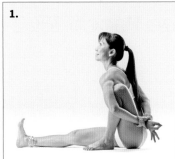

2.

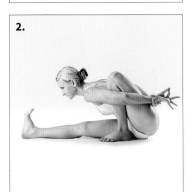

3.

Pose Dedicated to Sage Marichi 1

Marichyasana 1

(muh-ree-CHYAHS-uh-nuh)

Also Known As: Pose Dedicated to Sage Marichi A (Marichyasana A)

Modification: 1. spine straight

2. half forward bend

3. full forward bend, nose to the shin

Pose Type: seated, forward bend, binding

Drishti Point: 1. Bhrumadhye or Ajna Chakra (third eye, between the eyebrows)

2 & 3. Padhayoragrai or Padayoragre (toes/feet) or Nasagrai or Nasagre (nose)

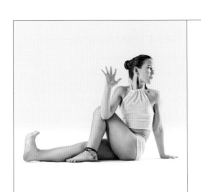

Pose Dedicated to Sage Marichi 2 Prep.

Marichyasana 2 Prep.

(muh-ree-CHYAHS-uh-nuh)

Also Known As: Pose Dedicated to Sage Marichi C (Marichyasana C)

Modification: elbow over the bent knee

Pose Type: seated, forward bend, twist

Drishti Point: Parshva Drishti (to the right), Parshva Drishti (to the left)

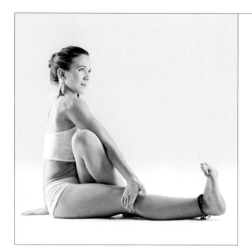

Pose Dedicated to Sage Marichi 2 Prep.

Marichyasana 2 Prep.

(muh-ree-CHYAHS-uh-nuh)

Also Known As: Pose Dedicated to Sage Marichi C (Marichyasana C)
Modification: grabbing onto the knee of the straight leg
Pose Type: seated, forward bend, twist, binding
Drishti Point: Bhrumadhye or Ajna Chakra (third eye, between the eyebrows) or Padhayoragrai or Padayoragre (toes/feet)

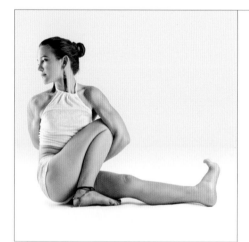

Pose dedicated to Sage Marichi 2

Marichyasana 2

(muh-ree-CHYAHS-uh-nuh)

Also Known As: Pose Dedicated to Sage Marichi C (Marichyasana C)
Pose Type: seated, forward bend, twist, binding
Drishti Point: Parshva Drishti (to the right), Parshva Drishti (to the left)

ONE LEG STRAIGHT & LIFTED, ONE LEG BENT

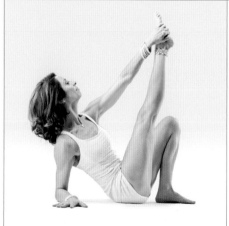

Seated Revolved Upward One Hand to Foot Pose

Upavishta Parivritta Urdhva Eka Pada Hastasana

(u-puh-VISH-tuh puh-ri-VRIT-tuh OORD-vuh EY-kuh PUH-duh huh-STAHS-uh-nuh)

Also Known As: Upavistha Parivritta Urdhva Eka Pada Hastasana
Modification: straight leg lifted, grabbing the foot with the opposite arm, other forearm on the floor
Pose Type: seated, forward bend
Drishti Point: Padhayoragrai or Padayoragre (toes/feet)

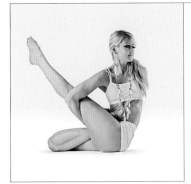

One Leg Extended Full Lord of the Fishes Pose

Utthita Eka Pada Paripurna Matsyendrasana
(UT-ti-tuh EY-kuh PUH-duh puh-ri-POOR-nuh muhts-yeyn-DRAHS-uh-nuh)
Pose Type: seated, forward bend, twist, binding
Drishti Point: Parshva Drishti (to the right), Parshva Drishti (to the left)

ONE LEG STRAIGHT, OTHER LEG CROSSED OVER: FOREARM & ELBOW TO THE FLOOR

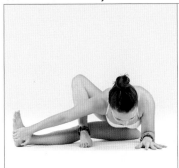

Revolved Western Intense Stretch Pose Hand to Foot Side Infinity Pose

Parivritta Paschimottana Hasta Pada Parshva Anantasana
(puh-ri-VRIT-tuh puhsh-chi-mo-TAHN-uh HUH-stuh PUH-duh PAHRSH-vuh uh-nuhn-TAHS-uh-nuh)
Also Known As: Revolved Seated Forward Bend Hand to Foot Side Infinity Pose
Pose Type: seated, forward bend, twist
Drishti Point: Angushtamadhye or Angushta Ma Dyai (thumbs), Nasagrai or Nasagre (nose)

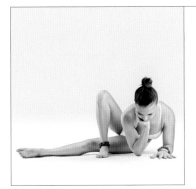

Revolved Western Intense Stretch Pose Uneven Arms Upward Side Infinity Pose

Parivritta Paschimottana Vishama Hasta Urdhva Parshva Anantasana
(puh-ri-VRIT-tuh puhsh-chi-mo-TAHN-uh VI-shuh-muh HUH-stuh OORD-vuh PAHRSH-vuh uh-nuhn-TAHS-uh-nuh)
Also Known As: Revolved Seated Forward Bend Uneven Arms Side Infinity Pose
Pose Type: seated, forward bend, twist
Drishti Point: Angushtamadhye or Angustha Ma Dyai (thumbs), Nasagrai or Nasagre (nose)

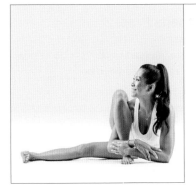

Revolved Western Intense Stretch Pose Bound Arms Upward Side Infinity Pose

Parivritta Paschimottana Baddha Hasta Urdhva Parshva Anantasana
(puh-ri-VRIT-tuh puhsh-chi-mo-TAHN-uh BUH-duh HUH-stuh OORD-vuh PAHRSH-vuh uh-nuhn-TAHS-uh-nuh)
Also Known As: Revolved Seated Forward Bend Bound Arms Upward Side Infinity Pose
Modification: arms wrapped around the foot, elbows toward the floor
Pose Type: seated, forward bend, twist
Drishti Point: Parshva Drishti (to the right), Parshva Drishti (to the left)

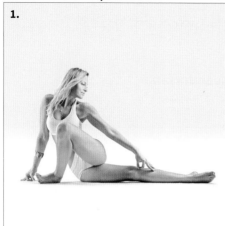

1.

Upward Side Infinity Pose

Urdhva Parshva Anantasana

(OORD-vuh PAHRSH-vuh uh-nuhn-TAHS-uh-nuh)

Modification: top leg crossed over, outside edge of the foot to the floor

1. looking to the side

2. head rolling back

Pose Type: 1. seated, side bend, twist

2. seated, side bend, twist, backbend

Drishti Point: 1. Hastagrai or Hastagre (hands), Padhayoragrai or Padayoragre (toes/feet)

2. Bhrumadhye or Ajna Chakra (third eye, between the eyebrows)

1.

2.

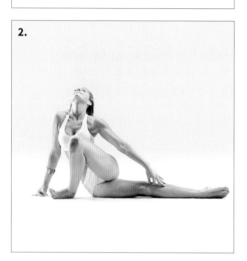

2.

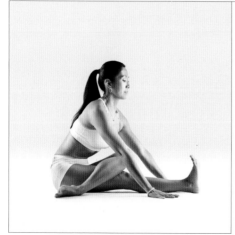

Half Cow Face Western Intense Stretch Pose Prep.

Ardha Gomukha Paschimottanasana Prep.

(UHR-duh GO-muk-uh puhsh-chi-mo-tahn-AHS-uh-nuh)

Also Known As: One-Legged Cow Face Western Intense Stretch Pose (Eka Pada Gomukha Paschimottanasana), Half Cow Face Seated Forward Bend

Modification: half forward bend

Pose Type: seated, forward bend

Drishti Point: Padhayoragrai or Padayoragre (toes/feet), Nasagrai or Nasagre (nose)

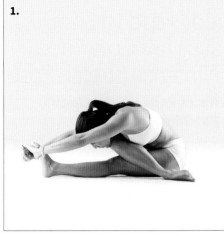

1.

Half Cow Face Western Intense Stretch Pose

Ardha Gomukha Paschimottanasana

(UHR-duh GO-muk-uh puhsh-chi-mo-tahn-AHS-uh-nuh)

Also Known As: One-Legged Cow Face Western Intense Stretch Pose (Eka Pada Gomukha Paschimottanasana), Half Cow Face Seated Forward Bend

Modification: 1. grabbing onto the wrist, chin to the knee

2. chin to the knee, arms straight, palms down in front of the foot

Pose Type: seated, forward bend

Drishti Point: Padhayoragrai or Padayoragre (toes/feet), Nasagrai or Nasagre (nose)

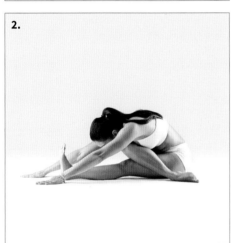

2.

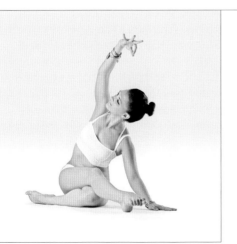

Revolved Sideways Half Cow Face Western Intense Stretch Pose

Parivritta Parshva Ardha Gomukha Paschimottanasana

(puh-ri-VRIT-tuh PAHRSH-vuh EY-kuh PUH-duh GO-muk-uh puhsh-chi-mo-tahn-AHS-uh-nuh)

Also Known As: Revolved Sideways One-Legged Cow Face Western Intense Stretch Pose (Parivritta Parshva Eka Pada Gomukha Paschimottanasana), Revolved Sideways Half Cow Face Seated Forward Bend

Modification: top leg straight

Pose Type: seated, forward bend, side bend, twist

Drishti Point: Padhayoragrai or Padayoragre (toes/feet), Hastagrai or Hastagre (hands), Parshva Drishti (to the right), Parshva Drishti (to the left)

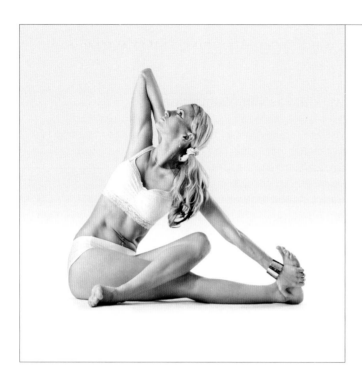

Revolved Hand to Foot Sideways Half Cow Face Western Intense Stretch Pose

Parivritta Hasta Pada Parshva Ardha Gomukha Paschimottanasana

(puh-ri-VRIT-tuh HUH-stuh PUH-duh PAHRSH-vuh UHR-duh GO-muk-uh puhsh-chi-mo-tahn-AHS-uh-nuh)

Also Known As: Revolved Hand to Foot Sideways One-Legged Cow Face Western Intense Stretch Pose (Parivritta Hasta Pada Parshva Eka Pada Gomukha Paschimottanasana), Revolved Hand to Foot Sideways Half Cow Face Seated Forward Bend

Modification: bottom leg straight, looking up to the sky

Pose Type: seated, forward bend, twist

Drishti Point: Urdhva or Antara Drishti (up to the sky)

HALF COW FACE POSE: LEG LIFTED

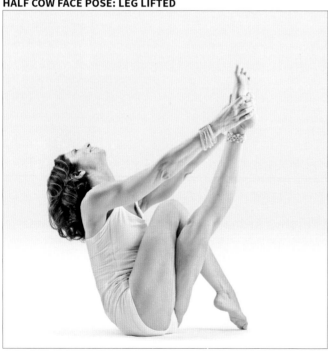

Upward Half Cow Face Western Intense Stretch Pose

Urdhva Ardha Gomukha Paschimottanasana

(OORD-vuh UHR-duh GO-muk-uh puhsh-chi-mo-tahn-AHS-uh-nuh)

Also Known As: Upward One-Legged Cow Face Western Intense Stretch Pose (Urdhva Eka Pada Gomukha Paschimottanasana), Upward Half Cow Face Seated Forward Bend

Modification: bottom leg straight, grabbing onto the foot

Pose Type: seated, forward bend, core

Drishti Point: Bhrumadhye or Ajna Chakra (third eye, between the eyebrows), Urdhva or Antara Drishti (up to the sky)

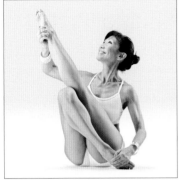

Upward Half Cow Face Western Intense Stretch Pose

Urdhva Ardha Gomukha Paschimottanasana

(OORD-vuh UHR-duh GO-muk-uh puhsh-chi-mo-tahn-AHS-uh-nuh)

Also Known As: Upward One-Legged Cow Face Western Intense Stretch Pose (Urdhva Eka Pada Gomukha Paschimottanasana), Upward Half Cow Face Seated Forward Bend
Modification: top leg straight, grabbing onto both feet
Pose Type: seated, forward bend, core
Drishti Point: Padhayoragrai or Padayoragre (toes/feet)

ONE LEG STRAIGHT, ONE LEG BENT: SHOULDER TO THE BACK OF THE KNEE

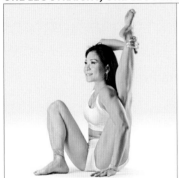

Sundial Pose 2

Surya Yantrasana 2

(SOOR-yuh yuhn-trahn-AHS-uh-nuh)
Pose Type: seated, forward bend
Drishti Point: Nasagrai or Nasagre (nose), Bhrumadhye or Ajna Chakra (third eye, between the eyebrows)

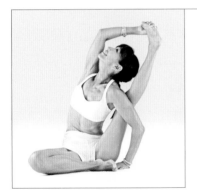

Sundial Pose 1

Surya Yantrasana 1

(SOOR-yuh yuhn-trahn-AHS-uh-nuh)
Pose Type: seated, twist
Drishti Point: Urdhva or Antara Drishti (up to the sky)

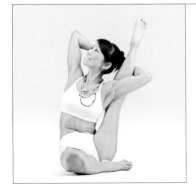

Upward Bound Hands Sundial Pose 1

Urdhva Baddha Hasta Surya Yantrasana 1

(OORD-vuh BUH-duh HUH-stuh SOOR-yuh yuhn-trahn-AHS-uh-nuh)
Pose Type: seated, twist, binding
Drishti Point: Urdhva or Antara Drishti (up to the sky)

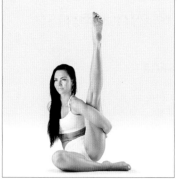

Downward Bound Hands Sundial Pose 1

Adho Baddha Hasta Surya Yantrasana 1

(uh-DO BUH-duh HUH-stuh SOOR-yuh yuhn-trahn-AHS-uh-nuh)

Pose Type: seated, forward bend, binding

Drishti Point: Nasagrai or Nasagre (nose), Bhrumadhye or Ajna Chakra (third eye, between the eyebrows)

ONE LEG STRAIGHT, ONE LEG BENT: HALF LOTUS & BINDING

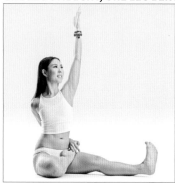

Half Bound Lotus Western Intense Stretch Pose Prep.

Ardha Baddha Padma Paschimottanasana Prep.

(UHR-duh BUH-duh PUHD-muh puhsh-chi-mo-tahn-AHS-uh-nuh)

Also Known As: Half Bound Lotus Seated Forward Bend Prep.

Modification: arm extended to the sky

Pose Type: seated, binding

Drishti Point: Nasagrai or Nasagre (nose), Bhrumadhye or Ajna Chakra (third eye, between the eyebrows)

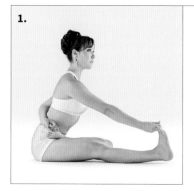

1.

Half Bound Lotus Western Intense Stretch Pose

Ardha Baddha Padma Paschimottanasana

(UHR-duh BUH-duh PUHD-muh puhsh-chi-mo-tahn-AHS-uh-nuh)

Also Known As: Half Bound Lotus Seated Forward Bend

Modification: 1. half forward bend

2. full forward bend

Pose Type: seated, forward bend, binding

Drishti Point: Padhayoragrai or Padayoragre (toes/feet), Nasagrai or Nasagre (nose), Bhrumadhye or Ajna Chakra (third eye, between the eyebrows)

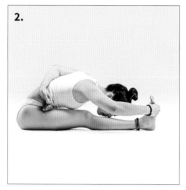

2.

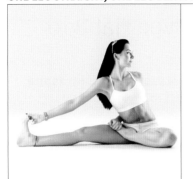

Revolved Half Bound Lotus Western Intense Stretch Pose

Parivritta Ardha Baddha Padma Paschimottanasana

(puh-ri-VRIT-tuh UHR-duh BUH-duh PUHD-muh puhsh-chi-mo-tahn-AHS-uh-nuh)

Also Known As: Revolved Half Bound Lotus Seated Forward Bend and Half Lord of the Fishes Pose (Ardha Matsyendrasana)

Modification: grabbing onto the big toe

Pose Type: seated, forward bend, twist, binding

Drishti Point: Parshva Drishti (to the right), Parshva Drishti (to the left)

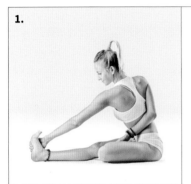

1.

Half Lord of The Fishes Pose 2

Ardha Matsyendrasana 2

(UHR-duh muhts-yeyn-DRAHS-uh-nuh)

Also Known As: Sage Warrior Bharadvaja Prep. (Bharadvajasana Prep.)

Modification: 1. looking toward the foot

2. looking over the shoulder

Pose Type: seated, forward bend, twist, binding

Drishti Point: 1. Padhayoragrai or Padayoragre (toes/feet)

2. Parshva Drishti (to the right), Parshva Drishti (to the left)

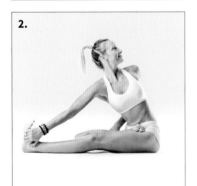

2.

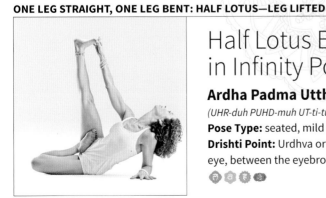

Half Lotus Extended Hand to Big Toe Pose in Infinity Pose

Ardha Padma Utthita Hasta Padangusthasana in Anantasana

(UHR-duh PUHD-muh UT-ti-tuh HUH-stuh puhd-ahng-goosh-TAHS-uh-nuh in uhn-uhnt-AHS-uh-nuh)

Pose Type: seated, mild backbend

Drishti Point: Urdhva or Antara Drishti (up to the sky), Bhrumadhye or Ajna Chakra (third eye, between the eyebrows)

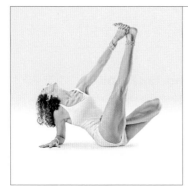

Half Lotus Extended Revolved Hand to Foot Pose in Infinity Pose

Ardha Padma Utthita Parivritta Pada Hastasana in Anantasana

(UHR-duh PUHD-muh UT-ti-tuh puh-ri-VRIT-tuh PUH-duh huh-STAHS-uh-nuh in uhn-uhnt-AHS-uh-nuh)

Modification: grabbing onto the foot on the opposite side

Pose Type: seated, mild backbend, forward bend

Drishti Point: Bhrumadhye or Ajna Chakra (third eye, between the eyebrows)

ONE LEG STRAIGHT, ONE LEG BENT: HALF LOTUS & BACKBEND—BINDING

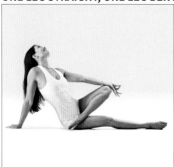

Half Lotus Upward Infinity Pose

Ardha Padma Urdhva Anantasana

(UHR-duh PUHD-muh OORD-vuh uhn-uhnt-AHS-uh-nuh)

Pose Type: seated

Drishti Point: Urdhva or Antara Drishti (up to the sky), Bhrumadhye or Ajna Chakra (third eye, between the eyebrows)

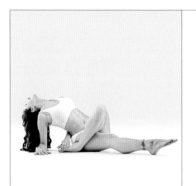

Half Bound Lotus Infinity Pose

Ardha Baddha Padma Anantasana

(UHR-duh BUH-duh PUHD-muh uhn-uhnt-AHS-uh-nuh)

Modification: Arm 1: forearm to the floor

Arm 2: grabbing onto the foot

Pose Type: seated, mild backbend, binding

Drishti Point: Bhrumadhye or Ajna Chakra (third eye, between the eyebrows)

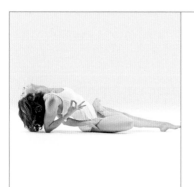

Half Bound Lotus Infinity Pose

Ardha Baddha Padma Anantasana

(UHR-duh BUH-duh PUHD-muh uhn-uhnt-AHS-uh-nuh)

Modification: Arm 1: elbow to the floor

Arm 2: hand to the hip socket

Pose Type: seated, mild backbend, binding

Drishti Point: Bhrumadhye or Ajna Chakra (third eye, between the eyebrows)

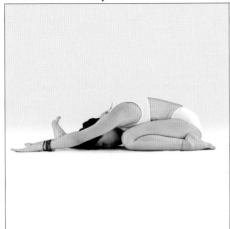

Three Limbed Face to Foot Western Intense Stretch Pose

Trianga Mukhaikapada Paschimottanasana

(tri-UHNG-uh muk-EYE-kuh-puh-duh puhsh-chi-mo-tahn-AHS-uh-nuh)
Also Known As: Three Limbed Face to Foot Seated Forward Bend
Pose Type: seated, forward bend
Drishti Point: Nasagrai or Nasagre (nose)

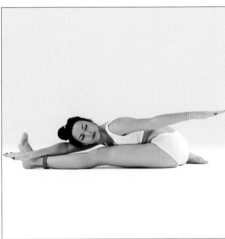

Churning Pose

Chalanasana

(chuh-luh-NAHS-uh-nuh)
Pose Type: seated, forward bend, twist
Drishti Point: Hastagrai or Hastagre (hands)

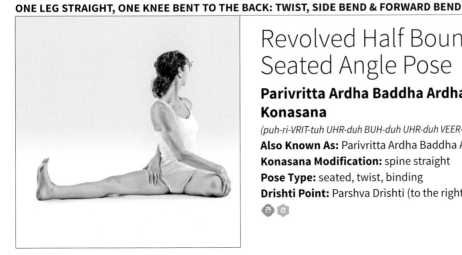

Revolved Half Bound Half Hero Half Seated Angle Pose

Parivritta Ardha Baddha Ardha Vira Ardha Upavishta Konasana

(puh-ri-VRIT-tuh UHR-duh BUH-duh UHR-duh VEER-uh UHR-duh u-puh-VISH-tuh ko-NAHS-uh-nuh)
Also Known As: Parivritta Ardha Baddha Ardha Vira Ardha Upavistha Konasana
Konasana Modification: spine straight
Pose Type: seated, twist, binding
Drishti Point: Parshva Drishti (to the right), Parshva Drishti (to the left)

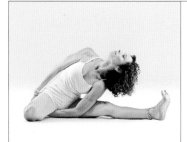

Gate Pose

Parighasana
(puh-ri-GAHS-uh-nuh)

Modification: side bend toward the straight leg; grabbing onto the heel of the bent leg with both hands
Pose Type: seated, side bend, forward bend, binding
Drishti Point: Urdhva or Antara Drishti (up to the sky)

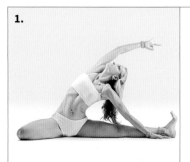

Gate Pose

Parighasana
(puh-ri-GAHS-uh-nuh)

Modification: seated: 1. palm to the floor by the ankle, other arm up over the head
2. elbow to the floor by the knee
3. both hands grabbing onto the foot, chest rotated up to the sky
Pose Type: 1 & 2. seated, side bend
3. seated, side bend, twist
Drishti Point: 1. Hastagrai or Hastagre (hands)
2 & 3. Urdhva or Antara Drishti (up to the sky)

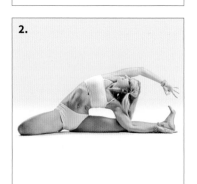

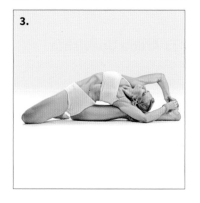

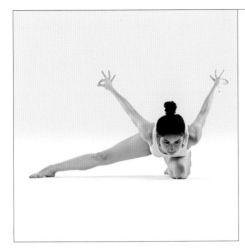

Benu Bird Pose 1

Benvasana 1

(ben-VAHS-uh-nuh)

Modification: seated; sitting bone on the heel, forward bend; arms to the side and to the back

Pose Type: seated, forward bend

Drishti Point: Nasagrai or Nasagre (nose)

ONE LEG STRAIGHT, ONE KNEE BENT TO THE BACK: LEG LIFTED—BACKBEND

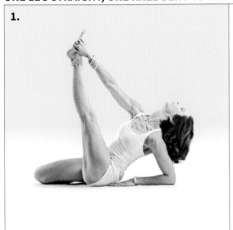

Reclined Half Hero Extended Hand to Foot Pose

Supta Ardha Vira Utthita Hasta Padasana

(SUP-tuh UHR-duh VEER-uh UT-ti-tuh HUH-stuh PUH-duhs-uh-nuh)

Modification: 1. right side view

2. left side view

Pose Type: seated, mild backbend, twist

Drishti Point: Urdhva or Antara Drishti (up to the sky), Bhrumadhye or Ajna Chakra (third eye, between the eyebrows)

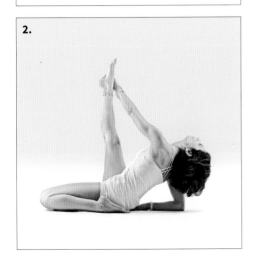

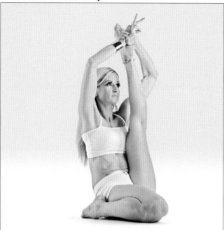

Heron Pose

Krounchasana

(crown-CHAHS-uh-nuh)
Modification: grabbing onto the wrist, toes pointed
Pose Type: seated, forward bend
Drishti Point: Nasagrai or Nasagre (nose), Bhrumadhye or Ajna Chakra (third eye, between the eyebrows)

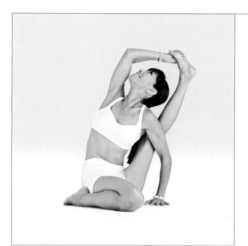

Sundial Pose 3

Surya Yantrasana 3

(SOOR-yuh yuhn-TRAHS-uh-nuh)
Modification: foot turned to the back
Pose Type: seated, twist
Drishti Point: Urdhva or Antara Drishti (up to the sky)

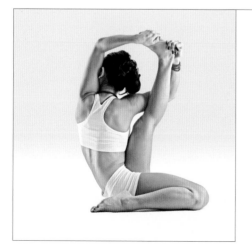

Revolved Heron Pose

Parivritta Krounchasana

(puh-ri-VRIT-tuh crown-CHAHS-uh-nuh)
Also Known As: Revolved Sundial Pose 3 (Parivritta Surya Yantrasana 3)
Pose Type: seated, forward bend, twist
Drishti Point: Parshva Drishti (to the right), Parshva Drishti (to the left)

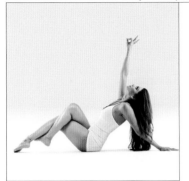

Seated Leg Position of the Pose Dedicated to Garuda

Upavishta Pada Garudasana
(u-puh-VISH-tuh PUH-duh guh-ru-DAHS-uh-nuh)

Also Known As: Upavistha Pada Garudasana
Modification: backbend, one hand to the sky
Pose Type: seated, backbend
Drishti Point: Hastagrai or Hastagre (hands)

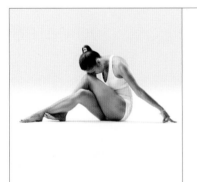

Revolved Hand to Foot Seated Leg Position of the Pose Dedicated to Garuda

Parivritta Hasta Pada Upavishta Pada Garudasana
(puh-ri-VRIT-tuh HUH-stuh PUH-duh u-puh-VISH-tuh PUH-duh guh-ru-DAHS-uh-nuh)

Also Known As: Parivritta Hasta Pada Upavistha Pada Garudasana
Pose Type: seated, forward bend, twist
Drishti Point: Hastagrai or Hastagre (hands)

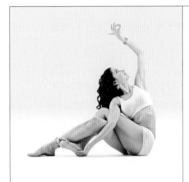

Seated Leg Position of the Pose Dedicated to Garuda

Upavishta Pada Garudasana
(u-puh-VISH-tuh PUH-duh guh-ru-DAHS-uh-nuh)

Also Known As: Upavistha Pada Garudasana
Modification: forehead to the knee
Pose Type: seated, forward bend
Drishti Point: Nasagrai or Nasagre (nose)

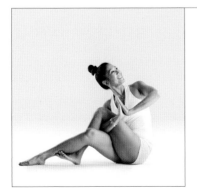

Revolved Seated Leg Position of the Pose Dedicated to Garuda

Parivritta Upavishta Pada Garudasana
(puh-ri-VRIT-tuh u-puh-VISH-tuh PUH-duh guh-ru-DAHS-uh-nuh)

Also Known As: Parivritta Upavistha Pada Garudasana
Modification: hands in Anjali Mudra (Hands in Prayer), one arm threaded through the legs
Pose Type: seated, forward bend, twist
Drishti Point: Parshva Drishti (to the right), Parshva Drishti (to the left)

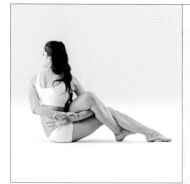

Bound Revolved Seated Leg Position of the Pose Dedicated to Garuda

Baddha Parivritta Upavishta Pada Garudasana

(BUH-duh puh-ri-VRIT-tuh u-puh-VISH-tuh PUH-duh guh-ru-DAHS-uh-nuh)

Also Known As: Baddha Parivritta Upavistha Pada Garudasana

Pose Type: seated, forward bend, twist, binding

Drishti Point: Parshva Drishti (to the right), Parshva Drishti (to the left)

GARUDA LEGS: KNEES TO THE FLOOR ON THE SIDE

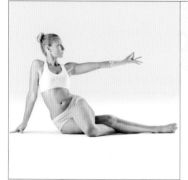

Seated Leg Position of the Pose Dedicated to Garuda in Upward Side Infinity Pose

Upavishta Pada Garudasana in Urdhva Parshva Anantasana

(u-puh-VISH-tuh PUH-duh guh-ru-DAHS-uh-nuh in OORD-vuh PAHRSH-vuh uhn-uhnt-AHS-uh-nuh)

Also Known As: Upavistha Pada Garudasana in Urdhva Parshva Anantasana

Modification: one hand to the floor, one arm extended out

Pose Type: seated, side bend

Drishti Point: Hastagrai or Hastagre (hands)

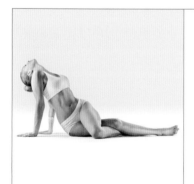

Seated Leg Position of the Pose Dedicated to Garuda in Upward Side Infinity Pose

Upavishta Pada Garudasana in Urdhva Parshva Anantasana

(u-puh-VISH-tuh PUH-duh guh-ru-DAHS-uh-nuh in OORD-vuh PAHRSH-vuh uhn-uhnt-AHS-uh-nuh)

Modification: palms flat on the floor, fingertips pointing away from the heels, backbend

Pose Type: seated, side bend, backbend

Drishti Point: Bhrumadhye or Ajna Chakra (third eye, between the eyebrows)

BOTH KNEES BENT: ANKLES HOOKED—TWIST & SIDE BEND

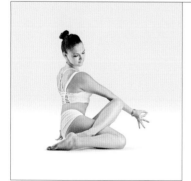

Twist Dedicated to Sage Bharadvaja 3

Bharadvajasana 3

(buh-ruhd-vahj-AHS-uh-nuh)

Pose Type: seated, forward bend, twist

Drishti Point: Padhayoragrai or Padayoragre (toes/feet)

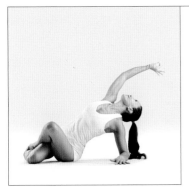

Sideways Twist Dedicated to Sage Bharadvaja 3

Parshva Bharadvajasana 3

(PAHRSH-vuh buh-ruhd-vahj-AHS-uh-nuh)

Modification: forearm to the floor
Pose Type: seated, mild backbend, side bend
Drishti Point: Hastagrai or Hastagre (hands)

LEG CRADLE: ONE LEG STRAIGHT

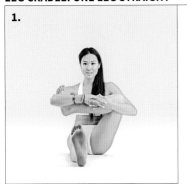

1.

Baby Cradle Pose

Hindolasana

(hin-do-LAHS-uh-nuh)

Also Known As: One Foot Behind the Head Pose A & B Prep. (Eka Pada Shirshasana A & B Prep.)
Modification: leg straight
1. spine straight, front view
2. half forward bend, side view
Pose Type: seated, forward bend
Drishti Point: Nasagrai or Nasagre (nose), Padhayoragrai or Padayoragre (toes/feet), Bhrumadhye or Ajna Chakra (third eye, between the eyebrows)

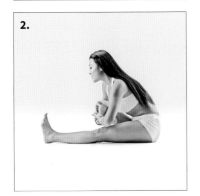

2.

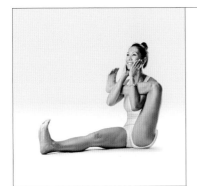

Baby Cradle Pose

Hindolasana

(hin-do-LAHS-uh-nuh)

Also Known As: One Foot Behind the Head Pose A Prep. (Eka Pada Shirshasana A Prep.)
Modification: leg straight, hands to the face
Pose Type: seated, forward bend
Drishti Point: Nasagrai or Nasagre (nose), Bhrumadhye or Ajna Chakra (third eye, between the eyebrows)

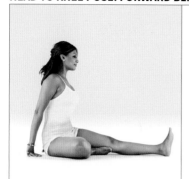

Head to Knee Pose Prep.

Janu Shirshasana Prep.

(JAH-nu sheer-SHAHS-uh-nuh)

Modification: palms to the floor by the hips, spine straight

Pose Type: seated

Drishti Point: Nasagrai or Nasagre (nose), Padhayoragrai or Padayoragre (toes/feet)

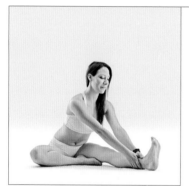

Both Hands to Ankle Head to Knee Pose

Dwi Hasta Kulpa Janu Shirshasana

(DWI-huh-stuh KUL-puh JAH-nu sheer-SHAHS-uh-nuh)

Pose Type: seated, forward bend

Drishti Point: Nasagrai or Nasagre (nose), Padhayoragrai or Padayoragre (toes/feet)

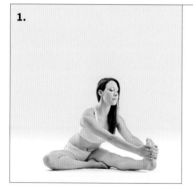
1.

Both Hands to Foot Head to Knee Pose

Dwi Hasta Pada Janu Shirshasana

(DWI-huh-stuh PUH-duh JAH-nu sheer-SHAHS-uh-nuh)

Modification: 1. grabbing onto the foot; fingers interlocked, half forward bend

2. grabbing onto the wrist, half forward bend

Pose Type: seated, forward bend

Drishti Point: Padhayoragrai or Padayoragre (toes/feet), Nasagrai or Nasagre (nose)

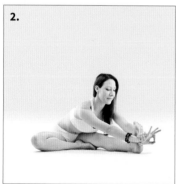
2.

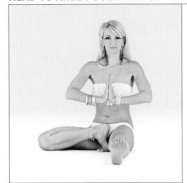

Head to Knee Pose C Prep.

Janu Shirshasana C Prep.

(JAH-nu sheer-SHAHS-uh-nuh)

Also Known As: Half Root Lock Pose (Ardha Mula Bandhasana)

Pose Type: seated

Drishti Point: Nasagrai or Nasagre (nose), Padhayoragrai or Padayoragre (toes/feet), Bhrumadhye or Ajna Chakra (third eye, between the eyebrows)

1.

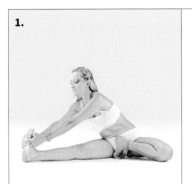

Head to Knee Pose C

Janu Shirshasana C

(JAH-nu sheer-SHAHS-uh-nuh)

Modification: 1. half forward bend

2. full forward bend

Pose Type: seated, forward bend

Drishti Point: Padhayoragrai or Padayoragre (toes/feet), Nasagrai or Nasagre (nose)

2.

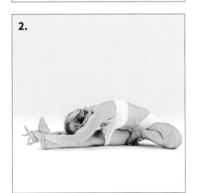

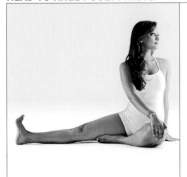

Revolved Half Bound Angle Pose

Parivritta Ardha Baddha Konasana

(puh-ri-VRIT-tuh UHR-duh BUH-duh ko-NAHS-uh-nuh)

Modification: hand to the knee, other hand to the floor behind the hips for support

Pose Type: seated, twist

Drishti Point: Parshva Drishti (to the right), Parshva Drishti (to the left)

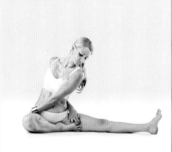

Revolved Half Bound Angle Pose

Parivritta Ardha Baddha Konasana

(puh-ri-VRIT-tuh UHR-duh BUH-duh ko-NAHS-uh-nuh)

Pose Type: seated, twist, binding

Drishti Point: Parshva Drishti (to the right), Parshva Drishti (to the left)

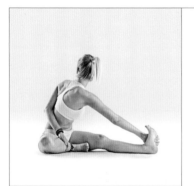

Revolved Sideways Half Bound Angle Pose

Parivritta Parshva Ardha Baddha Konasana

(puh-ri-VRIT-tuh PAHRSH-vuh UHR-duh BUH-duh ko-NAHS-uh-nuh)

Modification: grabbing onto the big toe of the bent leg

Pose Type: seated, twist, side bend, binding

Drishti Point: Padhayoragrai or Padayoragre (toes/feet)

Revolved Half Bound Angle Pose

Parivritta Ardha Baddha Konasana

(puh-ri-VRIT-tuh UHR-duh BUH-duh ko-NAHS-uh-nuh)

Modification: looking back

Arm 1: grabbing onto the outside edge of the opposite foot

Arm 2: grabbing onto the shin of the opposite leg behind the back

Pose Type: seated, forward bend, twist, binding

Drishti Point: Parshva Drishti (to the right), Parshva Drishti (to the left)

HEAD TO KNEE POSE— SIDE BENDS

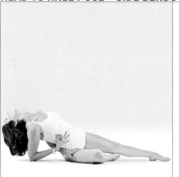

Half Bound Angle Pose in Infinity Pose

Ardha Baddha Konasana in Anantasana

(UHR-duh BUH-duh ko-NAHS-uh-nuh in uhn-uhnt-AHS-uh-nuh)

Modification: elbow to the floor, head rolling back

Pose Type: seated, mild backbend, side bend, binding

Drishti Point: Bhrumadhye or Ajna Chakra (third eye, between the eyebrows)

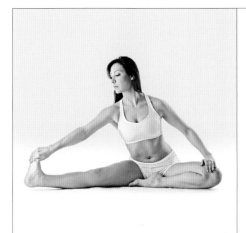

Revolved Head to Knee Pose Prep.

Parivritta Janu Shirshasana Prep.

(puh-ri-VRIT-tuh JAH-nu sheer-SHAHS-uh-nuh)

Modification: grabbing onto the foot, other hand to the knee

Pose Type: seated, forward bend

Drishti Point: Padhayoragrai or Padayoragre (toes/feet)

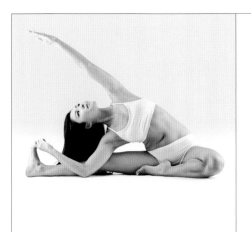

Sideways Head to Knee Pose

Parshva Janu Shirshasana

(PAHRSH-vuh JAH-nu sheer-SHAHS-uh-nuh)

Also Known As: Sideways Half Bound Angle Pose (Parshva Ardha Baddha Konasana)

Pose Type: seated, side bend

Drishti Point: Hastagrai or Hastagre (hands)

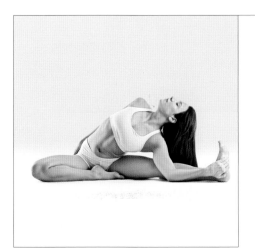

Sideways Head to Knee Pose

Parshva Janu Shirshasana

(PAHRSH-vuh JAH-nu sheer-SHAHS-uh-nuh)

Also Known As: Sideways Half Bound Angle Pose (Parshva Ardha Baddha Konasana)

Modification: elbow to the floor on the inside of the leg, other hand on the hip

Pose Type: seated, forward bend, side bend

Drishti Point: Urdhva or Antara Drishti (up to the sky)

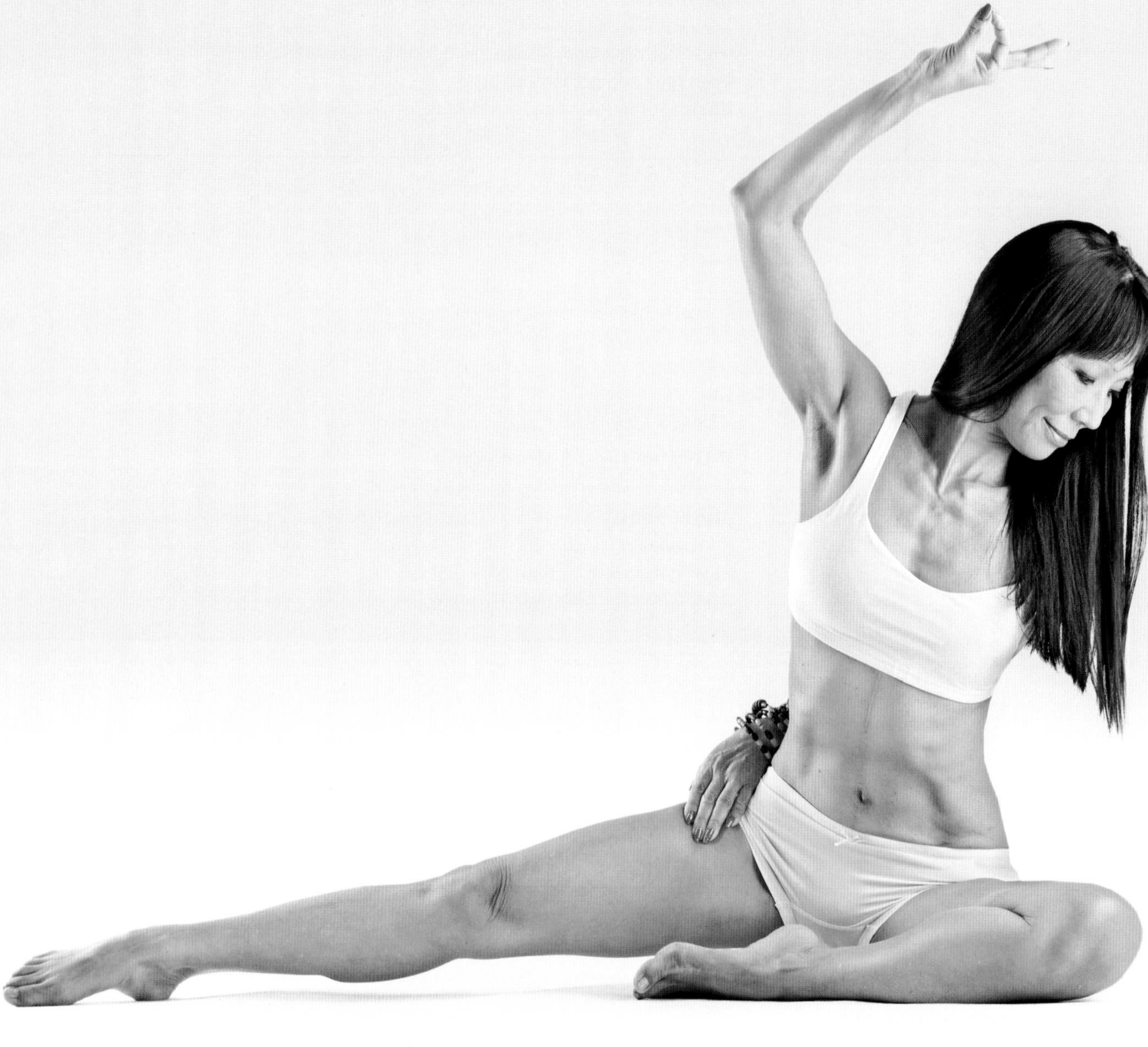

Half Bound
Half Seated Angle Pose

Ardha Baddha Ardha Upavishta Konasana
(UHR-duh BUH-duh UHR-duh u-puh-VISH-tuh ko-NAHS-uh-nuh)
Also Known As: Ardha Baddha Ardha Upavistha Konasana
Pose Type: seated, side bend, binding
Drishti Point: Nasagrai or Nasagre (nose)

Modification: side bend toward the bent knee

ardha = half
baddha = bound
ardha = half
upavishta = seated
kona = angle

How to Perform the Pose:

1. Begin by sitting on the floor with both your legs straight out in front of you. Engage your *mula bandha*, *uddhiyana bandha*, and *ujjayi* breathing.

2. Exhale as you bend your left knee and bring the sole of your left foot toward your right thigh.

3. On the next exhale, bring your right leg out to the right side, keeping it strong and straight by pulling up the kneecap and engaging the thigh muscles (quadriceps). Press your right toes and your right heel to the floor, lifting the right leg slightly on off the floor.

4. Inhale as you expand your chest and hold your arms straight out to the sides, parallel to the floor.

5. Exhale as you bend your left arm and reach your left hand behind the back to the inside of your right thigh to bind.

6. Inhale as you reach your right arm up to the sky. Exhale as you bend your right elbow and look toward your left knee.

7. Hold the pose for at least 30, and up to 90, seconds in order to receive full benefits of the stretch.

8. Inhale as you release the bind. Exhale as you bring both your legs straight out in front of you. Repeat on the other side.

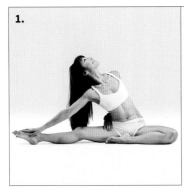

Half Bound Sideways Head to Knee Pose

Ardha Baddha Parshva Janu Shirshasana

(UHR-duh BUH-duh PAHRSH-vuh JAH-nu sheer-SHAHS-uh-nuh)

Also Known As: Sideways Half Bound Angle Pose (Parshva Ardha Baddha Konasana)

Modification: 1. toes pointed

2. toes flexed in

Pose Type: seated, forward bend, side bend, twist, binding

Drishti Point: Urdhva or Antara Drishti (up to the sky)

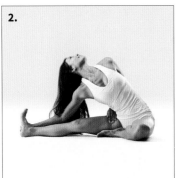

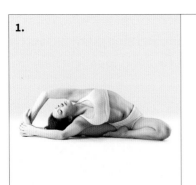

Revolved Head to Knee Pose

Parivritta Janu Shirshasana

(puh-ri-VRIT-tuh JAH-nu sheer-SHAHS-uh-nuh)

Modification: elbow to the floor

1. forearm to the floor, chest to the side

2. head on the knee, chest to the sky

Pose Type: seated, side bend, twist

Drishti Point: Urdhva or Antara Drishti (up to the sky)

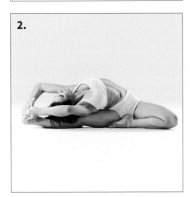

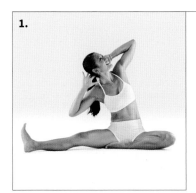

1.

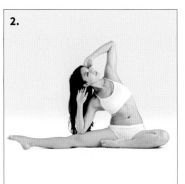

2.

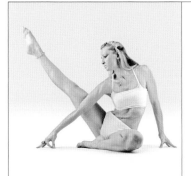

3.

Both Hands to the Head Sideways Head to Knee Pose

Dwi Hasta Shirsha Parshva Janu Shirshasana

(DWI-huh-stuh SHEER-shuh PAHRSH-vuh JAH-nu sheer-SHAHS-uh-nuh)

Also Known As: Sideways Half Bound Angle Pose (Parshva Ardha Baddha Konasana)

Modification: 1. slight side bend

2. elbow to the knee

3. elbow to the floor

Pose Type: seated, side bend

Drishti Point: Urdhva or Antara Drishti (up to the sky)

HEAD TO KNEE POSE: LEG LIFTED

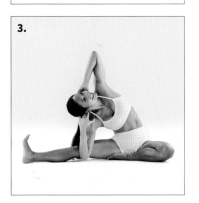

Hands Free Sundial Pose 1

Mukta Hasta Surya Yantrasana 1

(MUK-tuh HUH-stuh SOOR-yuh yuhn-TRAHS-uh-nuh)

Modification: foot to thigh, fingertips of both hands to the floor

Pose Type: seated, forward bend, side bend, core

Drishti Point: Hastagrai or Hastagre (hands)

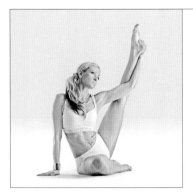

Sundial Pose 1

Surya Yantrasana 1

(SOOR-yuh yuhn-TRAHS-uh-nuh)

Modification: foot to thigh, grabbing onto the foot on the same side
Pose Type: seated, forward bend, side bend
Drishti Point: Parshva Drishti (to the right), Parshva Drishti (to the left)

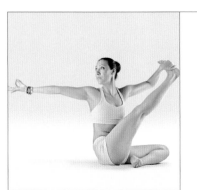

Unsupported Seated Revolved Upward One Hand to Foot Pose

Niralamba Upavishta Parivritta Urdhva Eka Pada Hastasana

(nir-AH-luhm-buh u-puh-VISH-tuh puh-ri-VRIT-tuh OORD-vuh EY-kuh PUH-duh huh-STAHS-uh-nuh)

Pose Type: seated, forward bend, twist, core
Drishti Point: Hastagrai or Hastagre (hands)

HERO POSE: TOES CURLED IN

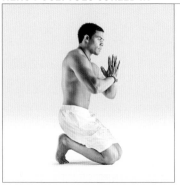

Tip Toe Hero Pose

Prapada Virasana

(PRUH-puh-duh veer-AHS-uh-nuh)

Also Known As: Thunderbolt Pose (Vajrasana)
Modification: toes curled in, hands in Anjali Mudra (Hands in Prayer)
Pose Type: seated
Drishti Point: Hastagrai or Hastagre (hands) or Nasagrai or Nasagre (nose)

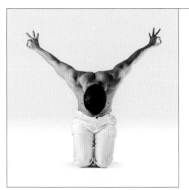

Tip Toe Hero Pose

Prapada Virasana

(PRUH-puh-duh veer-AHS-uh-nuh)

Also Known As: Thunderbolt Pose (Vajrasana)
Modification: head down, arms open wide
Pose Type: seated, forward bend
Drishti Point: Nasagrai or Nasagre (nose)

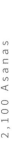

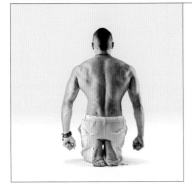

Hero Pose

Virasana

(veer-AHS-uh-nuh)

Also Known As: Thunderbolt Pose (Vajrasana)
Modification: arms to the sides; modified version for tight ankles
Pose Type: seated
Drishti Point: Nasagrai or Nasagre (nose)

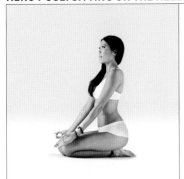

Hero Pose

Virasana

(veer-AHS-uh-nuh)

Also Known As: Thunderbolt Pose (Vajrasana)
Modification: hands on the knees, palms up
Pose Type: seated
Drishti Point: Nasagrai or Nasagre (nose), Bhrumadhye or Ajna Chakra (third eye, between the eyebrows)

1.

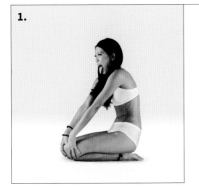

2.

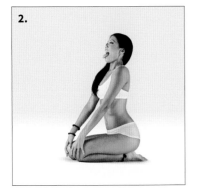

Lion Pose Dedicated to an Avatar of Lord Vishnu in Hero Pose

Narasimhasana in Virasana

(nuh-ruh-sim-HAHS-uh-nuh in veer-AHS-uh-nuh)

Also Known As: Lion Pose in Thunderbolt Pose (Simhasana in Vajrasana)
Modification: sitting on the heels
1. Cat Tilt
2. Dog Tilt
Pose Type: seated
1. forward bend
2. mild backbend
Drishti Point: Bhrumadhye or Ajna Chakra (third eye, between the eyebrows)

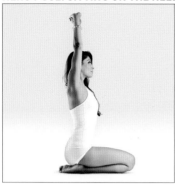

Hero Pose—Raised Bound Hands

Virasana Urdhva Baddha Hastasana

(veer-AHS-uh-nuh OORD-vuh BUH-duh huh-STAHS-uh-nuh)

Also Known As: Thunderbolt Pose Raised Bound Hands (Vajrasana Urdhva Baddha Hastasana)
Modification: palms facing up
Pose Type: seated
Drishti Point: Nasagrai or Nasagre (nose)

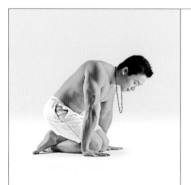

Hero Pose

Virasana

(veer-AHS-uh-nuh)

Also Known As: Thunderbolt Pose (Vajrasana)
Modification: forward bending, ankles crossed, palms to the floor by the knees
Pose Type: seated, forward bend
Drishti Point: Angushtamadhye or Angustha Ma Dyai (thumbs), Nasagrai or Nasagre (nose)

1.

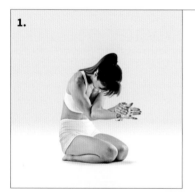

Hand Position of the Pose Dedicated to Garuda in Hero Pose

Hasta Garudasana in Virasana

(HUH-stuh guh-ru-DAHS-uh-nuh in veer-AHS-uh-nuh)

Also Known As: Hand Position of the Pose Dedicated to Garuda in Thunderbolt Pose (Hasta Garudasana in Vajrasana)
Modification: 1. half forward bend
2. spine straight
Pose Type: 1. seated, forward bend
2. seated
Drishti Point: Angushtamadhye or Angustha Ma Dyai (thumbs)

1.
2.

2.

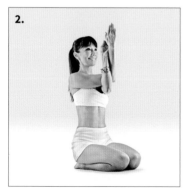

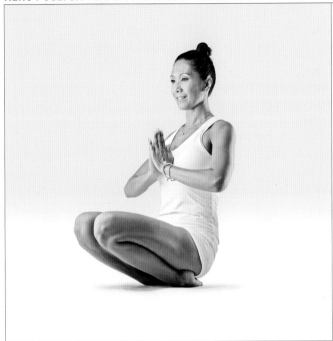

Hero Scale Pose with Hands in Prayer

Vira Tolasana Namaskar

(VEER-uh to-LAHS-uh-nuh nuh-muhs-KAHR)

Modification: hands in Anjali Mudra (Hands in Prayer)
Pose Type: seated, balance, core
Drishti Point: Nasagrai or Nasagre (nose) or Hastagrai or Hastagre (hands)

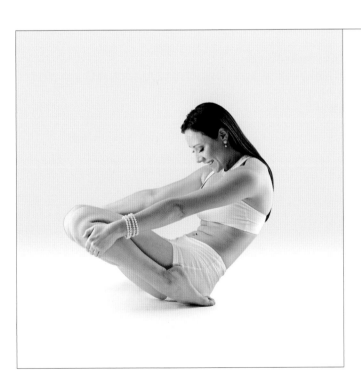

Hero Scale Pose

Vira Tolasana

(VEER-uh to-LAHS-uh-nuh)

Modification: grabbing onto the knees, Cat Tilt
Pose Type: seated, balance, core
Drishti Point: Nabhi, Nabhicakre, or Nabi Chakra (belly button)

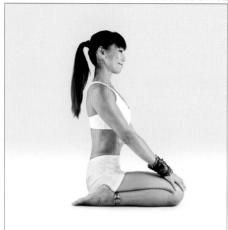

Hero Pose

Virasana

(veer-AHS-uh-nuh)

Also Known As: Thunderbolt Pose (Vajrasana)
Modification: sitting bones to the floor
Pose Type: seated
Drishti Point: Nasagrai or Nasagre (nose)

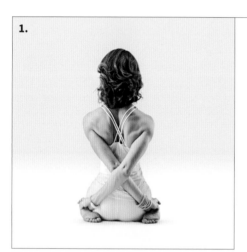

Both Hands to Feet Hero Pose

Dwi Hasta Pada Virasana

(DWI-huh-stuh PUH-duh veer-AHS-uh-nuh)

Also Known As: Both Hands to Feet Thunderbolt Pose (Dwi Hasta Pada Vajrasana)
Modification: sitting bones to the floor, arms crossed behind the back
1. back view
2. front view, mild backbend
Pose Type: 1. seated, binding
2. seated, mild backbend, binding
Drishti Point: Nasagrai or Nasagre (nose), Bhrumadhye or Ajna Chakra (third eye, between the eyebrows)

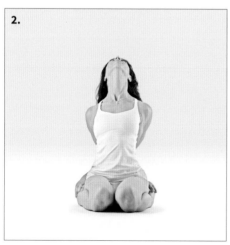

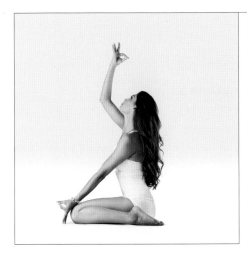

One Arm Upward Hero Pose

Eka Urdhva Hasta Virasana

(EY-kuh OORD-vuh HUH-stuh veer-AHS-uh-nuh)

Also Known As: One Arm Upward Thunderbolt Pose (Eka Urdhva Hasta Vajrasana)

Pose Type: seated

Drishti Point: Hastagrai or Hastagre (hands)

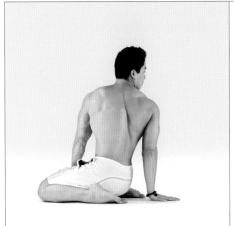

Hero Pose—Raised Bound Hands

Virasana Urdhva Baddha Hastasana

(veer-AHS-uh-nuh OORD-vuh BUH-duh huh-STAHS-uh-nuh)

Also Known As: Thunderbolt Pose Raised Bound Hands (Vajrasana Urdhva Baddha Hastasana)

Modification: palms facing up

Pose Type: seated

Drishti Point: Nasagrai or Nasagre (nose)

THUNDERBOLT POSE: SITTING BONES ON THE FLOOR—TWISTS & SIDE BEND

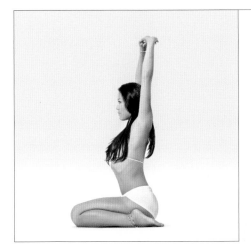

Revolved Hero Pose

Parivritta Virasana

(puh-ri-VRIT-tuh veer-AHS-uh-nuh)

Also Known As: Revolved Thunderbolt Pose (Parivritta Vajrasana)

Pose Type: seated, twist

Drishti Point: Parshva Drishti (to the right), Parshva Drishti (to the left)

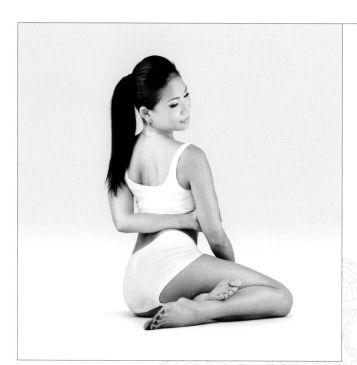

Pose Dedicated to Sage Bharadvaja 1

Bharadvajasana 1

(buh-ruhd-vuhj-AHS-uh-nuh)

Modification: ankles crossed, grabbing onto the bicep
Pose Type: seated, twist, binding
Drishti Point: Parshva Drishti (to the right), Parshva Drishti (to the left)

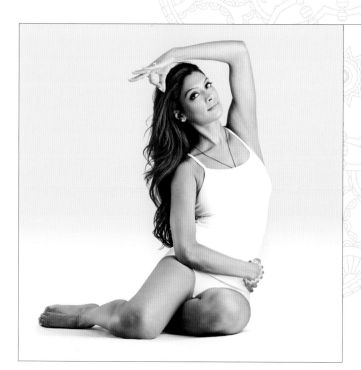

Sideways Pose Dedicated to Sage Bharadvaja 1

Parshva Bharadvajasana 1

(PAHRSH-vuh buh-ruhd-vuhj-AHS-uh-nuh)

Modification: one arm crossed in front; other arm over the head, elbow bent
Pose Type: seated, side bend
Drishti Point: Hastagrai or Hastagre (hands)

1.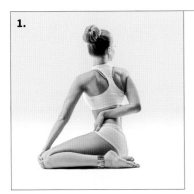

Pose Dedicated to Bharadvaja 1

Bharadvajasana 1

(buh-ruhd-vuhj-AHS-uh-nuh)

Modification: 1. grabbing onto the inside of the hip with opposite hand, other hand on the knee, looking over the shoulder
2. grabbing onto the tricep of the opposite arm, looking over the shoulder
Pose Type: seated, twist, binding
Drishti Point: Parshva Drishti (to the right), Parshva Drishti (to the left)

2.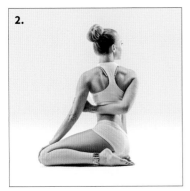

THUNDERBOLT POSE: SITTING BONES ON THE FLOOR—KNEES OPEN WIDE

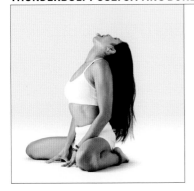

Lion Pose Dedicated to an Avatar of Lord Vishnu in Knees Spread Wide Hero Pose

Narasimhasana in Prasarita Janu Virasana

(nuh-ruh-sim-HAHS-uh-nuh in pruh-SAH-ri-tuh JAH-nu veer-AHS-uh-nuh)
Also Known As: Lion Pose (Simhasana)
Modification: sitting bones on the floor
Pose Type: seated, mild backbend
Drishti Point: Bhrumadhye or Ajna Chakra (third eye, between the eyebrows)

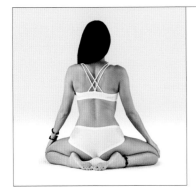

Knees Spread Wide Hero Pose

Prasarita Janu Virasana

(pruh-SAH-ri-tuh JAH-nu veer-AHS-uh-nuh)
Also Known As: Frog Pose (Mandukasana)
Modification: sitting bones off the floor
Pose Type: seated
Drishti Point: Nasagrai or Nasagre (nose)

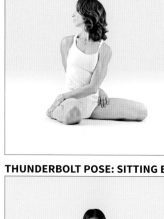

Half Bound Revolved Knees Spread Wide Hero Pose

Ardha Baddha Parivritta Prasarita Janu Virasana

(UHR-duh BUH-duh puh-ri-VRIT-tuh pruh-SAH-ri-tuh JAH-nu veer-AHS-uh-nuh)

Pose Type: seated, twist, binding

Drishti Point: Parshva Drishti (to the right), Parshva Drishti (to the left)

THUNDERBOLT POSE: SITTING BONES ON THE FLOOR—FEET TURNED OUT

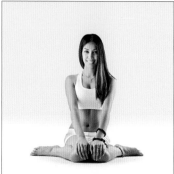

Complete Thunderbolt Pose

Paripurna Vajrasana

(puh-ri-POOR-nuh vuhj-RAHS-uh-nuh)

Pose Type: seated

Drishti Point: Nasagrai or Nasagre (nose)

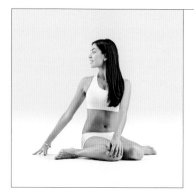

Revolved Complete Thunderbolt Pose

Parivritta Paripurna Vajrasana

(puh-ri-VRIT-uh puh-ri-POOR-nuh vuhj-RAHS-uh-nuh)

Pose Type: seated, twist

Drishti Point: Parshva Drishti (to the right), Parshva Drishti (to the left)

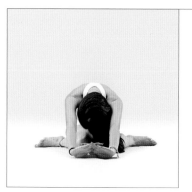

Western Intense Stretch Pose in Complete Thunderbolt Pose

Paschimottanasana in Paripurna Vajrasana

(puhsh-chi-mo-tahn-AHS-uh-nuh in puh-ri-POOR-nuh vuhj-RAHS-uh-nuh)

Also Known As: Seated Forward Bend in Complete Thunderbolt Pose

Modification: forward bend, toes turned out

Pose Type: seated, forward bend

Drishti Point: Nasagrai or Nasagre (nose)

1.

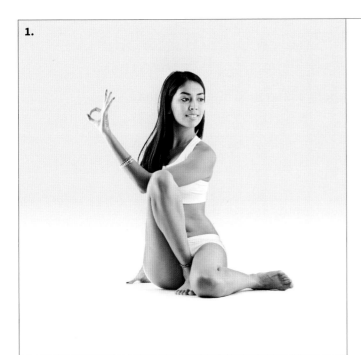

Half Pose Dedicated to Sage Marichi in Revolved Half Thunderbolt Pose

Ardha Marichyasana in Parivritta Ardha Vajrasana

(UHR-duh muh-ree-CHYAHS-uh-nuh in puh-ri-VRIT-uh UHR-duh vuhj-RAHS-uh-nuh)

Modification: 1. looking straight ahead
2. looking over the shoulder
Pose Type: seated, forward bend, twist
Drishti Point: Parshva Drishti (to the right), Parshva Drishti (to the left)

2.

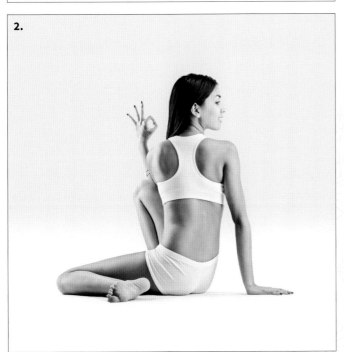

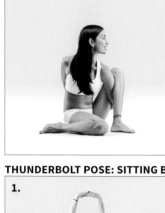

Half Bound Pose Dedicated to Sage Marichi in Half Thunderbolt Pose

Ardha Baddha Marichyasana in Ardha Vajrasana

(UHR-duh BUH-duh muh-ree-CHYAHS-uh-nuh in UHR-duh vuhj-RAHS-uh-nuh)

Pose Type: seated, forward bend, twist, binding

Drishti Point: Parshva Drishti (to the right), Parshva Drishti (to the left)

THUNDERBOLT POSE: SITTING BONES ON THE FLOOR—FEET TURNED OUT—ARMS UP OVER THE HEAD

1.

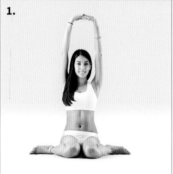

Complete Thunderbolt Pose—Raised Bound Hands

Paripurna Vajrasana—Urdhva Baddha Hastasana

(puh-ri-POOR-nuh vuhj-RAHS-uh-nuh OORD-vuh BUH-duh huh-STAHS-uh-nuh)

Modification: 1. looking straight ahead

2. head rolling back

Pose Type: 1. seated

2. seated, mild backbend

Drishti Point: 1. Nasagrai or Nasagre (nose)

2. Angushtamadhye (thumbs)

1.

2.

2.

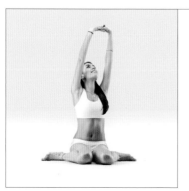

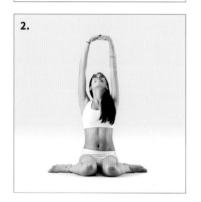

Revolved Complete Thunderbolt Pose—Raised Bound Hands

Parivritta Paripurna Vajrasana—Urdhva Baddha Hastasana

(puh-ri-VRIT-tuh puh-ri-POOR-nuh vuhj-RAHS-uh-nuh OORD-vuh BUH-duh huh-STAHS-uh-nuh)

Pose Type: seated, twist

Drishti Point: Angushtamadhye (thumbs)

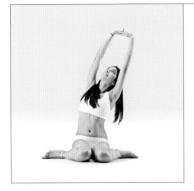

Sideways Complete Thunderbolt Pose— Raised Bound Hands

Parshva Paripurna Vajrasana—Urdhva Baddha Hastasana

(PAHRSH-vuh puh-ri-POOR-nuh vuhj-RAHS-uh-nuh OORD-vuh BUH-duh huh-STAHS-uh-nuh)
Pose Type: seated, side bend
Drishti Point: Angushtamadhye (thumbs)

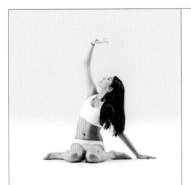

One Hand Sideways Complete Thunderbolt Pose

Eka Hasta Parshva Paripurna Vajrasana

(EY-kuh HUH-stuh PAHRSH-vuh puh-ri-POOR-nuh vuhj-RAHS-uh-nuh)
Pose Type: seated, side bend
Drishti Point: Hastagrai or Hastagre (hands)

THUNDERBOLT POSE: SITTING BONES ON THE FLOOR—FEET TURNED OUT—ONE-LEGGED & FORWARD BENDS

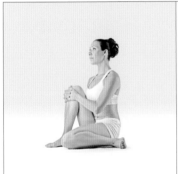

Half Pose Dedicated to Sage Marichi in Half Thunderbolt Pose

Ardha Marichyasana in Ardha Vajrasana

(UHR-duh muh-ree-CHYAHS-uh-nuh in UHR-duh vuhj-RAHS-uh-nuh)
Modification: grabbing onto the knee with both hands
Pose Type: seated, forward bend
Drishti Point: Nasagrai or Nasagre (nose)

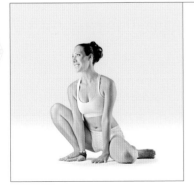

Half Pose Dedicated to Sage Marichi in Half Thunderbolt Pose

Ardha Marichyasana in Ardha Vajrasana

(UHR-duh muh-ree-CHYAHS-uh-nuh in UHR-duh vuhj-RAHS-uh-nuh)
Modification: palms to the floor in front of the hips
Pose Type: seated, forward bend
Drishti Point: Nasagrai or Nasagre (nose), Bhrumadhye or Ajna Chakra (third eye, between the eyebrows)

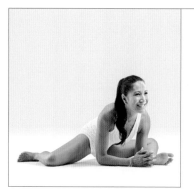

Half Star Pose in Half Frog Pose

Ardha Tarasana in Ardha Mandukasana

(UHR-duh tahr-AHS-uh-nuh in UHR-duh muhn-doo-KAHS-uh-nuh)

Pose Type: seated, forward bend

Drishti Point: Nasagrai or Nasagre (nose)

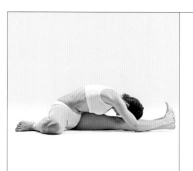

Pose Dedicated to Virancha (Brahma) 1 Prep.

Viranchyasana 1 Prep.

(vir-uhn-CHYAHS-uh-nuh)

Pose Type: seated, forward bend

Drishti Point: Nasagrai or Nasagre (nose)

ONE KNEE BENT TO THE BACK: OTHER FOOT TO THE THIGH—SPINE STRAIGHT, TWIST & SIDE BEND

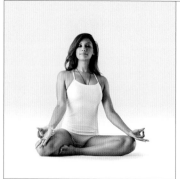

Easy Pose Dedicated to Sage Bharadvaja 2 Prep.

Sukha Bharadvajasana 2 Prep.

(SUK-uh buh-ruhd-vuhj-AHS-uh-nuh)

Modification: neutral spine, back of the hands on the knees

Pose Type: seated

Drishti Point: Nasagrai or Nasagre (nose)

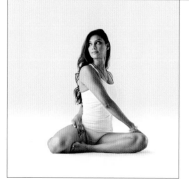

Easy Pose Dedicated to Sage Bharadvaja 2

Sukha Bharadvajasana 2

(SUK-uh buh-ruhd-vuhj-AHS-uh-nuh)

Modification: foot to the inside of the thigh

Pose Type: seated, twist, binding

Drishti Point: Parshva Drishti (to the right), Parshva Drishti (to the left)

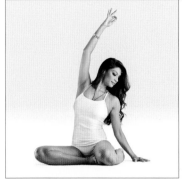

Sideways Easy Pose Dedicated to Sage Bharadvaja 2

Parshva Sukha Bharadvajasana 2

(PAHRSH-vuh SUK-uh buh-ruhd-vuhj-AHS-uh-nuh)

Modification: foot to the inside of the thigh, side bend
Pose Type: seated, side bend
Drishti Point: Hastagrai or Hastagre (hands)

ONE KNEE BENT TO THE BACK: OTHER FOOT TO THE THIGH—SIDE BEND

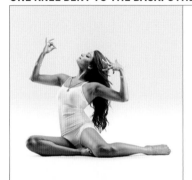

Easy One-Legged King Pigeon Pose 1

Sukha Eka Pada Raja Kapotasana 1

(SUK-uh EY-kuh PUH-duh RAH-juh kuh-po-TAHS-uh-nuh)

Pose Type: seated, side bend
Drishti Point: Hastagrai or Hastagre (hands)

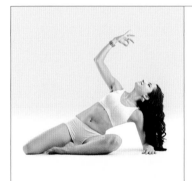

Sideways Half Hero Half Bound Angle Pose

Parshva Ardha Vira Ardha Baddha Konasana

(PAHRSH-vuh UHR-duh VEER-uh UHR-duh BUH-duh ko-NAHS-uh-nuh)

Modification: forearm to the floor
Pose Type: seated, side bend
Drishti Point: Hastagrai or Hastagre (hands)

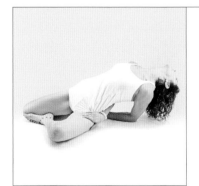

Half Hero Half Bound Angle Pose

Ardha Vira Ardha Baddha Konasana

(UHR-duh VEER-uh UHR-duh BUH-duh ko-NAHS-uh-nuh)

Modification: arm behind the back, hand to the hip; backbend
Pose Type: seated, backbend
Drishti Point: Bhrumadhye or Ajna Chakra (third eye, between the eyebrows)

1.

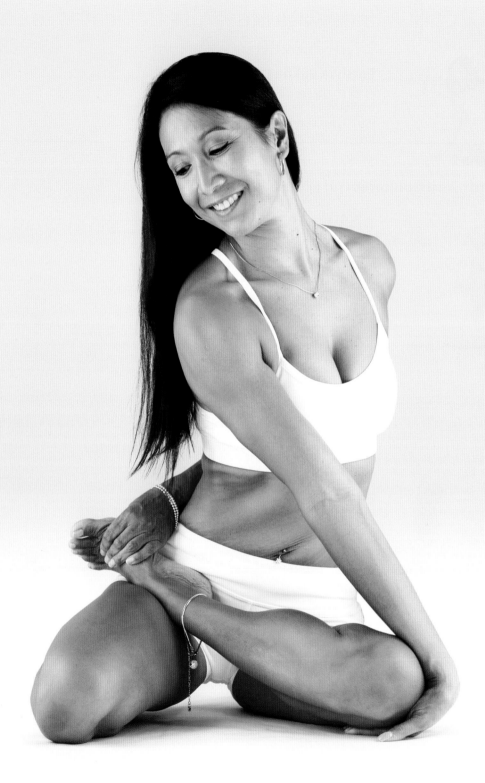

Twist Dedicated to Sage Bharadvaja 2

Bharadvajasana 2
(buh-ruhd-vuhj-AHS-uh-nuh)
Pose Type: seated, twist, binding
Drishti Point: Parsva Drishti (to the right), Parsva Drishti (to the left)

How to Perform the Pose:

1. Begin by sitting on the floor with both your legs straight out in front of you. Engage your *mula bandha*, *uddhiyana bandha*, and *ujjayi* breathing.

2. Inhale as you lean over to the left side, bending your right knee and bringing your right knee, shin, and ankle to the floor. Your right heel should be close to your right hip to protect the knee and your right knee should be open slightly to the side.

3. Exhale as you bend your left knee and bring your left foot to your right hip socket in the Half Lotus (*Ardha Padmasana*), rotating the sole of your left foot up to the sky. Try to keep both knees on the floor.

4. Inhale as you expand your chest and hold your arms straight out to the sides, parallel to the floor.

5. Exhale as you twist to the left, bringing your left arm behind your back and grabbing your left foot with your left hand to bind. Grab onto the left knee with your right hand and look over your left shoulder (Pose #2).

6. Inhale as you lengthen your spine. Exhale as you bring the back of your left hand under your right knee (Pose #1). On the next exhale, look over your right shoulder to deepen the twist (Pose #3).

7. Hold the pose for at least 30, and up to 90, seconds in order to receive the full benefits of the stretch.

8. Inhale as you release the bind and look forward. Exhale as you bring both your legs straight out in front of you. Repeat on the other side.

Modification:
1. palm under the knee, twisting to the inside of the body
2. hand on the knee, twisting to the inside of the body
3. palm under the knee, twisting to the outside of the body

Bharadvaja = Pindola Bharadvaja was one of four Arhats asked by Buddha to stay on earth to propagate Buddhist law or Dharma

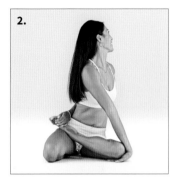
2.

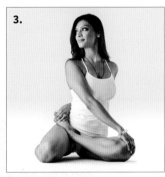
3.

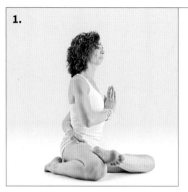

1.

Half Fire Log Pose in Half Bound Hero Pose

Ardha Agnistambhasana in Ardha Baddha Virasana
(UHR-duh uhg-ni-stuhm-BAHS-uh-nuh in UHR-duh BUH-duh veer-AHS-uh-nuh)
Modification: 1. grabbing onto the hip
2. grabbing onto the heel
Pose Type: seated, binding
Drishti Point: Nasagrai or Nasagre (nose), Hastagrai or Hastagre (hands)

2.

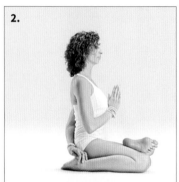

Pose Dedicated to Sage Bharadvaja 2 Prep.

Bharadvajasana 2 Prep.
(buh-ruhd-vuhj-AHS-uh-nuh)
Modification: palms together, heels of the palms resting on the crown of the head, neutral spine
Pose Type: seated
Drishti Point: Nasagrai or Nasagre (nose), Bhrumadhye or Ajna Chakra (third eye, between the eyebrows)

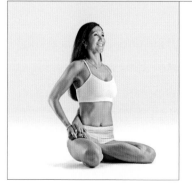

Pose Dedicated to Sage Bharadvaja 2 Prep.

Bharadvajasana 2 Prep.
(buh-ruhd-vuhj-AHS-uh-nuh)
Also Known As: Root Lock Pose (Mula Bandhasana)
Modification: sitting on the heel, both hands grabbing onto the foot, neutral spine
Pose Type: seated, binding
Drishti Point: Nasagrai or Nasagre (nose), Bhrumadhye or Ajna Chakra (third eye, between the eyebrows)

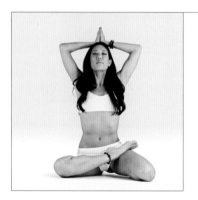

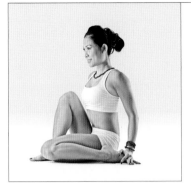

Pose Dedicated to Sage Marichi 5 & 6 Prep.

Marichyasana 5 & 6 Prep.

(muh-ree-CHYAHS-uh-nuh)

Also Known As: Pose Dedicated to Sage Marichi E & F Prep. (Marichyasana E & F Prep.)
Modification: spine straight
Pose Type: seated, forward bend
Drishti Point: Nasagrai or Nasagre (nose)

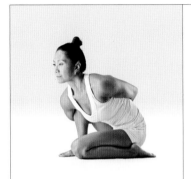

Pose Dedicated to Sage Marichi 5

Marichyasana 5

(muh-ree-CHYAHS-uh-nuh)

Also Known As: Pose Dedicated to Sage Marichi E (Marichyasana E)
Pose Type: seated, forward bend, binding
Drishti Point: Nasagrai or Nasagre (nose)

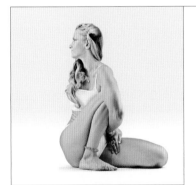

Pose Dedicated to Sage Marichi 6

Marichyasana 6

(muh-ree-CHYAHS-uh-nuh)

Also Known As: Pose Dedicated to Sage Marichi F (Marichyasana F)
Pose Type: seated, forward bend, twist, binding
Drishti Point: Parshva Drishti (to the right), Parshva Drishti (to the left)

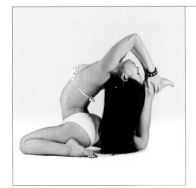

One-Legged King Pigeon Pose 3

Eka Pada Raja Kapotasana 3

(EY-kuh PUH-duh RAHJ-uh kuh-po-TAHS-uh-nuh)

Pose Type: seated, backbend
Drishti Point: Bhrumadhye or Ajna Chakra (third eye, between the eyebrows)

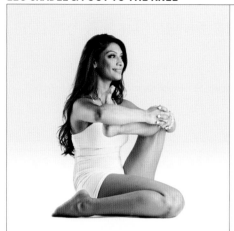

Baby Cradle Pose in Half Hero Pose

Hindolasana in Ardha Virasana

(hin-do-LAHS-uh-nuh in UHR-duh veer-AHS-uh-nuh)

Also Known As: Baby Cradle Pose in Half Thunderbolt Pose (Hindolasana in Ardha Vajrasana)

Pose Type: seated, forward bend

Drishti Point: Nasagrai or Nasagre (nose)

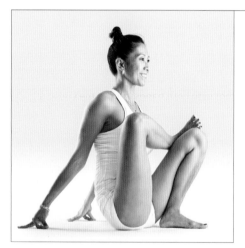

Baby Cradle Pose Prep.

Hindolasana Prep.

(hin-do-LAHS-uh-nuh)

Modification: palms to the floor behind the hips, heel of the bottom foot to the sitting bone

Pose Type: seated, forward bend

Drishti Point: Nasagrai or Nasagre (nose)

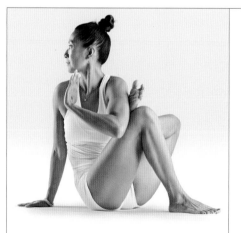

Half Fire Log Pose in Half Yogic Staff Pose Prep.

Ardha Agnistambhasana in Ardha Yogadandasana Prep.

(UHR-duh uhg-ni-stuhm-BAHS-uh-nuh in UHR-duh yo-guh-duhn-DAHS-uh-nuh)

Pose Type: seated, forward bend, twist

Drishti Point: Parshva Drishti (to the right), Parshva Drishti (to the left)

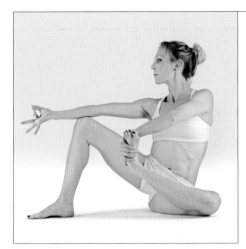

Yogic Staff Pose Prep.

Yogadandasana Prep.

(yo-guh-duhn-DAHS-uh-nuh)

Modification: grabbing onto the foot with one hand
Pose Type: seated, forward bend
Drishti Point: Hastagrai or Hastagre (hands)

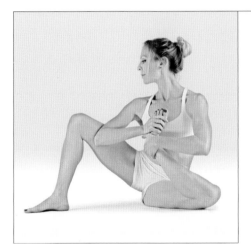

Yogic Staff Pose Prep.

Yogadandasana Prep.

(yo-guh-duhn-DAHS-uh-nuh)

Modification: grabbing onto the foot with both hands, foot to the chest
Pose Type: seated, forward bend
Drishti Point: Padhayoragrai or Padayoragre (toes/feet)

LEG CRADLE: FOOT TO THE HIP & HALF LOTUS

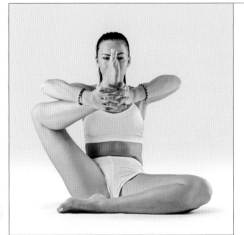

Baby Cradle Pose Prep.

Hindolasana Prep.

(hin-do-LAHS-uh-nuh)

Modification: both hands grabbing onto the foot, fingers interlocked
Pose Type: seated, forward bend
Drishti Point: Padhayoragrai or Padayoragre (toes/feet)

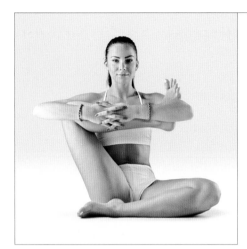

Baby Cradle Pose

Hindolasana

(hin-do-LAHS-uh-nuh)

Pose Type: seated, forward bend

Drishti Point: Nasagrai or Nasagre (nose)

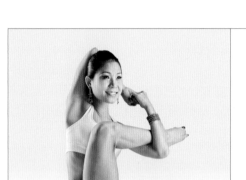

Four Corner Pose

Chatushkonasana

(chuh-tush-ko-NAHS-uh-nuh)

Pose Type: seated, forward bend, binding

Drishti Point: Nasagrai or Nasagre (nose)

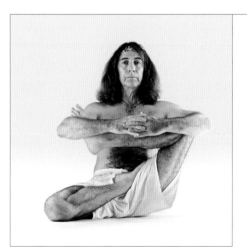

Half Lotus Baby Cradle Pose

Ardha Padma Hindolasana

(UHR-duh PUHD-muh hin-do-LAHS-uh-nuh)

Also Known As: Pose Dedicated to Virancha (Brahma) 1 or A Prep. (Viranchyasana 1 or A Prep.)

Pose Type: seated, forward bend

Drishti Point: Nasagrai or Nasagre (nose)

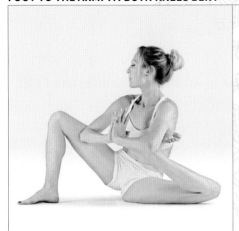

Yogic Staff Pose with Hands in Prayer

Yogadandasana Namaskar

(yo-guh-duhn-DAHS-uh-nuh nuh-muhs-KAHR)

Pose Type: seated, forward bend

Drishti Point: Nasagrai or Nasagre (nose), Hastagrai or Hastagre (hands)

Yogic Staff Pose

Yogadandasana

(yo-guh-duhn-DAHS-uh-nuh)

Pose Type: seated, forward bend

Drishti Point: Nasagrai or Nasagre (nose), Hastagrai or Hastagre (hands)

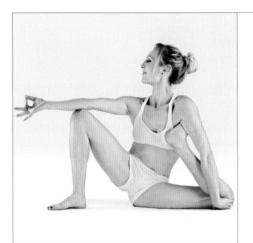

Half Bound Fire Log Pose in Half Yogic Staff Pose Prep.

Ardha Baddha Agnistambhasana in Ardha Yogadandasana Prep.

(UHR-duh BUH-duh uhg-ni-stuhm-BAHS-uh-nuh in UHR-duh yo-guh-duhn-DAHS-uh-nuh)

Pose Type: seated, forward bend, twist, binding

Drishti Point: Parshva Drishti (to the right), Parshva Drishti (to the left)

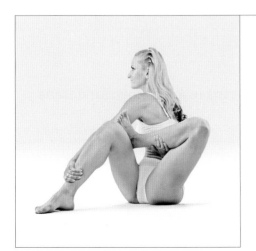

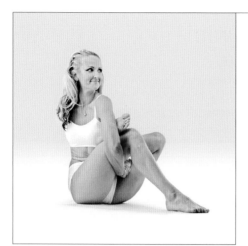

Bound Fire Log Pose in Half Yogic Staff Pose Prep.

Baddha Agnistambhasana in Ardha Yogadandasana Prep.

(BUH-duh uhg-ni-stuhm-BAHS-uh-nuh in UHR-duh yo-guh-duhn-DAHS-uh-nuh)

Pose Type: seated, forward bend, twist, binding

Drishti Point: Parshva Drishti (to the right), Parshva Drishti (to the left)

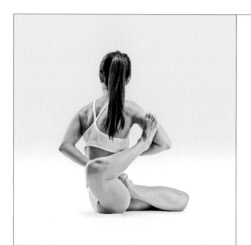

Hands Bound Half Lotus Pose in Half Yogic Staff Pose Prep.

Baddha Hasta Ardha Padmasana in Ardha Yogadandasana Prep.

(BUH-duh HUH-stuh UHR-duh puhd-MAHS-uh-nuh in UHR-duh yo-guh-duhn-DAHS-uh-nuh)

Pose Type: seated, twist, binding

Drishti Point: Parshva Drishti (to the right), Parshva Drishti (to the left)

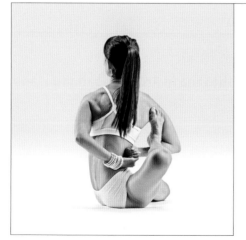

Hands Bound Half Hero Pose in Half Yogic Staff Pose Prep.

Baddha Hasta Ardha Virasana in Ardha Yogadandasana Prep.

(BUH-duh HUH-stuh UHR-duh veer-AHS-uh-nuh in UHR-duh yo-guh-duhn-DAHS-uh-nuh)

Pose Type: seated, twist, binding

Drishti Point: Parshva Drishti (to the right), Parshva Drishti (to the left)

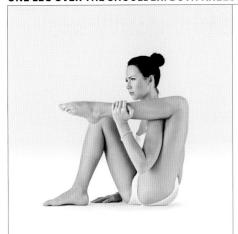

Sundial Pose 2 Prep.

Surya Yantrasana 2 Prep.

(SOOR-yuh yuhn-TRAHS-uh-nuh)

Modification: shoulder to the back of the knee, knee bent
Pose Type: seated, forward bend
Drishti Point: Padayoragrai or Padayoragre (toes/feet)

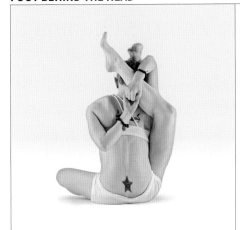

Pose Dedicated to Virancha (Brahma) 1

Viranchyasana 1

(vir-uhn-CHYAHS-uh-nuh)

Also Known As: Pose Dedicated to Virancha (Brahma) A (Viranchyasana A)
Pose Type: seated, binding
Drishti Point: Bhrumadhye or Ajna Chakra (third eye, between the eyebrows)

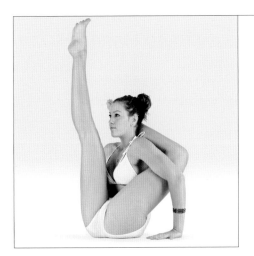

Seated Moonbird Pose

Upavishta Chakorasana

(u-puh-VISH-tuh chuh-kor-AHS-uh-nuh)

Also Known As: Upavistha Chakorasana
Pose Type: seated, forward bend
Drishti Point: Bhrumadhye or Ajna Chakra (third eye, between the eyebrows)

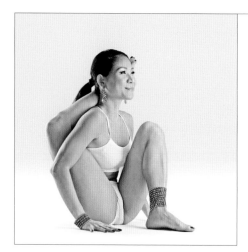

One Foot Behind the Head Pose

Eka Pada Shirshasana

(EY-kuh PUH-duh sheer-SHAHS-uh-nuh)

Modification: palms on the floor by the hips, knee bent toward the chest
Pose Type: seated, forward bend
Drishti Point: Bhrumadhye or Ajna Chakra (third eye, between the eyebrows)

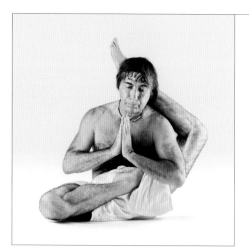

Pose Dedicated to Virancha (Brahma) 1

Viranchyasana 1

(vir-uhn-CHYAHS-uh-nuh)

Also Known As: Pose Dedicated to Virancha (Brahma) A (Viranchyasana A)
Modification: hands in Anjali Mudra (Hands in Prayer)
Pose Type: seated
Drishti Point: Bhrumadhye or Ajna Chakra (third eye, between the eyebrows)

COW FACE POSE: SPINE STRAIGHT

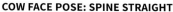

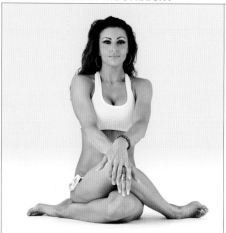

Leg Position of Cow Face Pose

Pada Gomukhasana

(PUH-duh go-muk-AHS-uh-nuh)

Modification: hands on the top knee, one palm on top of the other
Pose Type: seated
Drishti Point: Nasagrai or Nasagre (nose)

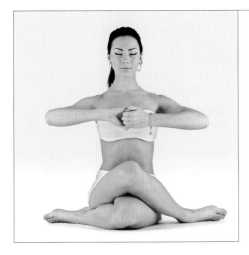

Ganesh Seal in Leg Position of Cow Face Pose

Ganesh Mudra in Pada Gomukhasana

(guh-NEYSH MU-druh in PUH-duh go-muk-AHS-uh-nuh)

Pose Type: seated

Drishti Point: Nasagrai or Nasagre (nose)

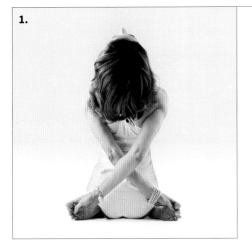

Both Hands to Feet Leg Position of Cow Face Pose

Dwi Hasta Pada Gomukhasana

(DWI-huh-stuh PUH-duh go-mu-KAHS-uh-nuh)

Modification: arms crossed behind the back, grabbing onto the feet

1. back view
2. front view

Pose Type: seated, backbend

Drishti Point: Bhrumadhye or Ajna Chakra (third eye, between the eyebrows)

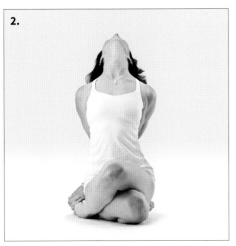

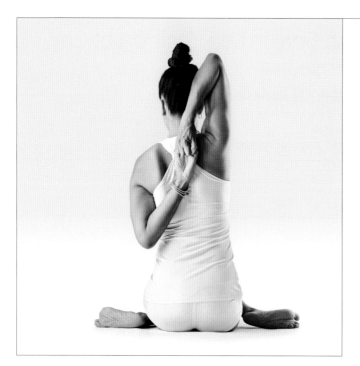

Cow Face Pose

Gomukhasana
(go-mu-KAHS-uh-nuh)
Pose Type: seated
Drishti Point: Nasagrai or Nasagre (nose)

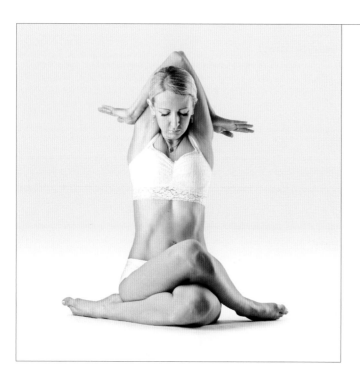

Leg Position of Cow Face Pose

Pada Gomukhasana
(PUH-duh go-mu-KAHS-uh-nuh)
Modification: elbows touching behind the head
Pose Type: seated
Drishti Point: Nasagrai or Nasagre (nose)

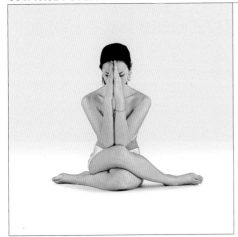

Leg Position of Cow Face Pose

Pada Gomukhasana

(PUH-duh go-mu-KAHS-uh-nuh)

Modification: hands in Anjali Mudra (Hands in Prayer), thumbs to third eye; elbows together

Pose Type: seated, forward bend

Drishti Point: Nasagrai or Nasagre (nose) or Angushtamadhye or Angustha Ma Dyai (thumbs)

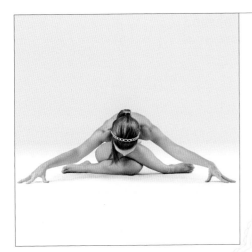

Western Intense Stretch Pose in Leg Position of Cow Face Pose

Paschimottanasana in Pada Gomukhasana

(puhsh-chi-mo-TAHS-uh-nuh in PUH-duh go-mu-KAHS-uh-nuh)

Also Known As: Seated Forward Bend in Leg Position of Cow Face Pose and Long Horn Pose (Dighasrngasana)

Pose Type: seated, forward bend

Drishti Point: Nasagrai or Nasagre (nose)

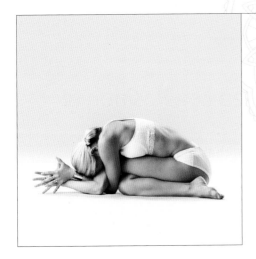

Hand Position of the Pose Dedicated to Garuda in Leg Position of Cow Face Pose

Hasta Garudasana in Pada Gomukhasana

(HUH-stuh guh-ru-DAHS-uh-nuh in PUH-duh go-mu-KAHS-uh-nuh)

Modification: forward bend

Pose Type: seated, forward bend

Drishti Point: Nasagrai or Nasagre (nose), Bhrumadhye or Ajna Chakra (third eye, between the eyebrows)

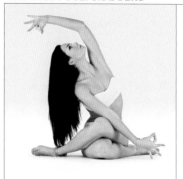

Sideways Leg Position of Cow Face Pose

Parshva Pada Gomukhasana

(PAHRSH-vuh PUH-duh go-mu-KAHS-uh-nuh)

Pose Type: seated, side bend

Drishti Point: Hastagrai or Hastagre (hands)

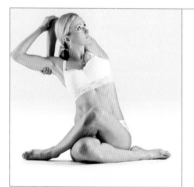

Hand to Foot Sideways Leg Position of Cow Face Pose

Hasta Pada Parshva Pada Gomukhasana

(HUH-stuh PUH-duh PAHRSH-vuh PUH-duh go-mu-KAHS-uh-nuh)

Pose Type: seated, side bend

Drishti Point: Hastagrai or Hastagre (hands)

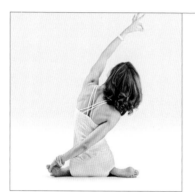

Sideways Leg Position of Cow Face Pose

Parshva Pada Gomukhasana

(PAHRSH-vuh PUH-duh go-mu-KAHS-uh-nuh)

Modification: intense shoulder stretch

Pose Type: seated, side bend

Drishti Point: Urdhva or Antara Drishti (up to the sky)

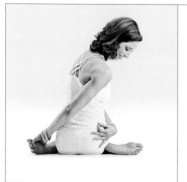

Hand to Foot Revolved Leg Position of Cow Face Pose

Hasta Pada Parivritta Pada Gomukhasana

(HUH-stuh PUH-duh puh-ri-VRIT-tuh PUH-duh go-mu-KAHS-uh-nuh)

Modification: grabbing onto the big toe, arm behind the back; other arm in front of the body, hand on the hip

Pose Type: seated, twist, binding

Drishti Point: Padayoragrai or Padayoragre (toes/feet)

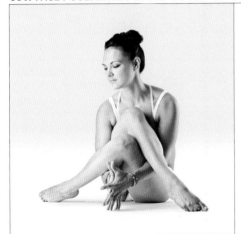

Upward Leg Position of Cow Face Pose

Urdhva Pada Gomukhasana

(OORD-vuh PUH-duh go-mu-KAHS-uh-nuh)

Modification: arms under the legs, knees lifted to the chest

Pose Type: seated, forward bend

Drishti Point: Padayoragrai or Padayoragre (toes/feet), Hastagrai or Hastagre (hands)

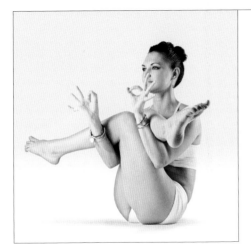

Upward Hands Upward Leg Position of Cow Face Pose

Urdhva Hasta Urdhva Pada Gomukhasana

(OORD-vuh HUH-stuh OORD-vuh PUH-duh go-mu-KAHS-uh-nuh)

Pose Type: seated, forward bend, core

Drishti Point: Hastagrai or Hastagre (hands), Nasagrai or Nasagre (nose)

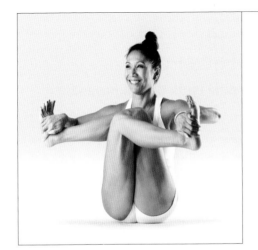

Both Hands to Feet Upward Leg Position of Cow Face Pose

Dwi Hasta Pada Urdhva Pada Gomukhasana

(DWI-huh-stuh PUH-duh OORD-vuh PUH-duh go-mu-KAHS-uh-nuh)

Modification: grabbing the outside edges of both feet

Pose Type: seated, forward bend, core

Drishti Point: Nasagrai or Nasagre (nose)

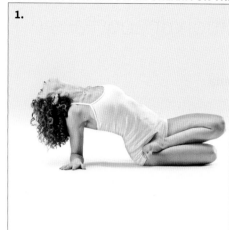

1.

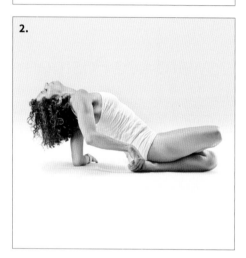

Half Bound Sideways Easy Leg Position of Cow Face Pose

Ardha Baddha Parshva Sukha Pada Gomukhasana

(UHR-duh BUH-duh PAHRSH-vuh SUK-uh PUH-duh go-mu-KAHS-uh-nuh)

Modification: forearm to the floor, sitting on the bottom heel

1. front view
2. back view

Pose Type: seated, backbend

Drishti Point: Bhrumadhye or Ajna Chakra (third eye, between the eyebrows)

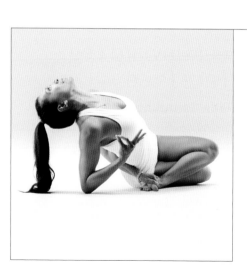

Half Bound Sideways Easy Leg Position of Cow Face Pose

Ardha Baddha Parshva Sukha Pada Gomukhasana

(UHR-duh BUH-duh PAHRSH-vuh SUK-uh PUH-duh go-mu-KAHS-uh-nuh)

Modification: elbow to the floor

Pose Type: seated, backbend, binding

Drishti Point: Bhrumadhye or Ajna Chakra (third eye, between the eyebrows)

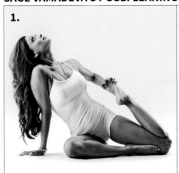

Pose Dedicated to Sage Vamadeva Prep.

Vamadevasana Prep.

(vahm-uh-dey-VAHS-uh-nuh)

Modification: 1. palm flat on the floor, chest rotating up

2. one arm crossed over in front, hand grabbing onto the back foot; top hand to the head

Pose Type: seated, side bend

Drishti Point: Bhrumadhye or Ajna Chakra (third eye, between the eyebrows)

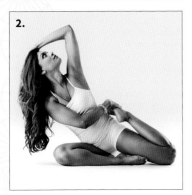

Pose Dedicated to Sage Vamadeva

Vamadevasana

(vahm-uh-dey-VAHS-uh-nuh)

Modification: binding:

1. hand to the hip socket

2. hand to the knee

Pose Type: seated, side bend, twist, binding

Drishti Point: 1. Urdhva or Antara Drishti (up to the sky)

2. Padayoragrai or Padayoragre (toes/feet)

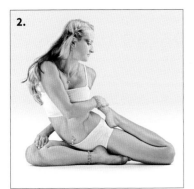

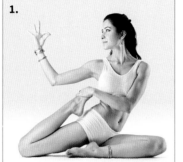

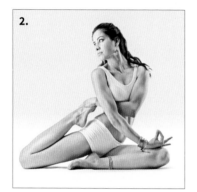

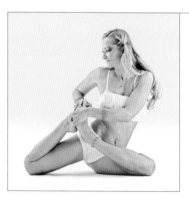

Revolved One-Legged King Pigeon Pose 1 Prep.

Parivritta Eka Pada Raja Kapotasana 1 Prep.
(puh-ri-VRIT-tuh EY-kuh PUH-duh RAH-juh kuh-po-TAHS-uh-nuh)
Modification: grabbing onto the back foot
1. one arm crossed over, other arm to the side, elbow bent
2. arms crossed in front of the body, free hand to the opposite knee
Pose Type: seated, side bend, twist
Drishti Point: Hastagrai or Hastagre (hands), Parshva Drishti (to the right), Parshva Drishti (to the left)

Pose Dedicated to Sage Vamadeva 2

Vamadevasana 2
(vahm-uh-dey-VAHS-uh-nuh)
Pose Type: seated, twist
Drishti Point: Padayoragrai or Padayoragre (toes/feet)

ONE-LEGGED KING PIGEON: HIPS OFF THE FLOOR

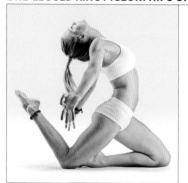

One-Legged King Pigeon Pose 1 Version B

Eka Pada Raja Kapotasana 1 B
(EY-kuh PUH-duh RAH-juh kuh-po-TAHS-uh-nuh)
Pose Type: standing (on the knees), backbend
Drishti Point: Bhrumadhye or Ajna Chakra (third eye, between the eyebrows)

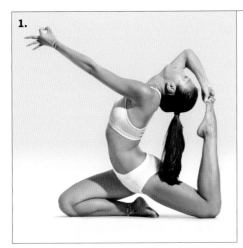

1.

Easy One-Legged King Pigeon Pose 1

Sukha Eka Pada Raja Kapotasana 1

(SUK-uh EY-kuh PUH-duh RAH-juh kuh-po-TAHS-uh-nuh)

Modification: hips lifted off the floor, grabbing onto the foot on the opposite side with overhead grip

1. free arm extended to the front
2. free hand to the floor by the opposite knee

Pose Type: standing (on the knees), backbend

Drishti Point: Bhrumadhye or Ajna Chakra (third eye, between the eyebrows)

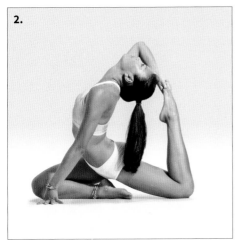

2.

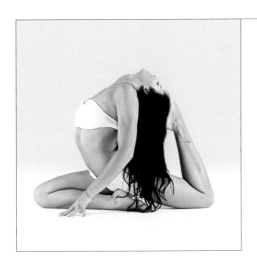

Easy One-Legged King Pigeon Pose 1

Sukha Eka Pada Raja Kapotasana 1

(SUK-uh EY-kuh PUH-duh RAH-juh kuh-po-TAHS-uh-nuh)

Modification: hips off the floor; fingertips to the floor by the hips, foot touching the head

Pose Type: seated, backbend

Drishti Point: Bhrumadhye or Ajna Chakra (third eye, between the eyebrows)

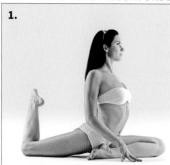

One-Legged King Pigeon Pose 1 Prep.

Eka Pada Raja Kapotasana 1 Prep.

(EY-kuh PUH-duh RAH-juh kuh-po-TAHS-uh-nuh)

Modification: 1. back knee bent

2. grabbing onto the back foot with one arm on the same side

Pose Type: seated, backbend

Drishti Point: Bhrumadhye or Ajna Chakra (third eye, between the eyebrows)

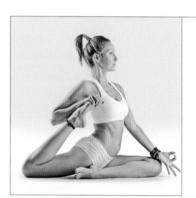

One-Legged King Pigeon Pose 1

Eka Pada Raja Kapotasana 1

(EY-kuh PUH-duh RAH-juh kuh-po-TAHS-uh-nuh)

Modification: one hand on the front knee on the same side, other hand pressing the back foot toward the hip

Pose Type: seated, backbend

Drishti Point: Nasagrai or Nasagre (nose), Hastagrai or Hastagre (hands)

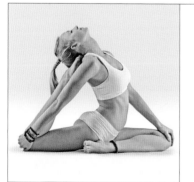

One-Legged King Pigeon Pose 1

Eka Pada Raja Kapotasana 1

(EY-kuh PUH-duh RAH-juh kuh-po-TAHS-uh-nuh)

Modification: one hand on the back knee, one hand on the front knee; foot to the back of the head

Pose Type: seated, backbend

Drishti Point: Bhrumadhye or Ajna Chakra (third eye, between the eyebrows)

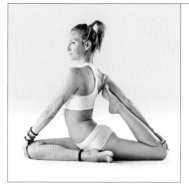

One-Legged King Pigeon Pose 1

Eka Pada Raja Kapotasana 1

(EY-kuh PUH-duh RAH-juh kuh-po-TAHS-uh-nuh)

Modification: foot to the opposite armpit
Pose Type: seated, backbend, twist
Drishti Point: Nasagrai or Nasagre (nose) or Hastagrai or Hastagre (hands)

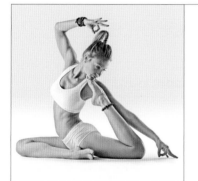

Revolved One-Legged King Pigeon Pose 1

Parivritta Eka Pada Raja Kapotasana 1

(puh-ri-VRIT-tuh EY-kuh PUH-duh RAH-juh kuh-po-TAHS-uh-nuh)

Modification: foot to the armpit on the same side
Pose Type: seated, backbend, twist
Drishti Point: Hastagrai or Hastagre (hands)

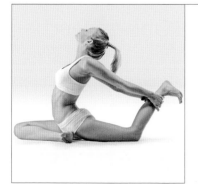

Revolved One-Legged King Pigeon Pose 1

Parivritta Eka Pada Raja Kapotasana 1

(puh-ri-VRIT-tuh EY-kuh PUH-duh RAH-juh kuh-po-TAHS-uh-nuh)

Modification: foot under the chin
Pose Type: seated, backbend, twist
Drishti Point: Hastagrai or Hastagre (hands)

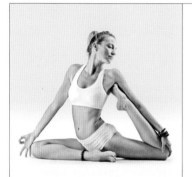

Pose of the Heavenly Spirits Prep.

Valakhilyasana Prep.

(vah-luh-kil-YAHS-uh-nuh)

Modification: under-head grip
Pose Type: seated, backbend
Drishti Point: Bhrumadhye or Ajna Chakra (third eye, between the eyebrows)

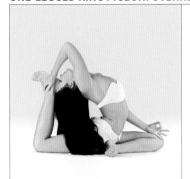

One-Legged King Pigeon Pose 1

Eka Pada Raja Kapotasana 1

(EY-kuh PUH-duh RAH-juh kuh-po-TAHS-uh-nuh)

Modification: grabbing onto the foot with one hand on the same side, overhead grip; other hand resting on the front knee

Pose Type: seated, backbend

Drishti Point: Bhrumadhye or Ajna Chakra (third eye, between the eyebrows)

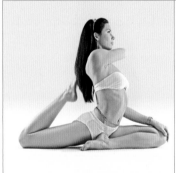

One-Legged King Pigeon Pose 1

Eka Pada Raja Kapotasana 1

(EY-kuh PUH-duh RAH-juh kuh-po-TAHS-uh-nuh)

Modification: grabbing onto the foot with both hands, overhead grip; heel of the back foot to the forehead

Pose Type: seated, backbend

Drishti Point: Bhrumadhye or Ajna Chakra (third eye, between the eyebrows)

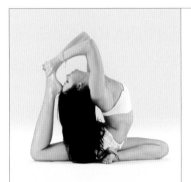

One Hand to Foot Bound One-Legged King Pigeon Pose 1

Eka Hasta Pada Baddha Eka Pada Raja Kapotasana 1

(EY-kuh HUH-stuh PUH-duh BUH-duh EY-kuh PUH-duh RAH-juh kuh-po-TAHS-uh-nuh)

Modification: arm crossed over in front of the neck, other hand on the knee

Pose Type: seated, backbend

Drishti Point: Nasagrai or Nasagre (nose)

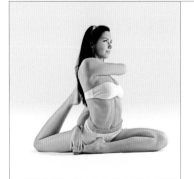

Both Hands to Feet Bound One-Legged King Pigeon Pose 1

Dwi Hasta Pada Baddha Eka Pada Raja Kapotasana 1

(DWI-huh-stuh PUH-duh BUH-duh EY-kuh PUH-duh RAH-juh kuh-po-TAHS-uh-nuh)

Modification: arm crossed over in front of the neck

Pose Type: seated, backbend, binding

Drishti Point: Nasagrai or Nasagre (nose)

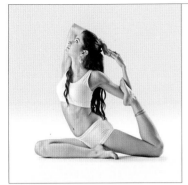

Mermaid Pose 1

Naginyasana 1

(nah-gin-YAHS-uh-nuh)

Pose Type: seated, backbend, binding

Drishti Point: Bhrumadhye or Ajna Chakra (third eye, between the eyebrows)

ONE-LEGGED KING PIGEON: ASYMMETRICAL ARMS—CROSS OVER & UNDER-HEAD/OVERHEAD GRIP

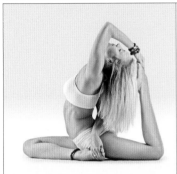

Both Hands to Feet Bound One-Legged King Pigeon Pose 1

Dwi Hasta Pada Baddha Eka Pada Raja Kapotasana 1

(DWI-huh-stuh PUH-duh BUH-duh EY-kuh PUH-duh RAH-juh kuh-po-TAHS-uh-nuh)

Modification: grabbing onto the opposite foot with overhead grip

Pose Type: seated, backbend, binding

Drishti Point: Bhrumadhye or Ajna Chakra (third eye, between the eyebrows)

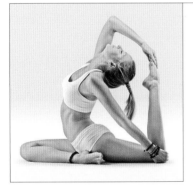

One-Legged King Pigeon Pose 1

Eka Pada Raja Kapotasana 1

(EY-kuh PUH-duh RAH-juh kuh-po-TAHS-uh-nuh)

Modification: one hand on the back knee, one hand grabbing onto the opposite foot with overhead grip

Pose Type: seated, backbend

Drishti Point: Bhrumadhye or Ajna Chakra (third eye, between the eyebrows)

ONE-LEGGED KING PIGEON: FOOT TO THE BACK OF THE HEAD

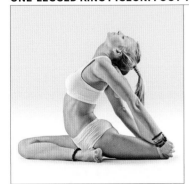

One-Legged King Pigeon Pose 1

Eka Pada Raja Kapotasana 1

(EY-kuh PUH-duh RAH-juh kuh-po-TAHS-uh-nuh)

Modification: grabbing onto the back knee with both hands under-head grip; foot to the back of the head

Pose Type: seated, backbend

Drishti Point: Bhrumadhye or Ajna Chakra (third eye, between the eyebrows)

1.

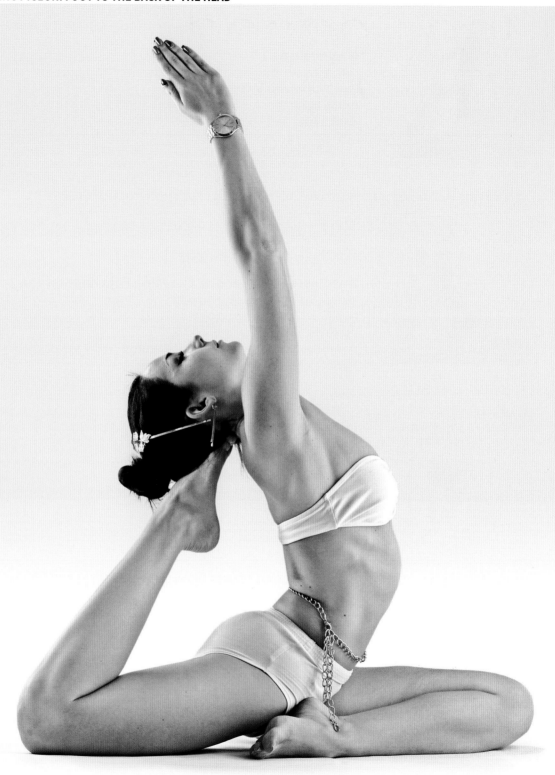

One Legged King Pigeon Pose 1

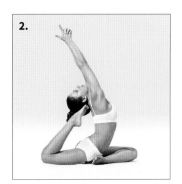

2.

Eka Pada Raja Kapotasana 1

(EY-kuh PUH-duh RAH-juh kuh-po-TAHS-uh-nuh)

Pose Type: seated, backbend

Drishti Point: Angusthamadhye or Angustha Ma Dyai (thumbs)

How to Perform the Pose:

1. Begin by sitting on the floor with both your legs straight out in front of you. Engage your *mula bandha*, *uddhiyana bandha*, and *ujjayi* breathing.

2. Exhale and bend your left knee, keeping the knee on the floor, and slide the left heel toward the inside of your right thigh.

3. Inhale as you lean forward. Exhale, extend the right leg straight out behind you with your right thigh, knee, shin, and front of the right foot on the floor. Square your hips by pulling the left hip to the back and right hip to the front.

4. Inhale as you lengthen the spine, pressing both hands to the floor by your hips for support. Exhale as you let your head roll back into a backbend.

5. Exhale as you bend your right knee, bringing your right foot toward your head. Once your right foot touches your head, slide your right foot under the back of your head and fix it in place.

6. Inhale as you stretch both arms up over your head. Exhale as you bring your palms together, keeping your arms straight and strong (Pose #1). Push through your chest. You can experiment with interlocking your fingers and letting your pointer fingers and thumbs be straight. You can also bring your foot to the side of your head (Pose #2).

7. Hold the pose for at least 30, and up to 90, seconds in order to receive the full benefits of the stretch.

8. Exhale as you release the right foot from under your head and lower it to the floor. Inhale and straighten your spine. Exhale as you bring both your legs straight out in front of you. Repeat on the other side.

Modification: both arms extended to the sky
1. foot to the back of the head, palms together
2. foot to the side of the head, fingers interlocked, pointer fingers free

eka = one
pada = foot or leg
raja = king, royal
kapota = pigeon

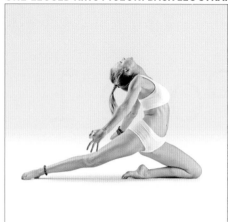

Easy One-Legged King Pigeon Pose 1
Sukha Eka Pada Raja Kapotasana 1
(SUK-uh EY-kuh PUH-duh RAH-juh kuh-po-TAHS-uh-nuh)
Modification: hips lifted, back leg straight, arms open wide
Pose Type: standing (on the knees), backbend
Drishti Point: Bhrumadhye or Ajna Chakra (third eye, between the eyebrows)

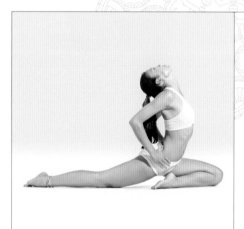

One-Legged King Pigeon Pose 1 Prep.
Eka Pada Raja Kapotasana 1 Prep.
(EY-kuh PUH-duh RAH-juh kuh-po-TAHS-uh-nuh)
Modification: hips off the floor, back leg straight; hands on the hips
Pose Type: seated, backbend
Drishti Point: Bhrumadhye or Ajna Chakra (third eye, between the eyebrows)

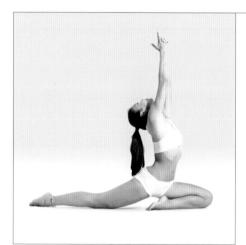

Upward Hands One-Legged King Pigeon Pose 1
Urdhva Hasta Eka Pada Raja Kapotasana 1
(OORD-vuh HUH-stuh EY-kuh PUH-duh RAH-juh kuh-po-TAHS-uh-nuh)
Modification: hips off the floor, back leg straight; arms extended to the sky
Pose Type: seated, backbend
Drishti Point: Angushtamadhye or Angustha Ma Dyai (thumbs)

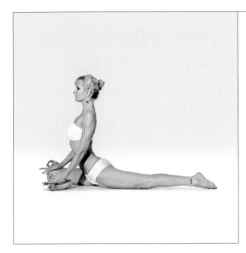

One-Legged King Pigeon Pose 1 Prep.

Eka Pada Raja Kapotasana 1 Prep.

(EY-kuh PUH-duh RAH-juh kuh-po-TAHS-uh-nuh)

Modification: back leg straight; palms facing up, back of the hand on the foot and the knee

Pose Type: seated, backbend

Drishti Point: Nasagrai or Nasagre (nose)

ONE-LEGGED KING PIGEON: BACK LEG STRAIGHT—FORWARD BEND & TWIST

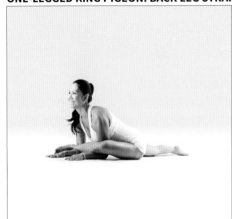

One-Legged King Pigeon Pose 1

Eka Pada Raja Kapotasana 1

(EY-kuh PUH-duh RAH-juh kuh-po-TAHS-uh-nuh)

Modification: back leg straight; forward bend, forearms to the floor, foot and knee to the elbow creases

Pose Type: seated, forward bend

Drishti Point: Nasagrai or Nasagre (nose)

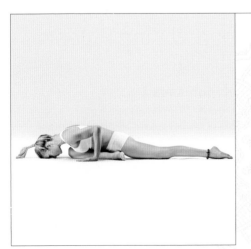

One-Legged King Pigeon Pose 1

Eka Pada Raja Kapotasana 1

(EY-kuh PUH-duh RAH-juh kuh-po-TAHS-uh-nuh)

Modification: back leg straight; forehead to the floor, palms to the floor, elbows on top of the wrists

Pose Type: seated, forward bend

Drishti Point: Nasagrai or Nasagre (nose)

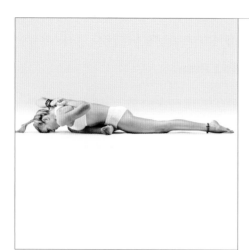

Hand Position of Cow Face Pose in One-Legged King Pigeon Pose 1

Hasta Gomukhasana in Eka Pada Raja Kapotasana 1

(HUH-stuh go-muk-AHS-uh-nuh in EY-kuh PUH-duh RAH-juh kuh-po-TAHS-uh-nuh)

Modification: back leg straight, forward bend with Gomukhasana Arms

Pose Type: seated, forward bend

Drishti Point: Nasagrai or Nasagre (nose)

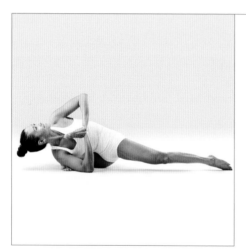

Revolved One-Legged King Pigeon Pose 1

Parivritta Eka Pada Raja Kapotasana 1

(puh-ri-VRIT-tuh EY-kuh PUH-duh RAH-juh kuh-po-TAHS-uh-nuh)

Modification: twisting to the inside of the body, back leg straight; foot to the armpit

Pose Type: seated, forward bend, twist

Drishti Point: Urdhva or Antara Drishti (up to the sky)

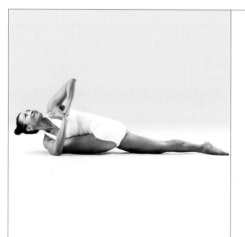

Revolved One-Legged King Pigeon Pose 1

Parivritta Eka Pada Raja Kapotasana 1

(puh-ri-VRIT-tuh EY-kuh PUH-duh RAH-juh kuh-po-TAHS-uh-nuh)

Modification: twisting to the outside of the body, back leg straight; knee to the armpit

Pose Type: seated, forward bend, twist

Drishti Point: Urdhva or Antara Drishti (up to the sky)

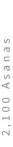

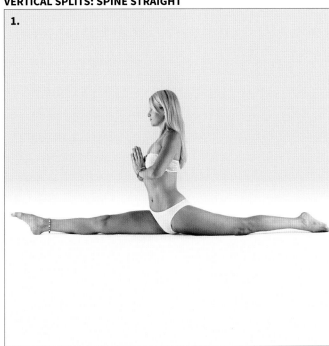

1.

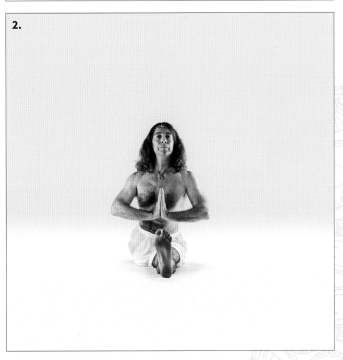

2.

Pose Dedicated to Hanuman

Hanumanasana

(huh-nu-mahn-AHS-uh-nuh)

Also Known As: Pose Dedicated to Hanuman A
(Hanumanasana A)
Modification: hands in Anjali Mudra (Hands in Prayer)
1. side view
2. front view
Pose Type: seated
Drishti Point: Nasagrai or Nasagre (nose) or Hastagrai or
Hastagre (hands)

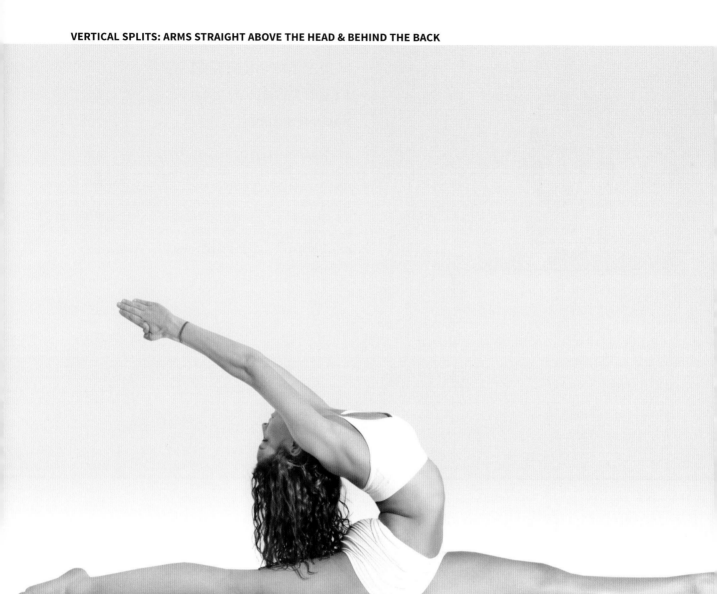

Upward Hands in
Pose Dedicated to Hanuman

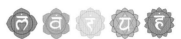

Urdhva Hasta Hanumanasana

(OORD-vuh HUH-stuh huh-nu-mahn-AHS-uh-nuh)
Also Known As: Pose Dedicated to Hanuman B (Hanumanasana B)
Pose Type: seated, backbend
Drishti Point: Angusthamadhye or Angustha Ma Dyai (thumbs)

Modification: deep backbend

urdhva = upward
hasta = hand
Hanuman = Hindu Deity, Lord of the Monkeys

How to Perform the Pose:

1. Begin by standing on your knees with sitting bones lifted off the heels. Engage your *mula bandha*, *uddhiyana bandha*, and *ujjayi* breathing.

2. Exhale, step your left foot to the front into a lunge. Keep your left knee on top of your left ankle and your right knee under your right hip.

3. Inhale as you slide your left foot out to the front, lifting your left toes off the floor until your left leg is straight.

4. Inhale and stretch your arms up to lengthen your spine. Exhale as you hinge forward from your hips, bringing your hands to the floor on either side of the left leg.

5. On your next exhale, start sliding your left foot out to the front and your right knee to the back, reaching your legs in two opposite directions, coming into a full vertical split. Keep your hips square by pulling your left hip back and your right hip forward.

6. Inhale and reach both your arms up to the sky. Exhale as you deepen the backbend by letting your head roll back and your arms reach in the direction of your back foot.

7. Hold the pose for at least 30, and up to 90, seconds in order to receive the full benefits of the stretch.

8. Inhale as you come out of the backbend. Exhale and place both your palms to the floor on the inside of the left leg. Inhale. As you exhale, swing your left leg back and bring your left knee to the floor by your right knee. Inhale and come up to the starting position with both knees on the floor. Repeat on the other side.

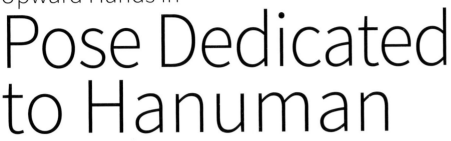

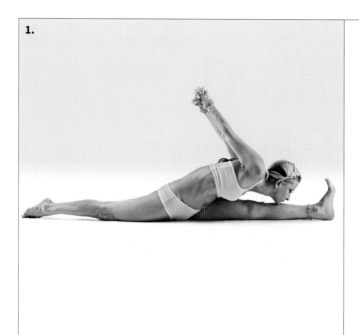

Hands Bound Pose Dedicated to Hanuman

Baddha Hasta Hanumanasana

(BUH-duh HUH-stuh huh-nu-mahn-AHS-uh-nuh)

Modification: forward bend

1. side view

2. front view

Pose Type: seated, forward bend

Drishti Point: Padayoragrai or Padayoragre (toes/feet), Nasagrai or Nasagre (nose)

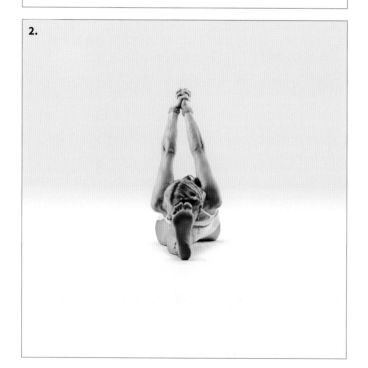

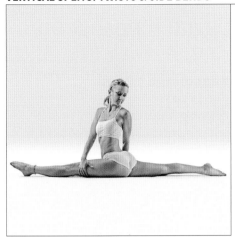

Revolved Pose Dedicated to Hanuman

Parivritta Hanumanasana
(puh-ri-VRIT-uh huh-nu-mahn-AHS-uh-nuh)
Pose Type: seated, twist
Drishti Point: Padayoragrai or Padayoragre (toes/feet)

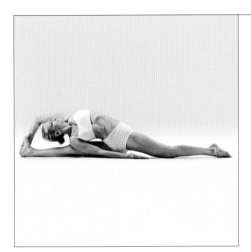

Revolved Sideways Pose Dedicated to Hanuman

Parivritta Parshva Hanumanasana
(puh-ri-VRIT-uh PAHRSH-vuh huh-nu-mahn-AHS-uh-nuh)
Modification: twisting to the inside of the body
Pose Type: seated, forward bend, twist, side bend
Drishti Point: Urdhva or Antara Drishti (up to the sky)

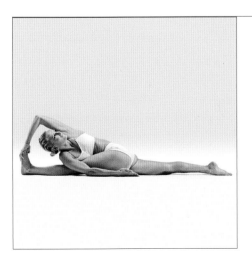

Revolved Sideways Pose Dedicated to Hanuman

Parivritta Parshva Hanumanasana
(puh-ri-VRIT-uh PAHRSH-vuh huh-nu-mahn-AHS-uh-nuh)
Modification: twisting to the outside of the body
Pose Type: seated, forward bend, twist, side bend
Drishti Point: Urdhva or Antara Drishti (up to the sky)

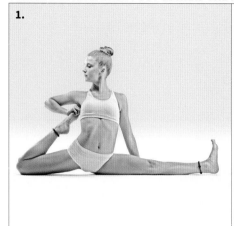

1.

Revolved One-Legged King Pigeon Pose 4 Prep.

Parivritta Eka Pada Raja Kapotasana 4 Prep.

(puh-ri-VRIT-tuh EY-kuh PUH-duh RAH-juh kuh-po-TAHS-uh-nuh)

Modification: 1. hand to the floor by the hip, other hand pressing the foot toward the hip

2. grabbing onto the big toe of the front foot on the same side, other hand pressing the back foot toward the hip

Pose Type: seated, backbend, twist

Drishti Point: Padayoragrai or Padayoragre (toes/feet), Parshva Drishti (to the right), Parshva Drishti (to the left)

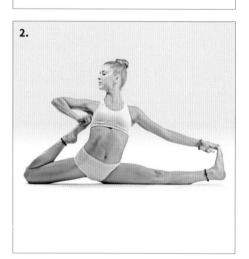

2.

Mermaid Pose 4

Naginyasana 4

(nuh-gin-YAHS-uh-nuh)

Pose Type: seated, backbend, binding

Drishti Point: Bhrumadhye or Ajna Chakra (third eye, between the eyebrows)

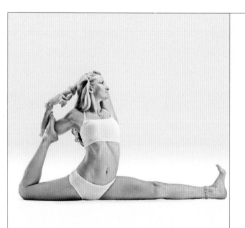

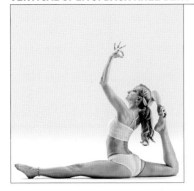

One-Legged King Pigeon Pose 4

Eka Pada Raja Kapotasana 4

(EY-kuh PUH-duh RAH-juh kuh-po-TAHS-uh-nuh)

Modification: one hand grabbing onto the back foot on the same side with overhead grip

Pose Type: seated, backbend

Drishti Point: Hastagrai or Hastagre (hands)

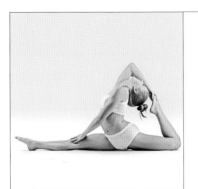

One-Legged King Pigeon Pose 4

Eka Pada Raja Kapotasana 4

(EY-kuh PUH-duh RAH-juh kuh-po-TAHS-uh-nuh)

Modification: one hand grabbing onto the back foot on the opposite side with overhead grip, foot reaching toward the head; other hand on the knee of the front leg

Pose Type: seated, backbend

Drishti Point: Bhrumadhye or Ajna Chakra (third eye, between the eyebrows)

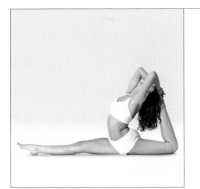

One-Legged King Pigeon Pose 4

Eka Pada Raja Kapotasana 4

(EY-kuh PUH-duh RAH-juh kuh-po-TAHS-uh-nuh)

Also Known As: One-Legged Stretched Out King Pigeon Pose (Prasarita Pada Raja Kapotasana), Pose of the Lord Kailasha (Kailashasana), Saw Pose A (Kroukachasana A)

Modification: both hands grabbing onto the back foot with overhead grip

Pose Type: seated, backbend

Drishti Point: Bhrumadhye or Ajna Chakra (third eye, between the eyebrows)

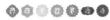

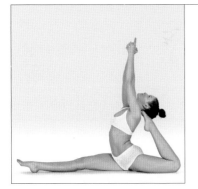

Foot to the Head One-Legged King Pigeon Pose 4

Shirsha Pada Eka Pada Raja Kapotasana 4

(SHEER-shuh PUH-duh EY-kuh PUH-duh RAH-juh kuh-po-TAHS-uh-nuh)

Also Known As: Hanuman Salutation Pose (Hanumana Namaskara)

Modification: both arms extended to the sky, back foot to the back of the head

Pose Type: seated, backbend

Drishti Point: Angushtamadhye or Angushta Ma Dyai (thumbs)

Core Poses

BOAT POSE

SIX TRIANGLES POSE

SUPINE POSES

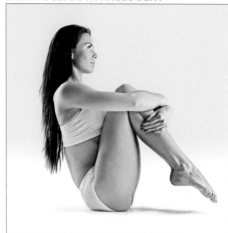

Easy Boat Pose

Sukha Navasana

(SUK-uh nah-VAHS-uh-nuh)

Modification: knees bent, arms wrapped around the shins
Pose Type: core, seated
Drishti Point: Nasagrai or Nasagre (nose)

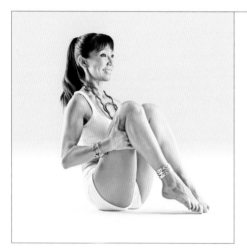

Easy Boat Pose

Sukha Navasana

(SUK-uh nah-VAHS-uh-nuh)

Modification: knees bent, grabbing the back of the thighs, toes touching the floor
Pose Type: core, seated
Drishti Point: Nasagrai or Nasagre (nose)

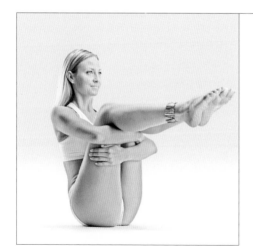

Easy Boat Pose

Sukha Navasana

(SUK-uh nah-VAHS-uh-nuh)

Modification: knees bent, arms wrapped around the back of the thighs, shins parallel to the floor
Pose Type: core, seated
Drishti Point: Padayoragrai or Padayoragre (toes/feet)

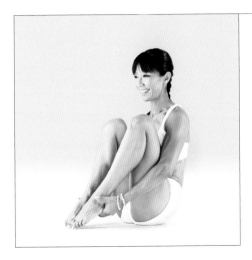

Easy Boat Pose

Sukha Navasana

(SUK-uh nah-VAHS-uh-nuh)

Modification: grabbing onto the heels, toes touching the floor
Pose Type: core, seated
Drishti Point: Nasagrai or Nasagre (nose)

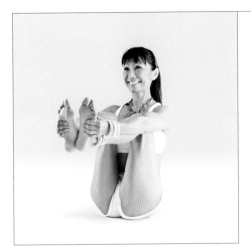

Easy Boat Pose

Sukha Navasana

(SUK-uh nah-VAHS-uh-nuh)

Modification: grabbing onto the outside edges of the feet, shins parallel to the floor
Pose Type: core, seated
Drishti Point: Nasagrai or Nasagre (nose)

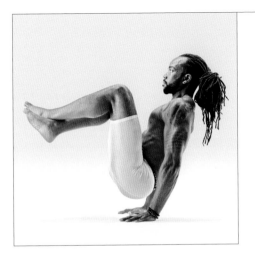

Pendant Pose

Lolasana

(lo-LAHS-uh-nuh)

Modification: knees in front of chest, ankles crossed
Pose Type: core, arm balance
Drishti Point: Nasagrai or Nasagre (nose)

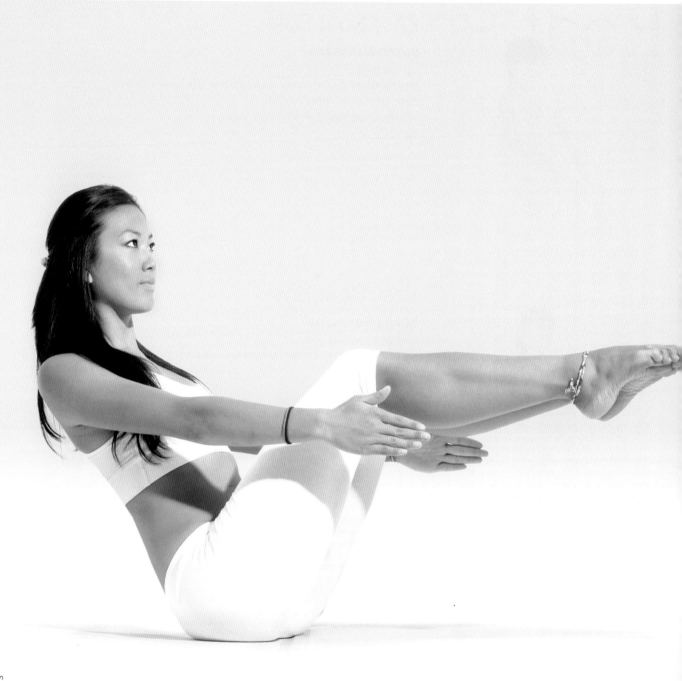

Boat Pose

Navasana

(nah-VAHS-uh-nuh)
Pose Type: core, seated
Drishti Point: Padhayoragrai or Padayoragre (toes/feet)

Variation: arms straight and parallel to the floor, knees bent, shins parallel to the floor

nava = boat

How to Perform the Pose:

1. Begin by sitting on the floor with both your legs straight out in front of you. Keep your hands on the floor at the sides of your hips for support. Engage your *mula bandha*, *uddhiyana bandha*, and *ujjayi* breathing.

2. Exhale, bend your knees, and slide your feet toward your sitting bones. Keep your feet and knees together.

3. Inhale as you lengthen your spine. Engage your core and lean back. Make sure your spine is straight and your lower back is off the floor.

4. Exhale and lift your feet off the floor until your shins are parallel to the floor.

5. Once you have your balance, exhale and lift your arms off the floor, keeping them parallel to the floor.

6. Hold the pose for at least 30, and up to 90, seconds in order to receive the full benefits of pose.

7. Inhale as you release the pose by lowering your hands and feet to the floor. Exhale and slide your feet out in front until your legs are straight to come back to the starting position.

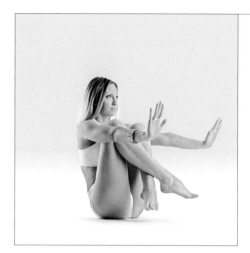

Easy Boat Pose

Sukha Navasana

(SUK-uh nah-VAHS-uh-nuh)

Modification: knees bent, ankles crossed, arms straight and parallel to the floor
Pose Type: core, seated
Drishti Point: Angushtamadhye or Angushta Ma Dyai (thumbs)

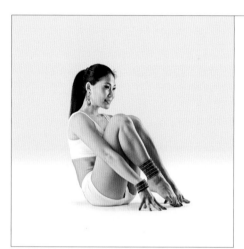

Easy Boat Pose

Sukha Navasana

(SUK-uh nah-VAHS-uh-nuh)

Modification: knees bent, fingertips to the floor, toes touching the floor
Pose Type: core, seated
Drishti Point: Nasagrai or Nasagre (nose)

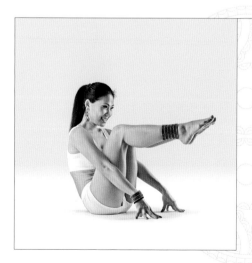

Easy Boat Pose

Sukha Navasana

(SUK-uh nah-VAHS-uh-nuh)

Modification: knees bent, fingertips to the floor, shins parallel to the floor
Pose Type: core, seated
Drishti Point: Padayoragrai or Padayoragre (toes/feet)

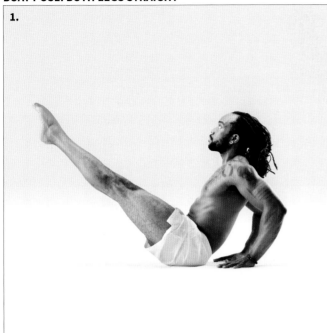

1.

Supported Boat Pose

Salamba Navasana

(SAH-luhm-buh nah-VAHS-uh-nuh)

Modification: palms to the floor behind the hips
1. both legs straight, fingertips pointing toward the hips
2. both legs straight, both arms straight, fingertips pointing to the back
Pose Type: core, seated
Drishti Point: Bhrumadhye or Ajna Chakra (third eye, between the eyebrows), Padayoragrai or Padayoragre (toes/feet)

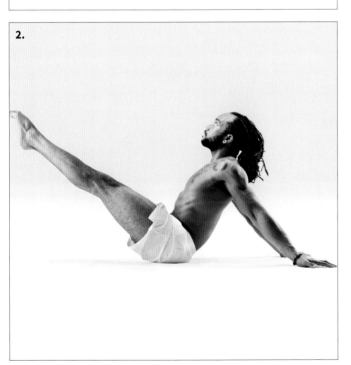

2.

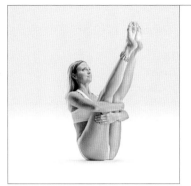

Supported Boat Pose

Salamba Navasana

(SAH-luhm-buh nah-VAHS-uh-nuh)

Modification: both arms wrapped around both legs, legs straight

Pose Type: core, seated

Drishti Point: Padayoragrai or Padayoragre (toes/feet)

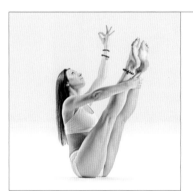

Supported Boat Pose—One-Handed

Eka Hasta Salamba Navasana

(EY-kuh HUH-stuh SAH-luhm-buh nah-VAHS-uh-nuh)

Modification: both legs straight; one arm straight, fingertips to the sky; other arm wrapping behind the ankles of both legs

Pose Type: core, seated

Drishti Point: Urdhva or Antara Drishti (up to the sky) or Hastagrai or Hastagre (hands)

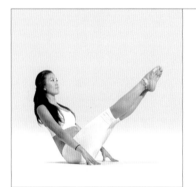

Supported Boat Pose

Salamba Navasana

(SAH-luhm-buh nah-VAHS-uh-nuh)

Modification: fingertips on the floor, pointing to the front

Pose Type: core, seated

Drishti Point: Padayoragrai or Padayoragre (toes/feet)

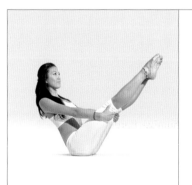

Supported Boat Pose

Salamba Navasana

(SAH-luhm-buh nah-VAHS-uh-nuh)

Modification: grabbing behind the knees, legs straight

Pose Type: core, seated

Drishti Point: Padayoragrai or Padayoragre (toes/feet)

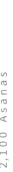

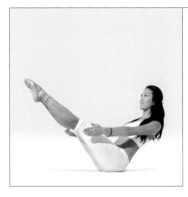

Complete Boat Pose

Paripurna Navasana

(puh-ri-POOR-nuh nah-VAHS-uh-nuh)

Modification: arms straight and parallel to the floor, legs straight
Pose Type: core, seated
Drishti Point: Padayoragrai or Padayoragre (toes/feet)

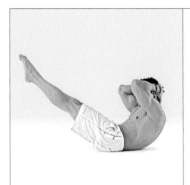

Half Boat Pose

Ardha Navasana

(UHR-duh nah-VAHS-uh-nuh)

Modification: fingers interlocked behind the head
Pose Type: core, seated
Drishti Point: Padayoragrai or Padayoragre (toes/feet)

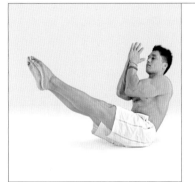

Boat Pose

Navasana

(nah-VAHS-uh-nuh)

Modification: palms and elbows together, elbows bent
Pose Type: core, seated
Drishti Point: Angushtamadhye or Angushta Ma Dyai (thumbs)

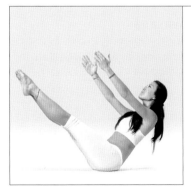

Unsupported Boat Pose

Niralamba Navasana

(nir-AH-luhm-buh nah-VAHS-uh-nuh)

Modification: arms shoulder width apart
Pose Type: core, seated
Drishti Point: Angushtamadhye or Angushta Ma Dyai (thumbs), Bhrumadhye or Ajna Chakra (third eye, between the eyebrows)

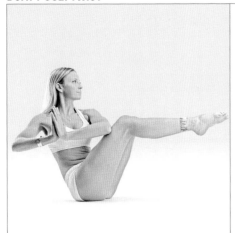

Revolved Boat Pose with Hands in Prayer

Parivritta Navasana Namaskar

(puh-ri-VRIT-tuh nah-VAHS-uh-nuh nuh-muhs-KAHR)

Pose Type: core, seated, twist

Drishti Point: Padayoragrai or Padayoragre (toes/feet)

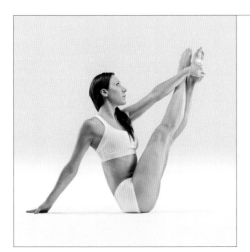

Supported Boat Pose—One-Handed

Eka Hasta Salamba Navasana

(EY-kuh HUH-stuh SAH-luhm-buh nah-VAHS-uh-nuh)

Modification: both legs straight, ankles crossed; one arm straight, palm to the floor behind the hips; other arm wrapping behind the ankles of both legs

Pose Type: core, seated

Drishti Point: Padayoragrai or Padayoragre (toes/feet)

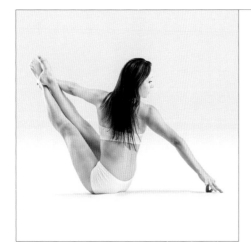

Revolved Supported Boat Pose— One-Handed

Parivritta Eka Hasta Salamba Navasana

(puh-ri-VRIT-tuh EY-kuh HUH-stuh SAH-luhm-buh nah-VAHS-uh-nuh)

Modification: both legs straight, ankles crossed; arms straight, fingertips to the floor behind the hips, one hand grabbing onto the heel

Pose Type: core, seated, twist

Drishti Point: Hastagrai or Hastagre (hands)

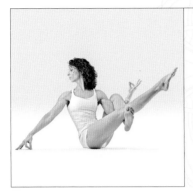

Revolved Supported Boat Pose—One-Handed

Parivritta Eka Hasta Salamba Navasana
(puh-ri-VRIT-tuh EY-kuh HUH-stuh SAH-luhm-buh nah-VAHS-uh-nuh)
Modification: one foot under the knee, other leg straight; one arm threaded under the bent leg, fingertips of the other hand on the floor
Pose Type: core, seated, twist
Drishti Point: Hastagrai or Hastagre (hands)

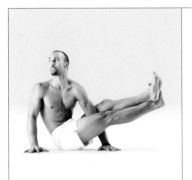

Revolved Supported Boat Pose

Parivritta Salamba Navasana
(puh-ri-VRIT-tuh SAH-luhm-buh nah-VAHS-uh-nuh)
Modification: ankles crossed, legs wrapped around the forearm
Pose Type: core, seated, twist
Drishti Point: Parshva (far to the right), Parshva (far to the left)

BOAT POSE: TWIST, SCISSOR LEGS

1.

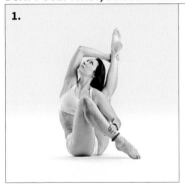

Revolved Boat Pose

Parivritta Navasana
(puh-ri-VRIT-tuh nah-VAHS-uh-nuh)
Modification: one leg over the shoulder, toes of the other leg to the floor
1. front view
2. back view
Pose Type: core, seated, twist
Drishti Point: Urdhva or Antara Drishti (up to the sky)

2.

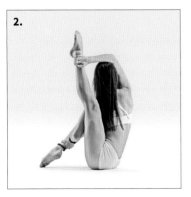

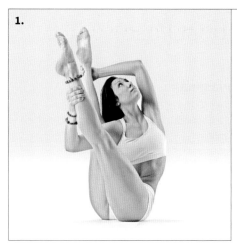

1.

Revolved Boat Pose

Parivritta Navasana

(puh-ri-VRIT-tuh nah-VAHS-uh-nuh)

Modification: one leg over the shoulder, both legs straight

1. front view
2. back view

Pose Type: core, seated, twist

Drishti Point: Urdhva or Antara Drishti (up to the sky)

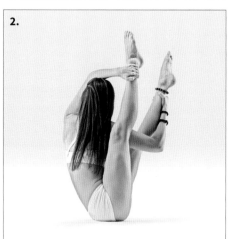

2.

BOAT POSE: ONE LEG STRAIGHT, ONE LEG BENT

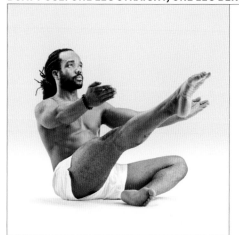

One-Legged Supported Boat Pose

Eka Pada Salamba Navasana

(EY-kuh PUH-duh SAH-luhm-buh nah-VAHS-uh-nuh)

Modification: one leg straight, one knee bent and dropped to the side for support

Pose Type: core, seated

Drishti Point: Bhrumadhye or Ajna Chakra (third eye, between the eyebrows) or Padayoragrai or Padayoragre (toes/feet)

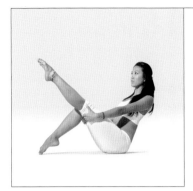

One-Legged Supported Boat Pose

Eka Pada Salamba Navasana

(EY-kuh PUH-duh SAH-luhm-buh nah-VAHS-uh-nuh)

Modification: grabbing onto the back of the thighs for support; one leg straight, one leg bent—toes touching the floor

Pose Type: core, seated

Drishti Point: Padayoragrai or Padayoragre (toes/feet)

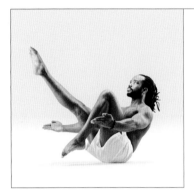

One-Legged Unsupported Boat Pose

Eka Pada Niralamba Navasana

(EY-kuh PUH-duh nir-AH-luhm-buh nah-VAHS-uh-nuh)

Modification: one leg straight; one knee bent toward the chest, foot off the floor

Pose Type: core, seated

Drishti Point: Padayoragrai or Padayoragre (toes/feet)

BOAT POSE: SCISSOR LEGS

1.

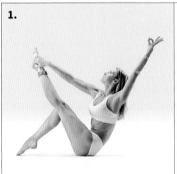

One-Legged Supported Boat Pose—One-Handed

Eka Pada Eka Hasta Salamba Navasana

(EY-kuh PUH-duh EY-kuh HUH-stuh SAH-luhm-buh nah-VAHS-uh-nuh)

Modification: grabbing the outside edge of the foot with the opposite hand for support, leg straight, other arm up to the sky

1. other leg bent, toes touching the floor

2. other leg straight, foot off the floor

Pose Type: core, seated

Drishti Point: Bhrumadhye or Ajna Chakra (third eye, between the eyebrows), Padayoragrai or Padayoragre (toes/feet)

2.

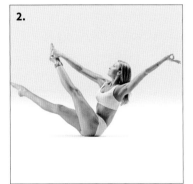

1.

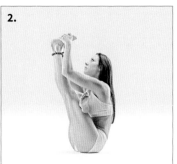

2.

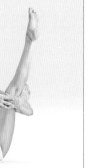

Upward Half Firelog Western Intense Stretch Pose

Urdhva Ardha Agnistambha Paschimottanasana

(OORD-vuh UHR-duh uhg-ni-STUHM-buh puhsh-chi-mo-tahn-AHS-uh-nuh)

Also Known As: Upward Half Firelog Seated Forward Bend

Modification: 1. forehead to the shin

2. forehead away from the shin

Pose Type: core, seated, forward bend

Drishti Point: Nasagrai or Nasagre (nose), Padayoragrai or Padayoragre (toes/feet)

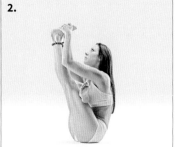

Baby Cradle Pose in Boat Pose

Hindolasana in Navasana

(hin-do-LAHS-uh-nuh in nah-VAHS-uh-nuh)

Modification: foot of the bent leg to the back of the knee of the straight leg

Pose Type: core, seated, forward bend

Drishti Point: Padayoragrai or Padayoragre (toes/feet)

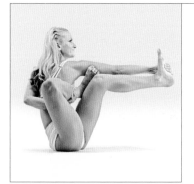

Revolved Yogic Staff Boat Pose

Parivritta Yogadanda Navasana

(puh-ri-VRIT-tuh yo-guh-DUHN-duh nah-VAHS-uh-nuh)

Modification: both knees bent; one arm behind the back, grabbing onto the ankle; other arm grabbing the outside edge of the foot

Pose Type: core, seated, twist, binding

Drishti Point: Padayoragrai or Padayoragre (toes/feet)

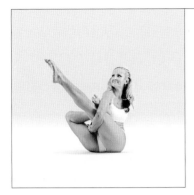

Revolved Bound Yogic Staff Boat Pose

Parivritta Baddha Yogadanda Navasana
(puh-ri-VRIT-tuh BUH-duh yo-guh-DUHN-duh nah-VAHS-uh-nuh)
Modification: binding around the straight leg
Pose Type: core, seated, twist, binding
Drishti Point: Padayoragrai or Padayoragre (toes/feet)

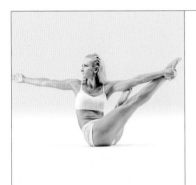

Revolved Yogic Staff Boat Pose

Parivritta Yogadanda Navasana
(puh-ri-VRIT-tuh yo-guh-DUHN-duh nah-VAHS-uh-nuh)
Modification: foot to the triceps; one arm grabbing onto the heel of the straight leg, other arm open to the side
Pose Type: core, seated, twist
Drishti Point: Hastagrai or Hastagre (hands)

BOAT POSE: ONE FOOT TO HIP SOCKET

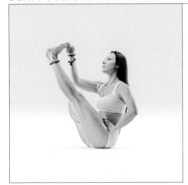

Upward One-Legged Half Lotus Western Intense Stretch Pose

Urdhva Eka Pada Ardha Padma Paschimottanasana
(OORD-vuh EY-kuh PUH-duh UHR-duh PUHD-muh puhsh-chi-mo-tahn-AHS-uh-nuh)
Also Known As: Upward One-Legged Half Lotus Seated Forward Bend
Modification: one hand grabbing onto the big toe, one hand on the hip
Pose Type: core, seated, forward bend
Drishti Point: Padayoragrai or Padayoragre (toes/feet)

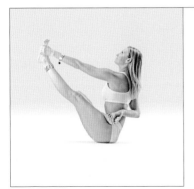

Upward One-Legged Half Bound Lotus Western Intense Stretch Pose

Urdhva Eka Pada Ardha Baddha Padma Paschimottanasana
(OORD-vuh EY-kuh PUH-duh UHR-duh BUH-duh PUHD-muh puhsh-chi-mo-tahn-AHS-uh-nuh)
Also Known As: Upward One-Legged Half Bound Lotus Seated Forward Bend
Pose Type: core, seated, forward bend, binding
Drishti Point: Padayoragrai or Padayoragre (toes/feet)

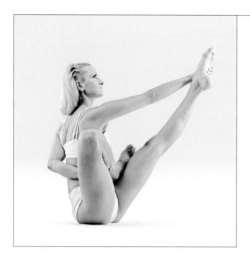

Upward One-Legged Half Bound Lotus Western Intense Stretch Pose

Urdhva Eka Pada Ardha Baddha Padma Paschimottanasana

(OORD-vuh EY-kuh PUH-duh UHR-duh BUH-duh PUHD-muh puhsh-chi-mo-tahn-AHS-uh-nuh)

Also Known As: Upward One-Legged Half Bound Lotus Seated Forward Bend
Modification: grabbing onto the foot, hand between the calf muscle and the hamstring
Pose Type: core, seated, forward bend, binding
Drishti Point: Padayoragrai or Padayoragre (toes/feet)

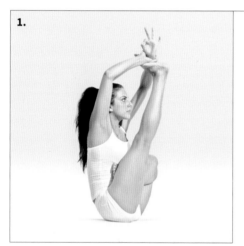

1.

Upward One-Legged Half Lotus Western Intense Stretch Pose

Urdhva Eka Pada Ardha Padma Paschimottanasana

(OORD-vuh EY-kuh PUH-duh UHR-duh PUHD-muh puhsh-chi-mo-tahn-AHS-uh-nuh)

Also Known As: Upward One-Legged Half Lotus Seated Forward Bend
Modification: 1. grabbing onto the wrist, hands over the foot
2. grabbing onto the foot, nose to the shin
Pose Type: core, seated, forward bend
Drishti Point: Padayoragrai or Padayoragre (toes/feet) or Nasagrai or Nasagre (nose)

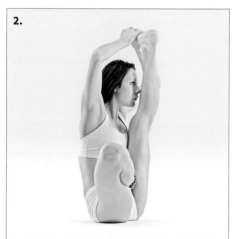

2.

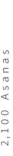

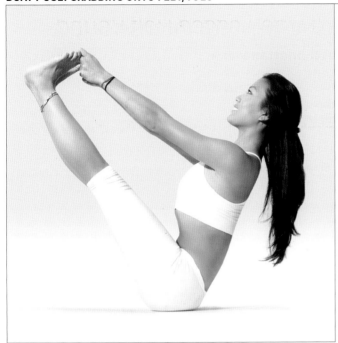

Big Toes Pose

Ubhaya Padangusthasana

(u-beye-uh puhd-ahng-goosh-TAHS-uh-nuh)

Modification: grabbing onto the big toes, toes flexed in

Pose Type: core, seated

Drishti Point: Padayoragrai or Padayoragre (toes/feet)

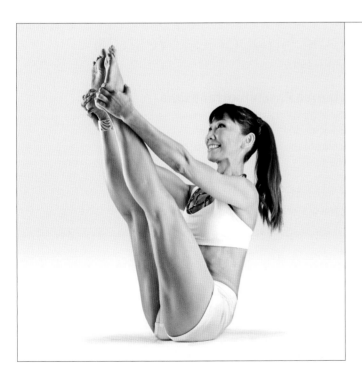

Upward Facing Western Intense Stretch

Urdhva Mukha Paschimottanasana

(OORD-vuh MUK-uh puhsh-chi-mo-tahn-AHS-uh-nuh)

Also Known As: Upward Facing Seated Forward Bend

Modification: grabbing onto the heels, arms straight

Pose Type: core, seated, forward bend, quadriceps to the chest

Drishti Point: Padayoragrai or Padayoragre (toes/feet)

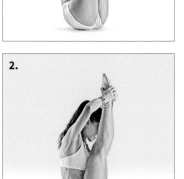

Upward Facing Western Intense Stretch

Urdhva Mukha Paschimottanasana

(OORD-vuh MUK-uh puhsh-chi-mo-tahn-AHS-uh-nuh)

Also Known As: Upward Facing Seated Forward Bend

Modification: grabbing onto the heels

1. forehead away from the shins

2. forehead to the shins

Pose Type: core, seated, forward bend

Drishti Point: Nasagrai or Nasagre (nose)

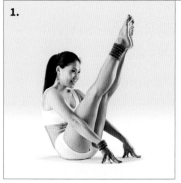

Upward Facing Supported Western Intense Stretch

Urdhva Mukha Salamba Paschimottanasana

(OORD-vuh MUK-uh SAH-luhm-buh puhsh-chi-mo-tahn-AHS-uh-nuh)

Also Known As: Upward Facing Seated Forward Bend

Modification: arms reaching to the front, fingertips to the floor,

1. forehead away from the shins

2. forehead to the shins

Pose Type: core, seated, forward bend

Drishti Point: Padayoragrai or Padayoragre (toes/feet) or Nasagrai or Nasagre (nose)

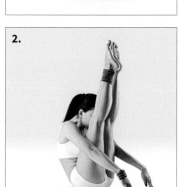

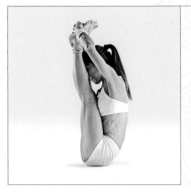

Bound Hands Upward Facing Western Intense Stretch

Baddha Hasta Urdhva Mukha Paschimottanasana

(BUH-duh HUH-stuh OORD-vuh MUK-uh puhsh-chi-mo-tahn-AHS-uh-nuh)

Also Known As: Bound Hands Upward Facing Seated Forward Bend

Pose Type: core, seated, forward bend

Drishti Point: Nasagrai or Nasagre (nose)

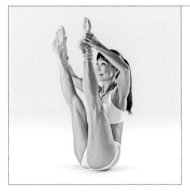

Upward Facing Western Intense Stretch

Urdhva Mukha Paschimottanasana

(OORD-vuh MUK-uh puhsh-chi-mo-tahn-AHS-uh-nuh)

Also Known As: Upward Facing Seated Forward Bend

Modification: grabbing onto the ankles, forehead to the shins

Pose Type: core, seated, forward bend

Drishti Point: Nasagrai or Nasagre (nose)

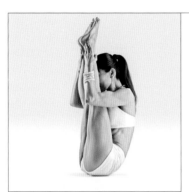

Upward Facing Western Intense Stretch

Urdhva Mukha Paschimottanasana

(OORD-vuh MUK-uh puhsh-chi-mo-tahn-AHS-uh-nuh)

Also Known As: Upward Facing Seated Forward Bend

Modification: grabbing onto the outside edges of the feet, feet hip distance apart, toes pointed

Pose Type: core, seated, forward bend

Drishti Point: Padayoragrai or Padayoragre (toes/feet)

ARM BALANCE: SITTING BONES & FEET OFF THE FLOOR

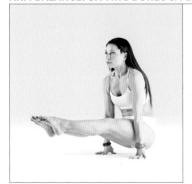

Celibate Pose

Brahmacharyasana

(bruh-muh-chahr-YAHS-uh-nuh)

Also Known As: Lifted Up Staff Pose (Dandasana Utpluti)

Modification: fingers to the floor, thumbs pointing to the back

Pose Type: core, arm balance

Drishti Point: Nasagrai or Nasagre (nose)

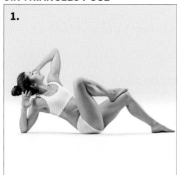

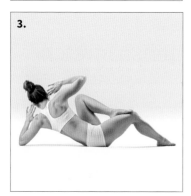

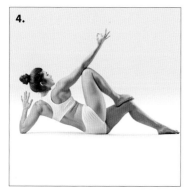

Six Triangles Pose

Shatkonasana

(shuht-ko-NAHS-uh-nuh)

Modification: top foot on the bottom knee

1. fingertips to the temples
2. one forearm to the floor, other arm wrapped around the top knee
3. fingertips to the temples, elbow toward the top knee
4. one elbow to the floor, other elbow to the top knee on the same side

Pose Type: core, seated, twist

Drishti Point: 1. Urdhva or Antara Drishti (up to the sky)

2. Nasagrai or Nasagre (nose)
3. Nasagrai or Nasagre (nose)
4. Hastagrai or Hastagre (hands)

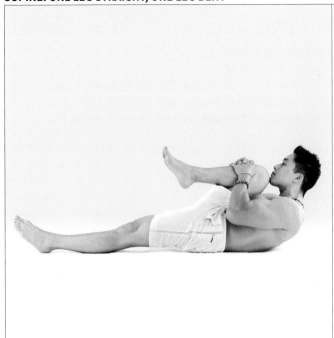

Half Wind Relieving Pose

Ardha Vayu Muktyasana
(UHR-duh VAH-yu muk-TYAHS-uh-nuh)

Also Known As: Wind-Relieving Pose (Pavana Muktasana)
Pose Type: core, supine
Drishti Point: Nasagrai or Nasagre (nose)

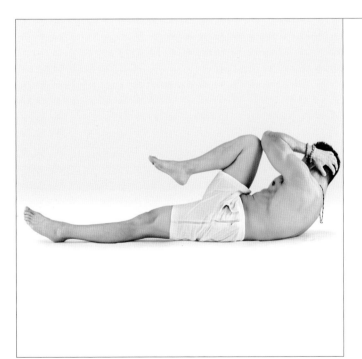

Revolved Half Wind Relieving Pose

Parivritta Ardha Vayu Muktyasana
(puh-ri-VRIT-tuh UHR-duh VAH-yu muk-TYAHS-uh-nuh)

Modification: one knee bent, one leg straight
Pose Type: core, supine, twist
Drishti Point: Nasagrai or Nasagre (nose), Bhrumadhye (third eye, between the eyebrows)

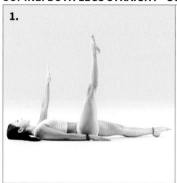

One-Legged Upward Extended Legs Pose

Eka Pada Urdhva Prasarita Padasana

(EY-kuh PUH-duh OORD-vuh pruh-SAH-ri-tuh puh-DAHS-uh-nuh)

Modification: 1. one arm extended to sky, other palm to the floor, head on the floor
2. one arm extended to sky, other palm to the floor, head and shoulders off the floor
3. fingers interlocked behind the back of the head, head and shoulders off the floor
Pose Type: core, supine
Drishti Point: Padayoragrai or Padayoragre (toes/feet)

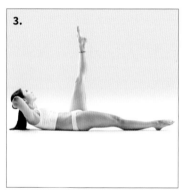

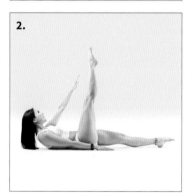

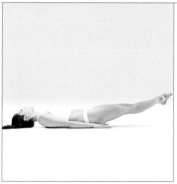

Abdominal Lift Pose

Jatharasana

(jah-tuh-RAHS-uh-nuh)

Modification: head on the floor, palms down by the hips
Pose Type: core, supine
Drishti Point: Bhrumadhye or Ajna Chakra (third eye, between the eyebrows)

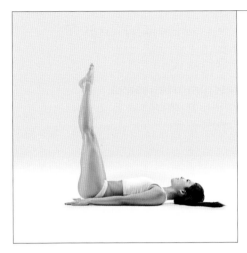

Upward Extended Legs Pose

Urdhva Prasarita Padasana

(OORD-vuh pruh-SAH-ri-tuh puh-DAHS-uh-nuh)

Pose Type: core, supine

Drishti Point: Bhrumadhye or Ajna Chakra (third eye, between the eyebrows)

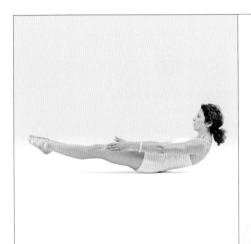

Abdominal Lift Pose

Jatharasana

(jah-tuh-RAHS-uh-nuh)

Modification: head and shoulders off the floor, feet off the floor

Pose Type: core, supine

Drishti Point: Padayoragrai or Padayoragre (toes/feet)

SUPINE: BOTH LEGS STRAIGHT

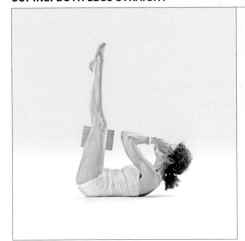

Two-Legged Abdominal Lift Upward Extended Legs Pose

Dwi Pada Jathara Urdhva Prasarita Padasana

(DWI-puh-duh JAH-tuh-ruh OORD-vuh pruh-SAH-ri-tuh puh-DAHS-uh-nuh)

Modification: with a yoga block

Pose Type: core, supine

Drishti Point: Urdhva or Antara Drishti (up to the sky), Padayoragrai or Padayoragre (toes/feet)

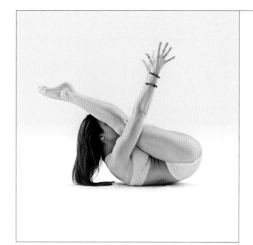

Abdominal Lift Upward Facing Western Intense Stretch

Jathara Urdhva Mukha Paschimottanasana
(JAH-tuh-ruh OORD-vuh MUK-uh puhsh-chi-mo-tahn-AHS-uh-nuh)
Also Known As: Abdominal Lift Upward Forward Bend
Modification: head lifted off the floor, forehead to the shins
Pose Type: core, supine
Drishti Point: Nasagrai or Nasagre (nose)

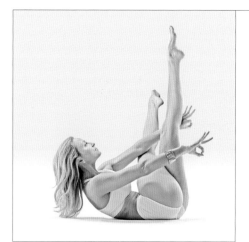

Abdominal Lift Upward Facing Western Intense Stretch

Jathara Urdhva Mukha Paschimottanasana
(JAH-tuh-ruh OORD-vuh MUK-uh puhsh-chi-mo-tahn-AHS-uh-nuh)
Also Known As: Abdominal Lift Upward Forward Bend
Modification: head lifted off the floor, legs crossed modification
Pose Type: core, supine
Drishti Point: Padayoragrai or Padayoragre (toes/feet)

SUPINE: ONE LEG STRAIGHT, ONE KNEE BENT

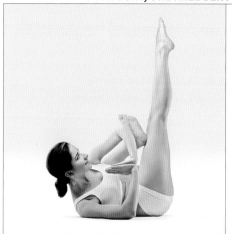

Revolved Stomach One Leg Extended Pose

Parivritta Jathara Utthita Eka Padasana
(puh-ri-VRIT-tuh JAH-tuh-tuh UT-ti-tuh EY-kuh puh-DAHS-uh-nuh)
Modification: foot to the elbow
Pose Type: core, supine, twist
Drishti Point: Padayoragrai or Padayoragre (toes/feet)

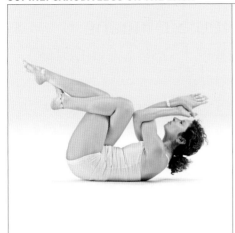

Reclining Abdominal Lift Pose Dedicated to Garuda

Supta Jathara Garudasana

(SUP-tuh JAH-tuh-ruh guh-ru-DAHS-uh-nuh)

Pose Type: core, supine

Drishti Point: Angushtamadhye or Angushta Ma Dyai (thumbs)

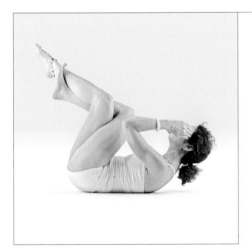

Reclining Abdominal Lift Pose Dedicated to Garuda

Supta Jathara Garudasana

(SUP-tuh JAH-tuh-ruh guh-ru-DAHS-uh-nuh)

Modification: fingers to the temples, elbows to the knees

Pose Type: core, supine

Drishti Point: Urdhva or Antara Drishti (up to the sky), Padayoragrai or Padayoragre (toes/feet)

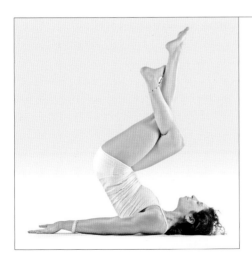

Abdominal Lift Pose Dedicated to Garuda

Jathara Garudasana

(JAH-tuh-ruh guh-ru-DAHS-uh-nuh)

Modification: palms to the floor, arms straight, sitting bones lifted off the floor

Pose Type: core, supine

Drishti Point: Urdhva or Antara Drishti (up to the sky), Padayoragrai or Padayoragre (toes/feet)

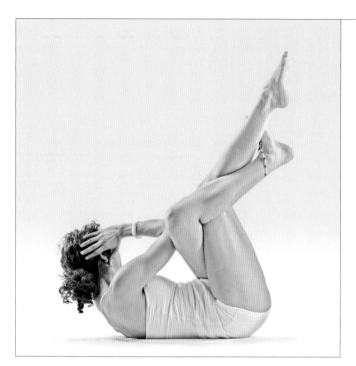

Revolved Stomach Reclining Pose Dedicated to Garuda

Parivritta Jathara Supta Garudasana
(puh-ri-VRIT-tuh JAH-tuh-ruh SUP-tuh guh-ru-DAHS-uh-nuh)

Modification: fingers to the temples, elbows out to the sides
Pose Type: core, supine, twist
Drishti Point: Parshva Drishti (to the right), Parshva Drishti (to the left)

SUPINE: FULL LOTUS

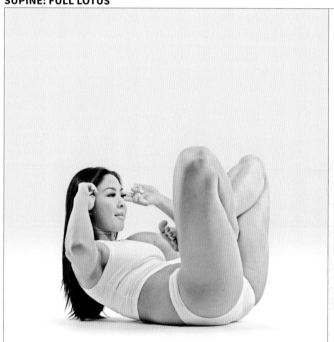

Reclining Abdominal Lift Lotus Pose

Supta Jathara Padmasana
(SUP-tuh JAH-tuh-ruh puhd-MAHS-uh-nuh)

Modification: fingers to the temples, knees up to the sky
Pose Type: core, supine
Drishti Point: Nasagrai or Nasagre (nose)

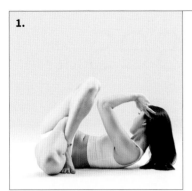

1.

Revolved Stomach Reclining Lotus Pose

Parivritta Jathara Supta Padmasana
(puh-ri-VRIT-tuh JAH-tuh-ruh SUP-tuh puhd-MAHS-uh-nuh)
Modification: fingers to the temples, elbows out to the sides
1. back view
2. front view
Pose Type: core, supine, twist
Drishti Point: Parshva Drishti (to the right), Parshva Drishti (to the left)

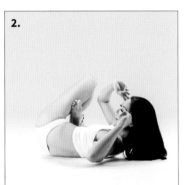

2.

Abdominal Lift Lotus Pose

Jathara Padmasana
(JAH-tuh-tuh puhd-MAHS-uh-nuh)
Modification: palms on the floor, arms straight, sitting bones lifted off the floor
Pose Type: core, supine
Drishti Point: Nasagrai or Nasagre (nose), Bhrumadhye or Ajna Chakra (third eye, between the eyebrows)

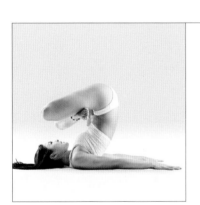

Unsupported Abdominal Lift Lotus Pose

Niralamba Jathara Padmasana
(nir-AH-luhm-buh JAH-tuh-tuh puhd-MAHS-uh-nuh)
Modification: arms extended in front, knees to the forearms
Pose Type: core, supine
Drishti Point: Nasagrai or Nasagre (nose)

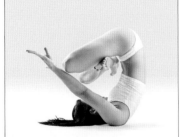

Quadruped Poses

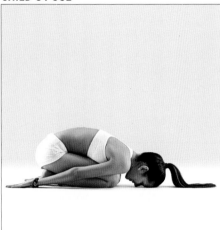

Child's Pose

Balasana

(bah-LAHS-uh-nuh)

Also Known As: Child's Pose (Garbhasana)
Modification: arms extended to the back, palms up; toes pointed to the back
Pose Type: forward bend
Drishti Point: Nasagrai or Nasagre (nose)

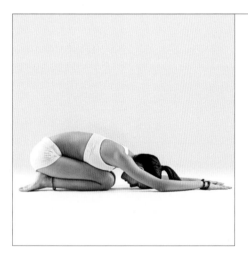

Child's Pose

Balasana

(bah-LAHS-uh-nuh)

Also Known As: Child's Pose (Garbhasana)
Modification: arms extended to the front, palms down; toes pointed to the back
Pose Type: forward bend
Drishti Point: Nasagrai or Nasagre (nose)

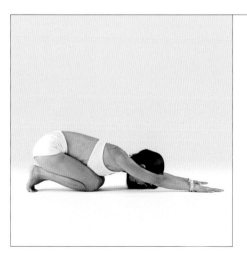

Child's Pose

Balasana

(bah-LAHS-uh-nuh)

Modification: arms extended to the front, palms down; toes curled in
Pose Type: forward bend
Drishti Point: Nasagrai or Nasagre (nose)

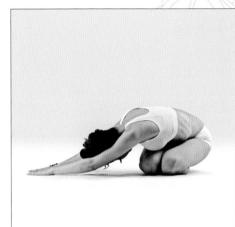

Hands to the Side Child's Pose

Parshva Hasta Balasana

(PAHRSH-vuh HUH-stuh bah-LAHS-uh-nuh)

Pose Type: forward bend, side bend

Drishti Point: Parshva Drishti (to the right), Parshva Drishti (to the left)

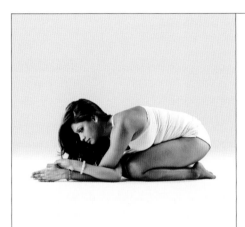

Hand Position of the Pose Dedicated to Garuda in Child's Pose

Hasta Garudasana in Balasana

(HUH-stuh guh-ru-DAHS-uh-nuh in bah-LAHS-uh-nuh)

Pose Type: forward bend

Drishti Point: Angushtamadhye or Angushta Ma Dyai (thumbs)

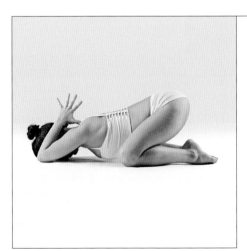

Child's Pose

Balasana

(bah-LAHS-uh-nuh)

Modification: knees open wide; palms pressed together, fingers spread wide, thumbs to the upper back

Pose Type: forward bend, mild backbend

Drishti Point: Nasagrai or Nasagre (nose)

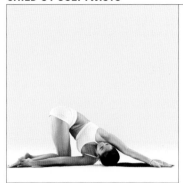

Revolved Side Child's Pose

Parivritta Parshva Balasana

(puh-ri-VRIT-tuh PAHRSH-vuh bah-LAHS-uh-nuh)
Pose Type: forward bend, twist
Drishti Point: Urdhva or Antara Drishti (up to the sky)

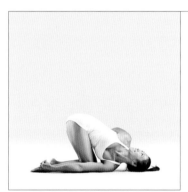

Both Hands to Legs Bound Revolved Child's Pose

Dwi Hasta Pada Baddha Parivritta Balasana

(DWI-huh-stuh PUH-duh BUH-duh puh-ri-VRIT-tuh bah-LAHS-uh-nuh)
Pose Type: forward bend, twist, binding
Drishti Point: Urdhva or Antara Drishti (up to the sky)

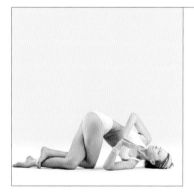

Leg Position of the Pose Dedicated to Garuda in Revolved Child's Pose

Pada Garudasana in Parivritta Balasana

(PUH-duh guh-ru-DAHS-uh-nuh in puh-ri-VRIT-tuh bah-LAHS-uh-nuh)
Modification: hands in Anjali Mudra (Hands in Prayer)
Pose Type: forward bend, twist
Drishti Point: Urdhva or Antara Drishti (up to the sky)

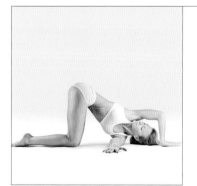

Revolved Child's Pose

Parivritta Balasana

(puh-ri-VRIT-tuh bah-LAHS-uh-nuh)
Also Known As: Turned Child's Pose (Parshva Balasana)
Modification: bottom arm straight out to the side; top arm bent at 90 degrees, palm to the floor overhead
Pose Type: forward bend, twist
Drishti Point: Urdhva or Antara Drishti (up to the sky)

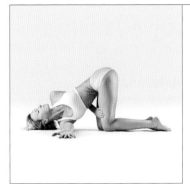

One Hand Bound Revolved Child's Pose

Eka Hasta Baddha Parivritta Balasana

(EY-kuh HUH-stuh BUH-duh puh-ri-VRIT-tuh bah-LAHS-uh-nuh)

Modification: grabbing onto the quadricep
Pose Type: forward bend, twist, binding
Drishti Point: Urdhva or Antara Drishti (up to the sky)

CHILD'S POSE: TWISTS & HALF LOTUS BINDING

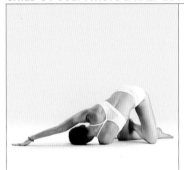

Hand to Foot Revolved Side Child's Pose

Hasta Pada Parivritta Parshva Balasana

(HUH-stuh PUH-duh puh-ri-VRIT-tuh PAHRSH-vuh bah-LAHS-uh-nuh)

Modification: foot resting on the back of the knee
Pose Type: forward bend, twist
Drishti Point: Urdhva or Antara Drishti (up to the sky)

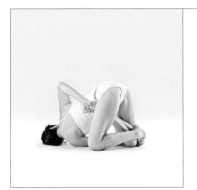

Both Hands to Feet Half Bound Lotus Revolved Child's Pose

Dwi Hasta Pada Ardha Baddha Padma Parivritta Balasana

(DWI-huh-stuh PUH-duh UHR-duh BUH-duh PUHD-muh puh-ri-VRIT-tuh bah-LAHS-uh-nuh)

Pose Type: forward bend, twist, binding
Drishti Point: Urdhva or Antara Drishti (up to the sky)

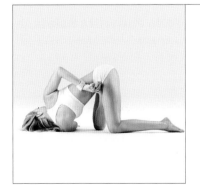

Half Bound Lotus Revolved Child's Pose

Ardha Baddha Padma Parivritta Balasana

(UHR-duh BUH-duh PUHD-muh puh-ri-VRIT-tuh bah-LAHS-uh-nuh)

Modification: torso twisting to the outside of the body, hand binding to the foot
Pose Type: forward bend, twist, binding
Drishti Point: Urdhva or Antara Drishti (up to the sky)

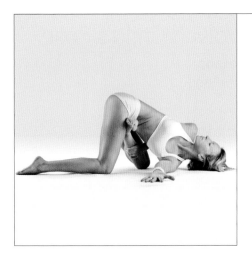

Half Bound Lotus Revolved Child's Pose

Ardha Baddha Padma Parivritta Balasana
(UHR-duh BUH-duh PUHD-muh puh-ri-VRIT-tuh bah-LAHS-uh-nuh)
Modification: torso twisting to the inside of the body, hand binding to the shin
Pose Type: forward bend, twist, binding
Drishti Point: Urdhva or Antara Drishti (up to the sky)

CHILD'S POSE: TWISTS—ONE-LEGGED—BACK FOOT IN THE AIR

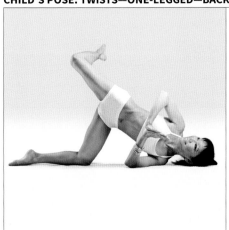

Equilibrium One-Legged Revolved Child's Pose with Hands in Prayer

Tulya Eka Pada Parivritta Balasana Namaskar
(TUL-yuh EY-kuh PUH-duh puh-ri-VRIT-tuh bah-LAHS-uh-nuh nuh-muhs-KAHR)
Modification: knee of the top leg bent
Pose Type: forward bend, twist
Drishti Point: Urdhva or Antara Drishti (up to the sky)

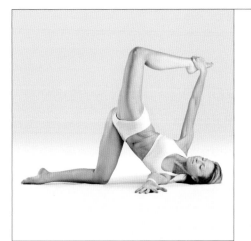

Half Bow Pose in Equilibrium One-Legged Revolved Child's Pose

Ardha Dhanurasana in Tulya Eka Pada Parivritta Balasana
(UHR-duh duh-nur-AHS-uh-nuh in TUL-yuh EY-kuh PUH-duh puh-ri-VRIT-tuh bah-LAHS-uh-nuh)
Pose Type: forward bend, twist, backbend
Drishti Point: Hastagrai or Hastagre (hands)

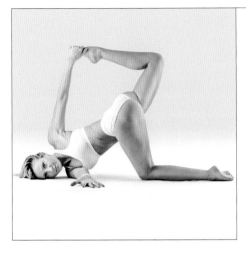

Revolved Half Bow Pose in Equilibrium One-Legged Revolved Child's Pose

Parivritta Ardha Dhanurasana in Tulya Eka Pada Parivritta Balasana

(puh-ri-VRIT-tuh UHR-duh duh-nur-AHS-uh-nuh in TUL-yuh EY-kuh PUH-duh puh-ri-VRIT-tuh bah-LAHS-uh-nuh)

Pose Type: forward bend, twist, backbend

Drishti Point: Hastagrai or Hastagre (hands)

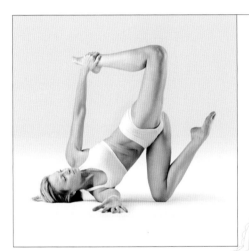

Half Bow Pose in Equilibrium One-Legged Revolved Child's Pose

Ardha Dhanurasana in Tulya Eka Pada Parivritta Balasana

(UHR-duh duh-nur-AHS-uh-nuh in TUL-yuh EY-kuh PUH-duh puh-ri-VRIT-tuh bah-LAHS-uh-nuh)

Modification: back heel toward the sitting bone

Pose Type: forward bend, twist, backbend

Drishti Point: Hastagrai or Hastagre (hands)

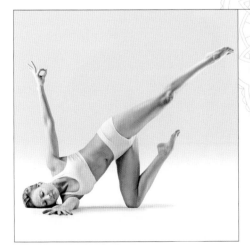

Equilibrium One-Legged Revolved Child's Pose

Tulya Eka Pada Parivritta Balasana

(TUL-yuh EY-kuh PUH-duh puh-ri-VRIT-tuh bah-LAHS-uh-nuh)

Modification: one leg straight, other knee bent, heel toward the sitting bone

Pose Type: forward bend, twist

Drishti Point: Hastagrai or Hastagre (hands)

1.

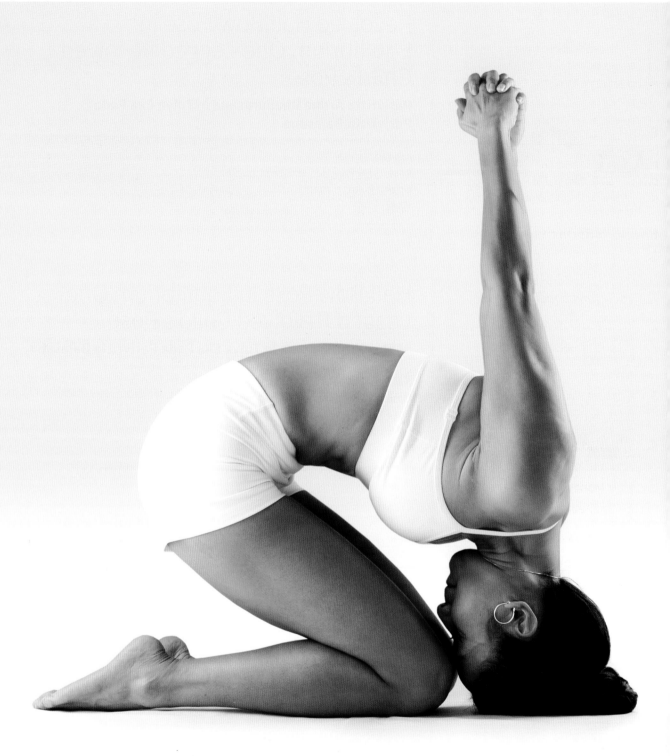

Hands Bound
Rabbit Pose

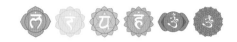

Baddha Hasta Sasangasana

(BUH-duh HUH-stuh shuh-shahng-AHS-uh-nuh)

Pose Type: forward bend

Drishti Point: Nasagrai or Nasagre (nose) or Nabhi, Nabhicakre, or Nabi Chakra (belly button)

How to Perform the Pose:

1. Begin by sitting on your heels in Hero Pose (*Virasana*). Engage your *mula bandha*, *uddhiyana bandha*, and *ujjayi* breathing.

Modification:

1. forehead to the knees, sitting bones lifted
2. forehead away from the knees, sitting bones to the heels

baddha = bound
hasta = hand
sasanga = rabbit

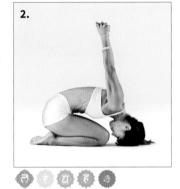
2.

2. Exhale and bend forward, letting the crown of your head touch the floor, and lift your sitting bones off your heels. Grab onto your heels with both your hands, keeping your arms on the outsides of your shins.

3. Exhale as you rock forward, bringing your forehead toward your knees. Feel the stretch in the upper back between your shoulder blades.

4. Inhale as you lift your hands off your heels and interlock your fingers behind your back. Try to press your palms together. Exhale and stretch your arms up to the sky behind your back. Feel the stretch in your front shoulder heads and your chest (Pose #1). You can experiment by leaving your sitting bones on the heels and moving your forehead away from your knees (Pose #2).

5. Hold the pose for at least 30, and up to 90, seconds in order to receive the full benefits of the stretch.

6. Inhale as you release the arms. Exhale as you straighten your spine, coming back to Hero Pose (*Virasana*).

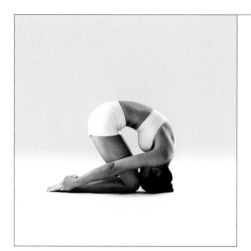

Rabbit Pose

Sasangasana

(shuh-shahn-GAHS-uh-nuh)

Also Known As: Rabbit Foot Pose

Pose Type: forward bend, inversion

Drishti Point: Nabhi, Nabhicakre, or Nabi Chakra (belly button)

COW POSE ON THE HEAD: HALF LOTUS & GARUDA LEGS

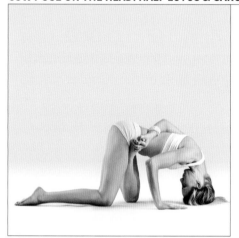

Half Bound Lotus Cow Pose on the Head

Ardha Baddha Padma Shirsha Bitilasana

(UHR-duh BUH-duh PUHD-muh SHEER-shuh bee-til-AHS-uh-nuh)

Also Known As: Ardha Baddha Padma Shirsha Gavasana*

Modification: crown of the head to the floor

Pose Type: forward bend, inversion, binding

Drishti Point: Nasagrai or Nasagre (nose), Nabhi, Nabhicakre, or Nabi Chakra (belly button)

* "Bitilisana" may also be translated as "Gavasana" in the following cow poses.

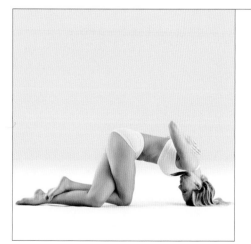

Reverse Prayer in Leg Position of the Pose Dedicated to Garuda in Cow Pose on the Head

Viparita Namaskar in Pada Garudasana in Shirsha Bitilasana

(vi-puh-REE-tuh nuh-muhs-KAHR in PUH-duh guh-ru-DAHS-uh-nuh in SHEER-shuh bee-til-AHS-uh-nuh)

Also Known As: Back of the Body Prayer Leg Position of the Pose Dedicated to Garuda in Cow Pose on the Head (Paschima Namaskara Pada Garudasana in Shirsha Bitilasana)

Pose Type: forward bend, inversion

Drishti Point: Nasagrai or Nasagre (nose), Nabhi, Nabhicakre, or Nabi Chakra (belly button)

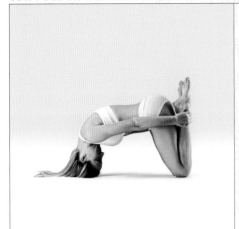

Both Hands to the Legs Cow Pose on the Head

Dwi Hasta Pada Shirsha Bitilasana

(DWI-huh-stuh PUH-duh SHEER-shuh bee-til-AHS-uh-nuh)

Modification: heels toward the sitting bones
Pose Type: forward bend, inversion
Drishti Point: Nabhi, Nabhicakre, or Nabi Chakra (belly button)

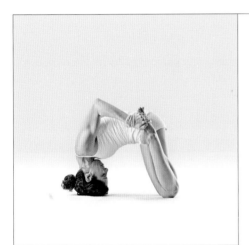

Both Hands to the Feet Cow Pose on the Head

Dwi Hasta Pada Shirsha Bitilasana

(DWI-huh-stuh PUH-duh SHEER-shuh bee-til-AHS-uh-nuh)

Modification: heels to the outside of the hips
Pose Type: forward bend, inversion
Drishti Point: Nabhi, Nabhicakre, or Nabi Chakra (belly button)

ALL FOURS: NEUTRAL SPINE

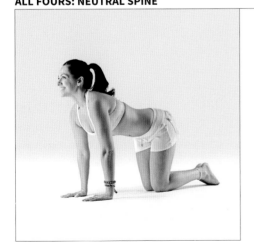

Cow Pose

Bitilasana

(bee-til-AHS-uh-nuh)

Also Known As: Table Pose (Bharmanasana)
Pose Type: standing (hands and knees)
Drishti Point: Nasagrai or Nasagre (nose), Bhrumadhye or Ajna Chakra (third eye, between the eyebrows)

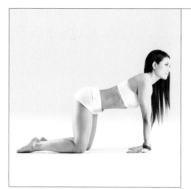

Intense Wrist Stretch Cow Pose

Uttana Manibandha Bitilasana

(ut-TAHN-uh muh-ni-BUHN-duh bee-til-AHS-uh-nuh)

Also Known As: Table Pose Modification (Bharmanasana)
Pose Type: standing (hands and knees)
Drishti Point: Nasagrai or Nasagre (nose), Bhrumadhye or Ajna Chakra (third eye, between the eyebrows)

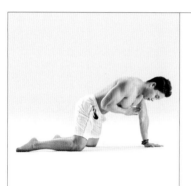

One Hand Cow Pose

Eka Hasta Bitilasana

(EY-kuh HUH-stuh bee-til-AHS-uh-nuh)

Also Known As: Table Pose (Bharmanasana)
Pose Type: standing (hands and knees)
Drishti Point: Nasagrai or Nasagre (nose), Bhrumadhye or Ajna Chakra (third eye, between the eyebrows)

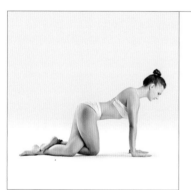

Leg Position of the Pose Dedicated to Garuda in Cow Pose

Pada Garudasana in Bitilasana

(PUH-duh guh-ru-DAHS-uh-nuh in bee-til-AHS-uh-nuh)

Also Known As: Table Pose Modification (Bharmanasana)
Pose Type: standing (on hands and knees)
Drishti Point: Angushtamadhye or Angushta Ma Dyai (thumbs), Nasagrai or Nasagre (nose)

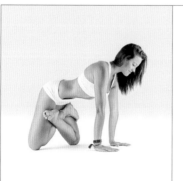

Lotus Pose in Cow Pose

Padmasana in Bitilasana

(puhd-MAHS-uh-nuh in bee-til-AHS-uh-nuh)

Also Known As: Table Pose Modification (Bharmanasana)
Pose Type: standing (on hands and knees)
Drishti Point: Angushtamadhye or Angushta Ma Dyai (thumbs), Nasagrai or Nasagre (nose)

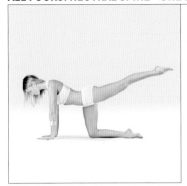

Tiger Pose

Vyaghrasana

(vyah-GRAHS-uh-nuh)

Also Known As: Table Pose Modification (Bharmanasana)

Modification: neutral spine

Pose Type: standing (hands and knees)

Drishti Point: Angushtamadhye or Angushta Ma Dyai (thumbs)

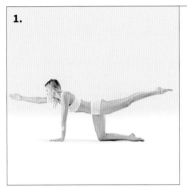

One Hand One-Legged Cow Pose

Eka Hasta Eka Pada Bitilasana

(EY-kuh HUH-stuh EY-kuh PUH-duh bee-til-AHS-uh-nuh)

Also Known As: Cat Pose (Marjarasana), Balancing Table Pose Modification (Dandayamana Bharmanasana)

Modification: neutral spine

1. arm reaching to the front, opposite leg reaching to the back
2. arm reaching to the back, opposite leg reaching to the back
3. arm reaching to the back, leg reaching to the back on the same side

Pose Type: standing (hands and knees)

Drishti Point: Angushtamadhye or Angushta Ma Dyai (thumbs)

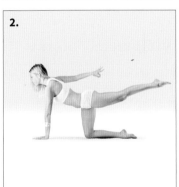

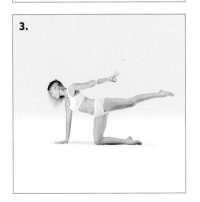

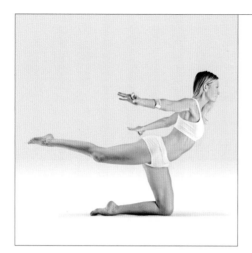

One Knee Cow Pose

Eka Janu Bitilasana

(EY-kuh JAH-nu bee-til-AHS-uh-nuh)

Also Known As: Unsupported Balancing Table Pose Modification (Niralamba Dandayamana Bharmanasana)

Pose Type: standing (on the knee), balance

Drishti Point: Bhrumadhye or Ajna Chakra (third eye, between the eyebrows), Nasagrai or Nasagre (nose)

ALL FOURS: NEUTRAL SPINE—ONE LEG EXTENDED TO THE BACK—HALF LOTUS

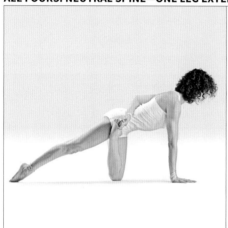

Downward Facing Pose Dedicated to Kashyapa

Adho Mukha Kashyapasana

(uh-DO MUK-uh kah-shyuh-PAHS-uh-nuh)

Modification: Leg 1: knee on the floor

Leg 2: foot on the floor

Pose Type: arm balance, binding

Drishti Point: Angushtamadhye or Angushta Ma Dyai (thumbs), Nasagrai or Nasagre (nose)

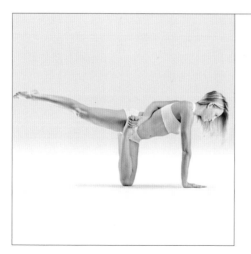

Downward Facing Pose Dedicated to Kasyapa

Adho Mukha Kasyapasana

(uh-DO MUK-uh kah-shyuh-PAHS-uh-nuh)

Modification: Leg 1: knee on the floor

Leg 2: foot off the floor

Pose Type: arm balance, binding

Drishti Point: Angushtamadhye or Angushta Ma Dyai (thumbs)

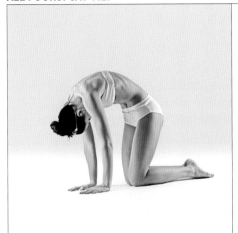

Downward Facing Cat Pose

Adho Mukha Marjarasana

(uh-DO MUK-uh mahr-jah-RAHS-uh-nuh)

Modification: toes pointing away from the head
Pose Type: standing (on hands and knees), forward bend
Drishti Point: Nabhi, Nabhicakre, or Nabi Chakra (belly button)

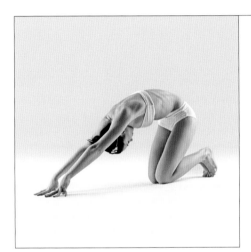

Downward Facing Cat Pose

Adho Mukha Marjarasana

(uh-DO MUK-uh mahr-jah-RAHS-uh-nuh)

Modification: arms straight to the front, fingertips to the floor; rocking back, toes curled in
Pose Type: standing (on hands and knees), forward bend
Drishti Point: Nabhi, Nabhicakre, or Nabi Chakra (belly button)

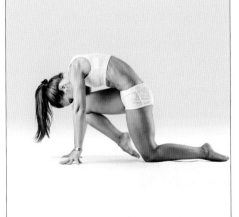

Tiger Pose

Vyaghrasana

(vyah-GRAHS-uh-nuh)

Also Known As: Cow Pose Modification (Bitilasana)
Modification: knee to the forehead
Pose Type: standing (on hands and knees), forward bend
Drishti Point: Nabhi, Nabhicakre, or Nabi Chakra (belly button)

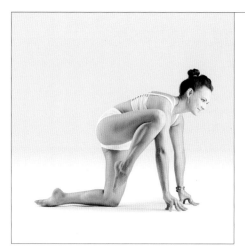

Tiger Pose

Vyaghrasana

(vyah-GRAHS-uh-nuh)

Also Known As: Cow Pose Modification (Bitilasana)

Modification: knee to the shoulder on the same side

Pose Type: standing (on hands and knees), forward bend

Drishti Point: Nasagrai or Nasagre (nose)

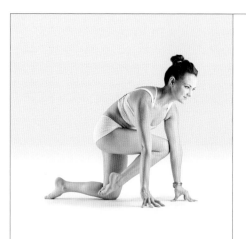

Tiger Pose

Vyaghrasana

(vyah-GRAHS-uh-nuh)

Also Known As: Cow Pose Modification (Bitilasana)

Modification: knee to the opposite tricep

Pose Type: standing (on hands and knees), forward bend, twist

Drishti Point: Nasagrai or Nasagre (nose)

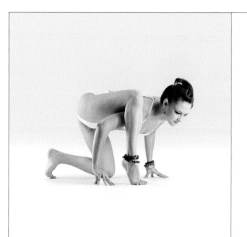

Tiger Pose

Vyaghrasana

(vyah-GRAHS-uh-nuh)

Also Known As: Cow Pose Modification (Bitilasana)

Modification: shoulder to the back of the knee; back leg, toes curled in

Pose Type: standing (on hands and knees), forward bend

Drishti Point: Nasagrai or Nasagre (nose), Padayoragrai or Padayoragre (toes/feet)

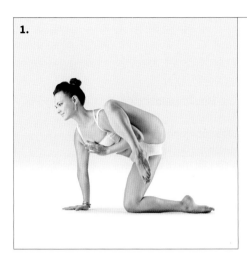

1.

Tiger Pose

Vyaghrasana

(vyah-GRAHS-uh-nuh)

Also Known As: Cow Pose Modification (Bitilasana)
Modification: one hand to the heart
1. back of the knee to the shoulder, leg bent
2. back of the knee to the shoulder, leg straight
Pose Type: standing (on hands and knees), forward bend
Drishti Point: Bhrumadhye or Ajna Chakra (third eye, between the eyebrows), Nasagrai or Nasagre (nose)

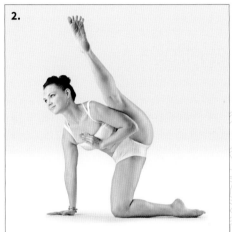

2.

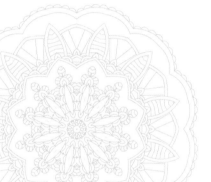

ALL FOURS: DOG TILT

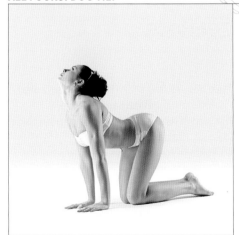

Upward Facing Dog Pose Tilt

Urdhva Mukha Shvanasana Tilt

(OORD-vuh MUK-uh shvuh-NAHS-uh-nuh)

Pose Type: standing (on hands and knees), backbend
Drishti Point: Bhrumadhye or Ajna Chakra (third eye, between the eyebrows

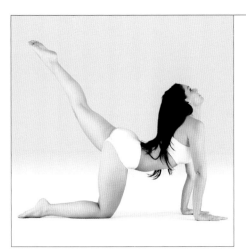

Tiger Pose

Vyaghrasana

(vyah-GRAHS-uh-nuh)

Also Known As: Balancing Table Pose Modification (Niralamba Dandayamana Bharmanasana)

Modification: one leg straight out, toes pointing away from the head

Pose Type: standing (on hands and knees), backbend

Drishti Point: Bhrumadhye or Ajna Chakra (third eye, between the eyebrows)

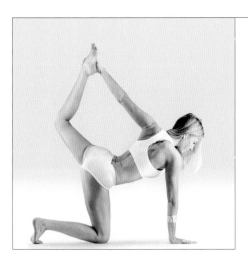

Unsupported Tiger Pose

Niralamba Vyaghrasana

(nir-AH-luhm-buh vyah-GRAHS-uh-nuh)

Also Known As: One-Legged Bow Pose from All Fours (Eka Pada Dhanurasana), Balancing Table Pose Modification (Dandayamana Bharmanasana)

Modification: grabbing onto the foot with under-head grip on the same side

Pose Type: standing (on hands and knees), backbend

Drishti Point: Angushtamadhye or Angushta Ma Dyai (thumbs)

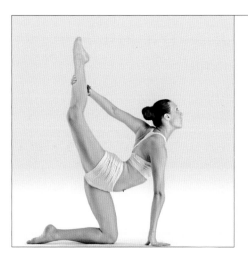

Unsupported Tiger Pose

Niralamba Vyaghrasana

(nir-AH-luhm-buh vyah-GRAHS-uh-nuh)

Also Known As: One-Legged Bow Pose from All Fours (Eka Pada Dhanurasana), Balancing Table Pose Modification (Dandayamana Bharmanasana)

Modification: grabbing onto the shin with under-head grip on the opposite side

Pose Type: standing (on hands and knees), backbend

Drishti Point: Bhrumadhye or Ajna Chakra (third eye, between the eyebrows)

1.

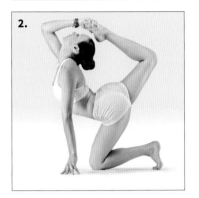

2.

Unsupported Tiger Pose

Niralamba Vyaghrasana

(nir-AH-luhm-buh vyah-GRAHS-uh-nuh)

Also Known As: Balancing Table Pose Modification (Dandayamana Bharmanasana)

Modification: grabbing onto the foot with overhead grip on the same side, foot toward the head

1. toes pointing away from the head
2. toes curled in

Pose Type: standing (on hands and knees), backbend

Drishti Point: Bhrumadhye or Ajna Chakra (third eye, between the eyebrows)

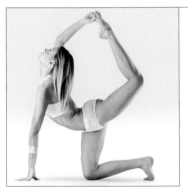

Unsupported Tiger Pose

Niralamba Vyaghrasana

(nir-AH-luhm-buh vyah-GRAHS-uh-nuh)

Also Known As: Balancing Table Pose Modification (Dandayamana Bharmanasana)

Modification: grabbing onto the foot with overhead grip on the opposite side, foot away from the head, toes curled in

Pose Type: standing (on hands and knees), backbend

Drishti Point: Bhrumadhye or Ajna Chakra (third eye, between the eyebrows)

ALL FOURS: FOREARMS

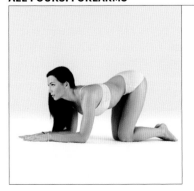

Cow Pose

Bitilasana

(bee-til-AHS-uh-nuh)

Also Known As: Table Pose Modification (Bharmanasana)

Modification: forearms to the floor

Pose Type: standing (on forearms and knees)

Drishti Point: Bhrumadhye or Ajna Chakra (third eye, between the eyebrows)

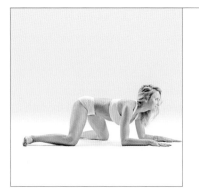

Frog Pose in Cow Pose

Mandukasana in Bitilasana
(muhn-doo-KAHS-uh-nuh in bee-til-AHS-uh-nuh)

Also Known As: Frog Pose in Table Pose Modification (Mandukasana in Bharmanasana)
Modification: forearms to the floor, knees open wider than hips
Pose Type: standing (on forearms and knees)
Drishti Point: Bhrumadhye or Ajna Chakra (third eye, between the eyebrows)

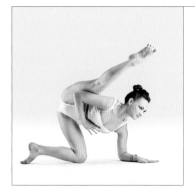

Uneven Wounded Duck Pose Prep.

Vishama Pungu Karandavasana Prep.
(VISH-uh-muh pung-u kahr-uhn-duh-VAHS-uh-nuh)

Modification: one forearm to the floor, toes of both feet on the floor
Pose Type: standing (on forearms and feet), forward bend
Drishti Point: Angushtamadhye or Angushta Ma Dyai (thumbs)

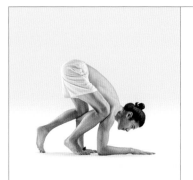

Supported Tiger Pose

Salamba Vyaghrasana *(SAH-luhm-buh vyah-GRAHS-uh-nuh)*

Also Known As: Cow Pose Modification (Bitilasana)
Modification: forearm on the floor, one hand to the heart; back of the knee to the shoulder, leg straight
Pose Type: standing (on forearms and knees), forward bend
Drishti Point: Bhrumadhye or Ajna Chakra (third eye, between the eyebrows), Nasagrai or Nasagre (nose)

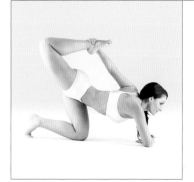

Supported Tiger Pose

Salamba Vyaghrasana *(SAH-luhm-buh-nuh vyah-GRAHS-uh-nuh)*

Also Known As: Cow Pose Modification (Bitilasana)
Modification: forearm on the floor, grabbing onto the foot with under-head grip on the opposite side
Pose Type: standing (on forearms and knees), backbend
Drishti Point: Bhrumadhye or Ajna Chakra (third eye, between the eyebrows), Nasagrai or Nasagre (nose)

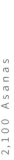

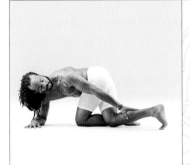

Hand to Leg Sideways Leg Position of Cow Face Pose in Cow Pose

Hasta Pada Parshva Pada Gomukhasana in Bitilasana

(HUH-stuh PUH-duh PAHRSH-vuh PUH-duh go-mu-KAHS-uh-nuh in bee-til-AHS-uh-nuh)

Modification: forearm to the floor

Pose Type: standing (on forearms and knees), twist

Drishti Point: Padayoragrai or Padayoragre (toes/feet)

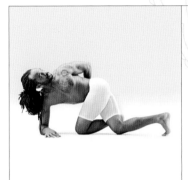

Half Bound Sideways Leg Position of Cow Face Pose in Cow Pose

Ardha Baddha Parshva Pada Gomukhasana in Bitilasana

(UHR-duh BUH-duh PAHRSH-vuh PUH-duh go-mu-KAHS-uh-nuh in bee-til-AHS-uh-nuh)

Modification: forearm to the floor

Pose Type: standing (on forearms and knees), twist, binding

Drishti Point: Urdhva or Antara Drishti (up to the sky)

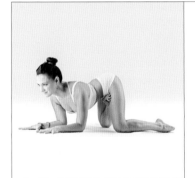

Half Lotus Cow Pose

Ardha Padma Bitilasana

(UHR-duh PUHD-muh bee-til-AHS-uh-nuh)

Also Known As: Half Lotus Table Pose Modification (Ardha Padma Bharmanasana)

Modification: forearms to the floor

Pose Type: standing (on forearms and knees)

Drishti Point: Bhrumadhye or Ajna Chakra (third eye, between the eyebrows)

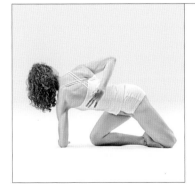

Revolved Half Lotus Cow Pose

Parivritta Ardha Padma Bitilasana

(puh-ri-VRIT-uh UHR-duh PUHD-muh bee-til-AHS-uh-nuh)

Also Known As: Revolved Half Lotus Table Pose Modification (Parivritta Ardha Padma Bharmanasana)

Modification: forearm on the floor, other hand behind the back

Pose Type: standing (on forearms and knees), twist

Drishti Point: Urdhva or Antara Drishti (up to the sky)

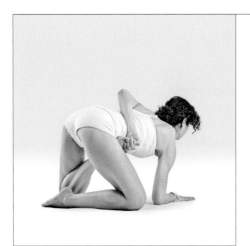

Half Bound Lotus Cow Pose

Ardha Baddha Padma Bitilasana

(UHR-duh PUHD-muh bee-til-AHS-uh-nuh)

Also Known As: Half Bound Lotus Table Pose Modification (Ardha Baddha Padma Bharmanasana)

Modification: forearm to the floor

Pose Type: standing (on forearms and knees), binding

Drishti Point: Bhrumadhye or Ajna Chakra (third eye, between the eyebrows)

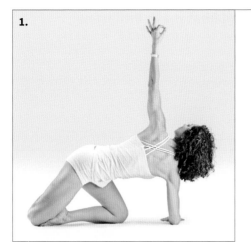

1.

Revolved Half Lotus Cow Pose

Parivritta Ardha Padma Bitilasana

(puh-ri-VRIT-uh UHR-duh PUHD-muh bee-til-AHS-uh-nuh)

Also Known As: Revolved Half Lotus Table Pose Modification (Parivritta Ardha Padma Bharmanasana)

Modification: forearm on the floor, top arm up to the sky

1. back view
2. front view

Pose Type: standing (on forearms and knees), twist

Drishti Point: Hastagrai or Hastagre (hands)

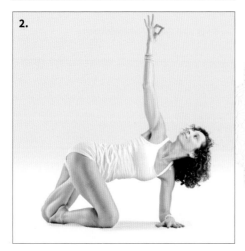

2.

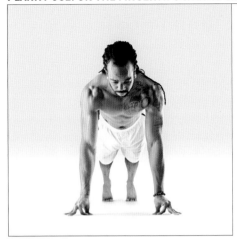

Extended Four Limbs Staff Pose

Utthita Chaturanga Dandasana

(UT-ti-tuh chuh-tur-UHNG-guh-uh duhn-DAHS-uh-nuh)

Also Known As: High Plank
Modification: on the fingertips
Pose Type: arm balance, core
Drishti Point: Nasagrai or Nasagre (nose)

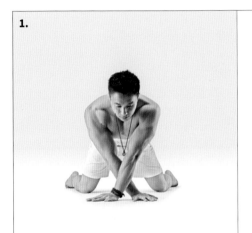

1.

Extended Four Limbs Staff Pose

Utthita Chaturanga Dandasana

(UT-ti-tuh chuh-tur-UHNG-guh duhn-DAHS-uh-nuh)

Also Known As: High Plank
Modification: arms crossed
1. knees on the floor
2. knees off the floor
Pose Type: arm balance, core
Drishti Point: Nasagrai or Nasagre (nose)

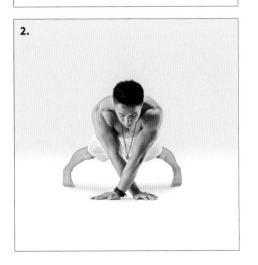

2.

1.

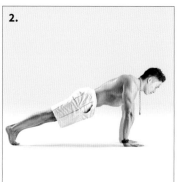

Extended Four Limbs Staff Pose

Utthita Chaturanga Dandasana

(UT-ti-tuh chuh-tur-UHNG-guh duhn-DAHS-uh-nuh)

Also Known As: High Plank Modification
Modification: 1. knees on the floor
2. knees off the floor
Pose Type: arm balance, core
Drishti Point: Nasagrai or Nasagre (nose)

2.

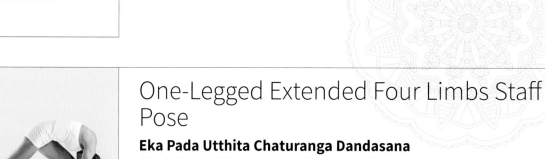

One-Legged Extended Four Limbs Staff Pose

Eka Pada Utthita Chaturanga Dandasana

(EY-kuh PUH-duh UT-ti-tuh chuh-tur-UHNG-guh duhn-DAHS-uh-nuh)

Also Known As: One-Legged High Plank Modification
Modification: knee to the nose
Pose Type: arm balance, forward bend, core
Drishti Point: Nabhi, Nabhicakre, or Nabi Chakra (belly button)

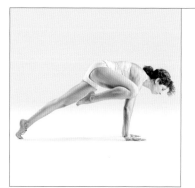

One-Legged Extended Four Limbs Staff Pose

Eka Pada Utthita Chaturanga Dandasana

(EY-kuh PUH-duh UT-ti-tuh chuh-tur-UHNG-guh duhn-DAHS-uh-nuh)

Also Known As: One-Legged High Plank Modification
Modification: knee to the shoulder on the same side
Pose Type: arm balance, forward bend, core
Drishti Point: Nasagrai or Nasagre (nose)

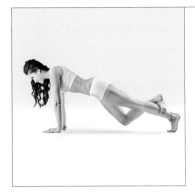

One-Legged Extended Four Limbs Staff Pose

Eka Pada Utthita Chaturanga Dandasana
(EY-kuh PUH-duh UT-ti-tuh chuh-tur-UHNG-guh duhn-DAHS-uh-nuh)
Also Known As: One-Legged High Plank Modification
Modification: foot wrapping around the calf muscle
Pose Type: arm balance, core
Drishti Point: Nasagrai or Nasagre (nose)

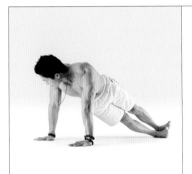

Revolved Extended Four Limbs Staff Pose

Parivritta Utthita Chaturanga Dandasana
(puh-ri-VRIT-tuh UT-ti-tuh chuh-tur-UHNG-guh duhn-DAHS-uh-nuh)
Also Known As: Revolved High Plank Modification
Pose Type: arm balance, twist, core
Drishti Point: Parshva Drishti (to the right), Parshva Drishti (to the left)

PLANK POSE: ARM AND LEG MODIFICATIONS

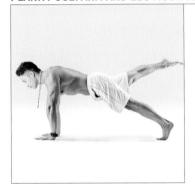

One-Legged Extended Four Limbs Staff Pose

Eka Pada Utthita Chaturanga Dandasana
(EY-kuh PUH-duh UT-ti-tuh chuh-tur-UHNG-guh duhn-DAHS-uh-nuh)
Also Known As: One-Legged High Plank Modification
Pose Type: arm balance, core
Drishti Point: Nasagrai or Nasagre (nose)

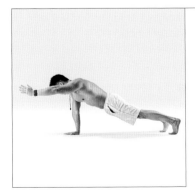

One Hand Extended Four Limbs Staff Pose

Eka Hasta Utthita Chaturanga Dandasana
(EY-kuh HUH-stuh UT-ti-tuh chuh-tur-UHNG-guh duhn-DAHS-uh-nuh)
Also Known As: One Hand High Plank Modification
Pose Type: arm balance, core
Drishti Point: Angushtamadhye or Angushta Ma Dyai (thumbs), Nasagrai or Nasagre (nose)

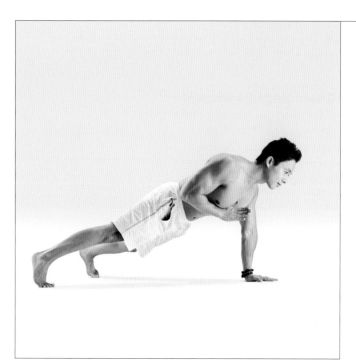

One Hand Extended Four Limbs Staff Pose

Eka Hasta Utthita Chaturanga Dandasana

(EY-kuh HUH-stuh UT-ti-tuh chuh-tur-UHNG-guh duhn-DAHS-uh-nuh)

Also Known As: One Hand High Plank Modification
Modification: hand to the heart
Pose Type: arm balance, core
Drishti Point: Angushtamadhye or Angushtha Ma Dyai (thumbs), Nasagrai or Nasagre (nose)

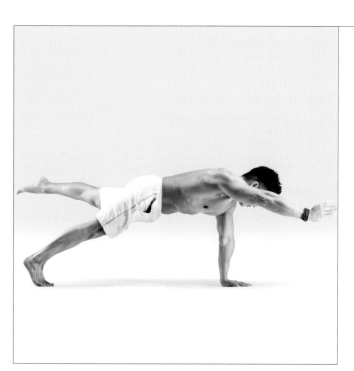

One Leg One Hand Extended Four Limbs Staff Pose

Eka Pada Eka Hasta Utthita Chaturanga Dandasana

(EY-kuh PUH-duh EY-kuh HUH-stuh UT-ti-tuh chuh-tur-UHNG-guh duhn-DAHS-uh-nuh)

Also Known As: One Hand High Plank Modification
Pose Type: arm balance, core
Drishti Point: Angushtamadhye or Angushta Ma Dyai (thumbs), Nasagrai or Nasagre (nose)

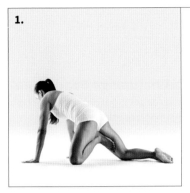

1.

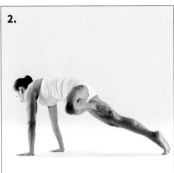

2.

Tree Pose in One-Legged Extended Four Limbs Staff Pose

Vrikshasana in Eka Pada Utthita Chaturanga Dandasana

(vrik-SHAHS-uh-nuh in EY-kuh PUH-duh UT-ti-tuh chuh-tur-UHNG-guh duhn-DAHS-uh-nuh)

Also Known As: Tree Pose in One-Legged High Plank Modification

Modification: 1. knees on the floor

2. knees off the floor

Pose Type: arm balance, core

Drishti Point: Nasagrai or Nasagre (nose)

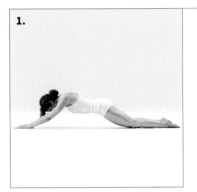

1.

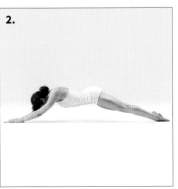

2.

Extended Four Limbs Staff Pose

Utthita Chaturanga Dandasana

(UT-ti-tuh chuh-tur-UHNG-guh duhn-DAHS-uh-nuh)

Also Known As: High Plank Modification

Modification: arms extended to the front, tops of the feet on the floor

1. knees on the floor

2. knees off the floor

Pose Type: arm balance, core

Drishti Point: Nasagrai or Nasagre (nose)

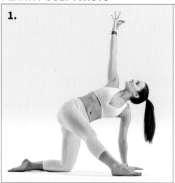

Leg to the Side Revolved One Hand Extended Four Limbs Staff Pose

Parshva Pada Parivritta Eka Hasta Utthita Chaturanga Dandasana

(PAHRSH-vuh PUH-duh puh-ri-VRIT-tuh EY-kuh HUH-stuh UT-ti-tuh chuh-tur-UHNG-guh duhn-DAHS-uh-nuh)

Also Known As: Leg to the Side Revolved One Hand High Plank Modification

Modification: 1. back knee on the floor

2. back knee off the floor, knee bent

3. back knee off the floor, both legs straight

4. back knee off the floor, knee bent, toes of the straight leg pointed

Pose Type: arm balance, twist, core

Drishti Point: Angushtamadhye or Angushta Ma Dyai (thumbs)

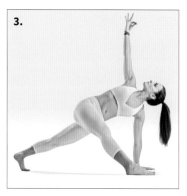

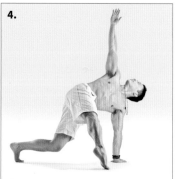

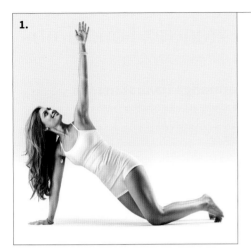

Revolved One Hand Extended Four Limbs Staff Pose

Parivritta Eka Hasta Utthita Chaturanga Dandasana
(puh-ri-VRIT-tuh EY-kuh HUH-stuh UT-ti-tuh chuh-tur-UHNG-guh duhn-DAHS-uh-nuh)
Also Known As: Revolved One Hand High Plank Modification
Modification: 1. knees on the floor
2. knees off the floor
Pose Type: arm balance, twist, core
Drishti Point: Angushtamadhye or Angushta Ma Dyai (thumbs)

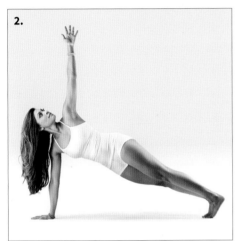

Revolved Leg to the Side Extended Four Limbs Staff Pose

Parivritta Parshva Pada Utthita Chaturanga Dandasana
(puh-ri-VRIT-tuh PAHRSH-vuh PUH-duh UT-ti-tuh chuh-tur-UHNG-guh duhn-DAHS-uh-nuh)
Also Known As: Revolved Leg to the Side High Plank Modification
Modification: leg sweeping under the torso
Pose Type: arm balance, twist, core
Drishti Point: Nasagrai or Nasagre (nose)

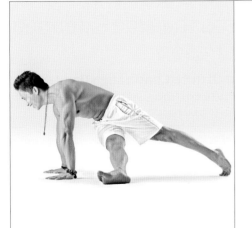

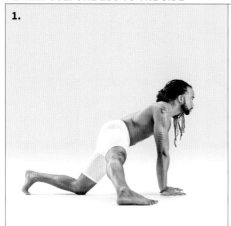

Leg to the Side Extended Four Limbs Staff Pose

Parshva Pada Utthita Chaturanga Dandasana

(PAHRSH-vuh PUH-duh UT-ti-tuh chuh-tur-UHNG-guh duhn-DAHS-uh-nuh)

Also Known As: Leg to the Side High Plank Modification
Modification: 1. back knee on the floor
2. back knee off the floor
Pose Type: arm balance, core
Drishti Point: Nasagrai or Nasagre (nose)

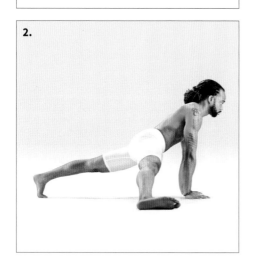

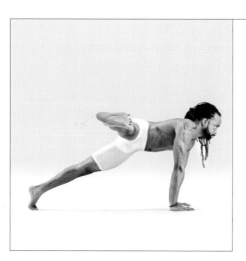

Upward One Leg to the Side Extended Four Limbs Staff Pose

Urdhva Parshva Eka Pada Utthita Chaturanga Dandasana

(OORD-vuh PAHRSH-vuh EY-kuh PUH-duh UT-ti-tuh chuh-tur-UHNG-guh duhn-DAHS-uh-nuh)

Also Known As: Leg to the Side One-Legged High Plank Modification
Modification: back knee off the floor, other leg off the floor
Pose Type: arm balance, core
Drishti Point: Nasagrai or Nasagre (nose)

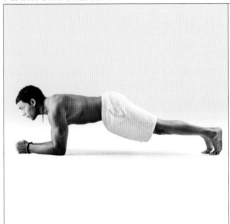

Staff Pose Dedicated to Makara

Makara Dandasana
(MUH-kuh-ruh duhn-DAHS-uh-nuh)
Also Known As: Dolphin Plank Modification
Pose Type: forearm balance, core
Drishti Point: Nasagrai or Nasagre (nose), Angushtamadhye or Angushta Ma Dyai (thumbs)

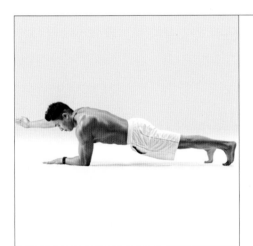

One Hand Staff Pose Dedicated to Makara

Eka Hasta Makara Dandasana
(EY-kuh HUH-stuh MUH-kuh-ruh duhn-DAHS-uh-nuh)
Also Known As: One Hand Dolphin Plank Modification
Pose Type: forearm balance, core
Drishti Point: Angushtamadhye or Angushta Ma Dyai (thumbs)

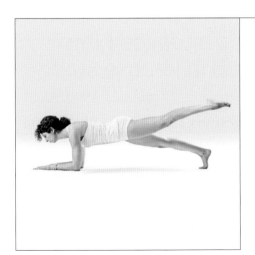

One-Legged Staff Pose Dedicated to Makara

Eka Pada Makara Dandasana
(EY-kuh PUH-duh MUH-kuh-ruh duhn-DAHS-uh-nuh)
Also Known As: One-Legged Dolphin Plank Modification
Pose Type: forearm balance, core
Drishti Point: Angushtamadhye or Angushta Ma Dyai (thumbs)

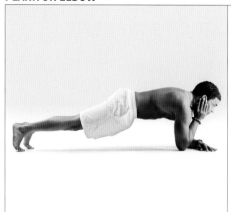

Uneven Repose Staff Pose

Vishama Sayana Dandasana

(VISH-uh-muh SHUH-yuh-nuh duhn-DAHS-uh-nuh)

Also Known As: Uneven Elbow Plank Pose Modification
Modification: one hand to the face, one forearm to the floor
Pose Type: forearm/elbow balance, core
Drishti Point: Bhrumadhye or Ajna Chakra (third eye, between the eyebrows)

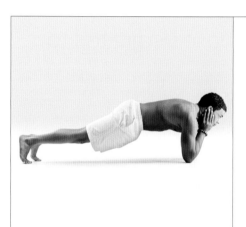

Repose Staff Pose

Sayana Dandasana

(SHUH-yuh-nuh duhn-DAHS-uh-nuh)

Also Known As: Elbow Plank
Pose Type: elbow balance, core
Drishti Point: Bhrumadhye or Ajna Chakra (third eye, between the eyebrows)

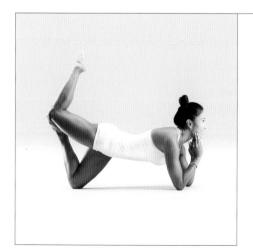

Leg Position of One-Legged King Pigeon 1 Version B in Repose Staff Pose

Pada Eka Pada Raja Kapotasana 1B in Sayana Dandasana

(PUH-duh EY-kuh PUH-duh RAH-juh kuh-po-TAHS-uh-nuh in SHUH-yuh-nuh duhn-DAHS-uh-nuh)

Pose Type: elbow balance, mild backbend
Drishti Point: Bhrumadhye or Ajna Chakra (third eye, between the eyebrows)

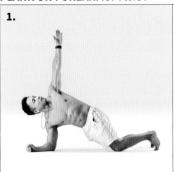

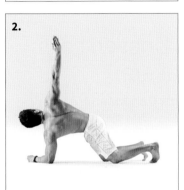

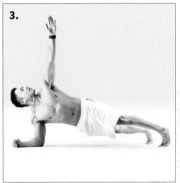

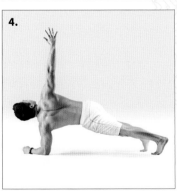

Revolved One Hand Staff Pose Dedicated to Makara

Parivritta Eka Hasta Makara Dandasana

(puh-ri-VRIT-tuh EY-kuh HUH-stuh MUH-kuh-ruh duhn-DAHS-uh-nuh)

Also Known As: Revolved Dolphin Plank Modification

Modification: 1 & 2. knees on the floor, front and back view

3 & 4. knees off the floor, front and back view

Pose Type: forearm balance, twist, core

Drishti Point: Angushtamadhye or Angushta Ma Dyai (thumbs)

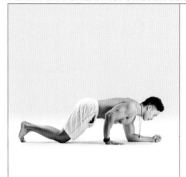

Uneven Staff Pose Dedicated to Makara

Vishama Makara Dandasana
(VISH-uh-muh MUH-kuh-ruh duhn-DAHS-uh-nuh)
Also Known As: Uneven Dolphin Plank Modification
Modification: one elbow bent at 90 degrees, other forearm to the floor, knees on the floor
Pose Type: arm/forearm balance, core
Drishti Point: Angushtamadhye or Angushta Ma Dyai (thumbs)

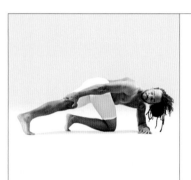

Hand to the Leg Sideways Uneven Legs Staff Pose Dedicated to Makara

Hasta Pada Parshva Vishama Pada Makara Dandasana
(HUH-stuh PUH-duh PAHRSH-vuh VISH-uh-muh PUH-duh MUH-kuh-ruh duhn-DAHS-uh-nuh)
Also Known As: Hand to the Leg Sideways Dolphin Plank Modification
Pose Type: forearm balance, twist, core
Drishti Point: Padayoragrai or Padayoragre (toes/feet)

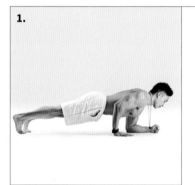

1.

Uneven Staff Pose Dedicated to Makara

Vishama Makara Dandasana
(VISH-uh-muh MUH-kuh-ruh duhn-DAHS-uh-nuh)
Also Known As: Uneven Dolphin Plank Modification
Modification: one elbow bent at 90 degrees, other forearm to the floor, knees off the floor
1. left forearm on the floor, right arm at 90 degrees
2. right forearm on the floor, left arm at 90 degrees
Pose Type: arm/forearm balance, core
Drishti Point: Angushtamadhye or Angushta Ma Dyai (thumbs)

2.

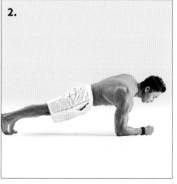

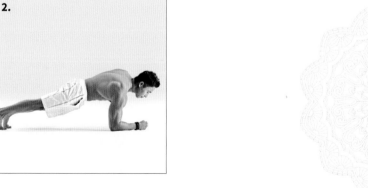

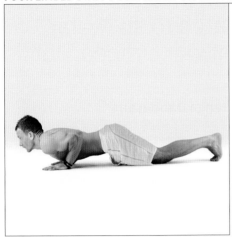

Four Limbed Staff Pose
Chaturanga Dandasana
(chuh-tur-UHNG-guh duhn-DAHS-uh-nuh)
Modification: knees on the floor
Pose Type: arm balance, core
Drishti Point: Nasagrai or Nasagre (nose)

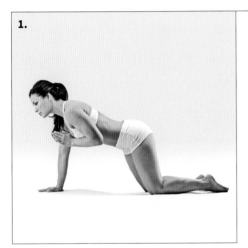

One Hand Four Limbed Staff Pose
Eka Hasta Chaturanga Dandasana
(EY-kuh HUH-stuh chuh-tur-UHNG-guh duhn-DAHS-uh-nuh)
Modification: knees on the floor
1. starting position
2. end position
Pose Type: arm balance, core
Drishti Point: Nasagrai or Nasagre (nose)

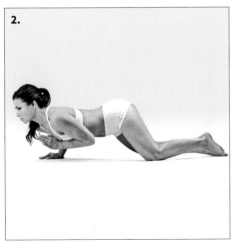

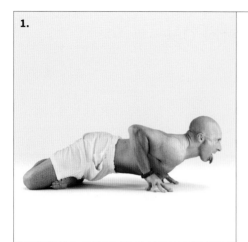

1.

Lion Pose Dedicated to an Avatar of Lord Vishnu in Four Limbed Staff Pose

Narasimhasana in Chaturanga Dandasana
(nuh-ruh-sim-HAHS-uh-nuh in chuh-tur-UHNG-guh duhn-DAHS-uh-nuh)
Also Known As: Lion Pose (Simhasana)
Modification: 1. on the fingertips
2. on the fists
Pose Type: arm balance, core
Drishti Point: Bhrumadhye or Ajna Chakra (third eye, between the eyebrows)

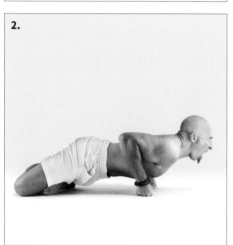

2.

Leg Position of One-Legged King Pigeon 1 Version B in Four Limbed Staff Pose

Pada Eka Pada Raja Kapotasana 1 B in Chaturanga Dandasana
(PUH-duh EY-kuh PUH-duh RAH-juh kuh-po-TAHS-uh-nuh in chuh-tur-UHNG-guh duhn-DAHS-uh-nuh)
Modification: bottom knee bent and on the floor; top leg straight—knee resting on the sole of the bottom foot
Pose Type: arm balance, core
Drishti Point: Nasagrai or Nasagre (nose)

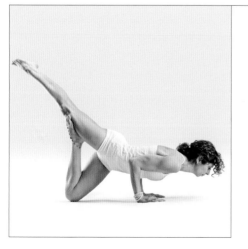

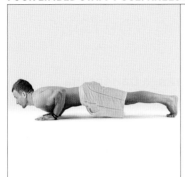

Four Limbed Staff Pose

Chaturanga Dandasana
(chuh-tur-UHNG-guh duhn-DAHS-uh-nuh)
Pose Type: arm balance, core
Drishti Point: Nasagrai or Nasagre (nose)

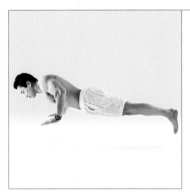

Crocodile Pose

Nakrasana
(nuh-KRAHS-uh-nuh)
Modification: feet and hands off the floor and up in the air
Pose Type: arm balance, core
Drishti Point: Nasagrai or Nasagre (nose)

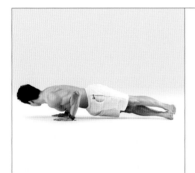

Revolved Four Limbed Staff Pose

Parivritta Chaturanga Dandasana
(puh-ri-VRIT-tuh chuh-tur-UHNG-guh duhn-DAHS-uh-nuh)
Pose Type: arm balance, twist, core
Drishti Point: Parshva Drishti (to the right), Parshva Drishti (to the left)

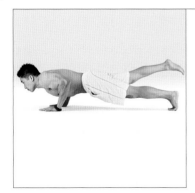

One-Legged Four Limbed Staff Pose

Eka Pada Chaturanga Dandasana
(EY-kuh PUH-duh chuh-tur-UHNG-guh duhn-DAHS-uh-nuh)
Pose Type: arm balance, core
Drishti Point: Bhrumadhye or Ajna Chakra (third eye, between the eyebrows), Nasagrai or Nasagre (nose)

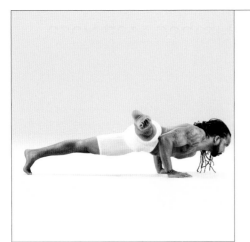

Upward One Leg to the Side Four Limbed Staff Pose

Urdhva Parshva Eka Pada Chaturanga Dandasana
(OORD-vuh PAHRSH-vuh EY-kuh PUH-duh chuh-tur-UHNG-guh duhn-DAHS-uh-nuh)
Pose Type: arm balance, core
Drishti Point: Bhrumadhye or Ajna Chakra (third eye, between the eyebrows), Nasagrai or Nasagre (nose)

FOUR LIMBED STAFF POSE: KNEE TO THE ARM

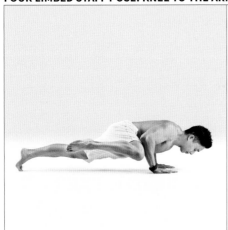

One-Legged Four Limbed Staff Pose

Eka Pada Chaturanga Dandasana
(EY-kuh PUH-duh chuh-tur-UHNG-guh duhn-DAHS-uh-nuh)
Modification: knee to the forearm
Pose Type: arm balance, forward bend, core
Drishti Point: Nasagrai or Nasagre (nose)

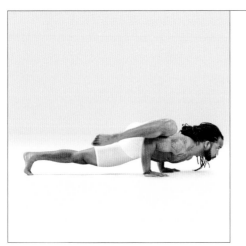

One-Legged Four Limbed Staff Pose

Eka Pada Chaturanga Dandasana
(EY-kuh PUH-duh chuh-tur-UHNG-guh duhn-DAHS-uh-nuh)
Modification: knee on top of the tricep
Pose Type: arm balance, forward bend, core
Drishti Point: Bhrumadhye or Ajna Chakra (third eye, between the eyebrows), Nasagrai or Nasagre (nose)

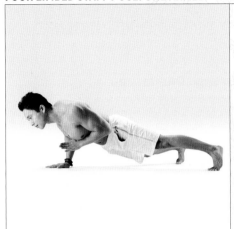

One Hand Four Limbed Staff Pose

Eka Hasta Chaturanga Dandasana

(EY-kuh HUH-stuh chuh-tur-UHNG-guh duhn-DAHS-uh-nuh)

Modification: hand to the heart

Pose Type: arm balance, core

Drishti Point: Hastagrai or Hastagre (hands) or Nasagrai or Nasagre (nose)

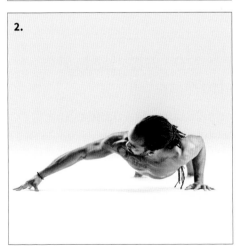

Hand to the Side Four Limbed Staff Pose

Parshva Hasta Chaturanga Dandasana

(PAHRSH-vuh HUH-stuh chuh-tur-UHNG-guh duhn-DAHS-uh-nuh)

Modification: 1. knees on the floor

2. knees off the floor

Pose Type: arm balance, core

Drishti Point: Hastagrai or Hastagre (hands) or Nasagrai or Nasagre (nose)

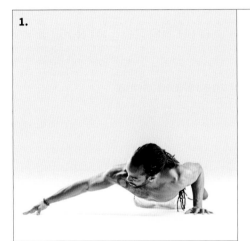

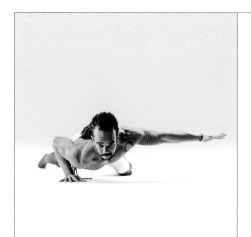

One Hand to the Side Four Limbed Staff Pose

Parshva Eka Hasta Chaturanga Dandasana

(PAHRSH-vuh EY-kuh HUH-stuh chuh-tur-UHNG-guh duhn-DAHS-uh-nuh)

Modification: one knee on the floor, other knee off the floor
Pose Type: arm balance, core
Drishti Point: Nasagrai or Nasagre (nose)

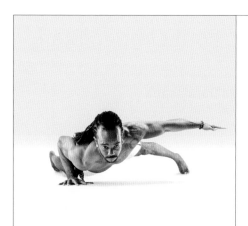

One Hand to the Side Four Limbed Staff Pose

Parshva Eka Hasta Chaturanga Dandasana

(PAHRSH-vuh EY-kuh HUH-stuh chuh-tur-UHNG-guh duhn-DAHS-uh-nuh)

Modification: knees off the floor
Pose Type: arm balance, core
Drishti Point: Nasagrai or Nasagre (nose)

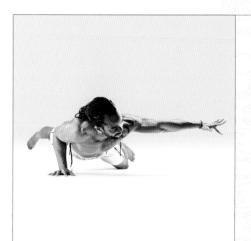

One Hand to the Side One-Legged Four Limbed Staff Pose

Parshva Eka Hasta Eka Pada Chaturanga Dandasana

(PAHRSH-vuh EY-kuh HUH-stuh EY-kuh PUH-duh chuh-tur-UHNG-guh duhn-DAHS-uh-nuh)

Modification: one knee on the floor
Pose Type: arm balance, core
Drishti Point: Hastagrai or Hastagre (hands)

1.

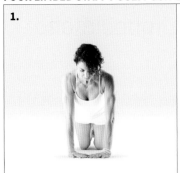

Diamond Four Limbed Staff Pose

Vajra Chaturanga Dandasana

(VAHJ-ruh chuh-tur-UHNG-guh duhn-DAHS-uh-nuh)

Modification: knees on the floor

1. start position
2. end position

Pose Type: arm balance, core

Drishti Point: Nasagrai or Nasagre (nose)

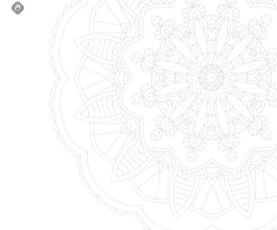

2.

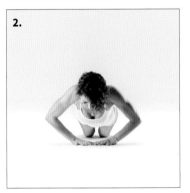

1.

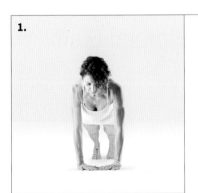

Diamond Four Limbed Staff Pose

Vajra Chaturanga Dandasana

(VAHJ-ruh chuh-tur-UHNG-guh duhn-DAHS-uh-nuh)

Modification: knees off the floor

1. start position
2. end position

Pose Type: arm balance, core

Drishti Point: Nasagrai or Nasagre (nose)

2.

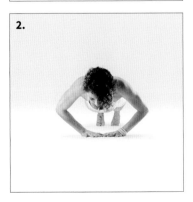

Hands Spread Wide Four Limbed Staff Pose

Prasarita Hasta Chaturanga Dandasana

(pruh-SAH-ri-tuh HUH-stuh chuh-tur-UHNG-guh duhn-DAHS-uh-nuh)

Modification: knees on the floor

1. start position
2. end position

Pose Type: arm balance, core

Drishti Point: Nasagrai or Nasagre (nose)

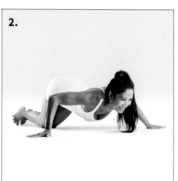

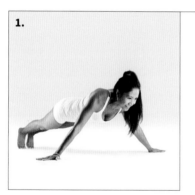

Hands Spread Wide Four Limbed Staff Pose

Prasarita Hasta Chaturanga Dandasana

(pruh-SAH-ri-tuh HUH-stuh chuh-tur-UHNG-guh duhn-DAHS-uh-nuh)

Modification: knees off the floor

1. start position
2. end position

Pose Type: arm balance, core

Drishti Point: Nasagrai or Nasagre (nose)

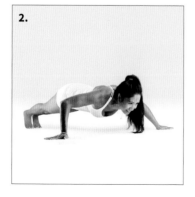

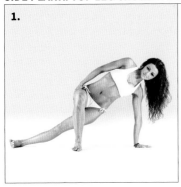

1.

Pose Dedicated to Sage Vasistha

Vasisthasana
(vuh-sish-TAHS-uh-nuh)
Also Known As: Side Plank Modification
Modification: top leg crossing over
1. arm alongside of the torso
2. arm extended up
Pose Type: arm balance, core
Drishti Point: Nasagrai or Nasagre (nose), Angushtamadhye or Angushta Ma Dyai (thumbs)

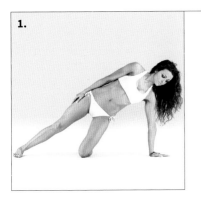

2.

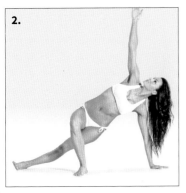

1.

Pose Dedicated to Sage Vasistha

Vasisthasana
(vuh-sish-TAHS-uh-nuh)
Also Known As: Side Plank Modification
Modification: bottom knee to the floor
1. arm alongside of the torso
2. arm extended up
Pose Type: arm balance, core
Drishti Point: Angushtamadhye or Angushtha Ma Dyai (thumbs)

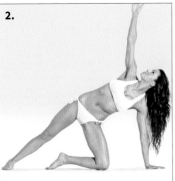

2.

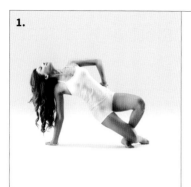

1.

Pose Dedicated to Sage Vasishta

Vasishtasana

(vuh-sish-TAHS-uh-nuh)

Also Known As: Side Plank Modification

Modification: both knees bent, shin of the top leg on the inside of the knee of the bottom leg

1. bottom leg bent at 90 degrees
2. bottom leg slightly bent

Pose Type: arm balance, core

Drishti Point: Urdhva or Antara Drishti (up to the sky)

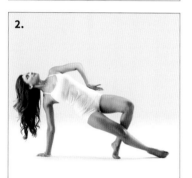

2.

SIDE PLANK: LEGS STRAIGHT

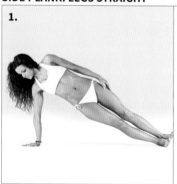

1.

Pose Dedicated to Sage Vasishta

Vasishtasana

(vuh-sish-TAHS-uh-nuh)

Also Known As: Side Plank Modification

Modification: both legs straight

1. arm alongside of the torso
2. arm extended up

Pose Type: arm balance, core

Drishti Point: Angushtamadhye or Angushta Ma Dyai (thumbs)

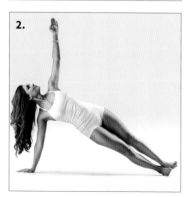

2.

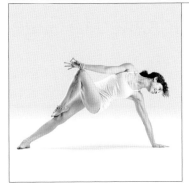

Revolved Pose Dedicated to Sage Vasistha

Parivritta Vasisthasana

(puh-ri-VRIT-tuh vuh-sish-TAHS-uh-nuh)

Also Known As: Revolved Side Plank Modification
Modification: bottom knee bent, foot resting on the thigh of the top leg; the wrist of the top arm to the knee of the bottom leg
Pose Type: arm balance, twist, forward bend, core
Drishti Point: Hastagrai or Hastagre (hands)

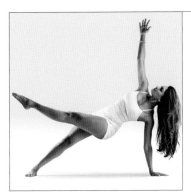

Revolved Leg to the Side Pose Dedicated to Sage Vasistha

Parivritta Parshva Pada Vasisthasana

(puh-ri-VRIT-tuh PAHRSH-vuh PUH-duh vuh-sish-TAHS-uh-nuh)

Also Known As: Revolved Leg to the Side Plank Modification
Modification: both legs straight, bottom foot lifted off the floor, leg crossing over in front of the body
Pose Type: arm balance, twist, core
Drishti Point: Angushtamadhye or Angushta Ma Dyai (thumbs), Padayoragrai or Padayoragre (toes/feet)

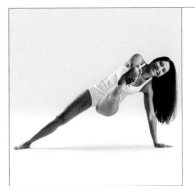

Hand to Foot Pose Dedicated to Sage Vasistha

Hasta Pada Vasisthasana

(HUH-stuh PUH-duh vuh-sish-TAHS-uh-nuh)

Also Known As: Hand to Foot Side Plank Modification
Modification: both legs straight; bottom leg crossing over in front of the body, foot in line with the center of the chest
Pose Type: arm balance, forward bend, core
Drishti Point: Padayoragrai or Padayoragre (toes/feet)

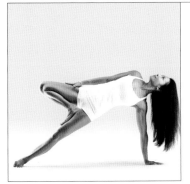

Tree Pose in Pose Dedicated to Sage Vasista

Vrikshasana in Vasishtasana

(vrik-SHAHS-uh-nuh in vuh-sish-TAHS-uh-nuh)

Also Known As: Tree Pose in Side Plank Modification
Modification: top foot to the inner thigh
Pose Type: arm balance, core
Drishti Point: Urdhva or Antara Drishti (up to the sky)

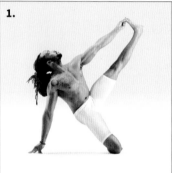

Half Lotus Pose in Pose Dedicated to Sage Vasishta

Ardha Padmasana in Vasishtasana

(UHR-duh puhd-MAHS-uh-nuh in vuh-sish-TAHS-uh-nuh)

Also Known As: Half Lotus Pose in Side Plank Modification
Modification: bottom knee on the floor
Pose Type: arm balance, core
Drishti Point: Hastagrai or Hastagre (hands)

SIDE PLANK: TOP LEG OFF THE FLOOR

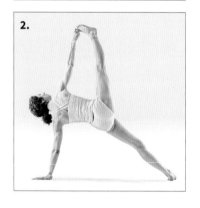

One Big Toe Pose Dedicated to Sage Vasishta

Eka Padangushta Vasisthasana

(EY-kuh puhd-ahng-GOOSH-tuh vuh-sish-TAHS-uh-nuh)

Also Known As: Big Toe Side Plank Modification
Modification: 1. bottom knee on the floor—leg bent, toes pointing to the back; on the fingertips
2. bottom knee off the floor; palm flat to the floor
Pose Type: arm balance, forward bend, core
Drishti Point: Urdhva or Antara Drishti (up to the sky), Padayoragrai or Padayoragre (toes/feet)

VISHVAMITRA'S POSE

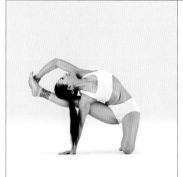

Pose Dedicated to Vishvamitra

Vishvamitrasana

(vish-vuh-mi-TRAHS-uh-nuh)

Modification: knee on the floor, grabbing onto the outside edge of the foot
Pose Type: arm balance, side bend, twist, core
Drishti Point: Urdhva or Antara Drishti (up to the sky)

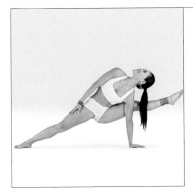

Pose Dedicated to Vishvamitra

Vishvamitrasana

(vish-vuh-mi-TRAHS-uh-nuh)

Modification: arm alongside of the torso
Pose Type: arm balance, core
Drishti Point: Urdhva or Antara Drishti (up to the sky)

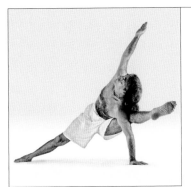

Pose Dedicated to Vishvamitra

Vishvamitrasana

(vish-vuh-mi-TRAHS-uh-nuh)

Modification: knee off the floor, top arm straight and extended up to the sky
Pose Type: arm balance, side bend, core
Drishti Point: Angushtamadhye or Angushta Ma Dyai (thumbs)

1.

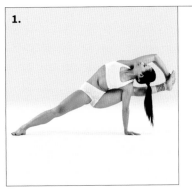

Pose Dedicated to Vishvamitra

Vishvamitrasana

(vish-vuh-mi-TRAHS-uh-nuh)

Modification: knee off the floor
1. grabbing onto the outside edge of the top foot
2. grabbing onto the ankle of the top leg
Pose Type: arm balance, side bend, twist, core
Drishti Point: Urdhva or Antara Drishti (up to the sky)

2.

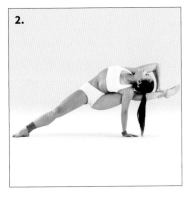

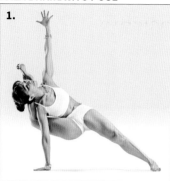

Pose Dedicated to Shiva the Destroyer

Kala Bhairavasana

(KAH-luh beye-ruh-VAHS-uh-nuh)

Modification: 1. arm extended up

2. top hand to the inside of the bottom thigh

Pose Type: arm balance, core

Drishti Point: Angushtamadhye or Angushta Ma Dyai (thumbs), Padayoragrai or Padayoragre (toes/feet)

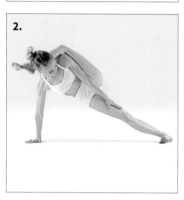

SIDE PLANK: TOP LEG OVERHEAD GRIP

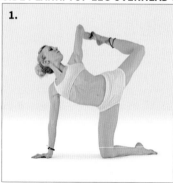

Partridge Pose

Kapinjalasana

(kuh-pinj-uh-LAHS-uh-nuh)

Modification: overhead grip

1. bottom knee on the floor

2. bottom knee off the floor

Pose Type: arm balance, backbend, core

Drishti Point: Bhrumadhye or Ajna Chakra (third eye, between the eyebrows)

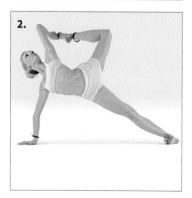

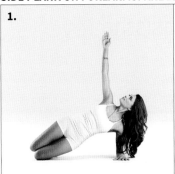

1.

Pose Dedicated to Sage Vasishta

Vasishtasana

(vuh-sish-TAHS-uh-nuh)

Also Known As: Dolphin Side Plank Modification

Modification: forearm on the floor, both knees to the floor

1. arm up to the sky
2. arm alongside the torso

Pose Type: forearm balance, core

Drishti Point: 1. Angushtamadhye or Angushta Ma Dyai (thumbs)

2. Nasagrai or Nasagre (nose)

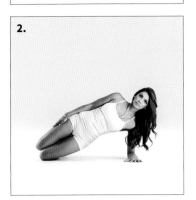

2.

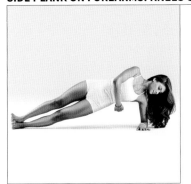

Pose Dedicated to Sage Vasishta

Vasishtasana

(vuh-sish-TAHS-uh-nuh)

Also Known As: Dolphin Side Plank Modification

Modification: forearm on the floor, arm crossed over in front of the chest, looking down

Pose Type: forearm balance, twist, core

Drishti Point: Angushtamadhye or Angushta Ma Dyai (thumbs)

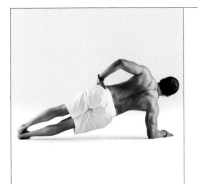

Pose Dedicated to Sage Vasishta

Vasishtasana

(vuh-sish-TAHS-uh-nuh)

Also Known As: Dolphin Side Plank Modification

Modification: forearm on the floor, top hand on the hip

Pose Type: forearm balance, core

Drishti Point: Nasagrai or Nasagre (nose)

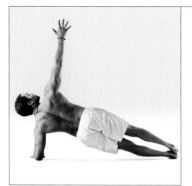

Pose Dedicated to Sage Vasistha

Vasishtasana

(vuh-sish-TAHS-uh-nuh)

Also Known As: Dolphin Side Plank Modification
Modification: forearm on the floor, top arm up to the sky
Pose Type: forearm balance, core
Drishti Point: Hastagrai or Hastagre (hands)

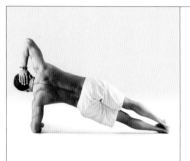

Pose Dedicated to Sage Vasishta

Vasishtasana

(vuh-sish-TAHS-uh-nuh)

Also Known As: Dolphin Side Plank Modification
Modification: forearm on the floor, top hand to the back of the head
Pose Type: forearm balance, core
Drishti Point: Nasagrai or Nasagre (nose)

SIDE PLANK ON FOREARMS: ONE LEG CROSSED OVER

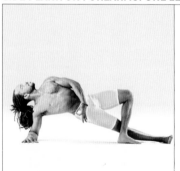

Pose Dedicated to Sage Vasishta

Vasishtasana

(vuh-sish-TAHS-uh-nuh)

Also Known As: Dolphin Side Plank Modification
Modification: forearm on the floor; top leg crossed over, foot flat on the floor; top hand by the bottom hip socket
Pose Type: forearm balance, core
Drishti Point: Urdhva or Antara Drishti (up to the sky)

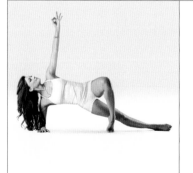

Pose Dedicated to Sage Vasishta

Vasishtasana

(vuh-sish-TAHS-uh-nuh)

Also Known As: Dolphin Side Plank Modification
Modification: forearm on the floor; top leg crossed over, heel lifted; top arm extended up to the sky
Pose Type: forearm balance, core
Drishti Point: Hastagrai or Hastagre (hands)

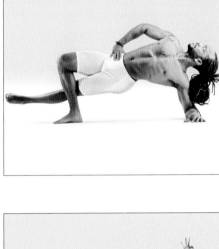

Pose Dedicated to Sage Vasishta

Vasishtasana

(vuh-sish-TAHS-uh-nuh)
Also Known As: Dolphin Side Plank Modification
Modification: forearm on the floor; top leg crossed over, foot flat on the floor, bottom leg lifted off the floor, top hand on the hip
Pose Type: forearm balance, core
Drishti Point: Urdhva or Antara Drishti (up to the sky)

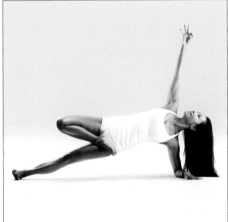

Half Lotus Pose in Pose Dedicated to Sage Vasishta

Ardha Padmasana in Vasishtasana

(UHR-duh puhd-MAHS-uh-nuh in vuh-sish-TAHS-uh-nuh)
Also Known As: Half Lotus Pose in Dolphin Side Plank Modification
Modification: forearm on the floor, top arm extended up to the sky
Pose Type: forearm balance, core
Drishti Point: Hastagrai or Hastagre (hands)

SIDE PLANK ON FOREARMS: TOP LEG LIFTED

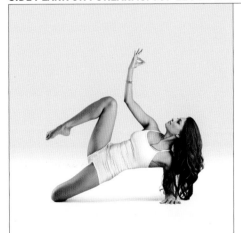

Pose Dedicated to Sage Vasishta

Vasishtasana

(vuh-sish-TAHS-uh-nuh)
Also Known As: Dolphin Side Plank Modification
Modification: forearm on the floor; top knee toward the top elbow, bottom knee on the floor; leg bent, toes pointing to the back
Pose Type: forearm balance, forward bend, core
Drishti Point: Hastagrai or Hastagre (hands)

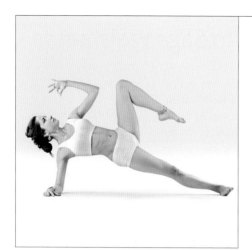

Pose Dedicated to Sage Vasishta

Vasishtasana

(vuh-sish-TAHS-uh-nuh)

Also Known As: Dolphin Side Plank Modification

Modification: forearm on the floor; top knee toward the top elbow; bottom leg straight, knee off floor

Pose Type: forearm balance, forward bend, core

Drishti Point: Hastagrai or Hastagre (hands)

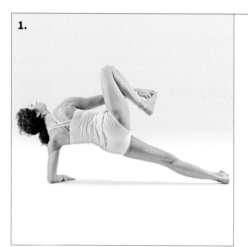

1.

One Big Toe Pose Dedicated to Sage Vasishta

Eka Padangushta Vasishtasana

(EY-kuh puhd-ahng-GOOSH-tuh vuh-sish-TAHS-uh-nuh)

Also Known As: Big Toe Dolphin Side Plank Modification

Modification: forearm on the floor

1. knee bent
2. leg straight

Pose Type: forearm balance, forward bend, core

Drishti Point: Padayoragrai or Padayoragre (toes/feet)

2.

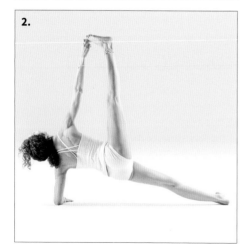

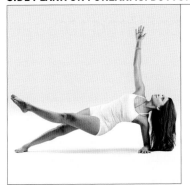

Revolved Leg to the Side Pose Dedicated to Sage Vasishta

Parivritta Parshva Pada Vasishtasana

(puh-ri-VRIT-tuh PAHRSH-vuh PUH-duh vuh-sish-TAHS-uh-nuh)

Also Known As: Revolved Leg to the Side Dolphin Side Plank Modification

Modification: forearm on the floor; both legs straight, bottom leg lifted in front of the body

Pose Type: forearm balance, twist, core

Drishti Point: Hastagrai or Hastagre (hands)

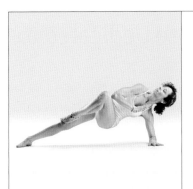

Revolved Pose Dedicated to Sage Vasishta

Parivritta Vasishtasana

(puh-ri-VRIT-tuh vuh-sish-TAHS-uh-nuh)

Also Known As: Revolved Dolphin Side Plank Modification

Modification: forearm on the floor; bottom knee bent, foot resting on the thigh of the top leg; the elbow of the top arm to the knee of the bottom leg

Pose Type: forearm balance, forward bend, twist, core

Drishti Point: Urdhva or Antara Drishti (up to the sky)

1.

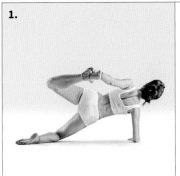

Partridge Pose

Kapinjalasana

(kuh-pinj-uh-LAHS-uh-nuh)

Modification: forearm on the floor, under-head grip:

1. knee on the floor
2. knee off the floor

Pose Type: forearm balance, backbend, core

Drishti Point: Bhrumadhye or Ajna Chakra (third eye, between the eyebrows)

2.

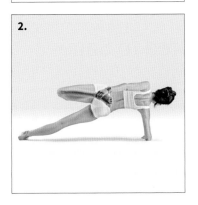

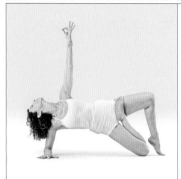

Half Lotus Pose in Pose Dedicated to Sage Vasistha

Ardha Padmasana in Vasishtasana

(UHR-duh puhd-MAHS-uh-nuh in vuh-sish-TAHS-uh-nuh)

Also Known As: Half Lotus Dolphin Side Plank Modification
Modification: forearm on the floor, bottom leg in half lotus, top knee bent, toes to the floor
Pose Type: forearm balance, core
Drishti Point: Hastagrai or Hastagre (hands)

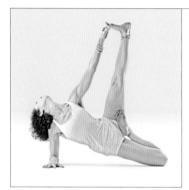

Half Lotus One Big Toe Pose Dedicated to Sage Vasistha

Ardha Padma Eka Padangushta Vasisthasana

(UHR-duh PUHD-muh EY-kuh puhd-ahng-GOOSH-tuh vuh-sish-TAHS-uh-nuh)

Also Known As: Half Lotus Big Toe Dolphin Side Plank Modification
Modification: forearm on the floor
Pose Type: forearm balance, forward bend, core
Drishti Point: Padayoragrai or Padayoragre (toes/feet), Urdhva or Antara Drishti (up to the sky)

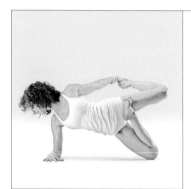

Half Lotus Half Bow Pose in Pose Dedicated to Sage Vasishta

Ardha Padma Dhanurasana in Vasishtasana

(UHR-duh PUHD-muh duh-nur-AHS-uh-nuh in vuh-sish-TAHS-uh-nuh)

Also Known As: Half Lotus Half Bow Pose in Dolphin Side Plank Modification
Modification: forearm on the floor, bottom leg in half lotus, grabbing onto the top foot with under-head grip
Pose Type: forearm balance, backbend, core
Drishti Point: Hastagrai or Hastagre (hands)

Lotus Pose in Pose Dedicated to Sage Vasishta

Padmasana in Vasisthasana

(puhd-MAHS-uh-nuh in vuh-sish-TAHS-uh-nuh)

Also Known As: Lotus Pose in Dolphin Side Plank Modification
Modification: forearm on the floor
Pose Type: forearm balance, core
Drishti Point: Hastagrai or Hastagre (hands)

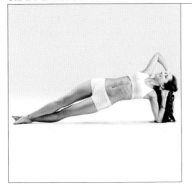

Pose Dedicated to Sage Vasishta

Vasishtasana

(vuh-sish-TAHS-uh-nuh)

Also Known As: Elbow Side Plank Modification
Modification: on the elbow; both legs straight, ankles crossed
Pose Type: elbow balance, core
Drishti Point: Urdhva or Antara Drishti (up to the sky)

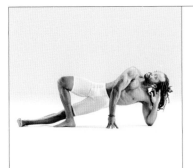

Pose Dedicated to Sage Vasishta

Vasishtasana

(vuh-sish-TAHS-uh-nuh)

Also Known As: Elbow Side Plank Modification
Modification: on the elbow; bottom leg straight; top leg crossed over, foot flat on the floor; fingertips of the top arm to the floor in front of the body
Pose Type: elbow balance, core
Drishti Point: Urdhva or Antara Drishti (up to the sky)

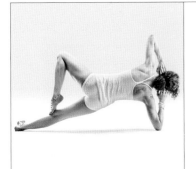

Pose Dedicated to Sage Vasishta

Vasishtasana

(vuh-sish-TAHS-uh-nuh)

Also Known As: Elbow Side Plank Modification
Modification: on the elbow, top foot to the side of the bottom leg
Pose Type: elbow balance, core
Drishti Point: Nasagrai or Nasagre (nose)

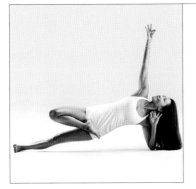

Half Lotus Pose in Pose Dedicated to Sage Vasistha

Ardha Padmasana in Vasisthasana

(UHR-duh puhd-MAHS-uh-nuh in vuh-sish-TAHS-uh-nuh)

Also Known As: Half Lotus Pose in Elbow Side Plank Modification
Modification: on the elbow
Pose Type: elbow balance, core
Drishti Point: Hastagrai or Hastagre (hands)

Backbends

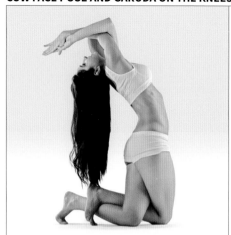

Pose Dedicated to Garuda on the Knees

Janu Garudasana

(JAH-nu guh-ru-DAHS-uh-nuh)

Pose Type: standing (on the knees), backbend

Drishti Point: Angushtamadhye or Angushta Ma Dyai (thumbs)

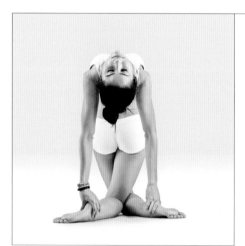

Leg Position of Cow Face Pose in Camel Pose

Pada Gomukhasana in Ushtrasana*

(PUH-duh go-moo-KAHS-uh-nuh in oosh-TRAHS-uh-nuh)

Modification: Gomukhasana legs modification

Pose Type: backbend, standing (on the knees)

Drishti Point: Bhrumadhye or Ajna Chakra (third eye, between the eyebrows)

* "Ushtrasana" may also be spelled as "Ustrasana" in the following camel poses.

KNEES ON THE FLOOR: LOTUS POSE

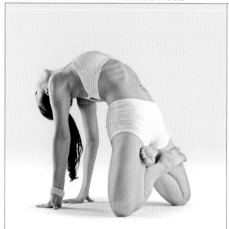

Half Pose Dedicated to Siddhar Kamalamuni

Ardha Kamalamunyasana

(UHR-duh KUH-muh-luhmoo-nyAHS-uh-nuh)

Also Known As: Upward Facing Lotus Pose (Urdhva Mukha Padmasana)

Modification: fingertips pointing to the back, thumbs pointing to the front, knees close to the hands

Pose Type: backbend, standing (on the knees)

Drishti Point: Bhrumadhye or Ajna Chakra (third eye, between the eyebrows)

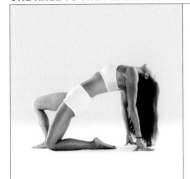

One-Legged Camel Pose

Eka Pada Ushtrasana

(EY-kuh PUH-duh oosh-TRAHS-uh-nuh)

Modification: Leg 1: knee to the floor

Leg 2: foot to the floor in semi-lunge position

Pose Type: backbend, standing (on the knees)

Drishti Point: Bhrumadhye or Ajna Chakra (third eye, between the eyebrows)

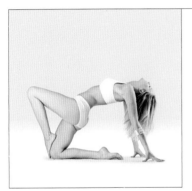

One-Legged Camel Pose

Eka Pada Ushtrasana

(EY-kuh PUH-duh oosh-TRAHS-uh-nuh)

Modification: Leg 1: knee to the floor

Leg 2: sole of the foot to the quadricep

Pose Type: backbend, standing (on the knees)

Drishti Point: Bhrumadhye or Ajna Chakra (third eye, between the eyebrows)

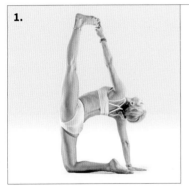

1.

Extended Hand to Big Toe Pose in Half Camel Pose

Utthita Hasta Padangushtasana in Ardha Ushtrasana

(UT-ti-tuh HUH-stuh puhd-AHNG-goosh-TAHS-uh-nuh in UHR-duh oosh-TRAHS-uh-nuh)

Modification: 1. toes pointed to the back

2. toes curled in

Pose Type: backbend, standing (on the knees)

Drishti Point: Bhrumadhye or Ajna Chakra (third eye, between the eyebrows)

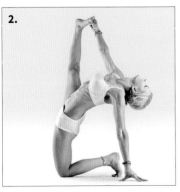

2.

1.

2.

Camel Pose Prep.

Ushtrasana Prep.

(oosh-TRAHS-uh-nuh)

Modification: 1. hands to the lower back

2. hands in Anjali Mudra (Hands in Prayer)

Pose Type: backbend, standing (on the knees)

Drishti Point: Bhrumadhye or Ajna Chakra (third eye, between the eyebrows)

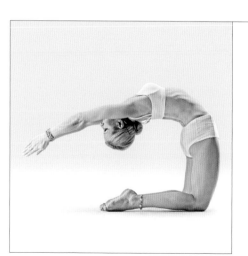

Upward Salute Pose in Camel Pose

Urdhva Hastasana in Ushtrasana

(OORD-vuh huh-STAHS-uh-nuh in oosh-TRAHS-uh-nuh)

Also Known As: Pigeon Pose Prep. (Kapotasana Prep.)

Modification: palms together

Pose Type: backbend, standing (on the knees)

Drishti Point: Bhrumadhye or Ajna Chakra (third eye, between the eyebrows), Angushtamadhye or Angushta Ma Dyai (thumbs)

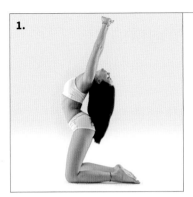

1.

Raised Bound Hands in Camel Pose

Urdhva Baddha Hastasana in Ushtrasana

(OORD-vuh BUH-duh huh-STAHS-uh-nuh in oosh-TRAHS-uh-nuh)

Modification: 1. hips pushed back

2. hips pushed forward

Pose Type: backbend, standing (on the knees)

Drishti Point: Bhrumadhye or Ajna Chakra (third eye, between the eyebrows)

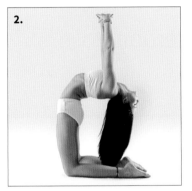

2.

KNEES ON THE FLOOR: BACKBEND—HANDS TO THE HEELS AND TO THE FLOOR

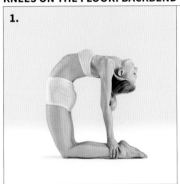

1.

Camel Pose

Ushtrasana

(oosh-TRAHS-uh-nuh)

Modification: 1. grabbing onto both ankles

2. palms to the heels, fingertips pointing to the back

Pose Type: backbend, standing (on the knees)

Drishti Point: Bhrumadhye or Ajna Chakra (third eye, between the eyebrows)

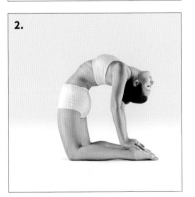

2.

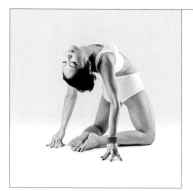

Pose Dedicated to King Nahusha

Nahushasana

(nuh-hu-SHAHS-uh-nuh)

Pose Type: backbend, standing (on the knees)

Drishti Point: Bhrumadhye or Ajna Chakra (third eye, between the eyebrows)

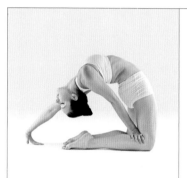

One Hand Graceful Thunderbolt Pose

Eka Hasta Laghuvajrasana

(EY-kuh huh-stuh luh-gu-vuhj-RAHS-uh-nuh)

Pose Type: backbend, standing (on the knees)

Drishti Point: Bhrumadhye or Ajna Chakra (third eye, between the eyebrows)

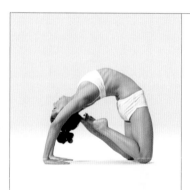

Pigeon Pose

Kapotasana

(kuh-po-TAHS-uh-nuh)

Also Known As: Sage Korakar Pose (Korakarasana), Graceful Thunderbolt Pose (Laghuvajrasana)

Modification: arms over the head, palms to the floor, feet toward the head

Pose Type: backbend, standing (on the knees)

Drishti Point: Bhrumadhye or Ajna Chakra (third eye, between the eyebrows)

KNEES ON THE FLOOR: ONE ARM EXTENDED

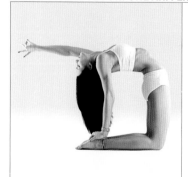

Half Camel Pose

Ardha Ushtrasana

(UHR-duh oosh-TRAHS-uh-nuh)

Also Known As: One Arm Camel Pose (Eka Hasta Ustrasana)

Pose Type: backbend, standing (on the knees)

Drishti Point: Bhrumadhye or Ajna Chakra (third eye, between the eyebrows), Hastagrai or Hastagre (hands)

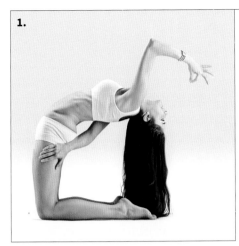

Half Camel Pose

Ardha Ushtrasana

(UHR-duh oosh-TRAHS-uh-nuh)

Modification: arm crossed behind the back to the opposite leg

1. hand to the outside of the hip

2. hand to the inside of the knee

Pose Type: backbend, standing (on the knees)

Drishti Point: Bhrumadhye or Ajna Chakra (third eye, between the eyebrows), Hastagrai or Hastagre (hands)

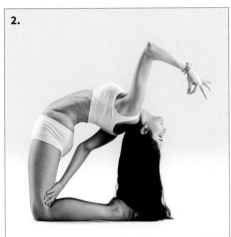

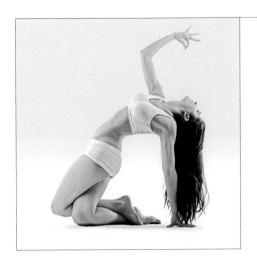

Leg Position of the Pose Dedicated to Garuda in Half Camel Pose

Pada Garudasana in Ardha Ushtrasana

(PUH-duh guh-ru-DAHS-uh-nuh in UHR-duh oosh-TRAHS-uh-nuh}

Modification: one hand to the floor; other arm up, elbow bent

Pose Type: backbend, standing (on the knees)

Drishti Point: Hastagrai or Hastagre (hands), Bhrumadhye or Ajna Chakra (third eye, between the eyebrows)

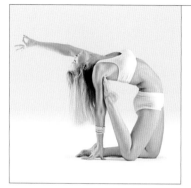

Half Camel Pose

Ardha Ushtrasana

(UHR-duh- oosh-TRAHS-uh-nuh)

Modification: one foot to the armpit on the same side; opposite arm straight up over the head

Pose Type: backbend, standing (on the knees)

Drishti Point: Hastagrai or Hastagre (hands), Bhrumadhye or Ajna Chakra (third eye, between the eyebrows)

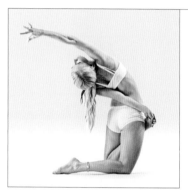

Half Bound Lotus Camel Pose

Ardha Baddha Padma Ushtrasana

(UHR-duh BUH-duh PUHD-muh oosh-TRAHS-uh-nuh)

Modification: free arm straight up over the head

Pose Type: backbend, standing (on the knees), binding

Drishti Point: Hastagrai or Hastagre (hands) or Bhrumadhye or Ajna Chakra (third eye, between the eyebrows)

ONE KNEE BENT TOWARD THE HIP: BACKBEND

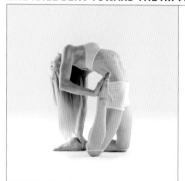

One-Legged Frog Pose in Camel Pose

Eka Pada Bhekasana in Ushtrasana

(EY-kuh PUH-duh bey-KAHS-uh-nuh in oosh-TRAHS-uh-nuh)

Pose Type: backbend, standing (on the knees)

Drishti Point: Bhrumadhye or Ajna Chakra (third eye, between the eyebrows)

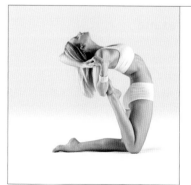

Mermaid Arm Position in Camel Pose

Hasta Naginyasana in Ushtrasana

(HUH-stuh nuh-gin-YAHS-uh-nuh in oosh-TRAHS-uh-nuh)

Pose Type: backbend, standing (on the knees)

Drishti Point: Bhrumadhye or Ajna Chakra (third eye, between the eyebrows)

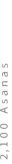

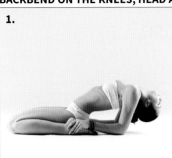

Bed Pose

Paryankasana

(puhr-yuhng-KAHS-uh-nuh)

Also Known As: Reclined Thunderbolt Pose (Supta Vajrasana)

Modification: 1. head off the floor

2. crown of the head on the floor

Pose Type: seated, backbend

Drishti Point: Bhrumadhye or Ajna Chakra (third eye, between the eyebrows)

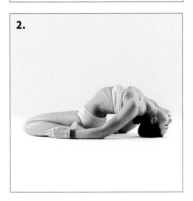

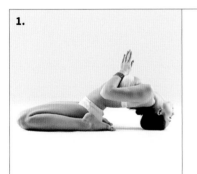

Bed Pose

Paryankasana

(puhr-yuhng-KAHS-uh-nuh)

Also Known As: Reclined Thunderbolt Pose (Supta Vajrasana)

Modification: 1. hands in Anjali Mudra (Hands in Prayer), fingertips pointing to the sky

2. grabbing onto the forearms, arms to the floor up over the head

Pose Type: seated, backbend

Drishti Point: Bhrumadhye or Ajna Chakra (third eye, between the eyebrows)

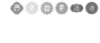

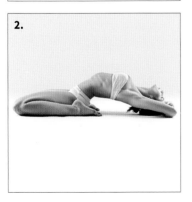

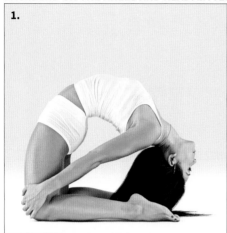

Little Thunderbolt Pose

Laghuvajrasana

(lluh-goo-vuhj-RAHS-uh-nuh)

Modification: 1. grabbing onto the knees, head off the floor

2. forehead to the floor, hands on the quadriceps

3. head to feet, grabbing onto the knees

Pose Type: backbend, standing (on the knees)

Drishti Point: Bhrumadhye or Ajna Chakra (third eye, between the eyebrows)

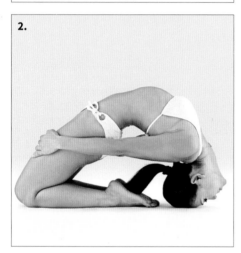

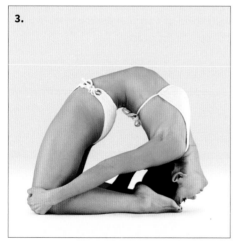

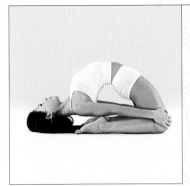

Little Thunderbolt Pose

Laghuvajrasana

(luh-goo-vuhj-RAHS-uh-nuh)

Modification: back of the head on the floor, grabbing onto the knees

Pose Type: backbend, standing (on the knees)

Drishti Point: Bhrumadhye or Ajna Chakra (third eye, between the eyebrows)

BACKBEND ON THE KNEES AND HEAD: PIGEON POSE

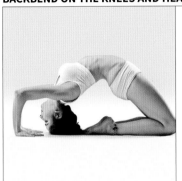

Little Thunderbolt Pose Prep.

Laghuvajrasana Prep.

(luh-goo-vuhj-RAHS-uh-nuh)

Modification: crown of the head to the floor, arms in Headstand 5 (see page 541) position

Pose Type: backbend, standing (on the knees)

Drishti Point: Bhrumadhye or Ajna Chakra (third eye, between the eyebrows)

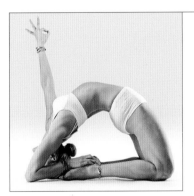

One Hand Pigeon Pose

Eka Hasta Kapotasana

(EY-kuh HUH-stuh kuh-po-TAHS-uh-nuh)

Pose Type: backbend, standing (on the knees)

Drishti Point: Bhrumadhye or Ajna Chakra (third eye, between the eyebrows)

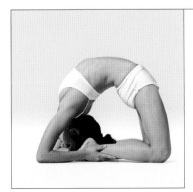

Pigeon Pose

Kapotasana

(kuh-po-TAHS-uh-nuh)

Modification: grabbing onto the ankles

Pose Type: backbend, standing (on the knees)

Drishti Point: Bhrumadhye or Ajna Chakra (third eye, between the eyebrows)

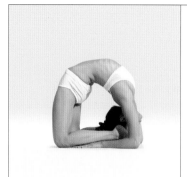

Pigeon Pose

Kapotasana

(kuh-po-TAHS-uh-nuh)

Modification: fingertips toward the knees, palms flat down
Pose Type: backbend, standing (on the knees)
Drishti Point: Bhrumadhye or Ajna Chakra (third eye, between the eyebrows)

PIGEON POSE: ONE-LEGGED

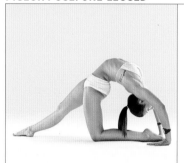

One-Legged Pigeon Pose Prep.

Eka Pada Kapotasana Prep.

(EY-kuh PUH-duh kuh-po-TAHS-uh-nuh)

Modification: arms over the head palms to the floor, head away from the foot
Pose Type: backbend, standing (on the knees)
Drishti Point: Bhrumadhye or Ajna Chakra (third eye, between the eyebrows)

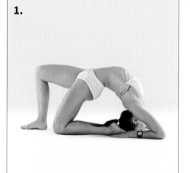

1.

One-Legged Pigeon Pose Prep.

Eka Pada Kapotasana Prep.

(EY-kuh PUH-duh kuh-po-TAHS-uh-nuh)

Modification: 1. knee bent, foot to the floor
2. leg straight, foot to the floor
Pose Type: backbend, standing (on the knees)
Drishti Point: Bhrumadhye or Ajna Chakra (third eye, between the eyebrows)

2.

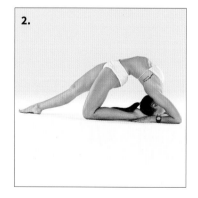

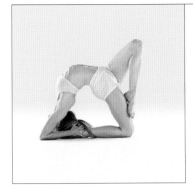

One-Legged Pigeon Pose

Eka Pada Kapotasana

(EY-kuh PUH-duh kuh-po-TAHS-uh-nuh)

Modification: foot to the quadriceps

Pose Type: backbend, standing (on the knees)

Drishti Point: Bhrumadhye or Ajna Chakra (third eye, between the eyebrows)

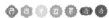

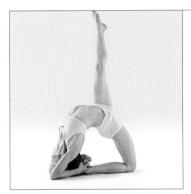

One-Legged Pigeon Pose

Eka Pada Kapotasana

(EY-kuh PUH-duh kuh-po-TAHS-uh-nuh)

Modification: leg straight

Pose Type: backbend, standing (on the knees)

Drishti Point: Bhrumadhye or Ajna Chakra (third eye, between the eyebrows)

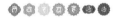

TOES CURLED IN: BACKBEND—SHOULDERS ON THE FLOOR & HEAD ON THE FLOOR

1.

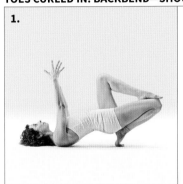

One-Legged Tip Toe Bridge Pose

Eka Pada Prapada Setu Bandhasana

(EY-kuh PUH-duh PRUH-puh-duh SEY-too buhn-DAHS-uh-nuh)

Modification: back of the head on the floor, arms up to the sky

1. knee bent, foot resting on the knee

2. leg straight and extended to the sky

Pose Type: supine, backbend

Drishti Point: Angushtamadhye or Angustha Ma Dyai (thumbs)

2.

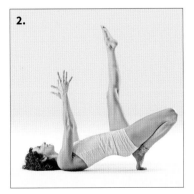

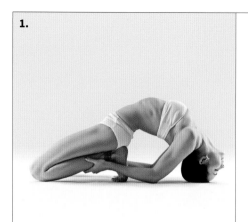

1.

Tip Toe Bridge Pose

Prapada Setu Bandhasana

(PRUH-puh-duh SEY-too buhn-DAHS-uh-nuh)

Also Known As: Tip Toe Bed Pose (Prapada Paryankasana), Big Toe Bridge Pose (Padangushta Setu Bandhasana)

Modification: 1. grabbing onto the shins, elbows to the floor

2. grabbing onto the shins, arms straight

3. hands on the quadriceps, arms straight

Pose Type: backbend, standing (on the knees)

Drishti Point: Bhrumadhye or Ajna Chakra (third eye, between the eyebrows)

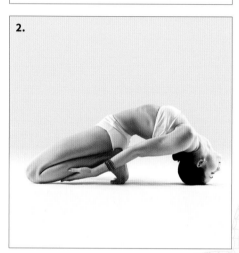

2.

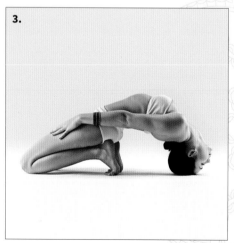

3.

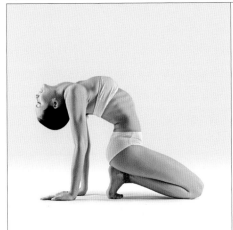

Thunderbolt Pose

Vajrasana

(vuhj-RAHS-uh-nuh)

Also Known As: Tip Toe Bed Pose Prep. (Prapada Paryankasana Prep.)

Modification: toes curled in, fingertips pointing away from the feet, intense backbend

Pose Type: backbend, standing (on the knees)

Drishti Point: Bhrumadhye or Ajna Chakra (third eye, between the eyebrows)

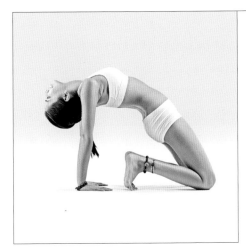

Tip Toe Camel Pose

Prapada Ushtrasana

(PRUH-puh-duh oosh-TRAHS-uh-nuh)

Modification: palms flat to the floor, fingertips pointing to the front

Pose Type: backbend, standing (on the knees)

Drishti Point: Bhrumadhye or Ajna Chakra (third eye, between the eyebrows)

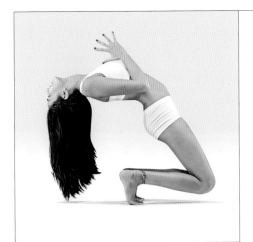

Unsupported Tip Toe Camel Pose

Niralamba Prapada Ushtrasana

(neer-AH-luhm-buh PRUH-puh-duh oosh-TRAHS-uh-nuh)

Modification: knees lifted off the floor, hands in Anjali Mudra (Hands in Prayer)

Pose Type: standing, balance, backbend

Drishti Point: Bhrumadhye or Ajna Chakra (third eye, between the eyebrows)

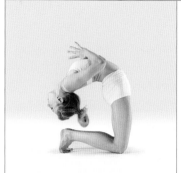

Tip Toe Camel Pose

Prapada Ushtrasana

(PRUH-puh-duh oosh-TRAHS-uh-nuh)

Modification: hands in Anjali Mudra (Hands in Prayer)

Pose Type: backbend, standing (on the knees)

Drishti Point: Bhrumadhye or Ajna Chakra (third eye, between the eyebrows)

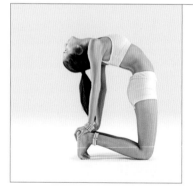

Half Tip Toe Camel Pose

Ardha Prapada Ushtrasana

(UHR-duh PRUH-puh-duh oosh-TRAHS-uh-nuh)

Pose Type: backbend, standing (on the knees)

Drishti Point: Bhrumadhye or Ajna Chakra (third eye, between the eyebrows), Hastagrai or Hastagre (hands)

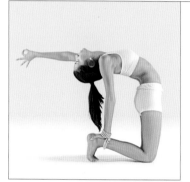

Tip Toe Camel Pose

Prapada Ushtrasana

(PRUH-puh-duh oosh-TRAHS-uh-nuh)

Pose Type: backbend, standing (on the knees)

Drishti Point: Bhrumadhye or Ajna Chakra (third eye, between the eyebrows)

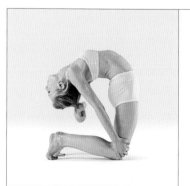

Tip Toe Camel Pose

Prapada Ushtrasana

(PRUH-puh-duh oosh-TRAHS-uh-nuh)

Modification: hands on the knees

Pose Type: backbend, standing (on the knees)

Drishti Point: Bhrumadhye or Ajna Chakra (third eye, between the eyebrows)

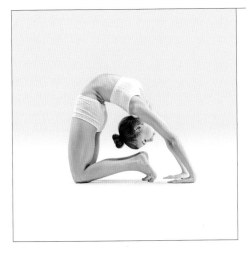

Tip Toe Pigeon Pose

Prapada Kapotasana
(PRUH-puh-duh kuh-po-TAHS-uh-nuh)

Also Known As: Big Toe Pigeon Pose (Padangushta Kapotasana)
Modification: arms straight up over the head, palms to the floor
Pose Type: backbend, standing (on the knees)
Drishti Point: Bhrumadhye or Ajna Chakra (third eye, between the eyebrows), Hastagrai or Hastagre (hands)

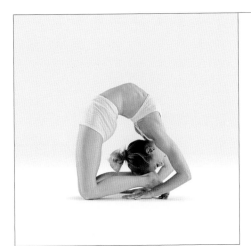

Tip Toe Pigeon Pose

Prapada Kapotasana
(PRUH-puh-duh kuh-po-TAHS-uh-nuh)

Also Known As: Big Toe Pigeon Pose (Padangustha Kapotasana), Little Wheel Pose (Laghu Chakrasana)
Modification: arms up over the head, elbows bent, palms to the floor, forehead to the heels
Pose Type: backbend, standing (on the knees)
Drishti Point: Bhrumadhye or Ajna Chakra (third eye, between the eyebrows)

TOES CURLED IN: BACKBEND—ARMS STRAIGHT, PALMS TOGETHER

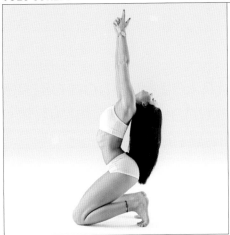

Raised Bound Hands in Tip Toe Camel Pose

Urdhva Baddha Hastasana in Prapada Ushtrasana
(OORD-vuh BUH-duh huh-STAHS-uh-nuh in PRUH-puh-duh oosh-TRAHS-uh-nuh)

Modification: hips pushing back
Pose Type: backbend, standing (on the knees)
Drishti Point: Bhrumadhye or Ajna Chakra (third eye, between the eyebrows), Angushtamadhye or Angushta Ma Dyai (thumbs)

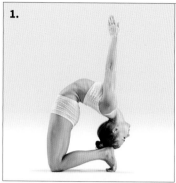

1.

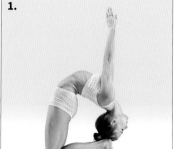

2.

Tip Toe Pigeon Pose

Prapada Kapotasana

(PRUH-puh-duh kuh-po-TAHS-uh-nuh)

Also Known As: Big Toe Pigeon Pose (Padangushta Kapotasana), Full Camel Pose (Purna Ushtrasana), or Little Wheel Pose (Laghu Chakrasana)

Modification: 1. arms extended to the sky

 2. arms parallel to the floor

Pose Type: backbend, standing (on the knees)

Drishti Point: Bhrumadhye or Ajna Chakra (third eye, between the eyebrows)

BACKBEND: HEADSTAND 5 ARM POSITION

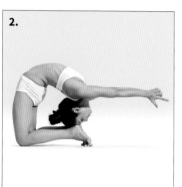

Upward Bow Pose in Headstand 5

Urdhva Dhanurasana in Shirshasana 5

(OORD-vuh duh-nur-AHS-uh-nuh in sheer-SHAS-uh-nuh)

Pose Type: backbend, inversion

Drishti Point: Bhrumadhye or Ajna Chakra (third eye, between the eyebrows)

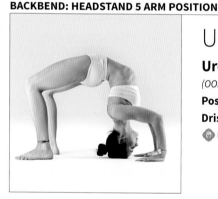

Upward Bow Pose with Leg Position of the Pose Dedicated to Garuda in Headstand 5

Urdhva Dhanurasana Pada Garudasana in Shirshasana 5

(OORD-vuh duh-nur-AHS-uh-nuh PUH-duh guh-ru-DAHS-uh-nuh in sheer-SHAHS-uh-nuh)

Pose Type: backbend, inversion

Drishti Point: Bhrumadhye or Ajna Chakra (third eye, between the eyebrows)

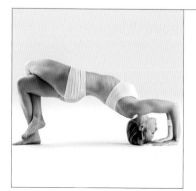

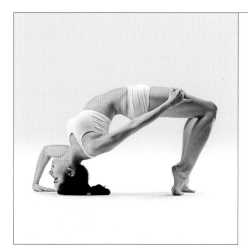

Upward Tip Toe Bow Pose in One Hand Headstand 5

Urdhva Prapada Dhanurasana in Eka Hasta Shirshasana 5

(OORD-vuh PRUH-puh-duh duh-nur-AHS-uh-nuh in EY-kuh HUH-stuh sheer-SHAHS-uh-nuh)

Pose Type: backbend, inversion

Drishti Point: Bhrumadhye or Ajna Chakra (third eye, between the eyebrows)

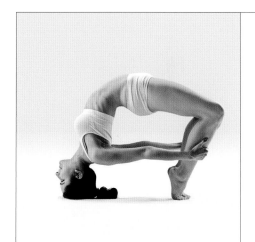

Inverted Tip Toe Bow Pose

Viparita Prapada Dhanurasana

(vi-puh-REE-tuh PRUH-puh-duh duh-nur-AHS-uh-nuh)

Also Known As: Headstand Bow Pose (Shirsha Dhanurasana)

Pose Type: backbend, inversion

Drishti Point: Bhrumadhye or Ajna Chakra (third eye, between the eyebrows)

BACKBEND: HEADSTAND 1 ARM POSITION—KNEE/KNEES BENT

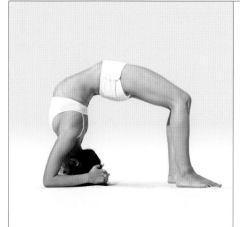

Upward Bow Pose in Headstand 1

Urdhva Dhanurasana in Shirshasana 1

(OORD-vuh duh-nur-AHS-uh-nuh in sheer-SHAHS-uh-nuh)

Pose Type: backbend, inversion

Drishti Point: Bhrumadhye or Ajna Chakra (third eye, between the eyebrows)

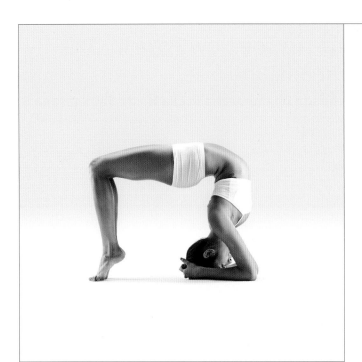

Upward Tip Toe Bow Pose in Headstand 1

Urdhva Prapada Dhanurasana in Shirshasana 1

(OORD-vuh PRUH-puh-duh duh-noor-AHS-uh-nuh in sheer-SHAHS-uh-nuh)

Pose Type: backbend, inversion

Drishti Point: Bhrumadhye or Ajna Chakra (third eye, between the eyebrows)

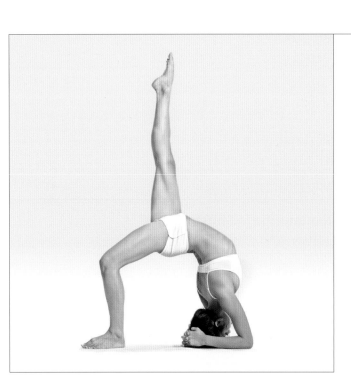

One-Legged Inverted Staff Pose

Eka Pada Viparita Dandasana

(EY-kuh PUH-duh vi-puh-REE-tuh duhn-DAHS-uh-nuh)

Modification: knee of the bottom leg bent

Pose Type: backbend, inversion

Drishti Point: Bhrumadhye or Ajna Chakra (third eye, between the eyebrows)

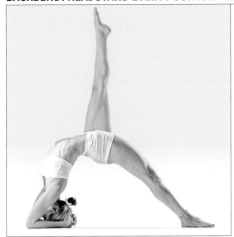

One-Legged Inverted Staff Pose

Eka Pada Viparita Dandasana

(EY-kuh PUH-duh vi-puh-REE-tuh duhn-DAHS-uh-nuh)

Also Known As: Inverted Staff Pose B (Viparita Dandasana B)

Modification: both legs straight

Pose Type: backbend, inversion

Drishti Point: Bhrumadhye or Ajna Chakra (third eye, between the eyebrows)

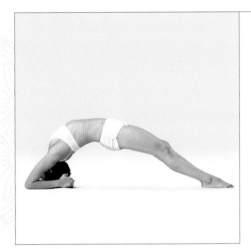

Two-Legged Inverted Staff Pose

Dwi Pada Viparita Dandasana

(DWI-puh-duh vi-puh-REE-tuh duhn-DAHS-uh-nuh)

Also Known As: Inverted Staff Pose A (Viparita Dandasana A)

Pose Type: backbend, inversion

Drishti Point: Bhrumadhye or Ajna Chakra (third eye, between the eyebrows)

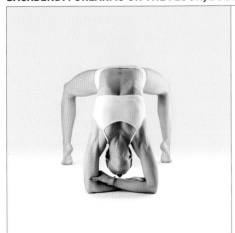

Bound Arms Tip Toe Bound Wheel Pose

Baddha Hasta Prapada Chakra Bandhasana

(BUH-duh HUH-stuh PRUH-puh-duh CHUHK-ruh buhn-DAHS-uh-nuh)

Pose Type: backbend, inversion

Drishti Point: Bhrumadhye or Ajna Chakra (third eye, between the eyebrows)

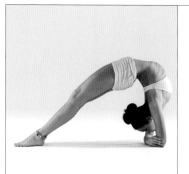

Bound Arms Both Legs Inverted Staff Pose

Baddha Hasta Dwi Pada Viparita Dandasana

(BUH-duh HUH-stuh DWI-puh-duh vi-puh-REE-tuh duhn-DAH-suh-nuh)

Pose Type: backbend, inversion

Drishti Point: Bhrumadhye or Ajna Chakra (third eye, between the eyebrows)

BACKBEND: FOREARMS ON THE FLOOR, HEELS DOWN

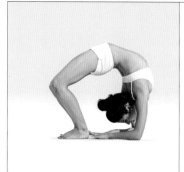

Bound Wheel Pose

Chakra Bandhasana

(CHUHK-ruh buhn-DAHS-uh-nuh)

Modification: forearms to the floor, heels down, fingertips touching the heels

Pose Type: backbend, inversion

Drishti Point: Bhrumadhye or Ajna Chakra (third eye, between the eyebrows)

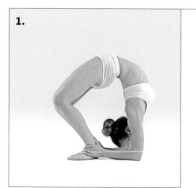

1.

Bound Wheel Pose

Chakra Bandhasana

(CHUHK-ruh buhn-DAHS-uh-nuh)

Also Known As: Bound Wheel Pose (Bandha Chakrasana)

Modification: grabbing onto ankles

1. looking straight ahead

2. head rolling back

Pose Type: backbend, inversion

Drishti Point: Bhrumadhye or Ajna Chakra (third eye, between the eyebrows)

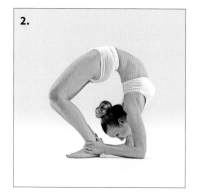

2.

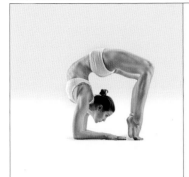

Tip Toe Bound Wheel Pose

Prapada Chakra Bandhasana

(PRUH-puh-duh CHUCK-ruh buhn-DAHS-uh-nuh)

Pose Type: backbend, inversion

Drishti Point: Bhrumadhye or Ajna Chakra (third eye, between the eyebrows)

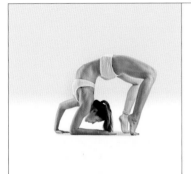

Uneven Tip Toe Bound Wheel Pose

Vishama Prapada Chakra Bandhasana

(VI-shuh-muh PRUH-puh-duh CHUCK-ruh buhn-DAHS-uh-nuh)

Pose Type: backbend, inversion

Drishti Point: Bhrumadhye or Ajna Chakra (third eye, between the eyebrows)

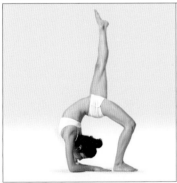

One-Legged Inverted Staff Pose

Eka Pada Viparita Dandasana

(EY-kuh PUH-duh vi-puh-REE-tuh duhn-DAHS-uh-nuh)

Modification: forearms to the floor, head off the floor

Pose Type: backbend, inversion

Drishti Point: Bhrumadhye or Ajna Chakra (third eye, between the eyebrows)

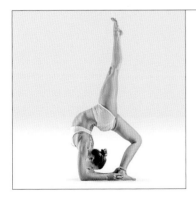

Bound Foot One-Legged Inverted Staff Pose

Baddha Pada Eka Pada Viparita Dandasana

(BUH-duh PUH-duh EY-kuh PUH-duh vi-puh-REE-tuh duhn-DAHS-uh-nuh)

Modification: forearms to the floor, head off the floor

Pose Type: backbend, inversion

Drishti Point: Bhrumadhye or Ajna Chakra (third eye, between the eyebrows)

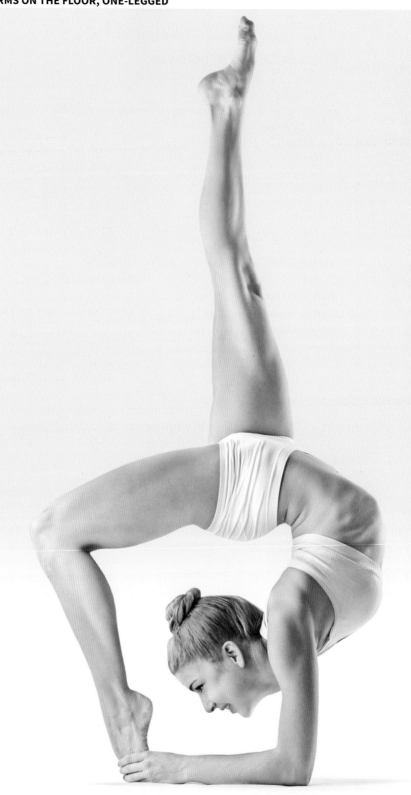

Tip Toe Bound Foot One-Legged Inverted
Staff Pose

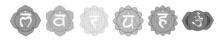

Prapada Baddha Pada Eka Pada Viparita Dandasana
(PRUH-puh-duh BUH-duh PUH-duh EY-kuh PUH-duh vi-puh-REE-tuh duhn-DAHS-uh-nuh)
Pose Type: backbend, inversion
Drishti Point: Bhrumadhye or Ajna Chakra (third eye, between the eyebrows)

Modification: forearms to the floor, head off the floor

prapada = tip of the feet
baddha = bound
pada = foot or leg
eka = one
pada = foot or leg
viparita = inverted
danda = stick or staff

How to Perform the Pose:

1. Begin by lying flat on your back. Engage your *mula bandha*, *uddhiyana bandha*, and *ujjayi* breathing. Inhale and bring your hands under your shoulders with elbows bent and close to your head, with the fingertips pointing away from your head.

2. Exhale and bend your knees, keep your feet flat on the floor and slide your heels toward your sitting bones. Keep your feet in line with your sitting bones and parallel to each other with your toes pointing straight ahead.

3. Exhale as you lift your sitting bones and your back off the floor. Place the crown of your head onto the floor, balancing on your hands, head, and feet.

4. Exhale as you slide your right palm in the direction of your feet until your forearm is flat on the floor. On the next exhale, slide your left palm to meet your right. Interlock your fingers at the back of your head.

5. Exhale and lift your head off the floor.

6. On the next exhale, walk your feet toward your hands. Grab onto your left ankle with both hands.

7. Exhale as you lift your right foot off the floor, keeping your right leg strong and straight with toes pointing up to the sky.

8. Inhale and lift your left heel, coming onto the toes of the left foot, while holding onto the left toes with both hands. Hold the pose for at least 30, and up to 90, seconds in order to receive the full benefits of the stretch on the right side.

9. Inhale and lower the left heel to the floor, followed by the right foot. Exhale and grab onto the right ankle with both hands. On the following exhale, lift your left foot off the floor, keeping your left leg strong and straight with toes pointing up to the sky.

10. Inhale and lift your right heel, coming onto the toes of the right foot while holding onto the right toes with both hands. Hold the pose for at least 30, and up to 90, seconds in order to receive the full benefits of the stretch on the left side.

11. Inhale and lower your right heel to the floor, followed by your left foot. Exhale and lower your head to the floor. Exhale and tuck your chin to your chest and lower your spine to the floor, coming out of the pose.

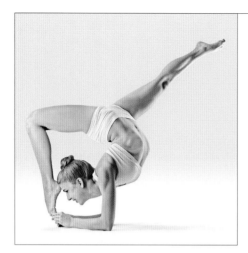

Foot to the Head One-Legged Inverted Staff Pose

Shirsha Pada Eka Pada Viparita Dandasana

(SHEER-shuh PUH-duh EY-kuh PUH-duh vi-puh-REE-tuh duhn-DAHS-uh-nuh)

Modification: forearms to the floor, head off the floor

Pose Type: backbend, inversion

Drishti Point: Bhrumadhye or Ajna Chakra (third eye, between the eyebrows)

UPWARD BOW POSE

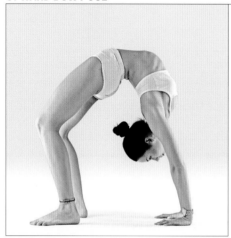

Upward Bow Pose

Urdhva Dhanurasana

(OORD-vuh duh-nur-AHS-uh-nuh)

Modification: heels down

Pose Type: backbend, inversion

Drishti Point: Bhrumadhye or Ajna Chakra (third eye, between the eyebrows)

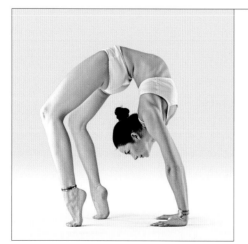

Tip Toe Upward Bow Pose

Prapada Urdhva Dhanurasana

(PRUH-puh-duh OORD-vuh duh-nur-AHS-uh-nuh)

Pose Type: backbend, inversion

Drishti Point: Bhrumadhye or Ajna Chakra (third eye, between the eyebrows)

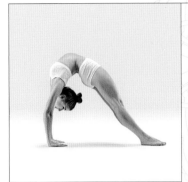

Elevated Both Legs Inverted Staff Pose

Utthita Dwi Pada Viparita Dandasana

(UT-ti-tuh DWI-puh-duh vi-puh-REE-tuh duhn-DAHS-uh-nuh)

Also Known As: Upward Bow Pose (Urdhva Dhanurasana)
Modification: head rolling back
Pose Type: backbend, inversion
Drishti Point: Bhrumadhye or Ajna Chakra (third eye, between the eyebrows)

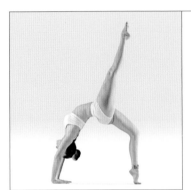

Tip Toe One-Legged Upward Bow Pose

Prapada Eka Pada Urdhva Dhanurasana

(PRUH-puh-duh EY-kuh PUH-duh OORD-vuh duh-nur-AHS-uh-nuh)

Pose Type: backbend, inversion
Drishti Point: Bhrumadhye or Ajna Chakra (third eye, between the eyebrows)

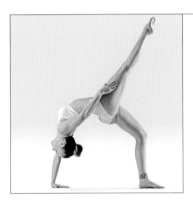

One-Legged Upward Bow Pose

Eka Pada Urdhva Dhanurasana

(EY-kuh PUH-duh OORD-vuh duh-nur-AHS-uh-nuh)

Also Known As: Two Limb Upward Bow Pose (Dwi Anga Urdhva Dhanurasana)
Modification: one hand to the thigh
Pose Type: backbend, inversion
Drishti Point: Bhrumadhye or Ajna Chakra (third eye, between the eyebrows)

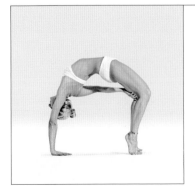

Tip Toe One Hand Upward Bow Pose

Prapada Eka Hasta Urdhva Dhanurasana

(PRUH-puh-duh EY-kuh HUH-stuh OORD-vuh duh-nur-AHS-uh-nuh)

Pose Type: backbend, inversion
Drishti Point: Bhrumadhye or Ajna Chakra (third eye, between the eyebrows)

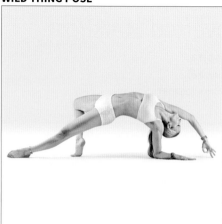

Wild Thing Pose

Chamatkarasana

(kuh-muht-kar-AHS-uh-nuh)

Modification: forearm to the floor

Pose Type: backbend

Drishti Point: Bhrumadhye or Ajna Chakra (third eye, between the eyebrows) or Hastagrai or Hastagre (hands)

See the glossary for a more precise translation of chamatkarasana.

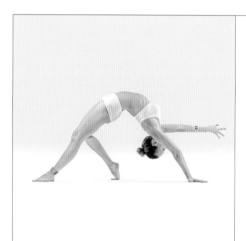

Wild Thing Pose

Chamatkarasana

(kuh-muht-kar-AHS-uh-nuh)

Pose Type: backbend, inversion

Drishti Point: Bhrumadhye or Ajna Chakra (third eye, between the eyebrows) or Hastagrai or Hastagre (hands)

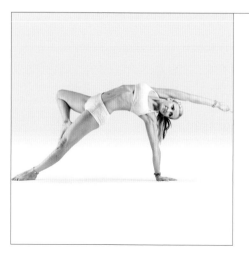

Wild Thing Pose

Chamatkarasana

(kuh-muht-kar-AHS-uh-nuh)

Modification: foot to inside of the thigh

Pose Type: backbend

Drishti Point: Hastagrai or Hastagre (hands)

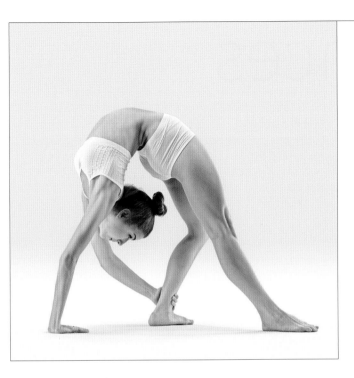

Wild Thing Pose

Chamatkarasana

(kuh-muht-kar-AHS-uh-nuh)

Modification: grabbing the ankle with overhead grip on the same side

Pose Type: backbend, inversion

Drishti Point: Bhrumadhye or Ajna Chakra (third eye, between the eyebrows) or Hastagrai or Hastagre (hands)

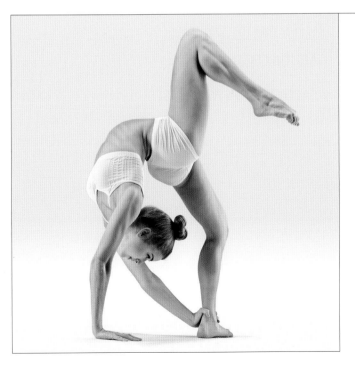

Wild Thing Pose

Chamatkarasana

(kuh-muht-kar-AHS-uh-nuh)

Modification: grabbing the ankle with overhead grip on the same side; other foot off the floor—knee bent

Pose Type: backbend, inversion

Drishti Point: Bhrumadhye or Ajna Chakra (third eye, between the eyebrows) or Hastagrai or

Arm Balances

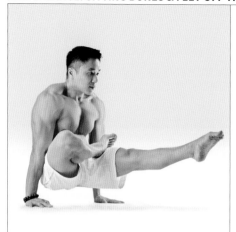

Half Fire Log Celibate Pose

Ardha Agnistambha Brahmacharyasana

(UHR_duh uhg-ni-STUHM-buh bruh-muh-chahr-YAHS-uh-nuh)
Pose Type: core, arm balance
Drishti Point: Padayoragrai or Padayoragre (toes/feet)

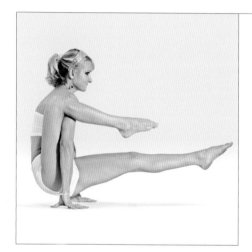

One Leg Over Shoulder Pose

Eka Hasta Bhujasana

(EY-kuh HUH-stuh buj-AHS-uh-nuh)
Also Known As: Comfortable Bird Pose (Sukha Chakorasana)
Pose Type: core, arm balance
Drishti Point: Padayoragrai or Padayoragre (toes/feet)

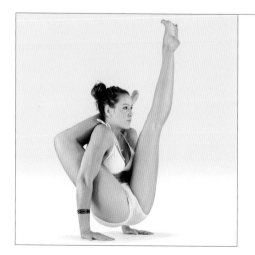

Moonbird Pose

Chakorasana

(chuh-kor-AHS-uh-nuh)
Pose Type: core, arm balance
Drishti Point: Bhrumadhye or Ajna Chakra (third eye, between the eyebrows)

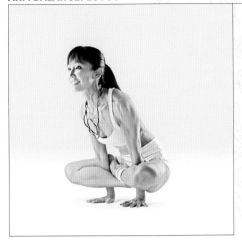

Rooster Pose

Kukkutasana

(ku-ku-TAHS-uh-nuh)
Pose Type: arm balance, forward bend
Drishti Point: Nasagrai or Nasagre (nose)

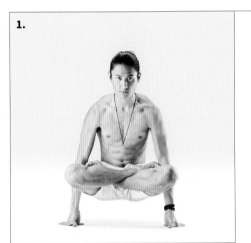

1.

Scales Pose

Tolasana

(to-LAHS-uh-nuh)
Modification: 1. fingertips pointing to the back, thumbs pointing to the front
2. palms flat on the floor, fingertips pointing to the front
Pose Type: arm balance, forward bend
Drishti Point: Nasagrai or Nasagre (nose)

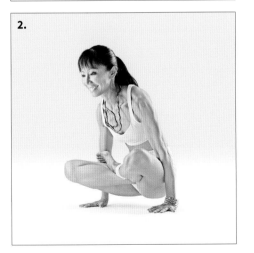

2.

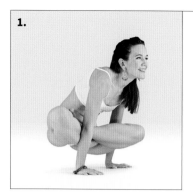

Pose Dedicated to Sage Galava

Galavasana

(gah-luh-VAHS-uh-nuh)

Modification: 1. hips low

2. hips high

Pose Type: arm balance, forward bend

Drishti Point: Nasagrai or Nasagre (nose)

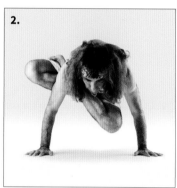

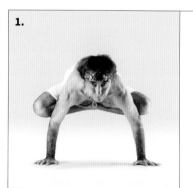

Upward Rooster Pose

Urdhva Kukkutasana

(OORD-vuh ku-ku-TAHS-uh-nuh)

Modification: 1. hips at shoulder height

2. hips higher than the shoulders

Pose Type: arm balance, forward bend

Drishti Point: Bhrumadhye or Ajna Chakra (third eye, between the eyebrows), Angushta-madhye or Angushta Ma Dyai (thumbs)

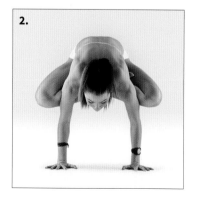

1.

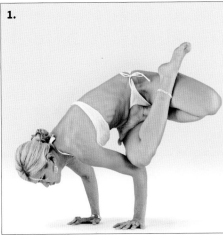

Side Rooster Pose

Parshva Kukkutasana

(PAHRSH-vuh ku-ku-TAHS-uh-nuh)

Also Known As: Revolved Rooster Pose (Parivritta Kukkutasana), Wounded Rooster Pose (Pungu Kukkutasana)

Modification: 1. elbows bent

2. arms straight

Pose Type: arm balance, forward bend, twist

Drishti Point: Nasagrai or Nasagre (nose)

2.

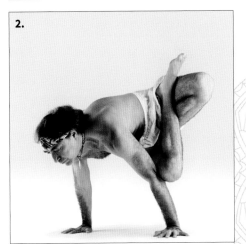

ARM BALANCE: PENDANT POSE

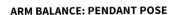

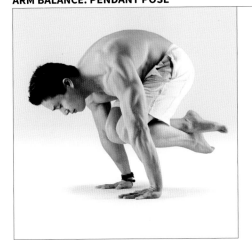

Pendant Pose

Lolasana

(lo-LAHS-uh-nuh)

Modification: ankles crossed

Pose Type: arm balance, forward bend, core

Drishti Point: Angushtamadhye or Angushta Ma Dyai (thumbs) or Nasagrai or Nasagre (nose)

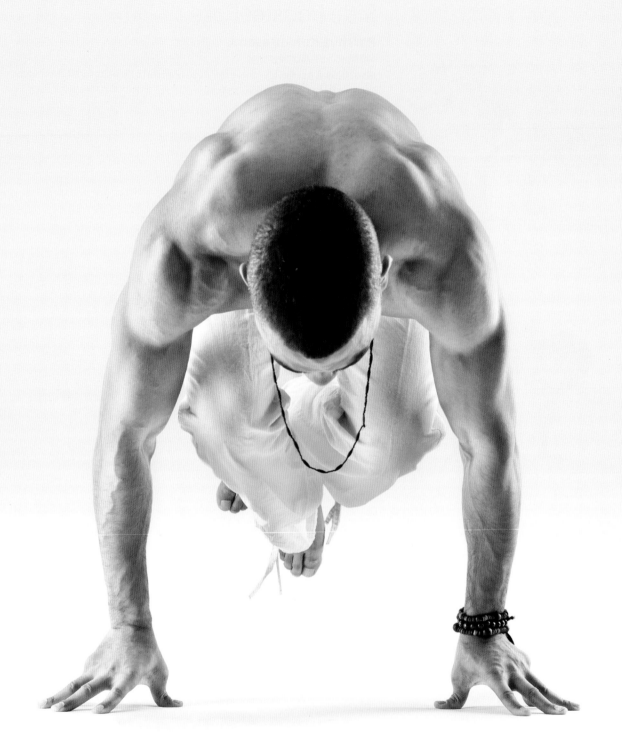

Pendant Pose

Lolasana
(lo-LAHS-uh-nuh)
Pose Type: arm balance, forward bend, core
Drishti Point: Angusthamadhye or Angustha Ma Dyai (thumbs) or Nasagrai or Nasagre (nose)

Modification: on the fingertips; ankles crossed

lola = pendant

How to Perform the Pose:

1. Begin by sitting on the floor with both your legs straight out in front of you. Keep your fingertips on the floor on the sides of your hips. Engage your *mula bandha*, *uddhiyana bandha*, and *ujjayi* breathing.

2. Exhale and lean forward, lifting your sitting bones off the floor. Bend your right knee, sliding your foot back. On the next exhale, bend your left knee, sliding your left foot back to meet your right. Your left shin should end up on top of your right calf muscle. Sit on your heels with ankles crossed under your sitting bones.

3. Inhale and rock forward. Exhale, engage your core, pull your quadriceps toward your chest, and lift your knees and feet off the floor, balancing on your fingertips. Make sure your arms are strong and straight and your shoulders are on top of your fingertips.

4. Aim to hold the pose for at least 30, and up to 90, seconds in order to receive the full benefits of the pose.

5. Inhale and lower your feet and knees to the floor. Exhale and bring both legs straight out in front of you. Repeat on the opposite side.

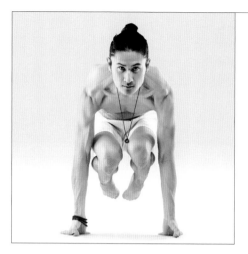

Pendant Pose

Lolasana

(lo-LAHS-uh-nuh)

Modification: fingertips pointing to the back, thumbs pointing to the front
Pose Type: arm balance, forward bend, core
Drishti Point: Bhrumadhye or Ajna Chakra (third eye, between the eyebrows), Nasagrai or Nasagre (nose)

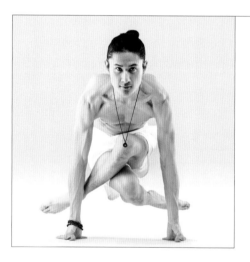

Leg Position of Cow Face Pose in Pendant Pose

Pada Gomukhasana in Lolasana

(PUH-duh go-muk-AHS-uh-nuh in lo-LAHS-uh-nuh)

Modification: fingertips pointing to the back, thumbs pointing to the front
Pose Type: arm balance, forward bend, core
Drishti Point: Bhrumadhye or Ajna Chakra (third eye, between the eyebrows), Nasagrai or Nasagre (nose)

ARM BALANCE: ONE LEG OVER THE SHOULDER

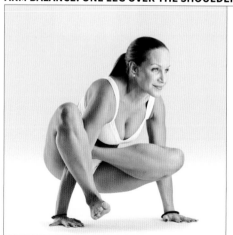

Pose Dedicated to Viranchi (Brahma) 1 Prep.

Viranchyasana 1 Prep.

(vir-uhn-CHYAHS-uh-nuh)

Modification: back of the knee toward the shoulder
Pose Type: arm balance, forward bend
Drishti Point: Nasagrai or Nasagre (nose)

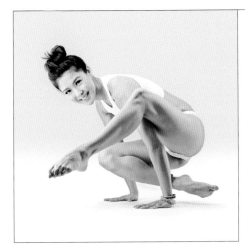

One-Legged Crane 2 Prep.

Eka Pada Bakasana 2 Prep.
(EY-kuh PUH-duh buh-KAHS-uh-nuh)

Modification: both knees bent, back of one knee over the shoulder, other knee toward the chest
Pose Type: arm balance, forward bend
Drishti Point: Padayoragrai or Padayoragre (toes/feet)

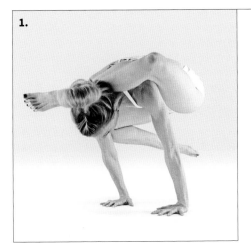
1.

One Foot Behind Head Crane Pose

Eka Pada Shirsha Bakasana
(EY-kuh PUH-duh SHEER-shuh buh-KAHS-uh-nuh)

Modification: 1. hips at shoulder height
2. hips at elbow height, head lifted
Pose Type: arm balance, forward bend
Drishti Point: Bhrumadhye or Ajna Chakra (third eye, between the eyebrows)

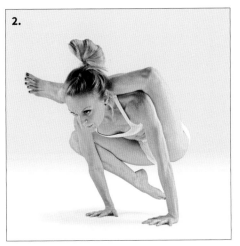
2.

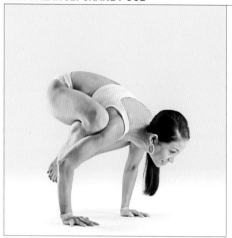

Crane Pose

Bakasana

(buh-KAHS-uh-nuh)

Also Known As: Crow Pose (Kakasana)
Modification: elbows bent
Pose Type: arm balance, forward bend
Drishti Point: Nasagrai or Nasagre (nose)

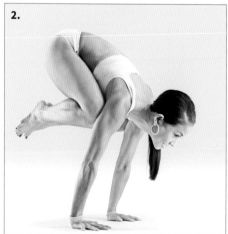

1.

Crane Pose

Bakasana

(buh-KAHS-uh-nuh)

Modification: 1. knees off the triceps
2. knees on the triceps
Pose Type: arm balance, forward bend
Drishti Point: Angushtamadhye or Angushta Ma Dyai (thumbs), Nasagrai or Nasagre (nose)

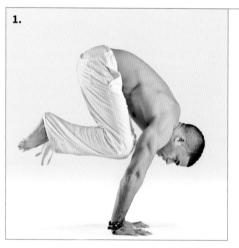

2.

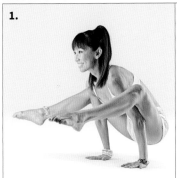

Two-Handed Arm Balance

Dwi Hasta Bhujasana

(DWI-huh-stuh buj-AHS-uh-nuh)

Modification: 1. feet off the floor

2. toes touching the floor

Pose Type: arm balance, forward bend

Drishti Point: Nasagrai or Nasagre (nose), Padayoragrai or Padayoragre (toes/feet)

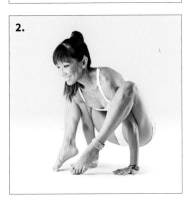

Shoulder Pressure Pose

Bhujapidasana

(buj-uh-peed-AHS-uh-nuh)

Also Known As: Shoulder Pressure Pose (Bhujapidasana A)

Modification: head off the floor

Pose Type: arm balance, forward bend

Drishti Point: Nasagrai or Nasagre (nose), Padayoragrai or Padayoragre (toes/feet)

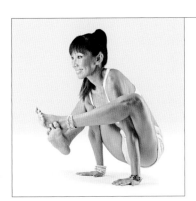

Firefly Pose 1

Tittibhasana 1

(ti-ti-BAHS-uh-nuh)

Also Known As: Firefly Pose A (Tittibhasana A)

Modification: elbows bent, legs on top of the shoulders

Pose Type: arm balance, forward bend

Drishti Point: Bhrumadhye or Ajna Chakra (third eye, between the eyebrows), or Nasagrai or Nasagre (nose)

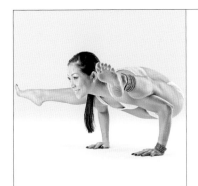

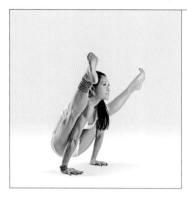

Firefly Pose 1

Tittibhasana 1

(ti-ti-BAHS-uh-nuh)

Also Known As: Firefly Pose A (Tittibhasana A)
Modification: arms straight, feet extended to the sky
Pose Type: arm balance, forward bend
Drishti Point: Bhrumadhye or Ajna Chakra (third eye, between the eyebrows) or Nasagrai or Nasagre (nose)

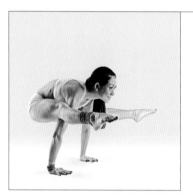

Firefly Pose 1

Tittibhasana 1

(ti-ti-BAHS-uh-nuh)

Also Known As: Firefly Pose A (Tittibhasana A), Raised Tortoise Pose (Utthita Kurmasana)
Modification: arms straight, legs parallel to the floor
Pose Type: arm balance, forward bend
Drishti Point: Nasagrai or Nasagre (nose)

ARM BALANCE: FIREFLY POSE

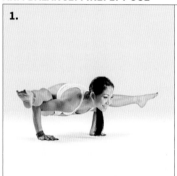

1.

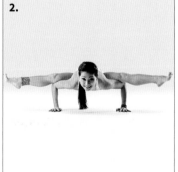

2.

Firefly Pose

Tittibhasana

(ti-ti-BAHS-uh-nuh)

Also Known As: Raised Up Feet Spread Out Resting on the Arms Pose (Utthita Dwi Pada Vrishtasana)
Modification: elbows bent, legs on triceps, wide legged
1. side view
2. front view
Pose Type: arm balance, forward bend
Drishti Point: Nasagrai or Nasagre (nose), Bhrumadhye or Ajna Chakra (third eye, between the eyebrows)

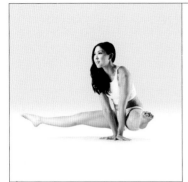

Lifted Feet Spread Out Pose

Utthita Dwi Pada Vrishtasana

(UT-ti-tuh DWI-puh-duh vrish-TAHS-uh-nuh)

Modification: arms straight, heels of the palms touching, fingertips pointing to the sides

Pose Type: arm balance, forward bend

Drishti Point: Nasagrai or Nasagre (nose)

ARM BALANCE: ONE LEG STRAIGHT, ONE KNEE BENT

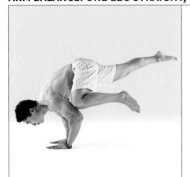

One-Legged Crane 1

Eka Pada Bakasana 1

(EY-kuh PUH-duh buh-KAHS-uh-nuh)

Modification: knee to the tricep

Pose Type: arm balance, forward bend

Drishti Point: Bhrumadhye or Ajna Chakra (third eye, between the eyebrows), Nasagrai or Nasagre (nose)

One-Legged Crane 1

Eka Pada Bakasana 1

(EY-kuh PUH-duh buh-KAHS-uh-nuh)

Modification: knee to the outside of the shoulder

Pose Type: arm balance, forward bend

Drishti Point: Bhrumadhye or Ajna Chakra (third eye, between the eyebrows), Nasagrai or Nasagre (nose)

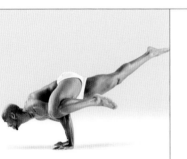

One-Legged Crane 2

Eka Pada Bakasana 2

(EY-kuh PUH-duh buh-KAHS-uh-nuh)

Modification: shin of the bent leg to the tricep

Pose Type: arm balance, forward bend

Drishti Point: Bhrumadhye or Ajna Chakra (third eye, between the eyebrows) or Nasagrai or Nasagre (nose)

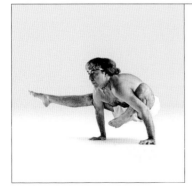

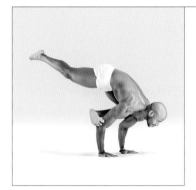

Pose Dedicated to Galava, One-Legged Modification

Eka Pada Galavasana

(EY-kuh PUH-duh gah-luh-VAHS-uh-nuh)

Pose Type: arm balance, forward bend

Drishti Point: Nasagrai or Nasagre (nose)

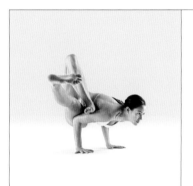

Dragonfly Pose 1

Maksikanagasana 1

(muhk-shi-kah-nah-GAHS-uh-nuh)

Also Known As: Stick Arm to the Side Grasshopper Pose (Parshva Bhuja Danda Salabhasana)

Pose Type: arm balance, forward bend, twist

Drishti Point: Nasagrai or Nasagre (nose)

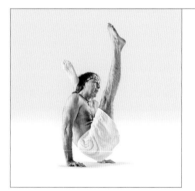

Moonbird Pose

Chakorasana

(chuh-kor-AHS-uh-nuh)

Pose Type: arm balance, forward bend

Drishti Point: Bhrumadhye or Ajna Chakra (third eye, between the eyebrows)

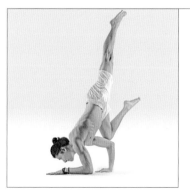

Uneven One-Legged Crane 1

Vishama Eka Pada Bakasana 1

(VISH-uh-muh EY-kuh PUH-duh buh-KAHS-uh-nuh)

Modification: one forearm to the floor, other elbow bent at 90 degrees

Pose Type: arm/forearm balance, forward bend, inversion

Drishti Point: Angushtamadhye or Angushta Ma Dyai (thumbs)

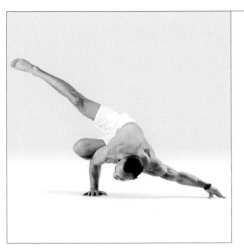

Arm to the Side Pose Dedicated to Sage Koundinya One-Legged Version 1

Parshva Hasta Eka Pada Koundinyasana 1

(PAHRSH-vuh HUH-stuh EY-kuh PUH-duh kown-din-YAHS-uh-nuh)

Modification: bottom knee bent
Pose Type: arm balance, forward bend, twist
Drishti Point: Parshva Drishti (to the right), Parshva Drishti (to the left)

ARM BALANCE: SCISSOR LEGS

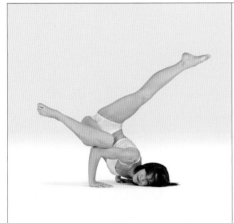

Pose Dedicated to Sage Koundinya One-Legged Version 1 Prep.

Eka Pada Koundinyasana 1 Prep.

(EY-kuh PUH-duh kown-din-YAHS-uh-nuh)

Modification: ear to the floor, bottom knee bent
Pose Type: arm balance, forward bend, twist
Drishti Point: Bhrumadhye or Ajna Chakra (third eye, between the eyebrows)

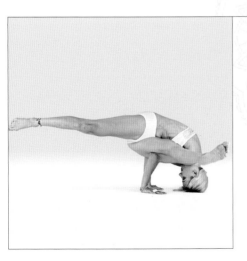

Pose Dedicated to Sage Koundinya One-Legged Version 1 Prep.

Eka Pada Koundinyasana 1 Prep.

(EY-kuh PUH-duh kown-din-YAHS-uh-nuh)

Modification: head on the floor
Pose Type: arm balance, forward bend, twist
Drishti Point: Nasagrai or Nasagre (nose)

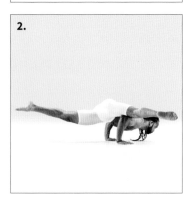

1.

2.

Pose Dedicated to Sage Koundinya One-Legged Version 2

Eka Pada Koundinyasana 2

(EY-kuh PUH-duh kown-din-YAHS-uh-nuh)

Modification: 1. prep. back foot on the floor, toes curled in
2. back foot lifted
Pose Type: arm balance, forward bend
Drishti Point: Bhrumadhye or Ajna Chakra (third eye, between the eyebrows), Nasagrai or Nasagre (nose)

ARM BALANCE: GARUDA LEGS

Revolved Leg Position of the Pose Dedicated to Garuda in Swan Pose

Parivritta Pada Garudasana in Hamsasana

(puh-ri-VRIT-tuh PUH-duh guh-ru-DAHS-uh-nuh in huhms-AHS-uh-nuh)
Pose Type: arm balance, forward bend, twist
Drishti Point: Padayoragrai or Padayoragre (toes/feet)

Revolved Leg Position of the Pose Dedicated to Garuda in Uneven Swan Pose

Parivritta Pada Garudasana in Vishama Hamsasana

(puh-ri-VRIT-tuh PUH-duh guh-ru-DAHS-uh-nuh in VISH-uh-muh huhms-AHS-uh-nuh)
Modification: forearm to the floor
Pose Type: arm balance, forward bend, twist
Drishti Point: Padayoragrai or Padayoragre (toes/feet)

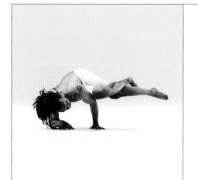

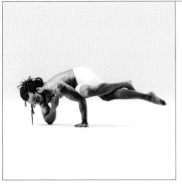

Revolved Leg Position of the Pose Dedicated to Garuda in Uneven Swan Pose

Parivritta Pada Garudasana in Vishama Hamsasana

(puh-ri-VRIT-tuh PUH-duh guh-ru-DAHS-uh-nuh in VISH-uh-muh huhms-AHS-uh-nuh)

Modification: elbow to the floor

Pose Type: arm balance, forward bend, twist

Drishti Point: Nasagrai or Nasagre (nose) or Padayoragrai or Padayoragre (toes/feet)

ARM BALANCE: BOTH LEGS TO THE SIDE

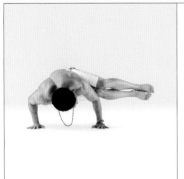

Two-Legged Pose Dedicated to Koundinya

Dwi Pada Koundinyasana

(DWI-puh-duh kown-din-YAHS-uh-nuh)

Pose Type: arm balance, forward bend, twist

Drishti Point: Padayoragrai or Padayoragre (toes/feet)

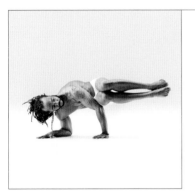

Uneven Two-Legged Pose Dedicated to Koundinya

Vishama Dwi Pada Koundinyasana

(VISH-uh-muh DWI-puh-duh kown-din-YAHS-uh-nuh)

Modification: one forearm to the floor, knees bent

Pose Type: arm balance, forward bend, twist

Drishti Point: Padayoragrai or Padayoragre (toes/feet)

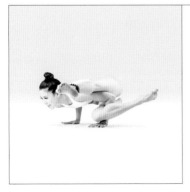

Pose Dedicated to Ashtavakra Prep.

Ashtavakrasana Prep.

(uh-shtuh-vuh-KRAHS-uh-nuh)

Also Known As: Eight Angle Pose Prep.

Modification: feet unhooked

Pose Type: arm balance, forward bend, twist

Drishti Point: Nasagrai or Nasagre (nose)

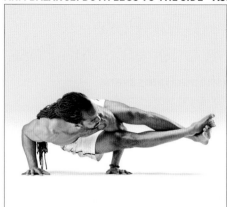

Pose Dedicated to Ashtavakra

Ashtavakrasana

(uh-shtuh-vuh-KRAHS-uh-nuh)

Also Known As: Eight Angle Pose

Pose Type: arm balance, forward bend, twist

Drishti Point: Padayoragrai or Padayoragre (toes/feet)

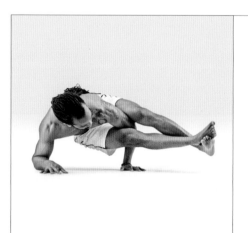

Uneven Pose Dedicated to Ashtavakra

Vishama Ashtavakrasana

(VISH-uh-muh uh-shtuh-vuh-KRAHS-uh-nuh)

Also Known As: Uneven Eight Angle Pose

Modification: one forearm to the floor

Pose Type: arm/forearm balance, forward bend, twist

Drishti Point: Padayoragrai or Padayoragre (toes/feet)

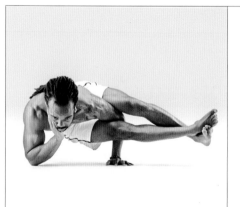

Uneven Half Repose Pose Dedicated to Ashtavakra

Vishama Ardha Shayana Ashtavakrasana

(VISH-uh-muh UHR-duh shuh-yuh-nuh uh-shtuh-vuh-KRAHS-uh-nuh)

Also Known As: Uneven Half Repose Eight Angle Pose

Modification: one elbow to the floor, hand to the face

Pose Type: arm/elbow balance, forward bend, twist

Drishti Point: Nasagrai or Nasagre (nose)

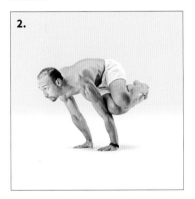

Side Crane Pose

Parshva Bakasana

(PAHRSH-vuh buh-KAHS-uh-nuh)

Also Known As: Revolved Crane Pose (Parivritta Bakasana), Sideways Crow Pose (Parshva Kakasana)

Modification: 1. elbows bent

2. arms straight

Pose Type: arm balance, forward bend, twist

Drishti Point: Bhrumadhye or Ajna Chakra (third eye, between the eyebrows), Nasagrai or Nasagre (nose)

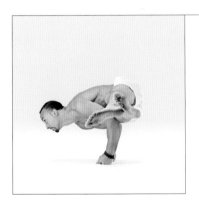

Two-Legged Pose Dedicated to Koundinya Modification on the Fists

Mushti Dwi Pada Koundinyasana

(mush-ti DWI-puh-duh kown-din-YAHS-uh-nuh)

Modification: ankles crossed

Pose Type: arm balance, forward bend, twist

Drishti Point: Bhrumadhye or Ajna Chakra (third eye, between the eyebrows)

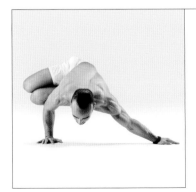

Uneven Arms Side Crane Pose

Vishama Hasta Parshva Bakasana

(VISH-uh-muh HUH-stuh PAHRSH-vuh buh-KAHS-uh-nuh)

Pose Type: arm balance, forward bend, twist

Drishti Point: Nasagrai or Nasagre (nose)

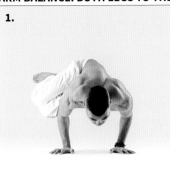

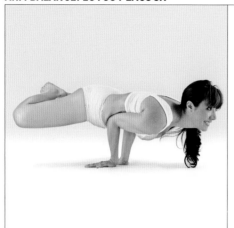

Bound Angle Pose in Peacock Pose

Baddha Konasana in Mayurasana

(BUH-duh ko-NAHS-uh-nuh in muh-yoor-AHS-uh-nuh)

Pose Type: arm balance

Drishti Point: Bhrumadhye or Ajna Chakra (third eye, between the eyebrows)

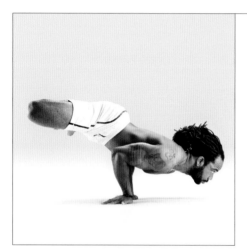

Lotus Pose in Peacock Pose

Padmasana in Mayurasana

(puhd-MAHS-uh-nuh in muh-yoor-AHS-uh-nuh)

Pose Type: arm balance, hip opener

Drishti Point: Bhrumadhye or Ajna Chakra (third eye, between the eyebrows)

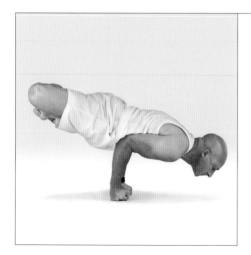

Fist Lotus Peacock Pose

Mushti Padma Mayurasana

(mush-ti PUHD-muh muh-yoor-AHS-uh-nuh)

Pose Type: arm balance

Drishti Point: Nasagrai or Nasagre (nose)

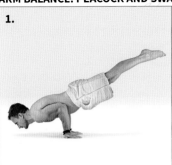

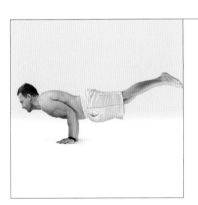

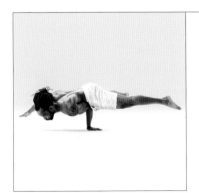

Peacock Pose

Mayurasana
(muh-yoor-AHS-uh-nuh)
Modification: 1. feet lifted higher than the hip level
2. body parallel to the floor
Pose Type: arm balance
Drishti Point: Bhrumadhye or Ajna Chakra (third eye, between the eyebrows), Nasagrai or Nasagre (nose)

Swan Pose

Hamsasana
(huhms-AHS-uh-nuh)
Also Known As: Swan Pose (Hansasana)
Pose Type: arm balance
Drishti Point: Nasagrai or Nasagre (nose)

One Hand Peacock Pose

Eka Hasta Mayurasana
(EY-kuh HUH-stuh muh-yoor-AHS-uh-nuh)
Also Known As: Wounded Peacock Pose (Pungu Mayurasana)
Pose Type: arm balance
Drishti Point: Nasagrai or Nasagre (nose)

Inversion Poses

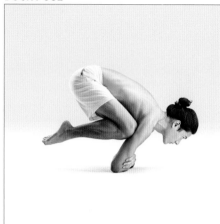

Duck Pose

Karandavasana

(kahr-uhn-duh-VAHS-uh-nuh)

Also Known As: Baby Duck Pose

Modification: thumbs grabbing onto the biceps, fingers grabbing onto the triceps; knees to the armpits, feet together

Pose Type: forearm balance, inversion

Drishti Point: Bhrumadhye or Ajna Chakra (third eye, between the eyebrows)

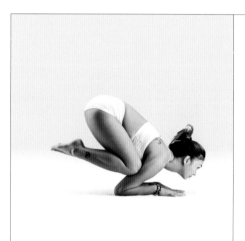

Duck Pose

Karandavasana

(kahr-uhn-duh-VAHS-uh-nuh)

Also Known As: Baby Duck Pose

Modification: forearms to the floor, knees to the armpits, feet together

Pose Type: forearm balance, inversion

Drishti Point: Bhrumadhye or Ajna Chakra (third eye, between the eyebrows)

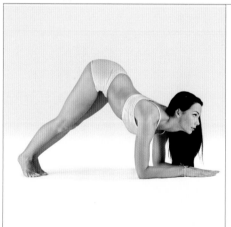

Downward Facing Pose Dedicated to Makara

Adho Mukha Makarasana

(uh-DO MUK-uh muh-kuh-RAHS-uh-nuh)

Also Known As: Dolphin Pose

Pose Type: forward bend, inversion, core

Drishti Point: Bhrumadhye or Ajna Chakra (third eye, between the eyebrows)

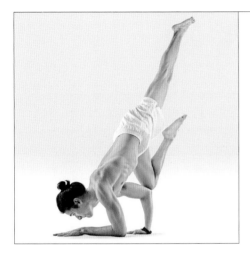

One-Legged Uneven Peacock Feather Pose

Eka Pada Vishama Picha Mayurasana

(EY-kuh PUH-duh VISH-uh-muh pich-chuh muh-yoor-AHS-uh-nuh)

Also Known As: Eka Pada Vishama Pincha Mayurasana
Pose Type: forearm balance, inversion, forward bend
Drishti Point: Angushtamadhye or Angushta Ma Dyai (thumbs)

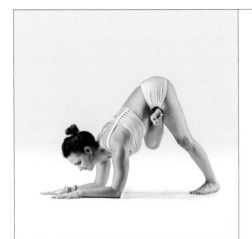

Half Lotus Downward Facing Pose Dedicated to Makara

Ardha Padma Adho Mukha Makarasana

(UHR-duh PUHD-muh uh-DO MUK-uh muh-kuh-RAHS-uh-nuh)

Also Known As: Half Lotus Dolphin Pose
Modification: heel down
Pose Type: forward bend, inversion, core
Drishti Point: Angushtamadhye or Angushta Ma Dyai (thumbs)

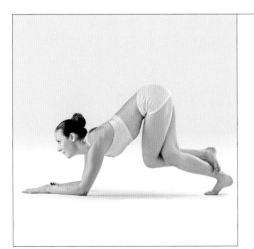

Leg Position of the Pose Dedicated to Garuda in Downward Facing Pose Dedicated to Makara

Pada Garudasana in Adho Mukha Makarasana

(PUH-duh guh-ru-DAHS-uh-nuh in uh-DO MUK-uh muh-kuh-RAHS-uh-nuh)

Also Known As: Leg Position of the Pose Dedicated to Garuda in Dolphin Pose
Pose Type: forward bend, inversion, core
Drishti Point: Bhrumadhye or Ajna Chakra (third eye, between the eyebrows)

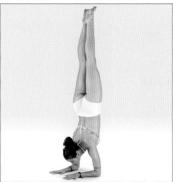

Peacock Feather Pose

Picha Mayurasana

(pich-chuh muh-yoor-AHS-uh-nuh)

Also Known As: Upright Scorpion Pose (Avakra Vrishchikasana), Pincha Mayurasana
Pose Type: forearm balance, inversion
Drishti Point: Angushtamadhye or Angushta Ma Dyai (thumbs)

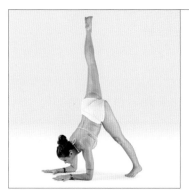

One-Legged Peacock Feather Pose

Eka Pada Picha Mayurasana

(EY-kuh PUH-duh pich-chuh muh-yoor-AHS-uh-nuh)

Also Known As: Eka Pada Pincha Mayurasana
Pose Type: forearm balance, inversion, forward bend
Drishti Point: Angushtamadhye or Angushta Ma Dyai (thumbs)

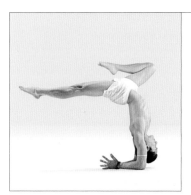

One-Legged Scorpion Pose

Eka Pada Vrishchikasana

(EY-kuh PUH-duh vrish-chi-KAHS-uh-nuh)

Modification: biceps in line with the ears
Pose Type: forearm balance, inversion, backbend
Drishti Point: Nasagrai or Nasagre (nose)

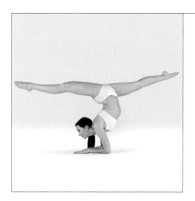

Pose Dedicated to Lord Hanuman in Peacock Feather Pose

Hanumanasana in Picha Mayurasana

(huh-nu-mahn-AHS-uh-nuh in pich-chuh muh-yoor-AHS-uh-nuh)

Also Known As: Hanumanasana in Pincha Mayurasana
Pose Type: forearm balance, inversion, backbend
Drishti Point: Bhrumadhye or Ajna Chakra (third eye, between the eyebrows)

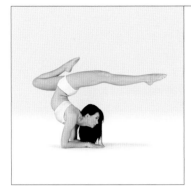

One-Legged Stretched Out Scorpion Pose

Eka Pada Paripurna Vrishchikasana
(EY-kuh PUH-duh puh-ri-POOR-nuh vrish-chi-KAHS-uh-nuh)

Pose Type: forearm balance, inversion, backbend

Drishti Point: Bhrumadhye or Ajna Chakra (third eye, between the eyebrows)

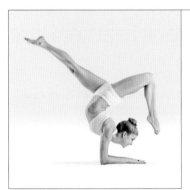

One-Legged Scorpion Pose

Eka Pada Vrishchikasana
(EY-kuh PUH-duh vrish-chi-KAHS-uh-nuh)

Modification: forearms to the floor, foot away from the head

Pose Type: forearm balance, inversion, backbend

Drishti Point: Bhrumadhye or Ajna Chakra (third eye, between the eyebrows)

BACKBENDS ON FOREARMS, LOTUS ON FOREARMS, AND ELBOW BALANCES

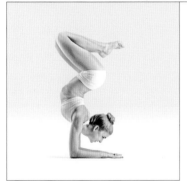

Inverted Puppy Dog Pose in Peacock Feather Pose

Viparita Shvanakasana in Picha Mayurasana
(vi-puh-REE-tuh shvuh-nuh-KAHS-uh-nuh in pich-chuh muh-yoor-AHS-uh-nuh)

Also Known As: Viparita Shvanakasana in Pincha Mayurasana

Modification: knees bent, backbend

Pose Type: forearm balance, inversion, backbend

Drishti Point: Angushtamadhye or Angushta Ma Dyai (thumbs)

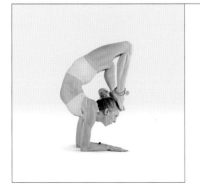

Scorpion Pose

Vrishchikasana
(vrish-chi-KAHS-uh-nuh)

Modification: forearms to the floor, feet to the head

Pose Type: forearm balance, inversion, backbend

Drishti Point: Bhrumadhye or Ajna Chakra (third eye, between the eyebrows)

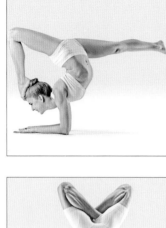

One-Legged Scorpion Pose

Eka Pada Vrishchikasana

(EY-kuh PUH-duh vrish-chi-KAHS-uh-nuh)

Modification: forearms to the floor, foot to the head, other leg parallel to the floor

Pose Type: forearm balance, inversion, backbend

Drishti Point: Bhrumadhye or Ajna Chakra (third eye, between the eyebrows)

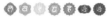

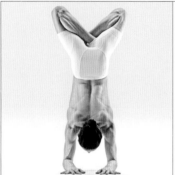

Upward Lotus Pose in Peacock Feather Pose

Urdhva Padmasana in Picha Mayurasana

(OORD-vuh puhd-MAHS-uh-nuh in pich-chuh muh-yoor-AHS-uh-nuh)

Also Known As: Raised Lotus Scorpion Pose (Urdhva Padma Vrishchikasana), Duck Pose (Karandavasana)

Pose Type: forearm balance, inversion

Drishti Point: Angushtamadhye or Angushta Ma Dyai (thumbs)

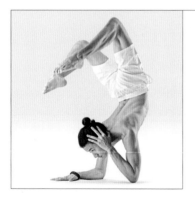

Uneven Repose Pose

Vishama Shayanasana

(VISH-uh-muh shuh-yuh-NAHS-uh-nuh)

Modification: both knees bent

Pose Type: forearm/elbow balance, inversion, backbend

Drishti Point: Bhrumadhye or Ajna Chakra (third eye, between the eyebrows)

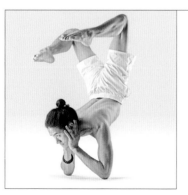

Repose Pose

Shayanasana

(shuh-yuh-NAHS-uh-nuh)

Modification: both knees bent

Pose Type: elbow balance, inversion, backbend

Drishti Point: Bhrumadhye or Ajna Chakra (third eye, between the eyebrows)

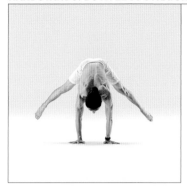

Feet Spread Intense Stretch Pose in Downward Facing Tree Pose

Prasarita Padottanasana in Adho Mukha Vrikshasana

(pruh-SAH-ri-tuh puh-do-tahn-AHS-uh-nuh in uh-DO MUK-uh vriks-SHAHS-anna)

Also Known As: Feet Spread Full Forward Bend Pose in Downward Facing Tree Pose, Prasarita Padottanasana in Adho Mukha Vrksasana

Pose Type: inversion, arm balance, forward bend

Drishti Point: Angushtamadhye or Angushta Ma Dyai (thumbs)

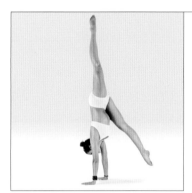

One-Legged Downward Facing Tree Pose

Eka Pada Adho Mukha Vrikshasana

(EY-kuh PUH-duh uh-DO MUK-uh vrik-SHAHS-uh-nuh)

Also Known As: Eka Pada Adho Mukha Vrksasana

Pose Type: inversion, arm balance, forward bend

Drishti Point: Angushtamadhye or Angushta Ma Dyai (thumbs)

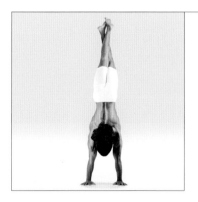

Downward Facing Tree Pose

Adho Mukha Vrikshasana

(uh-DO MUK-uh vrik-SHAHS-uh-nuh)

Also Known As: Adho Mukha Vrksasana

Modification: legs crossed

Pose Type: inversion, arm balance

Drishti Point: Angushtamadhye or Angushta Ma Dyai (thumbs)

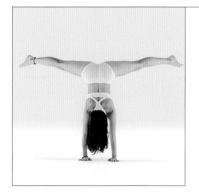

Seated Angle Pose in Downward Facing Tree Pose

Upavishta Konasana in Adho Mukha Vrikshasana

(u-puh-VISH-tuh ko-NAHS-uh-nuh in uh-DO MUK-uh vrik-SHAHS-uh-nuh)

Also Known As: Upward Spread Feet Pose A (Urdhva Prasarita Padasana A), Upavista Konasana in Adho Mukha Vrikshasana

Pose Type: inversion, arm balance

Drishti Point: Angushtamadhye or Angushta Ma Dyai (thumbs)

HANDSTAND, LEG CROSSED OVER: GARUDA LEGS & HALF LOTUS

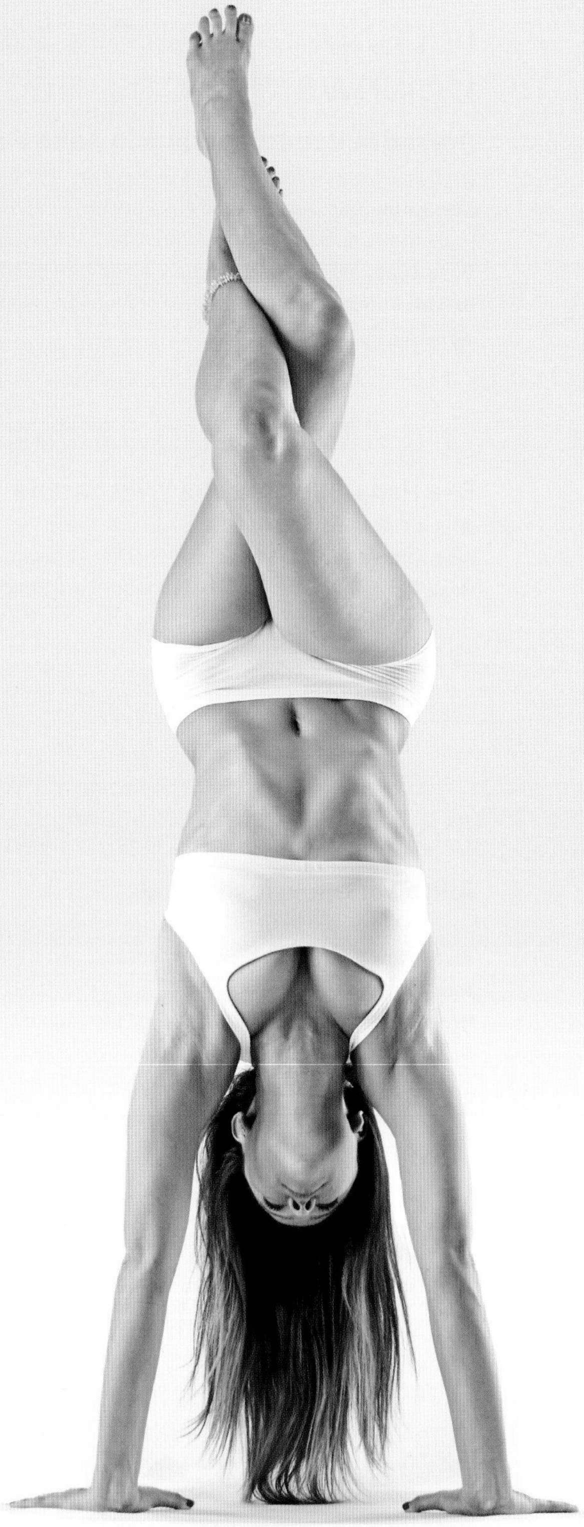

Leg Position of the Pose Dedicated to Garuda in
Downward Facing Tree Pose

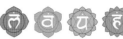

Pada Garudasana in Adho Mukha Vrikshasana
(PUH-duh guh-ru-DAHS-uh-nuh in uh-DO MUK-uh vrik-SHAHS-uh-nuh)
Also Known As: Pada Garudasana in Adho Mukha Vrksasana
Pose Type: inversion, arm balance
Drishti Point: Angusthamadhye or Angustha Ma Dyai (thumbs)

pada = foot or leg
Garuda = Hindu Deity, half-man half-
  eagle, carrier of Lord Vishnu
adho = downward
mukha = facing
vriksha = tree

How to Perform the Pose:

1. Begin by standing in Mountain Pose (*Tadasana*). Engage your *mula bandha*, *uddhiyana bandha*, and *ujjayi* breathing.

2. Exhale and hinge from the hips, coming into a forward bend, placing the palms on the floor on the outsides of your feet. Your hands should be shoulder width apart or slightly wider. Make sure your arms are straight and your shoulders are on top of your fingertips.

3. There are many ways to come into a handstand. When you start practicing handstands, make sure you can balance on your hands against the wall for at least 60 seconds. Then you can experiment with jumping into a handstand or lifting your legs using your core. Press strongly into your hands.

4. Once you find your balance in a Downward Facing Tree Pose (*Adho Mukha Vrikshasana*), also known as Handstand, exhale and bend your knees; cross your right leg over your left leg, hooking your right foot around your left calf muscle. Hold for 30, and up to 90, seconds to receive the full benefits of the stretch.

5. Inhale and bring your legs back to the straight position. Exhale and switch legs as you bend your knees and cross your left leg over your right leg, hooking your left foot around your right calf muscle. Hold for 30, and up to 90, seconds to receive the full benefits of the stretch.

6. Inhale and bring your legs back to the straight position. On the following inhale, lower your feet to the floor. Inhale as you come back to Mountain Pose (*Tadasana*).

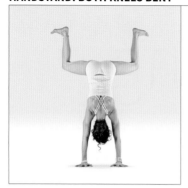

Frog Pose in Downward Facing Tree Pose

Mandukasana in Adho Mukha Vrikshasana

(muhn-doo-KAHS-uh-nuh in uh-DO MUK-uh vrik-SHAHS-uh-nuh)

Also Known As: Mandukasana in Adho Mukha Vrksasana

Pose Type: inversion, arm balance

Drishti Point: Nasagrai or Nasagre (nose) or Angusthamadhye or Angustha Ma Dyai (thumbs)

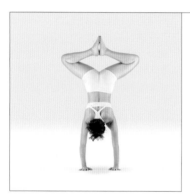

Bound Angle Pose in Downward Facing Tree Pose

Baddha Konasana in Adho Mukha Vrikshasana

(BUH-duh ko-NAHS-uh-nuh in uh-DO MUK-uh vrik-SHAHS-uh-nuh)

Also Known As: Baddha Konasana in Adho Mukha Vrksasana

Pose Type: inversion, arm balance

Drishti Point: Angushtamadhye or Angushta Ma Dyai (thumbs)

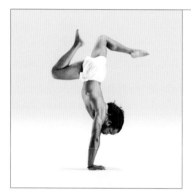

Svastika Legs in Downward Facing Tree Pose

Pada Svastikasana in Adho Mukha Vrikshasana

(PUH-duh svuh-sti-KAHS-uh-nuh in uh-DO MUK-uh vrik-SHAHS-uh-nuh)

Also Known As: Pada Svastikasana in Adho Mukha Vrksasana

Modification: both knees bent, one knee bent toward the chest, other foot pointing to the back

Pose Type: inversion, arm balance, mild backbend

Drishti Point: Angushtamadhye or Angushta Ma Dyai (thumbs)

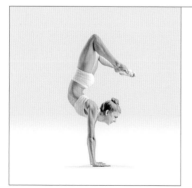

Scorpion Pose Prep.

Vrishchikasana Prep.

(vrish-chi-KAHS-uh-nuh)

Also Known As: Pose Dedicated to the Demon Taraka A (Tarakasana A)

Modification: knees bent, feet away from the head

Pose Type: inversion, arm balance, backbend

Drishti Point: Bhrumadhye or Ajna Chakra (third eye, between the eyebrows)

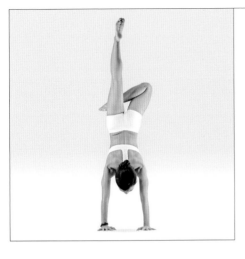

Half Lotus Pose in Downward Facing Tree Pose

Ardha Padmasana in Adho Mukha Vrikshasana

(UHR-duh puhd-MAHS-uh-nuh in uh-DO MUK-uh vrik-SHAHS-uh-nuh)

Also Known As: Ardha Padmasana in Adho Mukha Vrksasana

Pose Type: inversion, arm balance

Drishti Point: Angushtamadhye or Angushta Ma Dyai (thumbs)

HANDSTAND, LEGS CROSSED: GARUDA LEGS & LOTUS

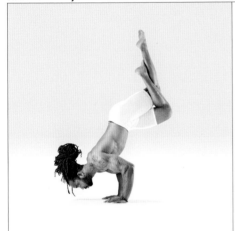

Leg Position of the Pose Dedicated to Garuda in Downward Facing Tree Pose

Pada Garudasana in Adho Mukha Vrikshasana

(PUH-duh guh-ru-DAHS-uh-nuh in uh-DO MUK-uh vrik-SHAHS-uh-nuh)

Also Known As: Pada Garudasana in Adho Mukha Vrksasana

Modification: arms bent at 90 degrees

Pose Type: inversion, arm balance

Drishti Point: Nasagrai or Nasagre (nose)

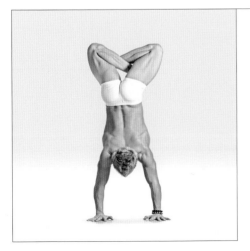

Upward Lotus Pose in Downward Facing Tree Pose

Urdhva Padmasana in Adho Mukha Vrikshasana

(OORD-vuh puhd-MAHS-uh-nuh in uh-DO MUK-uh vrik-SHAHS-uh-nuh)

Also Known As: Urdhva Padmasana in Adho Mukha Vrksasana

Pose Type: inversion, arm balance

Drishti Point: Angushtamadhye or Angushta Ma Dyai (thumbs)

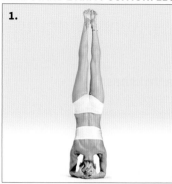

1.

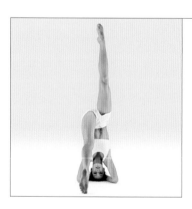

2.

Headstand 1

Shirshasana 1

(sheer-SHAHS-uh-nuh)

Also Known As: Supported Headstand (Salamba Shirshasana*), Bound Hands Headstand A (Baddha Hasta Shirshasana A)

Modification: 1. back view

2. side view

Pose Type: inversion

Drishti Point: Nasagrai or Nasagre (nose)

* "Shirshasana" may also be spelled as "Sirsasana" in the following headstand poses.

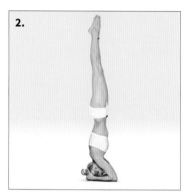

One-Legged Headstand 1

Eka Pada Shirshasana 1

(EY-kuh PUH-duh sheer-SHAHS-uh-nuh)

Pose Type: inversion, forward bend

Drishti Point: Nasagrai or Nasagre (nose), Padayoragrai or Padayoragre (toes/feet)

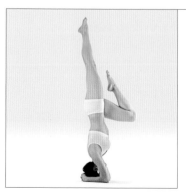

Leg Contraction Knee Bend Pose in Headstand 1

Pada Akunchanasana in Shirshasana 1

(PUH-duh uh-kunch-uh-NAHS-uh-nuh in sheer-SHAHS-uh-nuh)

Modification: one knee bent toward the chest

Pose Type: inversion, forward bend

Drishti Point: Nasagrai or Nasagre (nose)

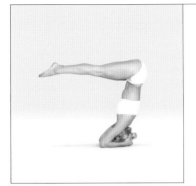

Upward Staff Pose in Headstand 1

Urdhva Dandasana in Shirshasana 1

(OORD-vuh duhn-DAHS-uh-nuh in sheer-SHAHS-uh-nuh)

Also Known As: Half Headstand Pose (Ardha Shirshasana), Headstand B (Shirshana B)

Pose Type: inversion, forward bend

Drishti Point: Nasagrai or Nasagre (nose)

HEADSTAND 1 ARM POSITION: VARIOUS LEG POSITIONS

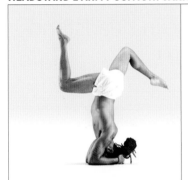

Svastika Legs in Headstand 1

Pada Svastikasana in Shirshasana 1

(PUH-duh svuh-sti-KAHS-uh-nuh in sheer-SHAHS-uh-nuh)

Pose Type: inversion, mild backbend

Drishti Point: Nasagrai or Nasagre (nose)

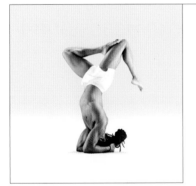

Leg Position of One-Legged King Pigeon 1 Version B in Headstand 1

Pada Eka Pada Raja Kapotasana 1 B in Shirshasana 1

(PUH-duh EY-kuh PUH-duh RAH-juh kuh-po-TAHS-uh-nuh in sheer-SHAHS-uh-nuh)

Modification: both knees bent, one knee to the sky, other foot to the knee

Pose Type: inversion, mild backbend

Drishti Point: Nasagrai or Nasagre (nose)

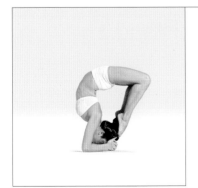

Feet to Head Pose

Shirsha Padasana

(SHEER-shuh puh-DAHS-uh-nuh)

Pose Type: inversion, backbend

Drishti Point: Bhrumadhye or Ajna Chakra (third eye, between the eyebrows)

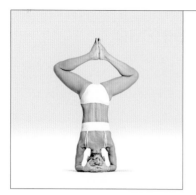

Bound Angle Pose in Headstand 1

Baddha Konasana in Shirshasana 1

(BUH-duh ko-NAHS-uh-nuh in sheer-SHAHS-uh-nuh)

Pose Type: inversion

Drishti Point: Nasagrai or Nasagre (nose)

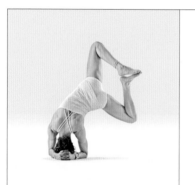

Sideways Bound Angle Pose in Headstand 1

Parshva Baddha Konasana in Shirshasana 1

(PAHRSH-vuh BUH-duh ko-NAHS-uh-nuh in sheer-SHAHS-uh-nuh)

Pose Type: inversion, side bend

Drishti Point: Nasagrai or Nasagre (nose)

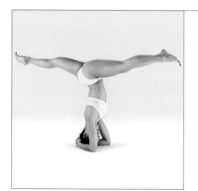

Pose Dedicated to Hanuman in Headstand 1

Hanumanasana in Shirshasana 1

(huh-nu-mahn-AHS-uh-nuh in sheer-SHAH-suh-nuh)

Pose Type: inversion

Drishti Point: Nasagrai or Nasagre (nose)

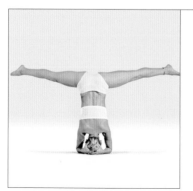

Seated Angle Pose in Headstand 1

Upavishta Konasana in Shirshasana 1

(u-puh-VISH-tuh ko-NAHS-uh-nuh in sheer-SHAHS-uh-nuh)

Also Known As: Upavista Konasana in Adho Mukha Vrikshasana, Upavista Konasana in Adho Mukha Vrksasana

Pose Type: inversion

Drishti Point: Nasagrai or Nasagre (nose)

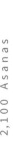

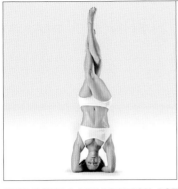

Leg Position of the Pose Dedicated to Garuda in Headstand 1

Pada Garudasana in Shirshasana 1

(PUH-duh guh-ru-DAHS-uh-nuh in sheer-SHAHS-uh-nuh)

Pose Type: inversion

Drishti Point: Nasagrai or Nasagre (nose)

HEADSTAND 1 ARM POSITION: LOTUS LEG POSITION

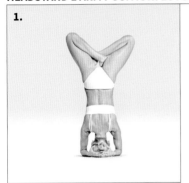

1.

Upward Lotus in Headstand 1

Urdhva Padmasana in Shirshasana 1

(OORD-vuh puhd-MAHS-uh-nuh in sheer-SHAHS-uh-nuh)

Modification: 1. back view

2. side view

Pose Type: inversion

Drishti Point: Nasagrai or Nasagre (nose)

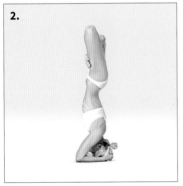

2.

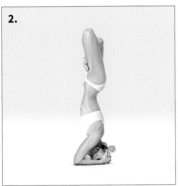

Sideways Upward Lotus in Headstand 1

Parshva Urdhva Padmasana in Shirshasana 1

(PAHRSH-vuh OORD-vuh puhd-MAHS-uh-nuh in sheer-SHAHS-uh-nuh)

Pose Type: inversion, twist

Drishti Point: Nasagrai or Nasagre (nose)

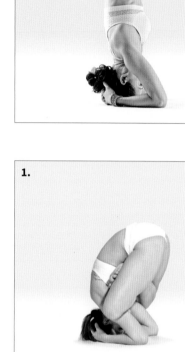

Embryo Pose in Headstand 1 Prep.

Pindasana in Shirshasana 1 Prep.

(pin-DAHS-uh-nuh in sheer-SHAHS-uh-nuh)
Modification: thighs parallel to the floor
Pose Type: inversion, forward bend
Drishti Point: Nasagrai or Nasagre (nose)

Embryo Pose in Headstand 1

Pindasana in Shirshasana 1

(pin-DAHS-uh-nuh in sheer-SHAHS-uh-nuh)
Modification: 1. knees to the triceps
2. knees to the chest
Pose Type: inversion, forward bend
Drishti Point: Nasagrai or Nasagre (nose)

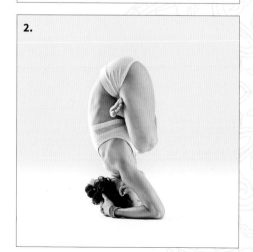

1.

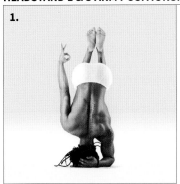

One Hand Headstand 1

Eka Hasta Shirshasana 1

(EY-kuh HUH-stuh sheer-SHAHS-uh-nuh)

Modification: both knees bent toward the chest, one forearm on the floor

1. other arm straight, fingertips to the sky
2. other arm behind the back, fingertips pointing to the upper back

Pose Type: inversion, forward bend

Drishti Point: Nasagrai or Nasagre (nose)

2.

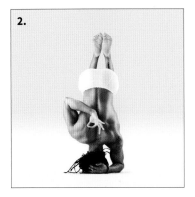

Sideways Uneven Upward Staff Pose

Parshva Vishama Urdhva Dandasana

(PAHRSH-vuh VISH-uh-muh OORD-vuh duhn-DAHS-uh-nuh)

Modification: forearm to the floor in front of the face, palm down; legs parallel to the floor

Pose Type: inversion, forward bend, twist

Drishti Point: Hastagrai or Hastagre (hands)

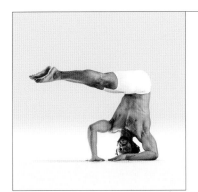

Leg Contraction Pose in Headstand 3

Pada Akunchanasana in Shirshasana 3

(PUH-duh uh-kunch-AHS-uh-nuh in sheer-SHAHS-uh-nuh)

Modification: one leg straight and out to the side, other knee to the chest

Pose Type: inversion, forward bend

Drishti Point: Nasagrai or Nasagre (nose)

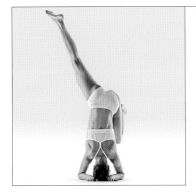

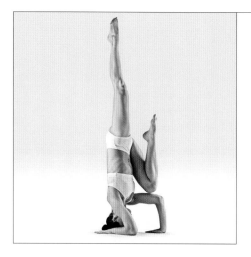

Leg Contraction Pose in Uneven Headstand (Fusion of Headstand 5 and Headstand 3 Arm Position)

Pada Akunchanasana in Vishama Shirshasana

(PUH-duh uh-kunch-AHS-uh-nuh in VISH-uh-muh sheer-SHAHS-uh-nuh)

Modification: one forearm to the floor, other elbow on top of the wrist, knee to the tricep on the same side

Pose Type: inversion, forward bend

Drishti Point: Nasagrai or Nasagre (nose)

HEADSTAND 5 ARM POSITION: VARIOUS LEG POSITIONS

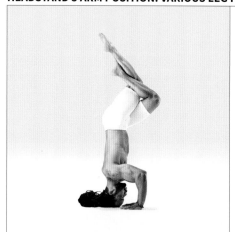

Leg Position of the Pose Dedicated to Garuda in Headstand 5

Pada Garudasana in Shirshasana 5

(PUH-duh guh-ru-AHS-uh-nuh in sheer-SHAHS-uh-nuh)

Pose Type: inversion

Drishti Point: Nasagrai or Nasagre (nose)

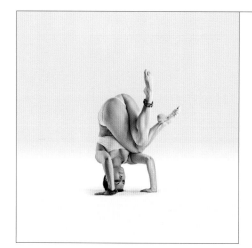

Leg Position of Cow Face Pose in Headstand 5

Pada Gomukhasana in Shirshasana 5

(PUH-duh go-muk-AHS-uh-nuh in sheer-SHAHS-uh-nuh)

Modification: bottom knee to the opposite tricep

Pose Type: inversion, forward bend

Drishti Point: Nasagrai or Nasagre (nose)

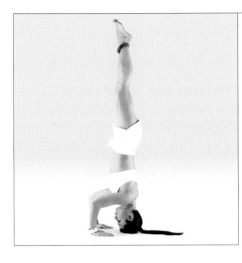

Headstand 5

Shirshasana 5

(sheer-SHAHS-uh-nuh)

Also Known As: Tripod Headstand
Pose Type: inversion
Drishti Point: Nasagrai or Nasagre (nose)

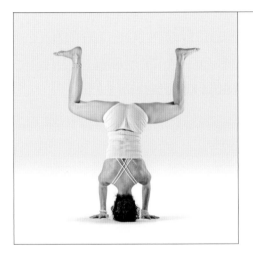

Frog Pose in Headstand 5

Mandukasana in Shirshasana 5

(muhn-doo-KAHS-uh-nuh in sheer-SHAHS-uh-nuh)

Pose Type: inversion
Drishti Point: Nasagrai or Nasagre (nose)

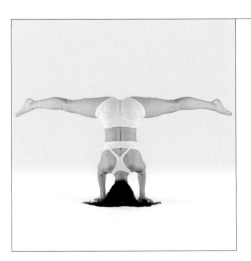

Seated Angle Pose in Headstand 5

Upavishta Konasana in Shirshasana 5

(u-puh-VISH-tuh ko-NAHS-uh-nuh in sheer-SHAHS-uh-nuh)

Also Known As: Tripod Headstand Same Angle Pose (Utripada Shirsha
Samakonasana), Upavista Konasana in Shirshasana
Pose Type: inversion
Drishti Point: Nasagrai or Nasagre (nose)

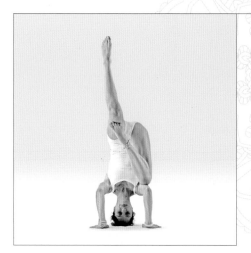

Leg Position of One-Legged King Pigeon 1 Version B in Headstand 5

Pada Eka Pada Raja Kapotasana 1 B in Shirshasana 5

(PUH-duh EY-kuh PUH-duh RAH-juh kuh-po-TAHS-uh-nuh in sheer-SHAHS-uh-nuh)

Modification: knee to the tricep on the same side, other knee resting on the foot

Pose Type: inversion, forward bend

Drishti Point: Nasagrai or Nasagre (nose)

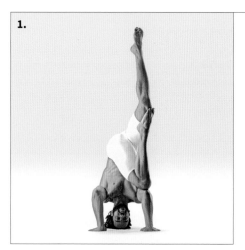

1.

Revolved Leg Position of One-Legged King Pigeon 1 Version B in Headstand 5

Parivritta Pada Eka Pada Raja Kapotasana 1 B in Shirshasana 5

(puh-ri-VRIT-tuh PUH-duh EY-kuh PUH-duh RAH-juh kuh-po-TAHS-uh-nuh in sheer-SHAHS-uh-nuh)

Modification: knee resting on the foot

1. top leg straight
2. top knee bent at 90 degrees

Pose Type: inversion, forward bend, twist

Drishti Point: Nasagrai or Nasagre (nose)

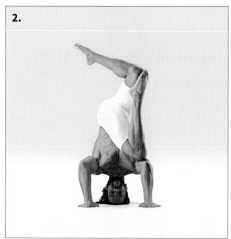

2.

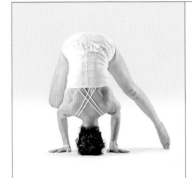

Headstand 5 Prep.

Shirshasana 5 Prep.

(sheer-SHAHS-uh-nuh)

Modification: one knee to the tricep, other foot to the floor on the side

Pose Type: inversion, forward bend

Drishti Point: Nasagrai or Nasagre (nose)

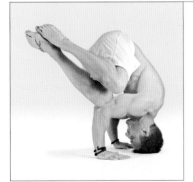

Crane Pose in Headstand 5 Prep.

Bakasana in Shirshasana 5 Prep.

(buh-KAHS-uh-nuh in sheer-SHAHS-uh-nuh)

Modification: knees on the triceps

Pose Type: inversion, forward bend

Drishti Point: Nasagrai or Nasagre (nose)

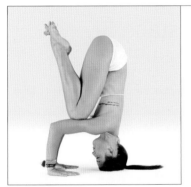

Side Crane Pose in Headstand 5

Parshva Bakasana in Shirshasana 5

(PAHRSH-vuh buh-KAHS-uh-nuh in sheer-SHAHS-uh-nuh)

Modification: knees together, knee to the opposite tricep

Pose Type: inversion, forward bend, twist

Drishti Point: Nasagrai or Nasagre (nose)

Embryo in the Womb Pose in Headstand 5

Garba Pindasana in Shirshasana 5

(guhr-buh-pin-DAHS-uh-nuh in sheer-SHAHS-uh-nuh)

Pose Type: inversion, forward bend

Drishti Point: Nasagrai or Nasagre (nose)

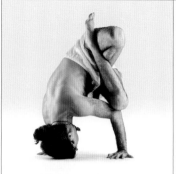

Side Rooster Pose in Headstand 5 Prep.

Parshva Kukkutasana in Shirshasana 5 Prep.

(PAHRSH-vuh ku-ku TAHS-uh-nuh in sheer-SHAHS-uh-nuh)

Modification: crown of the head on the floor
Pose Type: inversion, forward bend, twist
Drishti Point: Nasagrai or Nasagre (nose)

HEADSTAND 5 ARM POSITION: VARIOUS ARM POSITIONS BASED ON HEADSTAND 5 & VARIOUS LEG POSITIONS

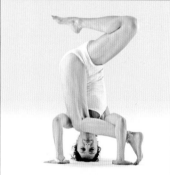

Baby Cradle Pose in Headstand 5

Hindolasana in Shirshasana 5

(hin-do-LAHS-uh-nuh in sheer-SHAHS-uh-nuh)

Modification: Side 1: ankle to the inside of the elbow joint of the opposite arm, knee bent to the inside of the same arm, toes touching the floor.
Side 2: other knee bent to the side, heel toward the sitting bone
Pose Type: inversion, forward bend
Drishti Point: Nasagrai or Nasagre (nose)

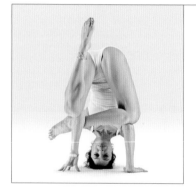

Baby Cradle Pose in Headstand 5

Hindolasana in Shirshasana 5

(hin-do-LAHS-uh-nuh in sheer-SHAHS-uh-nuh)

Modification: Side 1: arm bent at 90 degrees, fingertips to the floor, knee to the elbow on the same side.
Side 2: arm bent at 90 degrees, palm flat on the floor, ankle to the inside of the elbow joint, toes lifted off the floor
Pose Type: inversion, forward bend
Drishti Point: Nasagrai or Nasagre (nose)

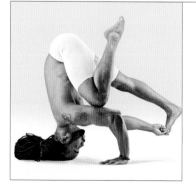

Extended Hand to Big Toe Pose in One Hand Headstand 5

Utthita Hasta Padangushtasana in Eka Hasta Shirshasana 5

(UT-ti-tuh HUH-stuh puhd-ahng-goosh-TAHS-uh-nuh in EY-kuh HUH-stuh sheer-SHAHS-uh-nuh)

Modification: Side 1: arm and leg straight out, grabbing onto the big toe.
Side 2: arm bent 90 degrees, knee resting on the tricep on the same side
Pose Type: inversion, forward bend
Drishti Point: Nasagrai or Nasagre (nose), Hastagrai or Hastagre (hands)

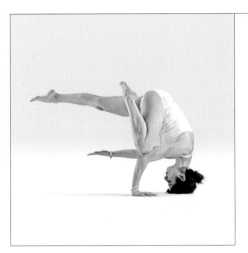

One-Legged Crane Pose 1 in One Hand Headstand 5

Eka Pada Bakasana 1 in Eka Hasta Shirshasana 5

(EY-kuh PUH-duh buh-KAHS-uh-nuh in EY-kuh HUH-stuh sheer-SHAHS-uh-nuh)

Modification: Side 1: arm and leg straight out.
Side 2: arm bent 90 degrees, knee resting on the tricep on the same side

Pose Type: inversion, forward bend

Drishti Point: Nasagrai or Nasagre (nose), Hastagrai or Hastagre (hands)

HEADSTAND 6 ARM POSITION: VARIOUS ARM POSITIONS BASED OFF HEADSTAND 6 & VARIOUS LEG POSITIONS

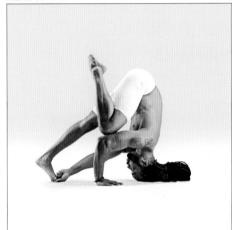

Extended Hand to Big Toe Pose in Uneven Headstand (Fusion of Headstand 5 and Headstand 6 Arm Position)

Utthita Hasta Padangushtasana in Vishama Shirshasana 5 & 6

(UT-ti-tuh HUH-stuh puhd-ahng-goosh-TAHS-uh-nuh in VISH-uh-muh sheer-SHAHS-uh-nuh)

Modification: Side 1: arm and leg straight out, grabbing onto the big toe
Side 2: arm bent 90 degrees, knee bent to the tricep on the same side

Pose Type: inversion, forward bend

Drishti Point: Padayoragrai or Padayoragre (toes/feet), Hastagrai or Hastagre (hands)

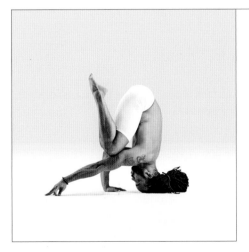

Crane Pose in Uneven Headstand (Fusion of Headstand 5 and Headstand 6 Arm Position)

Bakasana in Vishama Shirshasana 5 & 6

(buh-KAHS-uh-nuh in VISH-uh-muh sheer-SHAHS-uh-nuh)

Modification: Side 1: arm straight out, fingertips to the floor, knee to the tricep.
Side 2: arm bent 90 degrees, knee bent to the tricep on the same side

Pose Type: inversion, forward bend

Drishti Point: Hastagrai or Hastagre (hands)

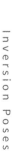

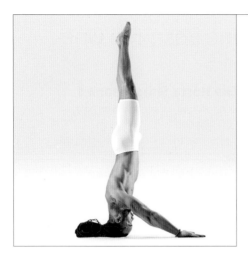

Headstand 6

Shirshasana 6

(sheer-SHAHS-uh-nuh)

Also Known As: Hands Free Headstand (Mukta Hasta Shirshasana)
Pose Type: inversion
Drishti Point: Nasagrai or Nasagre (nose), Hastagrai or Hastagre (hands)

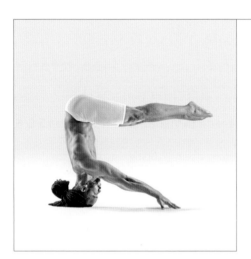

Upward Staff Pose in Headstand 6

Urdhva Dandasana in Shirshasana 6

(OORD-vuh duhn-DAHS-uh-nuh in sheer-SHAHS-uh-nuh)

Modification: on the fingertips
Pose Type: inversion, forward bend
Drishti Point: Nasagrai or Nasagre (nose), Hastagrai or Hastagre (hands)

HEADSTAND 7 ARM POSITION: VARIOUS ARM POSITIONS BASED OFF HEADSTAND 7 & VARIOUS LEG POSITIONS

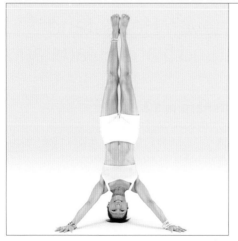

Headstand 7A

Shirshasana 7A

(sheer-SHAHS-uh-nuh)

Also Known As: Spread Hands Headstand (Prasarita Hasta Shirshasana), Hands Free Headstand C (Mukta Hasta Shirshasana C)
Pose Type: inversion
Drishti Point: Nasagrai or Nasagre (nose)

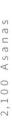

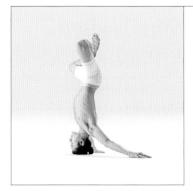

Bound Angle Pose in Headstand 7B

Baddha Konasana in Shirshasana 7B

(BUH-duh ko-NAHS-uh-nuh in sheer-SHAHS-uh-nuh)

Also Known As: Bound Angle Pose in Free Hands Headstand (Baddha Konasana in Mukta Hasta Shirshasana)
Pose Type: inversion
Drishti Point: Nasagrai or Nasagre (nose)

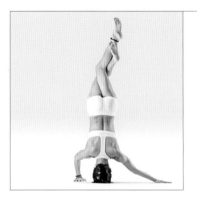

Leg Position of the Pose Dedicated to Garuda in Uneven Headstand (Fusion of Headstand 5 and Headstand 7 Arm Positions)

Pada Garudasana in Vishama Shirshasana 5 & 7A

(PUH-duh guh-ru-DAHS-uh-nuh in VISH-uh-muh sheer-SHAHS-uh-nuh)

Pose Type: inversion
Drishti Point: Nasagrai or Nasagre (nose)

1.

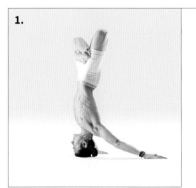

Upward Lotus Pose in Headstand 7B

Urdhva Padmasana in Shirshasana 7B

(OORD-vuh puhd-MAHS-uh-nuh in sheer-SHAHS-uh-nuh)

Also Known As: Supported Lotus Headstand Pose (Salamba Padma Shirshasana), Upward Lotus Pose in Spread Hands Headstand (Urdhva Padmasana in Prasarita Hasta Shirshasana), Upward Lotus in Hands Free Headstand (Urdhva Padmasana in Mukta Hasta Shirshasana)
Modification: 1. neutral spine
2. backbend
Pose Type: 1. inversion
2. inversion, backbend
Drishti Point: Nasagrai or Nasagre (nose)

2.

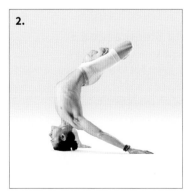

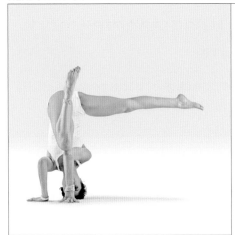

Leg to the Side Revolved Uneven Headstand (Fusion of Headstand 5 and Headstand 8 Arm Positions)

Parshva Pada Parivritta Vishama Shirshasana 5 & 8

(PAHRSH-vuh PUH-duh puh-ri-VRIT-tuh VISH-uh-muh sheer-SHAHS-uh-nuh)

Modification: Side 1: arm bent at 90 degrees, palm flat on the floor, knee resting on the opposite elbow

Side 2: arm bent at 90 degrees, fingertips to the floor, leg straight out to the side

Pose Type: inversion, forward bend, twist

Drishti Point: Hastagrai or Hastagre (hands)

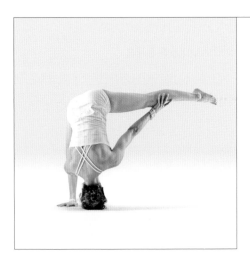

Leg to the Side One Hand Headstand 5

Parshva Pada Eka Hasta Shirshasana 5

(PAHRSH-vuh PUH-duh EY-kuh HUH-stuh sheer-SHAHS-uh-nuh)

Modification: Side 1: arm bent at 90 degrees, palm flat on the floor, knee resting on the same elbow

Side 2: arm straight, grabbing onto the shin of the leg, leg straight out to the side

Pose Type: inversion, forward bend

Drishti Point: Nasagrai or Nasagre (nose)

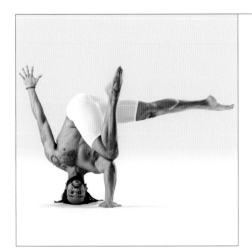

Leg to the Side Revolved One Hand Headstand 5

Parshva Pada Parivritta Eka Hasta Shirshasana 5

(PAHRSH-vuh PUH-duh puh-ri-VRIT-tuh EY-kuh HUH-stuh sheer-SHAHS-uh-nuh)

Modification: Side 1: arm bent at 90 degrees, palm flat to the floor, leg straight out to the side

Side 2: arm straight up to the sky, knee resting on the opposite tricep

Pose Type: inversion, forward bend, twist

Drishti Point: Hastagrai or Hastagre (hands), Nasagrai or Nasagre (nose)

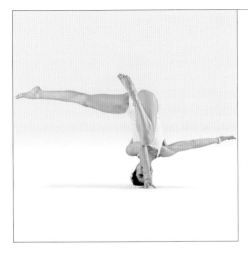

Leg to the Side Revolved One Hand Headstand 8

Parshva Pada Parivritta Eka Hasta Shirshasana 8

(PAHRSH-vuh PUH-duh puh-ri-VRIT-tuh EY-kuh HUH-stuh sheer-SHAHS-uh-nuh)

Modification: Side 1: arm bent at 90 degrees, fingertips to the floor, leg straight out to the side
Side 2: arm straight out to the side, knee resting on the opposite tricep
Pose Type: inversion, forward bend, twist
Drishti Point: Hastagrai or Hastagre (hands), Nasagrai or Nasagre (nose)

HEADSTAND 8 ARM POSITION: VARIOUS LEG POSITIONS

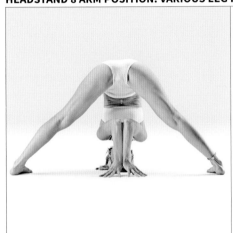

Feet Spread Intense Stretch Pose in Headstand 8

Prasarita Padottanasana in Shirshasana 8

(pruh-SAH-ri-tuh puh-do-tahn-AHS-uh-nuh in sheer-SHAHS-uh-nuh)

Also Known As: Feet Spread Full Forward Bend in Headstand 8
Modification: fingertips on the floor
Pose Type: inversion, forward bend
Drishti Point: Nasagrai or Nasagre (nose), Hastagrai or Hastagre (hands)

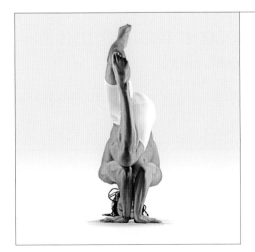

Revolved Leg Position of One-Legged King Pigeon 1 Version B in Headstand 8

Parivritta Pada Eka Pada Raja Kapotasana 1 B in Shirshasana 8

(puh-ri-VRIT-tuh PUH-duh EY-kuh PUH-duh RAH-juh kuh-po-TAHS-uh-nuh in sheer-SHAHS-uh-nuh)

Modification: palms flat on the floor
Pose Type: inversion, forward bend, twist
Drishti Point: Nasagrai or Nasagre (nose), Hastagrai or Hastagre (hands)

1.

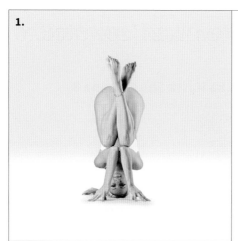

Headstand 8

Shirshasana 8

(sheer-SHAHS-uh-nuh)

Modification: knees resting on the triceps, ankles crossed

1. hands apart, elbows touching, fingertips to the floor

2. hands together, elbows together, palms flat on the floor

Pose Type: inversion, forward bend

Drishti Point: Nasagrai or Nasagre (nose), Hastagrai or Hastagre (hands)

2.

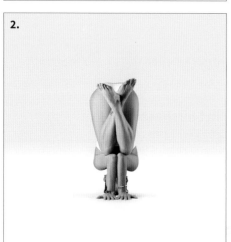

HEADSTAND 2 ARM POSITION: LOTUS

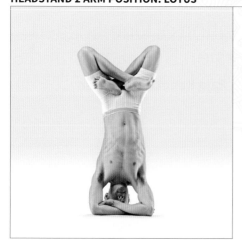

Upward Lotus Pose in Headstand 2

Urdhva Padmasana in Shirshasana 2

(OORD-vuh puhd-MAHS-uh-nuh in sheer-SHAHS-uh-nuh)

Also Known As: Upward Lotus in Hands Bound Headstand (Urdhva Padmasana in Baddha Hasta Shirshasana)

Pose Type: inversion

Drishti Point: Nasagrai or Nasagre (nose)

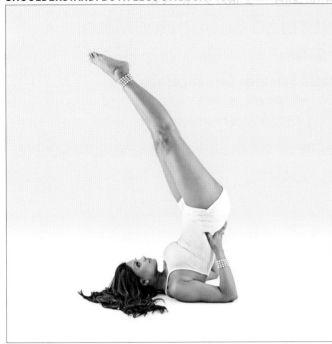

Inverted Pose Dedicated to Mythological Khimi Karani Pond

Viparita Khimi Karanyasana

(vi-puh-REE-tuh kuh-HEE-mee kuh-ruh-NEE-uhs-uh-nuh)

Also Known As: Inverted Lake Seal (Viparita Karani Mudra), Half Whole Body Pose (Ardha Sarvangasana)

Pose Type: inversion

Drishti Point: Bhrumadhye or Ajna Chakra (third eye, between the eyebrows)

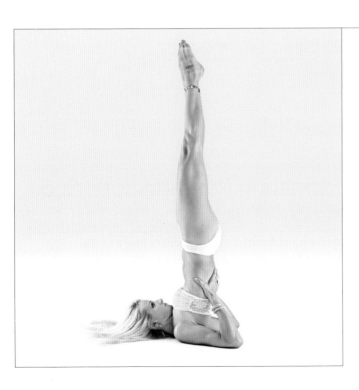

Supported Whole Body Pose

Salamba Sarvangasana

(SAH-luhm-buh suhr-vuhng-GAHS-uh-nuh)

Also Known As: Shoulderstand

Pose Type: inversion

Drishti Point: Bhrumadhye or Ajna Chakra (third eye, between the eyebrows)

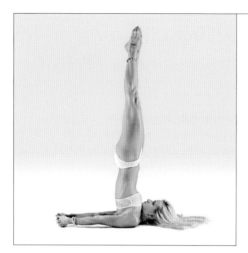

Hands Bound Supported Whole Body Pose

Baddha Hasta Salamba Sarvangasana

(BUH-duh HUH-stuh SAH-luhm-buh suhr-vuhng-GAHS-uh-nuh)

Also Known As: Shoulderstand
Pose Type: inversion
Drishti Point: Bhrumadhye or Ajna Chakra (third eye, between the eyebrows)

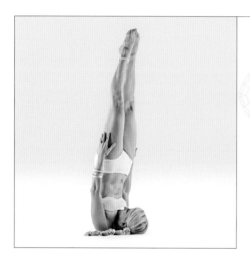

Unsupported Whole Body Pose

Niralamba Sarvangasana

(nir-AH-luhm-buh suhr-vuhng-GAHS-uh-nuh)

Also Known As: Shoulderstand
Pose Type: inversion
Drishti Point: Bhrumadhye or Ajna Chakra (third eye, between the eyebrows),
Nabhi, Nabhicakre, or Nabi Chakra (belly button)

SHOULDERSTAND: ONE LEG UP, ONE LEG DOWN

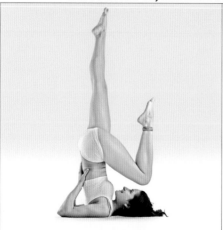

Leg Contraction Pose in Supported Whole Body Pose

Pada Akunchanasana in Salamba Sarvangasana

(PUH-duh uh-kunch-AHS-uh-nuh in SAH-luhm-buh suhr-vuhng-GAHS-uh-nuh)

Also Known As: Shoulderstand
Modification: one knee bent toward the forehead
Pose Type: inversion, forward bend
Drishti Point: Bhrumadhye or Ajna Chakra (third eye, between the eyebrows)

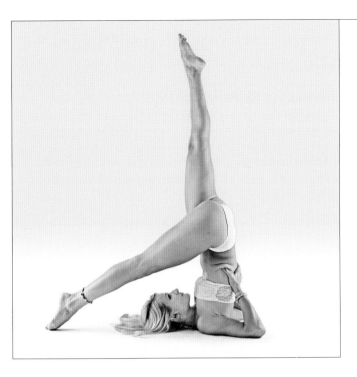

One-Legged Supported Whole Body Pose

Eka Pada Salamba Sarvangasana

(EY-kuh PUH-duh SAH-luhm-buh suhr-vuhng-GAHS-uh-nuh)

Also Known As: One-Legged Plow Pose (Eka Pada Halasana), Shoulderstand

Pose Type: inversion, forward bend

Drishti Point: Bhrumadhye or Ajna Chakra (third eye, between the eyebrows)

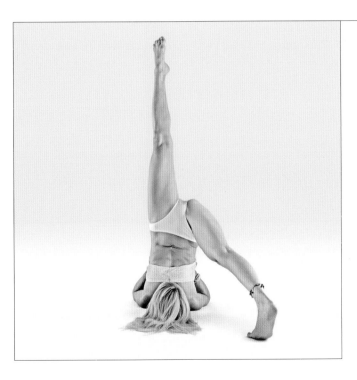

One-Legged Sideways Supported Whole Body Pose

Parshva Eka Pada Salamba Sarvangasana

(PAHRSH-vuh EY-kuh PUH-duh SAH-luhm-buh suhr-vuhng-GAHS-uh-nuh)

Also Known As: Shoulderstand

Pose Type: inversion, forward bend

Drishti Point: Bhrumadhye or Ajna Chakra (third eye, between the eyebrows)

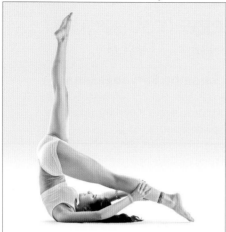

One-Legged Unsupported Whole Body Pose

Eka Pada Niralamba Sarvangasana

(EY-kuh PUH-duh nir-AH-luhm-buh suhr-vuhng-GAHS-uh-nuh)

Also Known As: Shoulderstand
Modification: both hands to the calf of the bottom leg
Pose Type: inversion, forward bend
Drishti Point: Bhrumadhye or Ajna Chakra (third eye, between the eyebrows)

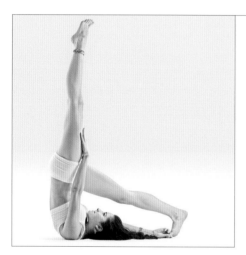

Extended Hand to Big Toe Pose in Unsupported Whole Body Pose

Utthita Hasta Padangushtasana in Niralamba Sarvangasana

(UT-ti-tuh HUH-stuh puhd-ahng-goosh-tahn-AHS-uh-nuh in nir-AH-luhm-buh suhr-vuhng-GAHS-uh-nuh)

Also Known As: Shoulderstand
Pose Type: inversion, forward bend
Drishti Point: Bhrumadhye or Ajna Chakra (third eye, between the eyebrows)

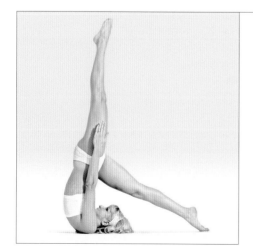

One-Legged Unsupported Whole Body Pose

Eka Pada Niralamba Sarvangasana

(EY-kuh PUH-duh nir-AH-luhm-buh suhr-vuhng-GAHS-uh-nuh)

Also Known As: Shoulderstand
Modification: both arms along the sides of the torso
Pose Type: inversion, forward bend
Drishti Point: Bhrumadhye or Ajna Chakra (third eye, between the eyebrows)

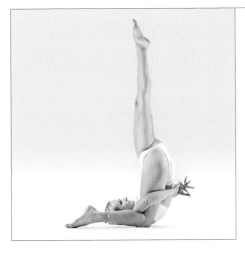

Half Bound Inverted Tortoise Pose

Ardha Baddha Viparita Kurmasana

(UHR-duh BUH-duh vi-puh-REE-tuh koor-MAHS-uh-nuh)

Pose Type: inversion, forward bend, binding

Drishti Point: Bhrumadhye or Ajna Chakra (third eye, between the eyebrows)

SHOULDERSTAND: GARUDA LEGS

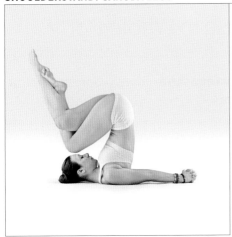

Leg Position of the Pose Dedicated to Garuda in Hands Bound Supported Whole Body Pose

Pada Garudasana in Baddha Hasta Salamba Sarvangasana

(PUH-duh guh-ru-DAHS-uh-nuh in BUH-duh HUH-stuh SAH-luhm-buh suhr-vuhng-GAHS-uh-nuh)

Also Known As: Shoulderstand

Modification: knees toward the forehead

Pose Type: inversion, forward bend

Drishti Point: Nasagrai or Nasagre (nose), Bhrumadhye or Ajna Chakra (third eye, between the eyebrows)

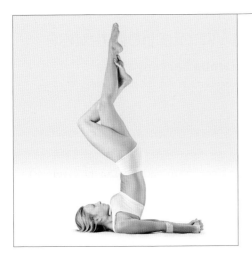

Leg Position of the Pose Dedicated to Garuda in Hands Bound Supported Whole Body Pose

Pada Garudasana in Baddha Hasta Salamba Sarvangasana

(PUH-duh guh-ru-DAHS-uh-nuh in BUH-duh HUH-stuh SAH-luhm-buh suhr-vuhng-GAHS-uh-nuh)

Also Known As: Shoulderstand

Modification: legs extended toward the sky

Pose Type: inversion, forward bend

Drishti Point: Nasagrai or Nasagre (nose), Bhrumadhye or Ajna Chakra (third eye, between the eyebrows)

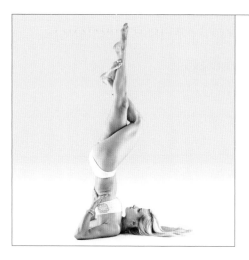

Leg Position of the Pose Dedicated to Garuda in Supported Whole Body Pose

Pada Garudasana in Salamba Sarvangasana

(PUH-duh guh-ru-DAHS-uh-nuh in SAH-luhm-buh suhr-vuhng-GAHS-uh-nuh)

Also Known As: Shoulderstand
Pose Type: inversion
Drishti Point: Bhrumadhye or Ajna Chakra (third eye, between the eyebrows)

SHOULDERSTAND: BOUND ANGLE & LOTUS

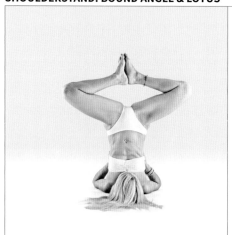

Bound Angle Pose in Whole Body Pose

Baddha Konasana in Sarvangasana

(BUH-duh ko-NAHS-uh-nuh in suhr-vuhng-GAHS-uh-nuh)

Also Known As: Shoulderstand
Pose Type: inversion
Drishti Point: Bhrumadhye or Ajna Chakra (third eye, between the eyebrows)

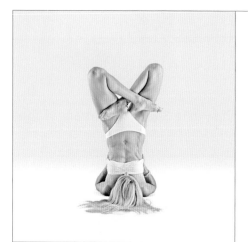

Upward Lotus in Whole Body Pose

Urdhva Padmasana in Salamba Sarvangasana

(OORD-vuh puhd-MAHS-uh-nuh in SAH-luhm-buh suhr-vuhng-GAHS-uh-nuh)

Also Known As: Shoulderstand
Pose Type: inversion
Drishti Point: Bhrumadhye or Ajna Chakra (third eye, between the eyebrows)

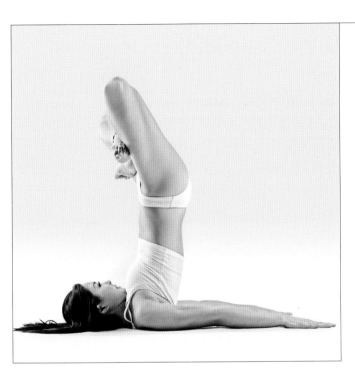

Upward Lotus in Whole Body Pose

Urdhva Padmasana in Salamba Sarvangasana

(OORD-vuh puhd-MAHS-uh-nuh in SAH-luhm-buh suhr-vuhng-GAHS-uh-nuh)

Also Known As: Shoulderstand
Modification: arms straight to the back, palms on the floor
Pose Type: inversion
Drishti Point: Bhrumadhye or Ajna Chakra (third eye, between the eyebrows)

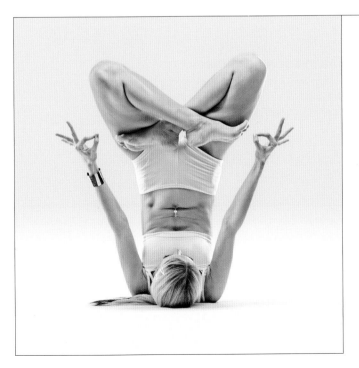

Upward Lotus in Unsupported Whole Body Pose

Urdhva Padmasana in Niralamba Sarvangasana

(OORD-vuh puhd-MAHS-uh-nuh in nir-AH-luhm-buh suhr-vuhng-GAHS-uh-nuh)

Also Known As: Shoulderstand
Pose Type: inversion
Drishti Point: Bhrumadhye or Ajna Chakra (third eye, between the eyebrows)

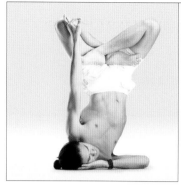

Inverted Ear Pressure Raised Up Lotus Pose

Viparita Karnapida Urdhva Padmasana

(vi-puh-REE-tuh kuhr-nah-PEED-uh OORD-vuh puhd-MAHS-uh-nuh)

Pose Type: inversion
Drishti Point: Nasagrai or Nasagre (nose)

SHOULDERSTAND: LOTUS—BACKBEND & FORWARD BEND

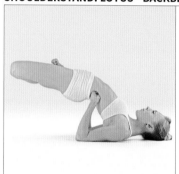

Intense Lotus Peacock Prep.

Uttana Padma Mayurasana Prep.

(ut-TAHN-uh PUHD-muh muh-yoor-AHS-uh-nuh)

Also Known As: Intense Front Body Stretching and Rejuvenating Lotus Pose (Purvottana Padma Sarvangasana)
Modification: knees off the floor, fists to the lower back
Pose Type: inversion, backbend
Drishti Point: Bhrumadhye or Ajna Chakra (third eye, between the eyebrows)

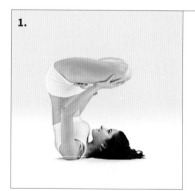

1.

Upward Lotus Pose in Whole Body Pose

Urdhva Padmasana in Sarvangasana

(OORD-vuh puhd-MAHS-uh-nuh in suhr-vuhng-GAHS-uh-nuh)

Also Known As: Shoulderstand
Modification: 1. thighs parallel to the floor, elbows bent
2. arms straight
Pose Type: inversion
Drishti Point: Bhrumadhye or Ajna Chakra (third eye, between the eyebrows)

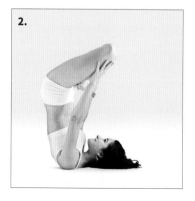

2.

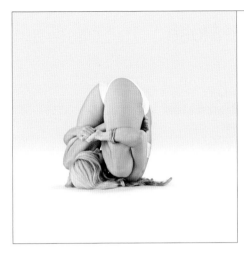

Embryo Pose in Whole Body Pose

Pindasana in Sarvangasana

(pin-DAHS-uh-nuh in suhr-vuhng-GAHS-uh-nuh)

Also Known As: Inverted Embryo Pose (Viparita Pindasana), Embryo Pose in Plow Pose (Pindasana in Halasana), Shoulderstand

Pose Type: inversion, forward bend

Drishti Point: Bhrumadhye or Ajna Chakra (third eye, between the eyebrows)

SHOULDERSTAND: LOTUS—KNEES ON THE FLOOR

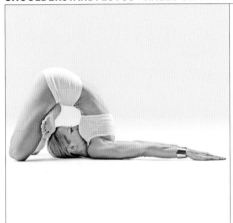

Lotus Pose in Plow Pose

Padmasana in Halasana

(puhd-MAHS-uh-nuh in hul-AHS-uh-nuh)

Pose Type: inversion, forward bend

Drishti Point: Nabhi, Nabhicakre, or Nabi Chakra (belly button)

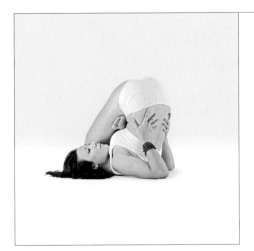

Sideways Embryo Pose in Whole Body Pose

Parshva Pindasana in Sarvangasana

(PAHRSH-vuh pin-DAHS-uh-nuh in suhr-vuhng-GAHS-uh-nuh)

Also Known As: Side Embryo Pose (Parshva Pindasana), Embryo Pose in Plow Pose (Pindasana in Halasana), Shoulderstand

Pose Type: inversion, forward bend, twist

Drishti Point: Nasagrai or Nasagre (nose)

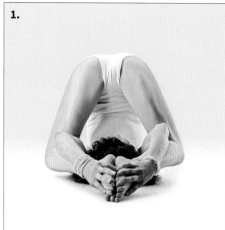

Inverted Tortoise Pose

Viparita Kurmasana

(vi-puh-REE-tuh koor-MAHS-uh-nuh)

Modification: 1. grabbing onto the feet

2. palms to the floor, fingertips facing to the back

Pose Type: inversion, forward bend

Drishti Point: Nabhi, Nabhicakre, or Nabi Chakra (belly button)

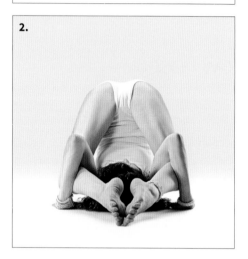

Bound Inverted Tortoise Pose

Baddha Viparita Kurmasana

(BUH-duh vi-puh-REE-tuh koor-MAHS-uh-nuh)

Pose Type: inversion, forward bend, binding

Drishti Point: Nabhi, Nabhicakre, or Nabi Chakra (belly button)

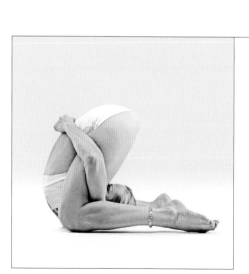

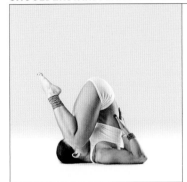

Ear Pressure Pose Prep.

Karnapidasana Prep.

(kuhr-nah-pee-DAHS-uh-nuh)

Modification: knees to the temples, palms to the lower back
Pose Type: inversion, forward bend
Drishti Point: Nabhi, Nabhicakre, or Nabi Chakra (belly button)

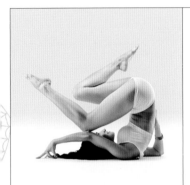

Ear Pressure Pose Prep.

Karnapidasana Prep.

(kuhr-nah-pee-DAHS-uh-nuh)

Modification: one hand to the lower back; other arm up over the head, elbow bent, fingertips to the floor; both knees bent, one knee to the elbow of the front arm, heel of the other foot toward the sitting bone
Pose Type: inversion, forward bend
Drishti Point: Nabhi, Nabhicakre, or Nabi Chakra (belly button)

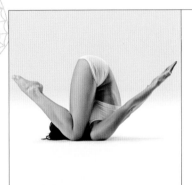

Ear Pressure Pose

Karnapidasana

(kuhr-nah-pee-DAHS-uh-nuh)

Modification: both knees bent, feet off the floor; arms straight behind the back and off the floor, palms up
Pose Type: inversion, forward bend, balance
Drishti Point: Nabhi, Nabhicakre, or Nabi Chakra (belly button)

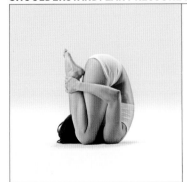

Ear Pressure Pose

Karnapidasana

(kuhr-nah-pee-DAHS-uh-nuh)

Modification: both heels to the sitting bones, grabbing onto the ankles, elbows bent
Pose Type: inversion, forward bend
Drishti Point: Nabhi, Nabhicakre, or Nabi Chakra (belly button)

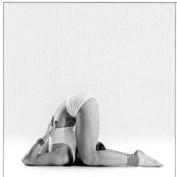

Ear Pressure Pose

Karnapidasana

(kuhr-nah-pee-DAHS-uh-nuh)

Modification: palms to the lower back
Pose Type: inversion, forward bend
Drishti Point: Nabhi, Nabhicakre, or Nabi Chakra (belly button)

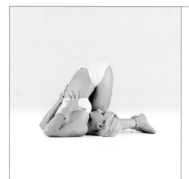

Sideways Ear Pressure Pose

Parshva Karnapidasana

(PAHRSH-vuh kuhr-nah-pee-DAHS-uh-nuh)

Also Known As: Side Contraction Pose (Parshva Akunchanasana)
Modification: palms to the lower back
Pose Type: inversion, forward bend, twist
Drishti Point: Nabhi, Nabhicakre, or Nabi Chakra (belly button)

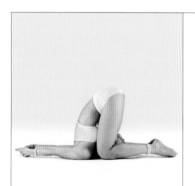

Hands Bound Ear Pressure Pose

Baddha Hasta Karnapidasana

(BUH-duh HUH-stuh kuhr-nah-pee-DAHS-uh-nuh)

Modification: fingers interlocked
Pose Type: inversion, forward bend
Drishti Point: Nabhi, Nabhicakre, or Nabi Chakra (belly button)

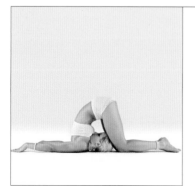

Shivalinga Pose

Lingasana

(ling-GAHS-uh-nuh)

Also Known As: Ear Pressure Pose (Karnapidasana)
Pose Type: inversion, forward bend
Drishti Point: Nabhi, Nabhicakre, or Nabi Chakra (belly button)

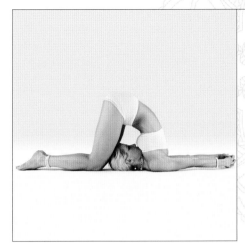

Bound Hands Shivalinga Pose

Baddha Hasta Lingasana

(BUH-duh HUH-stuh ling-GAHS-uh-nuh)

Also Known As: Ear Pressure Pose (Karna Pidasana)

Pose Type: inversion, forward bend

Drishti Point: Nabhi, Nabhicakre, or Nabi Chakra (belly button)

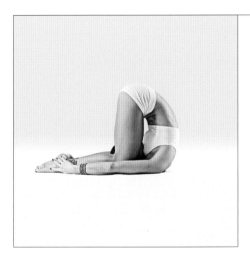

Ear Pressure Pose

Karnapidasana

(kuhr-nah-pee-DAHS-uh-nuh)

Modification: grabbing onto the heels

Pose Type: inversion, forward bend

Drishti Point: Nabhi, Nabhicakre, or Nabi Chakra (belly button)

PLOW POSE: LEGS STRAIGHT AND TOGETHER—DIFFERENT ARM POSITIONS

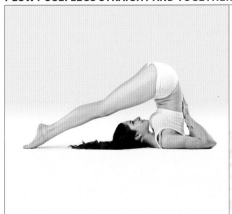

Plow Pose

Halasana

(huh-LAHS-uh-nuh)

Modification: palms to the lower back, toes pointed to the front

Pose Type: inversion, forward bend

Drishti Point: Bhrumadhye or Ajna Chakra (third eye, between the eyebrows)

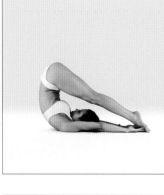

Plow Pose

Halasana

(huh-LAHS-uh-nuh)

Modification: fingers to the toes, palms up
Pose Type: inversion, forward bend
Drishti Point: Nabhi, Nabhicakre, or Nabi Chakra (belly button)

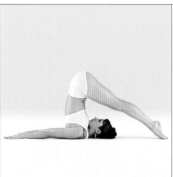

Plow Pose

Halasana

(huh-LAHS-uh-nuh)

Modification: arms straight to the back, palms on the floor
Pose Type: inversion, forward bend
Drishti Point: Bhrumadhye or Ajna Chakra (third eye, between the eyebrows)

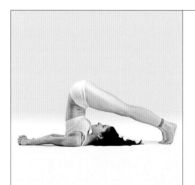

Bound Hands Plow Pose

Baddha Hasta Halasana

(BUH-duh HUH-stuh huh-LAHS-uh-nuh)

Pose Type: inversion, forward bend
Drishti Point: Bhrumadhye or Ajna Chakra (third eye, between the eyebrows)

PLOW POSE: LEGS TO THE SIDE & LEGS WIDE APART

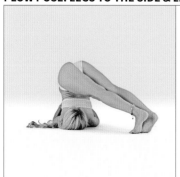

Sideways Plow Pose

Parshva Halasana

(PAHRSH-vuh huh-LAHS-uh-nuh)

Modification: palms to the lower back
Pose Type: inversion, forward bend, twist
Drishti Point: Nabhi, Nabhicakre, or Nabi Chakra (belly button)

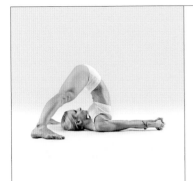

Hands Bound Feet Spread Wide Intense Stretch Pose in Plow Pose

Baddha Hasta Prasarita Padottanasana in Halasana
(BUH-duh HUH-stuh pruh-SAH-ri-tuh puh-do-tahn-AHS-uh-nuh in huh-LAHS-uh-nuh)
Also Known As: Hands Bound Feet Spread Wide Full Forward Bend in Plow Pose
Pose Type: inversion, forward bend
Drishti Point: Bhrumadhye or Ajna Chakra (third eye, between the eyebrows)

PLOW POSE: ONE LEG STRAIGHT, ONE LEG BENT

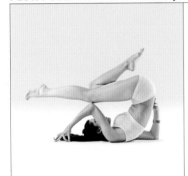

One-Legged Elbow to Knee Plow Pose

Eka Pada Kurpara Janu Halasana
(EY-kuh PUH-duh kuhr-PAH-ruh JAH-nu hul-AHS-uh-nuh)
Modification: one hand to the lower back; other arm up over the head, elbow bent, fingertips to the floor; knees together, one leg straight; knee to the elbow, other knee bent, heel to the sitting bone
Pose Type: inversion, forward bend
Drishti Point: Bhrumadhye or Ajna Chakra (third eye, between the eyebrows)

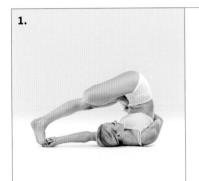

1.

Reclined Upward Foot Thunderbolt Pose

Supta Urdhva Pada Vajrasana
(SUP-tuh OORD-vuh PUH-duh vuhj-RAHS-uh-nuh)
Also Known As: Half Bound Lotus Pose in Whole Body Pose (Ardha Baddha Padmasana in Sarvangasana), Shoulderstand
Modification: 1. front side view
2. back side view
Pose Type: inversion, forward bend, binding
Drishti Point: Bhrumadhye or Ajna Chakra (third eye, between the eyebrows)

2.

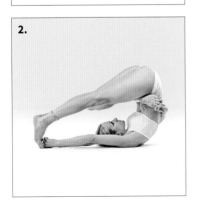

Prone Poses

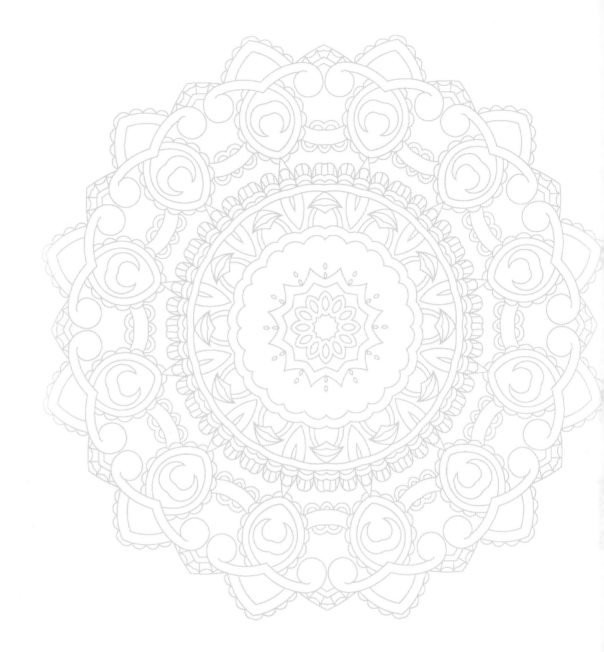

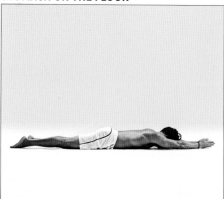

Pose Dedicated to Makara—Prone Modification

Makarasana

(muh-kuh-RAHS-uh-nuh)

Also Known As: Crocodile Pose

Modification: whole body flat on the floor; arms straight out in front, palms together

Pose Type: prone

Drishti Point: Nasagrai or Nasagre (nose)

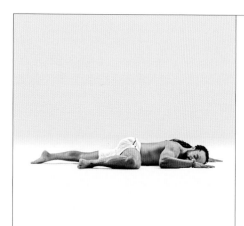

Side Corpse Pose

Parshva Shavasana

(PAHRSH-vuh shuh-VAHS-uh-nuh)

Pose Type: prone

Drishti Point: Angushtamadhye or Angushta Ma Dyai (thumbs)

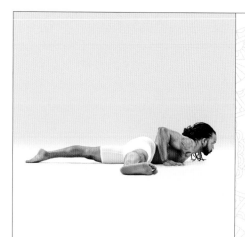

Downward Facing One Leg to the Side Pose

Adho Mukha Parshva Eka Padasana

(uh-DO MUK-uh PAHRSH-vuh EY-kuh puh-DAHS-uh-nuh)

Pose Type: prone

Drishti Point: Nasagrai or Nasagre (nose)

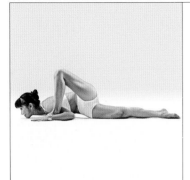

Intense Stretch Slithering Lizard Lunge Pose

Utthana Sarpa Godhasana

(ut-TAHN-uh SUHR-puh go-DAHS-uh-nuh)

Also Known As: Extended Lizard Tail Lunge Pose (Uttana Pristhasana)

Modification: foot to the elbow crease

Pose Type: prone

Drishti Point: Bhrumadhye or Ajna Chakra (third eye, between the eyebrows)

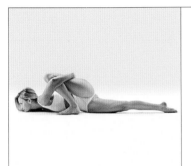

Intense Stretch Slithering Lizard Lunge Pose

Utthan Sarpa Godhasana

(ut-TAHN-uh SUHR-puh go-DAHS-uh-nuh)

Also Known As: Extended Lizard Tail Lunge Pose (Uttana Pristhasana)

Modification: foot to the outside of the rib cage, arm binds around the leg

Pose Type: prone

Drishti Point: Bhrumadhye or Ajna Chakra (third eye, between the eyebrows), Nasagrai or Nasagre (nose)

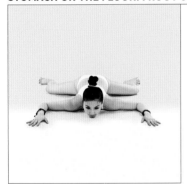

Frog Pose

Mandukasana

(muhn-doo-KAHS-uh-nuh)

Also Known As: Thavaliasana

Pose Type: prone

Drishti Point: Nasagrai or Nasagre (nose)

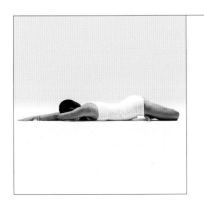

Lotus Staff Surrender Salutation Pose

Padma Danda Namaskarasana

(PUHD-muh DUHN-duh nuh-muhs-kahr-AHS-uh-nuh)

Modification: arms straight in front, palms down to the floor

Pose Type: prone

Drishti Point: Nasagrai or Nasagre (nose)

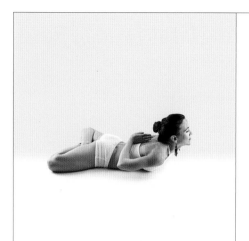

Hidden Lotus Pose

Gupta Padmasana

(GUP-tuh puhd-MAHS-uh-nuh)

Pose Type: prone, mild backbend

Drishti Point: Bhrumadhye or Ajna Chakra (third eye, between the eyebrows)

CHEST FACING THE FLOOR: TWISTS

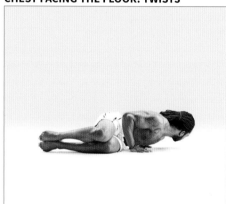

Downward Facing Twisted Stomach Pose

Adho Mukha Jatara Parivartanasana

(uh-DO MUK-uh JAHT-uh-ruh puh-ri-vuhr-tuh-NAHS-uh-nuh)

Modification: knees together, legs bent

Pose Type: prone, twist

Drishti Point: Parshva Drishti (to the right), Parshva Drishti (to the left)

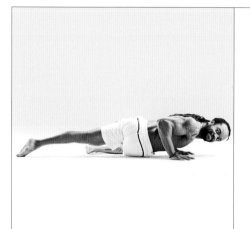

Downward Facing Twisted Stomach Pose

Adho Mukha Jatara Parivartanasana

(uh-DO MUK-uh JAHT-uh-ruh puh-ri-vuhr-tuh-NAHS-uh-nuh)

Modification: top leg straight, bottom knee bent

Pose Type: prone, twist

Drishti Point: Parshva Drishti (to the right), Parshva Drishti (to the left)

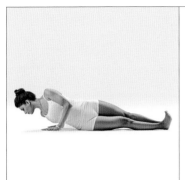

Downward Facing Twisted Stomach Pose

Adho Mukha Jatara Parivartanasana

(uh-DO MUK-uh JAHT-uh-ruh puh-ri-vuhr-tuh-NAHS-uh-nuh)

Modification: legs straight
Pose Type: prone, twist
Drishti Point: Nasagrai or Nasagre (nose)

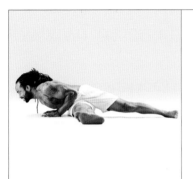

Pose Dedicated to St. Brighid of Kildare

Brighidasana

(bree-gid-AHS-uh-nuh)

Modification: bottom leg crossed under, looking straight ahead
Pose Type: prone, twist
Drishti Point: Nasagrai or Nasagre (nose)

CHEST FACING THE FLOOR: TWISTS—LEGS TO THE SIDE

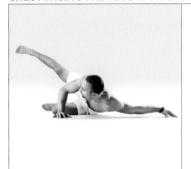

Pose Dedicated to Sage Koundinya One-Legged Version 1—Prone Modification

Eka Pada Koundinyasana 1

(EY-kuh PUH-duh kown-din-YAHS-uh-nuh)

Modification: one arm straight to the side, bottom knee bent
Pose Type: arm balance, forward bend, twist
Drishti Point: Parshva Drishti (to the right), Parshva Drishti (to the left)

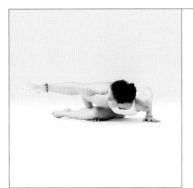

Pose Dedicated to Ashtavakra— Prone Modification

Ashtavakrasana

(uh-shtuh-vuh-KRAHS-uh-nuh)

Also Known As: Eight Angle Pose—Prone Modification
Modification: legs unhooked, bottom knee wrapped around the opposite forearm, top leg straight
Pose Type: arm balance, forward bend, twist
Drishti Point: Padayoragrai or Padayoragre (toes/feet)

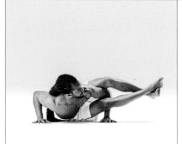

Pose Dedicated to Ashtavakra—Prone Modification

Ashtavakrasana

(uh-shtuh-vuh-KRAHS-uh-nuh)

Also Known As: Eight Angle Pose—Prone Modification
Pose Type: arm balance, forward bend, twist
Drishti Point: Padayoragrai or Padayoragre (toes/feet)

CHEST FACING THE FLOOR: TWIST & VERTICAL SPLITS

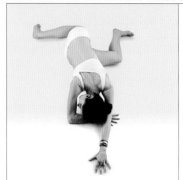

Svastika Legs in Downward Facing Twisted Stomach Pose

Pada Svastikasana in Adho Mukha Jatara Parivartanasana

(PUH-duh svuh-sti-KAHS-uh-nuh in uh-DO MUK-uh JAHT-uh-ruh puh-ri-vuhr-tuh-NAHS-uh-nuh)

Modification: one arm straight out in front, palm down to the floor; other elbow bent, temple resting on the forearm of the bent arm
Pose Type: prone, twist
Drishti Point: Parshva Drishti (to the right), Parshva Drishti (to the left)

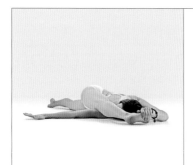

Downward Facing Pose Dedicated to Trivikrama—Prone Modification

Adho Mukha Trivikramasana

(uh-DO MUK-uh tri-vi-kruhm-AHS-uh-nuh)

Pose Type: prone
Drishti Point: Hastagrai or Hastagre (hands)

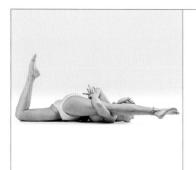

Bound Downward Facing Pose Dedicated to Trivikrama—Prone Modification

Baddha Adho Mukha Trivikramasana

(BUH-duh uh-DO MUK-uh tri-vi-kruhm-AHS-uh-nuh)

Modification: back leg bent—toes pointing to the sky
Pose Type: prone, binding
Drishti Point: Bhrumadhye or Ajna Chakra (third eye, between the eyebrows)

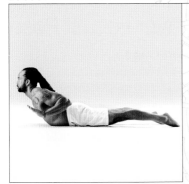

Cobra Pose 1

Bhujangasana 1

(buj-uhng-GAHS-uh-nuh)

Modification: palms lifted off the floor, elbows bent

Pose Type: prone, backbend

Drishti Point: Bhrumadhye or Ajna Chakra (third eye, between the eyebrows)

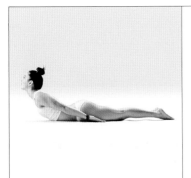

Locust Pose

Shalabhasana

(shuh-luh-BAHS-uh-nuh)

Modification: arms straight, palms facing up by the hips; feet on the floor

Pose Type: prone, backbend

Drishti Point: Bhrumadhye or Ajna Chakra (third eye, between the eyebrows)

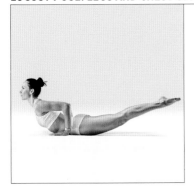

Locust Pose

Shalabhasana

(shuh-luh-BAHS-uh-nuh)

Also Known As: Locust Pose B (Shalabhasana B)

Modification: palms to the floor by the bottom of the ribs, elbows bent at 90 degrees

Pose Type: prone, backbend

Drishti Point: Bhrumadhye or Ajna Chakra (third eye, between the eyebrows)

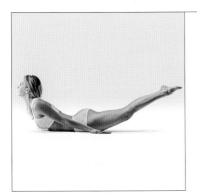

Locust Pose

Shalabhasana

(shuh-luh-BAHS-uh-nuh)

Also Known As: Locust Pose A (Salabhasana A)

Modification: palms to the floor by the hips, arms straight, legs and chest lifted

Pose Type: prone, backbend

Drishti Point: Bhrumadhye or Ajna Chakra (third eye, between the eyebrows)

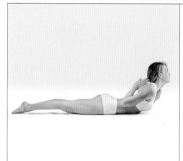

Fingers to Head Reverse Prayer Locust Pose

Anguli Shirsha Viparita Namaskar Shalabhasana

(UHNG-goo-lee SHEER-shuh vi-puh-REE-tuh nuh-muhs-KAHR shuh-luh-BAHS-uh-nuh)

Also Known As: Back of the Body Prayer Fingers to Head Locust Pose (Paschima Namaskara Anguli Shirsha Shalabhasana)

Modification: feet on the floor

Pose Type: prone, backbend

Drishti Point: Bhrumadhye or Ajna Chakra (third eye, between the eyebrows)

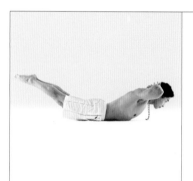

Pose Dedicated to Makara

Makarasana

(muh-kuh-RAHS-uh-nuh)

Also Known As: Crocodile Pose

Pose Type: prone, backbend

Drishti Point: Bhrumadhye or Ajna Chakra (third eye, between the eyebrows)

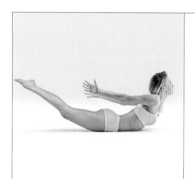

Locust Pose

Shalabhasana

(shuh-luh-BAHS-uh-nuh)

Modification: arms open wide, fingertips pointing to the toes

Pose Type: prone, backbend

Drishti Point: Bhrumadhye or Ajna Chakra (third eye, between the eyebrows)

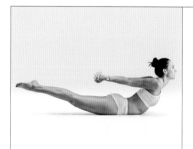

Hands Bound Locust Pose

Baddha Hasta Shalabhasana

(BUH-duh HUH-stuh shuh-luh-BAHS-uh-nuh)

Pose Type: prone, backbend

Drishti Point: Bhrumadhye or Ajna Chakra (third eye, between the eyebrows)

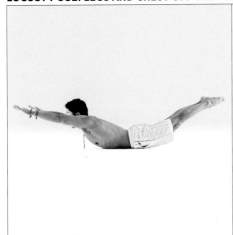

Locust Pose

Shalabhasana

(shuh-luh-BAHS-uh-nuh)

Also Known As: Crocodile Pose (Makarasana), Boat Pose (Navasana)
Modification: both arms straight in front, palms facing down
Pose Type: prone, backbend
Drishti Point: Bhrumadhye or Ajna Chakra (third eye, between the eyebrows) or Angushtamadhye or Angushta Ma Dyai (thumbs)

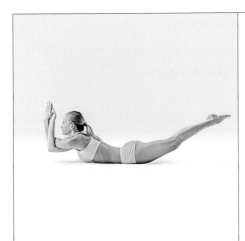

Hand Position of the Pose Dedicated to Garuda in Locust Pose

Hasta Garudasana in Shalabhasana

(HUH-stuh guh-ru-DAHS-uh-nuh in shuh-luh-BAHS-uh-nuh)

Pose Type: prone, backbend
Drishti Point: Angushtamadhye or Angushta Ma Dyai (thumbs)

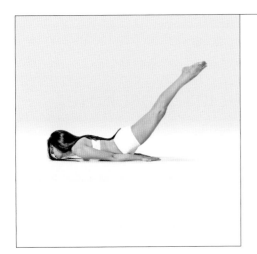

Inverted Locust Pose

Viparita Shalabhasana

(vi-puh-REE-tuh shuh-luh-BAHS-uh-nuh)

Modification: chin to the floor, legs lifted
Pose Type: prone, backbend
Drishti Point: Bhrumadhye or Ajna Chakra (third eye, between the eyebrows)

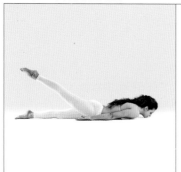

Half Locust Pose

Ardha Shalabhasana

(UHR-duh shuh-luh-BAHS-uh-nuh)

Modification: hands to the floor by the hips, palms facing up, arms straight
Pose Type: prone, backbend
Drishti Point: Nasagrai or Nasagre (nose), Bhrumadhye or Ajna Chakra (third eye, between the eyebrows)

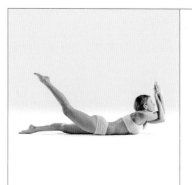

Hand Position of the Pose Dedicated to Garuda in Half Locust Pose

Hasta Garudasana in Ardha Shalabhasana

(HUH-stuh guh-ruh-DAHS-uh-nuh in UHR-duh shuh-luh-BAHS-uh-nuh)

Pose Type: prone, backbend
Drishti Point: Angushtamadhye or Angushta Ma Dyai (thumbs)

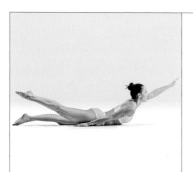

Half Locust Pose

Ardha Shalabhasana

(UHR-duh shuh-luh-BAHS-uh-nuh)

Also Known As: Crocodile Pose (Makarasana)
Modification: one arm straight to the front—palm facing down, other hand to the floor by the hip—palm down
Pose Type: prone, backbend
Drishti Point: Angushtamadhye or Angushta Ma Dyai (thumbs)

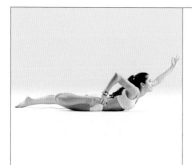

One-Legged Frog Pose in Locust Pose

Eka Pada Bhekasana in Shalabhasana

(EY-kuh PUH-duh bey-KAHS-uh-nuh in shuh-luh-BAHS-uh-nuh)

Pose Type: prone, backbend
Drishti Point: Bhrumadhye or Ajna Chakra (third eye, between the eyebrows) or Hastagrai or Hastagre (hands)

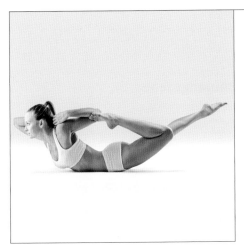

Mermaid Pose in Locust Pose

Naginyasana in Shalabhasana

(nuh-gin-YAHS-uh-nuh in shuh-luh-BAHS-uh-nuh)

Pose Type: prone, backbend, binding

Drishti Point: Bhrumadhye or Ajna Chakra (third eye, between the eyebrows)

SPHINX POSE: BOTH AND ONE LEG STRAIGHT

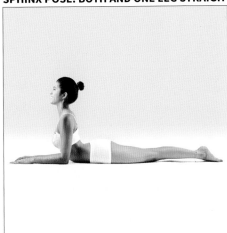

Supported Cobra Pose

Salamba Bhujangasana

(SAH-luhm-buh buj-uhng-GAHS-uh-nuh)

Also Known As: Sphinx Pose or Crocodile Pose (Makarasana)

Pose Type: prone, backbend

Drishti Point: Bhrumadhye or Ajna Chakra (third eye, between the eyebrows)

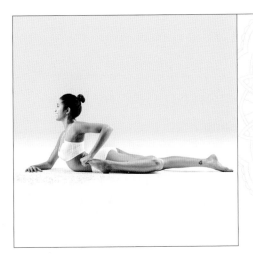

One-Legged Frog Pose

Eka Pada Bhekasana

(EY-kuh PUH-duh bey-KAHS-uh-nuh)

Modification: open ankles modification, heel to the floor by the hip socket

Pose Type: prone, backbend

Drishti Point: Nasagrai or Nasagre (nose), Bhrumadhye or Ajna Chakra (third eye, between the eyebrows)

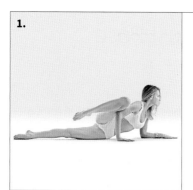

1.

Leg Extended Uneven Supported Cobra Pose

Utthita Pada Vishama Salamba Bhujangasana

(UT-ti-tuh PUH-duh VISH-uh-muh SAH-luhm-buh buj-ung-GAHS-uh-nuh)

Also Known As: Uneven Sphinx Pose
Modification: 1. knee bent
 2. leg straight
Pose Type: prone
Drishti Point: Bhrumadhye or Ajna Chakra (third eye, between the eyebrows)

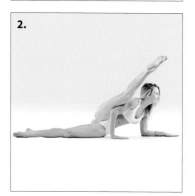

2.

SPHINX POSE: BOTH KNEES BENT

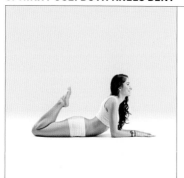

Supported Cobra Pose

Salamba Bhujangasana

(SAH-luhm-buh buj-uhng-GAHS-uh-nuh)

Also Known As: Sphinx Pose or Crocodile Pose (Makarasana)
Modification: knees bent
Pose Type: prone, backbend
Drishti Point: Bhrumadhye or Ajna Chakra (third eye, between the eyebrows)

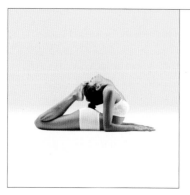

Feet to the Head Supported Cobra Pose

Shirsha Pada Salamba Bhujangasana

(SHEER-shuh PUH-duh SAH-luhm-buh buj-uhng-GAHS-uh-nuh)

Also Known As: Feet to the Head Sphinx Pose
Modification: toes to the forehead
Pose Type: prone, backbend
Drishti Point: Bhrumadhye or Ajna Chakra (third eye, between the eyebrows)

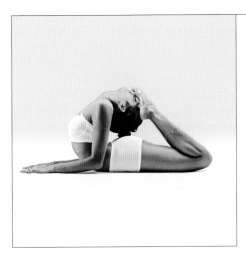

Feet to the Face Supported Cobra Pose

Mukha Pada Salamba Bhujangasana

(MUK-uh PUH-duh SAH-luhm-buh buj-uhng-GAHS-uh-nuh)

Also Known As: Feet to the Face Sphinx Pose
Modification: heels to the forehead
Pose Type: prone, backbend
Drishti Point: Bhrumadhye or Ajna Chakra (third eye, between the eyebrows), Padayoragrai or Padayoragre (toes/feet)

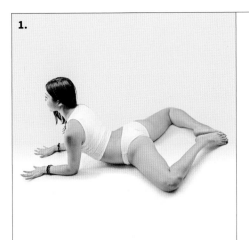

1.

Downward Facing Bound Angle Pose

Adho Mukha Baddha Konasana

(uh-DO MUK-uh BUH-duh ko-NAHS-uh-nuh)

Modification: forearms to the floor
1. top view
2. side view
Pose Type: prone, backbend
Drishti Point: Nasagrai or Nasagre (nose)

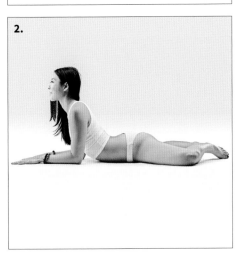

2.

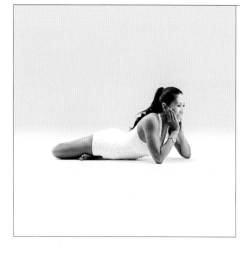

Hidden Lotus Pose

Gupta Padmasana

(GUP-tuh puhd-MAHS-uh-nuh)

Modification: hands to the face on the elbows

Pose Type: prone, backbend

Drishti Point: Nasagrai or Nasagre (nose)

COBRA POSE

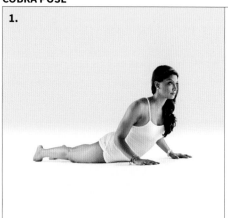

Cobra Pose

Bhujangasana

(buj-uhng-GAHS-uh-nuh)

Modification: palms on the floor, elbows bent

1. mild backbend

2. intense backbend

Pose Type: prone, backbend

Drishti Point: Nasagrai or Nasagre (nose), Bhrumadhye or Ajna Chakra (third eye, between the eyebrows)

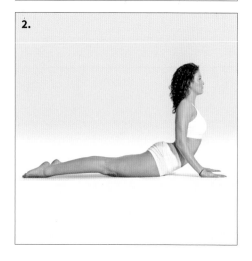

1.

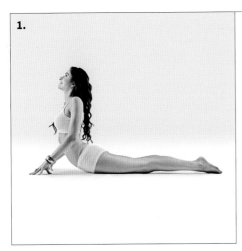

Cobra Pose

Bhujangasana

(buj-uhng-GAHS-uh-nuh)

Modification: 1. elbows bent, fingertips to the floor

2. arms straight, palms to the floor

Pose Type: prone, backbend

Drishti Point: Bhrumadhye or Ajna Chakra (third eye, between the eyebrows), Nasagrai or Nasagre (nose)

2.

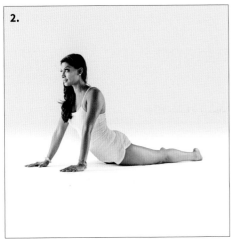

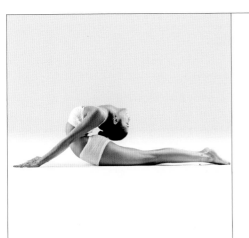

Cobra Pose

Bhujangasana

(buj-uhng-GAHS-uh-nuh)

Modification: palms on the floor, arms straight, head to the glutes

Pose Type: prone, backbend

Drishti Point: Bhrumadhye or Ajna Chakra (third eye, between the eyebrows)

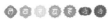

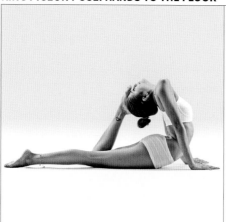

Half King Pigeon Pose

Ardha Raja Kapotasana

(UHR-duh RAH-juh kuh-po-TAHS-uh-nuh)

Modification: palms to the floor, one foot to the head
Pose Type: prone, backbend
Drishti Point: Bhrumadhye or Ajna Chakra (third eye, between the eyebrows)

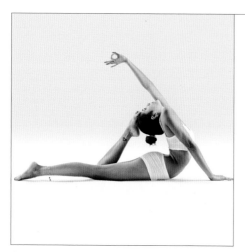

One-Legged One Hand King Pigeon Pose

Eka Pada Eka Hasta Raja Kapotasana

(EY-kuh PUH-duh EY-kuh HUH-stuh RAH-juh kuh-po-TAHS-uh-nuh)

Pose Type: prone, backbend
Drishti Point: Bhrumadhye or Ajna Chakra (third eye, between the eyebrows), Hastagrai or Hastagre (hands)

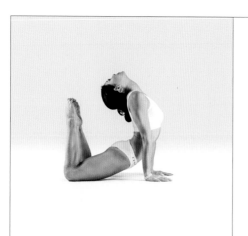

King Pigeon Pose

Raja Kapotasana

(RAH-juh kuh-po-TAHS-uh-nuh)

Modification: palms to the floor, feet away from the head
Pose Type: prone, backbend
Drishti Point: Bhrumadhye or Ajna Chakra (third eye, between the eyebrows)

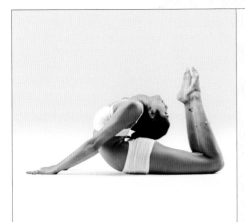

King Pigeon Pose

Raja Kapotasana

(RAH-juh kuh-po-TAHS-uh-nuh)

Modification: head touching the glutes, knees bent, feet away from the head
Pose Type: prone, backbend
Drishti Point: Bhrumadhye or Ajna Chakra (third eye, between the eyebrows),
Padayoragrai or Padayoragre (toes/feet)

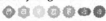

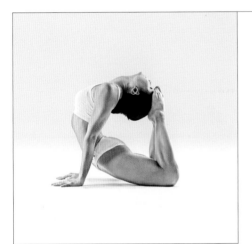

King Pigeon Pose

Raja Kapotasana

(RAH-juh kuh-po-TAHS-uh-nuh)

Modification: palms to the floor, feet to the head
Pose Type: prone, backbend
Drishti Point: Bhrumadhye or Ajna Chakra (third eye, between the eyebrows)

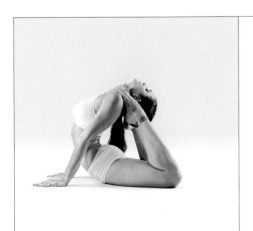

King Pigeon Pose

Raja Kapotasana

(RAH-juh kuh-po-TAHS-uh-nuh)

Modification: palms to the floor, feet to the shoulders
Pose Type: prone, backbend
Drishti Point: Bhrumadhye or Ajna Chakra (third eye, between the eyebrows)

1.

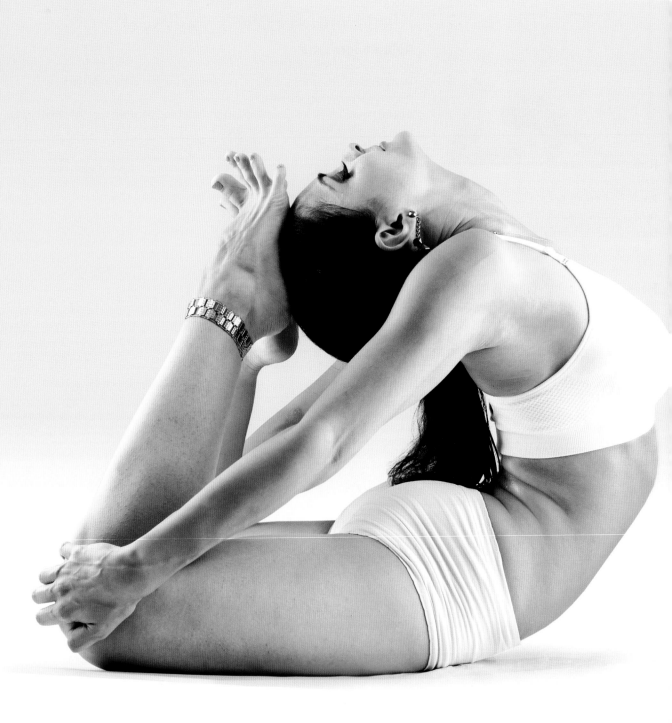

King Pigeon Pose

Raja Kapotasana

(RAH-juh kuh-po-TAHS-uh-nuh)
Pose Type: prone, backbend
Drishti Point: Bhrumadhye or Ajna Chakra (third eye, between the eyebrows)

Modification: grabbing onto the knees
1. feet to the head
2. feet to the shoulders

raja = king, royal
kapota = pigeon

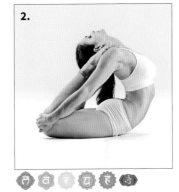

How to Perform the Pose:

1. Begin by lying flat on your stomach with your legs straight out behind you. Engage your *mula bandha*, *uddhiyana bandha*, and *ujjayi* breathing.

2. Exhale and bring your forearms to the floor with your shoulders on top of your elbows. Inhale, lengthen your neck, roll your shoulder blades down, and feel the backbend in your upper back.

3. On the next exhale, press strongly into your hands and straighten your arms. Walk your hands as close as you can toward you.

4. Exhale and bend both your knees, reaching your feet toward your head.

5. Inhale and shift your weight to your left hand. Exhale, bring your right arm behind you, and grab onto your right knee. On the next exhale, bring your left arm behind you and grab onto your left knee.

6. Exhale as you push through your chest, keeping the backbend in the upper back and pressing your feet to the crown of your head (Pose #1).

7. To deepen the pose, exhale and bring your feet to your shoulders (Pose #2).

8. Hold the pose for at least 30, and up to 90, seconds in order to receive the full benefits of the stretch.

9. Inhale as you release the pose, letting go of your knees. Bring your hands to the front and lower your chest and feet to the floor.

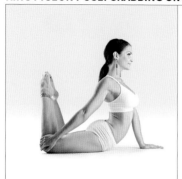

King Pigeon Pose Prep.

Raja Kapotasana Prep.

(RAH-juh kuh-po-TAHS-uh-nuh)

Modification: one hand to the floor, other hand grabbing onto the knee

Pose Type: prone, backbend

Drishti Point: Nasagrai or Nasagre (nose)

1.

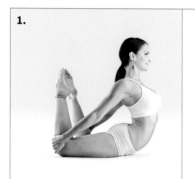

King Pigeon Pose Prep.

Raja Kapotasana Prep.

(RAH-juh kuh-po-TAHS-uh-nuh)

Modification: both hands grabbing onto the knees

1. looking straight ahead
2. head rolling back

Pose Type: prone, backbend

Drishti Point: 1. Nasagrai or Nasagre (nose)

2. Bhrumadhye or Ajna Chakra (third eye, between the eyebrows)

2.

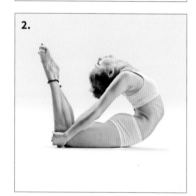

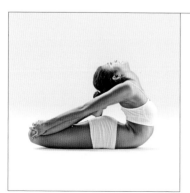

Feet to the Back King Pigeon Pose

Pada Paschima Raja Kapotasana

(PUH-duh PUHSH-chi-muh RAH-juh kuh-po-TAHS-uh-nuh)

Pose Type: prone, backbend

Drishti Point: Bhrumadhye or Ajna Chakra (third eye, between the eyebrows)

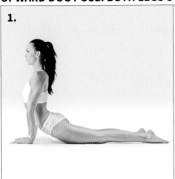

Upward Facing Dog Pose

Urdhva Mukha Shvanasana

(OORD-vuh MUK-uh shvuh-NAHS-uh-nuh)

Modification: toes pointed to the back, knees on the floor

1. looking straight ahead
2. head rolling back

Pose Type: prone, backbend

Drishti Point: Bhrumadhye or Ajna Chakra (third eye, between the eyebrows)

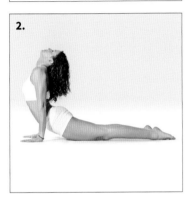

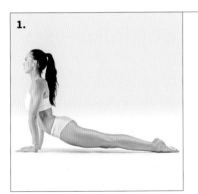

Upward Facing Dog Pose

Urdhva Mukha Shvanasana

(OORD-vuh MUK-uh shvuh-NAHS-uh-nuh)

Modification: toes pointed to the back, knees off the floor

1. looking straight ahead
2. head rolling back

Pose Type: prone, backbend

Drishti Point: Nasagrai or Nasagre (nose), Bhrumadhye or Ajna Chakra (third eye, between the eyebrows)

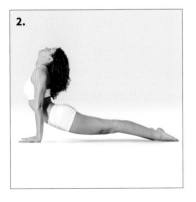

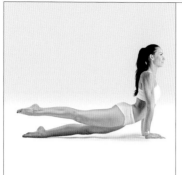

Uneven One-Legged Upward Facing Dog Pose

Vishama Eka Pada Urdhva Mukha Shvanasana

(VISH-uh-muh EY-kuh PUH-duh OORD-vuh MUK-uh shvuh-NAHS-uh-nuh)

Modification: both toes pointed

Pose Type: prone, backbend

Drishti Point: Bhrumadhye or Ajna Chakra (third eye, between the eyebrows)

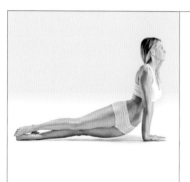

Sideways Upward Facing Dog Pose

Parshva Urdhva Mukha Shvanasana

(PAHRSH-vuh OORD-vuh MUK-uh shvuh-NAHS-uh-nuh)

Pose Type: prone, backbend, side bend

Drishti Point: Bhrumadhye or Ajna Chakra (third eye, between the eyebrows)

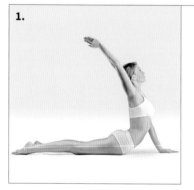

1.

One Hand Upward Facing Dog Pose

Eka Hasta Urdhva Mukha Shvanasana

(EY-kuh HUH-stuh OORD-vuh MUK-uh shvuh-NAHS-uh-nuh)

Modification: toes pointed to the back

1. knees on the floor

2. knees off the floor

Pose Type: prone, backbend

Drishti Point: Bhrumadhye or Ajna Chakra (third eye, between the eyebrows)

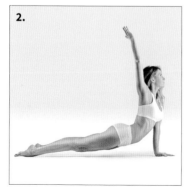

2.

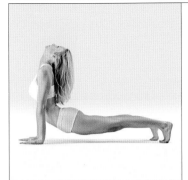

Upward Facing Dog Pose

Urdhva Mukha Shvanasana

(OORD-vuh MUK-uh shvuh-NAHS-uh-nuh)

Modification: toes curled in
Pose Type: prone, backbend
Drishti Point: Bhrumadhye or Ajna Chakra (third eye, between the eyebrows)

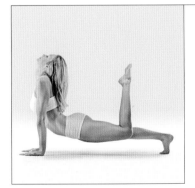

Sideways One-Legged Upward Facing Dog Pose

Parshva Eka Pada Urdhva Mukha Shvanasana

(PAHRSH-vuh EY-kuh PUH-duh OORD-vuh MUK-uh shvuh-NAHS-uh-nuh)

Modification: toes curled in
Pose Type: prone, backbend, twist
Drishti Point: Bhrumadhye or Ajna Chakra (third eye, between the eyebrows)

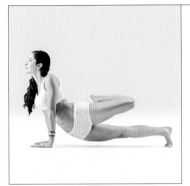

One-Legged Upward Facing Dog Pose

Eka Pada Urdhva Mukha Shvanasana

(EY-kuh PUH-duh OORD-vuh MUK-uh shvuh-NAHS-uh-nuh)

Modification: toes of the straight leg curled in; knee of the other leg bent, toes pointing up to the sky
Pose Type: prone, backbend
Drishti Point: Bhrumadhye or Ajna Chakra (third eye, between the eyebrows)

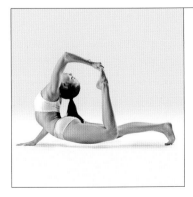

Half Big Toe Bow Pose in One-Legged Upward Facing Dog Pose

Ardha Padangushta Dhanurasana in Eka Pada Urdhva Mukha Shvanasana

(UHR-duh puhd-ahng-GOOSH-tuh duh-nur-AHS-uh-nuh in EY-kuh PUH-duh OORD-vuh MUK-uh shvuh-NAHS-uh-nuh)

Modification: grabbing onto the foot with overhead grip on the same side
Pose Type: prone, backbend
Drishti Point: Bhrumadhye or Ajna Chakra (third eye, between the eyebrows)

Prone Poses

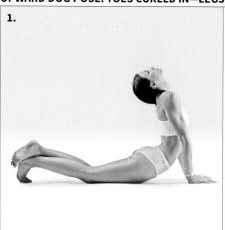

Upward Facing Dog Pose

Urdhva Mukha Shvanasana

(OORD-vuh MUK-uh shvuh-NAHS-uh-nuh)

Modification: toes curled in, ankles crossed

1. knees on the floor
2. knees off the floor, looking straight ahead
3. knees off the floor, head rolling back

Pose Type: prone, backbend

Drishti Point: Bhrumadhye or Ajna Chakra (third eye, between the eyebrows)

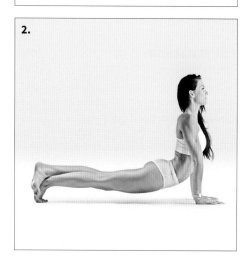

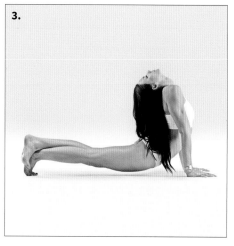

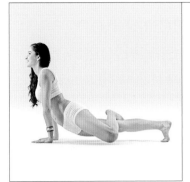

One-Legged Upward Facing Dog Pose

Eka Pada Urdhva Mukha Shvanasana

(EY-kuh PUH-duh OORD-vuh MUK-uh shvuh-NAHS-uh-nuh)

Modification: toes curled in, foot of the bent leg to the inside of the knee of the straight leg

Pose Type: prone, backbend

Drishti Point: Bhrumadhye or Ajna Chakra (third eye, between the eyebrows)

UPWARD DOG POSE: ONE LEG BENT

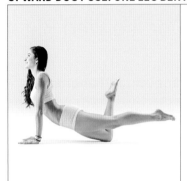

Uneven One-Legged Upward Facing Dog Pose

Vishama Eka Pada Urdhva Mukha Shvanasana

(VISH-uh-muh EY-kuh PUH-duh OORD-vuh MUK-uh shvuh-NAHS-uh-nuh)

Modification: Leg 1: knee bent and on the floor, toes pointed to the sky

Leg 2: straight and off the floor, toes pointed away

Pose Type: prone, backbend

Drishti Point: Bhrumadhye or Ajna Chakra (third eye, between the eyebrows)

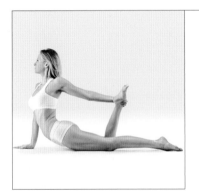

Half Bow Pose in One-Legged Upward Facing Dog Pose

Ardha Dhanurasana in Eka Pada Urdhva Mukha Shvanasana

(UHR-duh duh-nur-AHS-uh-nuh in EY-kuh PUH-duh OORD-vuh MUK-uh shvuh-NAHS-uh-nuh)

Modification: grabbing onto the opposite foot with under-head grip

Pose Type: prone, backbend

Drishti Point: Bhrumadhye or Ajna Chakra (third eye, between the eyebrows)

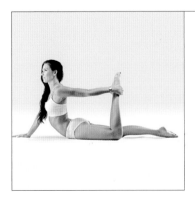

Half Bow Pose in One-Legged Upward Facing Dog Pose

Ardha Dhanurasana in Eka Pada Urdhva Mukha Shvanasana

(UHR-duh duh-nur-AHS-uh-nuh in EY-kuh PUH-duh OORD-vuh MUK-uh shvuh-NAHS-uh-nuh)

Modification: under-head grip on the same side

Pose Type: prone, backbend

Drishti Point: Nasagrai or Nasagre (nose), Bhrumadhye or Ajna Chakra (third eye, between the eyebrows)

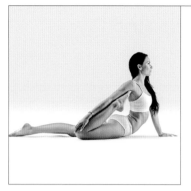

Half Pose Dedicated to Siddhar Konganar in One-Legged Upward Facing Dog Pose

Ardha Konganarasana in Eka Pada Urdhva Mukha Shvanasana

(UHR-duh kong-guh-nuh-RAHS-uh-nuh in EY-kuh PUH-duh OORD-vuh MUK-uh shvuh-NAHS-uh-nuh)

Modification: grabbing onto the knee with under-head grip on the same side—foot to the armpit

Pose Type: prone, backbend

Drishti Point: Nasagrai or Nasagre (nose), Bhrumadhye or Ajna Chakra (third eye, between the eyebrows)

COBRA POSE: UNDER-HEAD GRIP

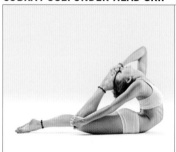

Half King Pigeon Pose in One-Legged Big Toe Bow Pose

Ardha Raja Kapotasana in Eka Pada Padangushta Dhanurasana

(UHR-duh RAH-juh kuh-po-TAHS-uh-nuh in EY-kuh PUH-duh puhd-ahng-GOOSH-tuh duh-nur-AHS-uh-nuh)

Modification: Hand 1: grabbing onto the knee on the same side.

Hand 2: grabbing onto the big toe of the opposite foot with overhead grip

Pose Type: prone, backbend

Drishti Point: Bhrumadhye or Ajna Chakra (third eye, between the eyebrows)

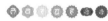

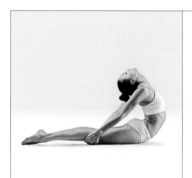

Cobra Pose

Bhujangasana

(buj-uhng-GAHS-uh-nuh)

Also Known As: Supported Cobra Pose (Alamba Bhujangasana), King Pigeon Pose Prep. (Raja Kapotasana Prep.)

Modification: grabbing onto the knees with under-head grip

Pose Type: prone, backbend

Drishti Point: Bhrumadhye or Ajna Chakra (third eye, between the eyebrows)

COBRA POSE: OVERHEAD GRIP

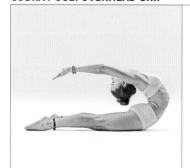

Upward Facing Unsupported Cobra Pose

Urdhva Mukha Niralamba Bhujangasana

(OORD-vuh MUK-uh nir-AH-luhm-buh buj-uhng-GAHS-uh-nuh)

Pose Type: prone, backbend

Drishti Point: Angushtamadhye or Angushta Ma Dyai (thumbs), Bhrumadhye or Ajna Chakra (third eye, between the eyebrows)

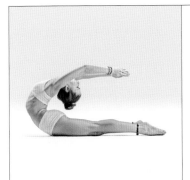

Unsupported Complete Cobra Pose

Niralamba Paripurna Bhujangasana

(nir-AH-luhm-buh puh-ri-POOR-nuh buj-uhng-GAHS-uh-nuh)

Pose Type: prone, backbend

Drishti Point: Angushtamadhye or Angushta Ma Dyai (thumbs), Bhrumadhye or Ajna Chakra (third eye, between the eyebrows)

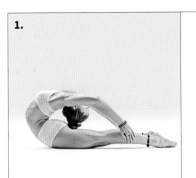

Complete Cobra Pose

Paripurna Bhujangasana

(puh-ri-POOR-nuh buj-uhng-GAHS-uh-nuh)

Modification: 1. grabbing onto the shins with overhead grip

2. grabbing onto the knees with overhead grip

3. grabbing onto the shins with overhead grip, toes curled in

Pose Type: prone, backbend

Drishti Point: Bhrumadhye or Ajna Chakra (third eye, between the eyebrows)

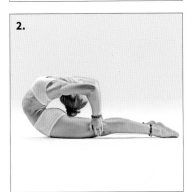

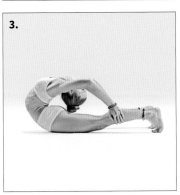

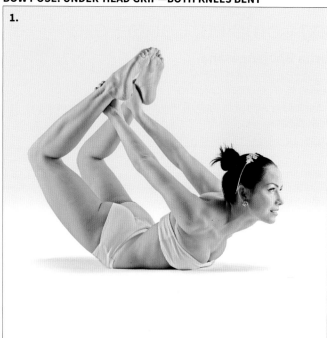

1.

Bow Pose

Dhanurasana

(duh-nur-AHS-uh-nuh)

Modification: hands grabbing onto the ankles

1. on the inside of the ankles
2. on the outside of the ankles

Pose Type: prone, backbend

Drishti Point: Bhrumadhye or Ajna Chakra (third eye, between the eyebrows)

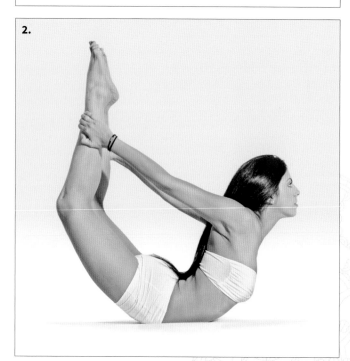

2.

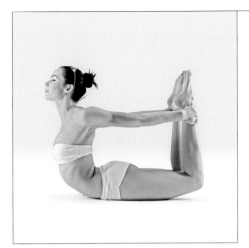

Bow Pose

Dhanurasana

(duh-nur-AHS-uh-nuh)

Modification: legs bent at 90 degrees; ankles and knees together, toes pointed to the sky

Pose Type: prone, backbend

Drishti Point: Bhrumadhye or Ajna Chakra (third eye, between the eyebrows)

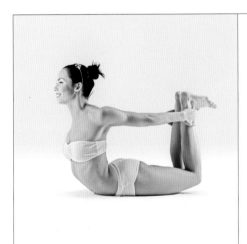

Bow Pose

Dhanurasana

(duh-nur-AHS-uh-nuh)

Modification: legs bent at 90 degrees; ankles and knees together, toes flexed away from the head

Pose Type: prone, backbend

Drishti Point: Bhrumadhye or Ajna Chakra (third eye, between the eyebrows), Nasagrai or Nasagre (nose)

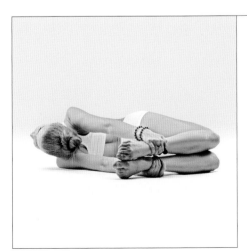

Sideways Bow Pose

Parshva Dhanurasana

(PAHRSH-vuh duh-nur-AHS-uh-nuh)

Pose Type: supine, prone, backbend

Drishti Point: Bhrumadhye or Ajna Chakra (third eye, between the eyebrows)

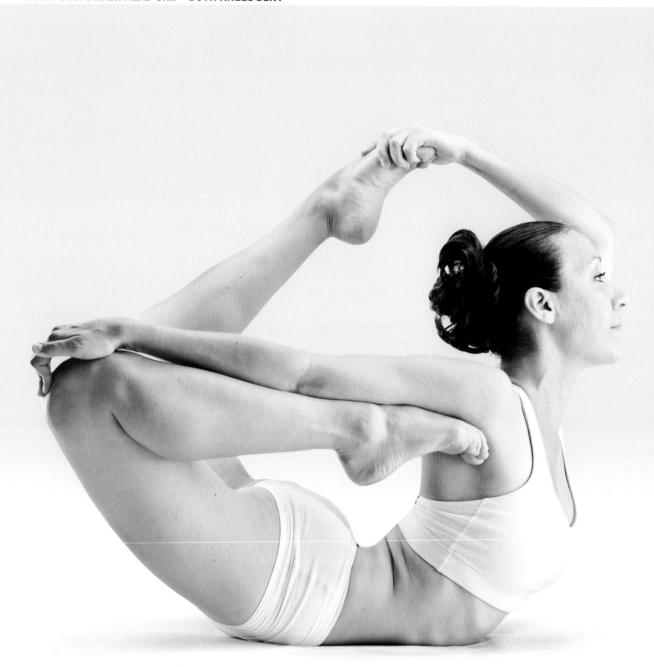

One-Legged
Pose Dedicated to Siddhar Konganar

Eka Pada Konganarasana
(EY-kuh PUH-duh kong-guh-nuh-RAHS-uh-nuh)
Pose Type: prone, backbend
Drishti Point: Nasagrai or Nasagre (nose) or Bhrumadhye or Ajna Chakra (third eye, between the eyebrows)

eka = one
pada = foot or leg
Konganar = one of the Siddhars

How to Perform the Pose:

1. Begin by lying flat on your stomach with your legs straight out behind you. Engage your *mula bandha*, *uddhiyana bandha*, and *ujjayi* breathing.

2. Exhale and bring your forearms to the floor with your shoulders on top of your elbows. Inhale, lengthen your neck, roll your shoulder blades down, and feel the backbend in your upper back.

3. On the next exhale, press strongly into your hands and straighten your arms.

4. Exhale and bend both your knees, reaching your feet toward your head.

5. On the next exhale, reach your right hand behind you and grab onto your right shin. Keep sliding your right hand until your right foot reaches your right armpit and your right hand rests on your right knee.

6. Inhale and reach your left arm up and over your head. Exhale and grab onto your left foot with your left hand, keeping your left elbow close to your ear.

7. Hold the pose for at least 30, and up to 90, seconds in order to receive the full benefits of the stretch.

8. Inhale, let go of your legs one by one, and lower your chest and feet to the floor to come back to the starting position. Repeat on the opposite side.

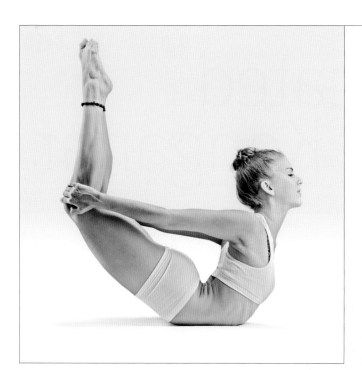

Little Bow Pose

Laghu Dhanurasana

(LUH-gu duh-nur-AHS-uh-nuh)

Pose Type: prone, backbend

Drishti Point: Nasagrai or Nasagre (nose), Bhrumadhye or Ajna Chakra (third eye, between the eyebrows)

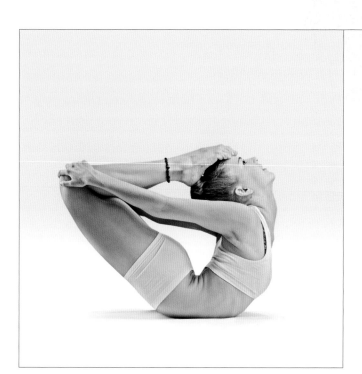

Feet to the Head Little Bow Pose

Shirsha Pada Laghu Dhanurasana

(SHEER-suh PUH-duh LUH-gu duh-nur-AHS-uh-nuh)

Pose Type: prone, backbend

Drishti Point: Bhrumadhye or Ajna Chakra (third eye, between the eyebrows)

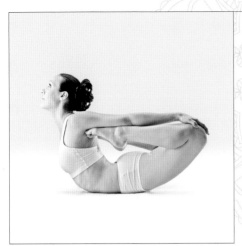

Pose Dedicated to Siddhar Konganar

Konganarasana

(kong-guh-nuh-RAHS-uh-nuh)
Pose Type: prone, backbend
Drishti Point: Bhrumadhye or Ajna Chakra (third eye, between the eyebrows)

BOW POSE: OVERHEAD GRIP—BOTH KNEES BENT

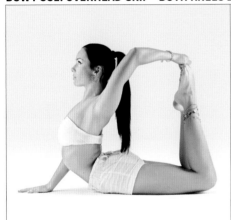

One Hand Both Feet Big Toe Bow Pose

Eka Hasta Dwi Pada Padangushta Dhanurasana

(EY-kuh HUH-stuh DWI-puh-duh puhd-ahng-GOOSH-tuh duh-nur-AHS-uh-nuh)
Modification: grabbing onto the toes of both feet with one hand, other palm to the floor
Pose Type: prone, backbend
Drishti Point: Bhrumadhye or Ajna Chakra (third eye, between the eyebrows)

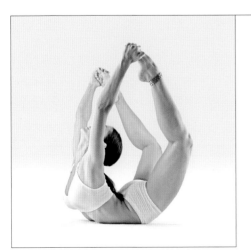

Big Toe Bow Pose

Padangushta Dhanurasana

(puhd-ahng-GOOSH-tuh duh-nur-AHS-uh-nuh)
Modification: head rolling back
Pose Type: prone, backbend
Drishti Point: Bhrumadhye or Ajna Chakra (third eye, between the eyebrows)

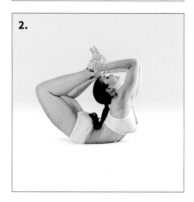

Big Toe Bow Pose

Padangushta Dhanurasana

(puhd-ahng-GOOSH-tuh duh-nur-AHS-uh-nuh)

Modification: 1. feet to the face

2. heels to the forehead

Pose Type: prone, backbend

Drishti Point: Bhrumadhye or Ajna Chakra (third eye, between the eyebrows)

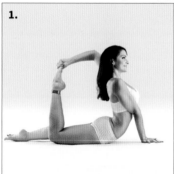

BOW POSE: OVERHEAD GRIP—ONE KNEE BENT, ONE LEG STRAIGHT

One Hand One-Legged Big Toe Bow Pose

Eka Hasta Eka Pada Padangushta Dhanurasana

(EY-kuh HUH-stuh EY-kuh PUH-duh puhd-ahng-GOOSH-tuh duh-nur-AHS-uh-nuh)

Modification: 1. one hand grabbing onto the foot on the opposite side with overhead grip

2. with backbend

Pose Type: prone, backbend

Drishti Point: Nasagrai or Nasagre (nose), Bhrumadhye or Ajna Chakra (third eye, between the eyebrows)

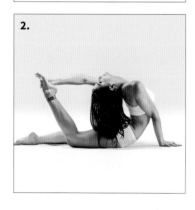

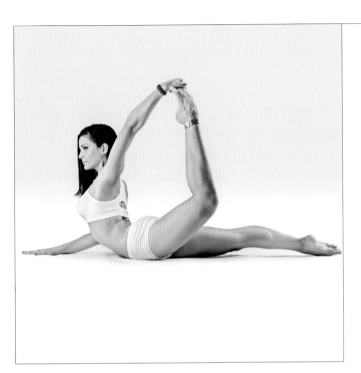

One Hand One-Legged Big Toe Bow Pose

Eka Hasta Eka Pada Padangushta Dhanurasana

(EY-kuh HUH-stuh PUH-duh puhd-ahng-GOOSH-tuh duh-nur-AHS-uh-nuh)

Modification: one hand grabbing onto the foot on the same side with overhead grip

Pose Type: prone, backbend

Drishti Point: Nasagrai or Nasagre (nose), Bhrumadhye or Ajna Chakra (third eye, between the eyebrows)

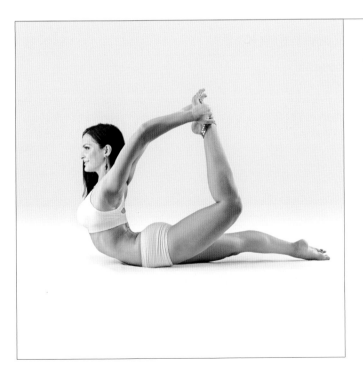

Both Hand One-Legged Big Toe Bow Pose

Dwi Hasta Eka Pada Padangushta Dhanurasana

(DWI-huh-stuh EY-kuh PUH-duh puhd-ahng-GOOSH-tuh duh-nur-AHS-uh-nuh)

Modification: both hands grabbing onto the foot with overhead grip

Pose Type: prone, backbend

Drishti Point: Nasagrai or Nasagre (nose), Bhrumadhye or Ajna Chakra (third eye, between the eyebrows)

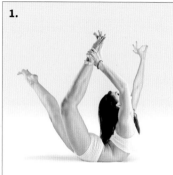

Pose Dedicated to Goddess Kamala

Kamalasana

(kuh-muh-LAHS-uh-nuh)

Also Known As: Upward Facing One-Handed Big Toe Boat Pose (Urdhva Mukha Eka Hasta Padangushta Navasana)

Modification: 1: grabbing onto the ankle

2. foot to the shoulder

Pose Type: prone, backbend

Drishti Point: Bhrumadhye or Ajna Chakra (third eye, between the eyebrows)

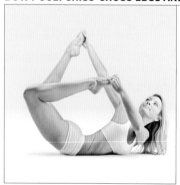

Revolved Bow Pose

Parivritta Dhanurasana

(puh-ri-VRIT-tuh duh-nur-AHS-uh-nuh)

Pose Type: prone, backbend, twist

Drishti Point: Bhrumadhye or Ajna Chakra (third eye, between the eyebrows), Padhayora-grai or Padayoragre (toes/feet)

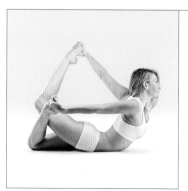

Bow Pose

Dhanurasana

(duh-nur-AHS-uh-nuh)

Modification: legs crossed

Pose Type: prone, backbend

Drishti Point: Bhrumadhye or Ajna Chakra (third eye, between the eyebrows)

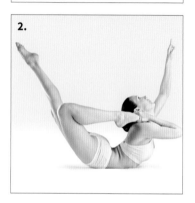

1.

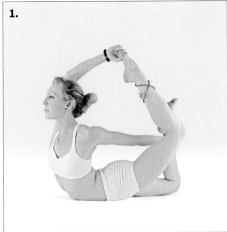

Big Toe Bow Pose

Padangushta Dhanurasana

(puhd-ahng-GOOSH-tuh duh-nur-AHS-uh-nuh)

Also Known As: Difficult Bow Pose (Dur Dhanurasana)

Modification: one hand grabbing opposite ankle with under-head grip, other hand grabbing the opposite foot with overhead grip

1. one knee on the floor
2. both knees off the floor

Pose Type: prone, backbend

Drishti Point: Nasagrai or Nasagre (nose), Bhrumadhye or Ajna Chakra (third eye, between the eyebrows)

2.

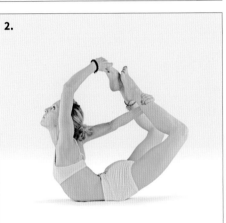

Big Toe Bow Pose

Padangushta Dhanurasana

(puhd-ahng-GOOSH-tuh duh-nur-AHS-uh-nuh)

Modification: one foot toward the shoulder

Pose Type: prone, backbend

Drishti Point: Bhrumadhye or Ajna Chakra (third eye, between the eyebrows)

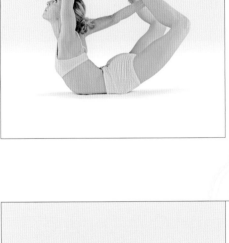

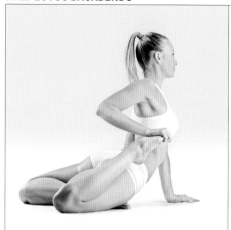

Half Lotus Frog Pose

Ardha Padma Bhekasana

(UHR-duh PUHD-muh bey-KAHS-uh-nuh)

Pose Type: prone, backbend

Drishti Point: Bhrumadhye or Ajna Chakra (third eye, between the eyebrows)

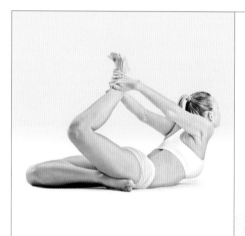

Half Lotus Bow Pose

Ardha Padma Dhanurasana

(UHR-duh PUHD-muh duh-nur-AHS-uh-nuh)

Modification: both hands grabbing onto the ankle with under-head grip

Pose Type: prone, backbend

Drishti Point: Bhrumadhye or Ajna Chakra (third eye, between the eyebrows)

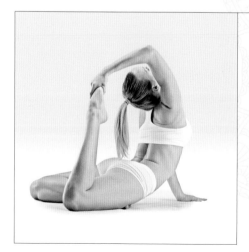

Half Lotus One Hand One-Legged Big Toe Bow Pose

Ardha Padma Eka Hasta Eka Pada Padangushta Dhanurasana

(UHR-duh PUHD-muh EY-kuh HUH-stuh EY-kuh PUH-duh puhd-ahng-GOOSH-tuh duh-nur-AHS-uh-nuh)

Modification: grabbing onto the foot with overhead grip on the same side, other hand to the floor

Pose Type: prone, backbend

Drishti Point: Bhrumadhye or Ajna Chakra (third eye, between the eyebrows)

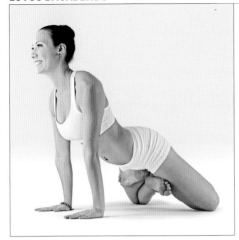

Lotus Cobra Pose

Padma Bhujangasana

(PUHD-muh buj-uhng-GAHS-uh-nuh)

Modification: both hands to the floor, hips off the floor, arms straight
Pose Type: prone, backbend
Drishti Point: Bhrumadhye or Ajna Chakra (third eye, between the eyebrows)

1.

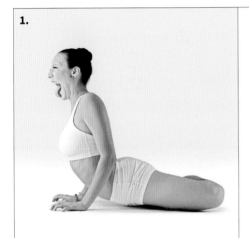

Lion Pose Dedicated to an Avatar of Lord Vishnu

Narasimhasana

(nuh-ruh-sim-HAHS-uh-nuh)

Also Known As: Lion Pose (Simhasana)
Modification: full lotus leg position
1. elbows bent, fingers in lion claw
2. arms straight, palms flat on the floor
Pose Type: prone, backbend
Drishti Point: Bhrumadhye or Ajna Chakra (third eye, between the eyebrows)

2.

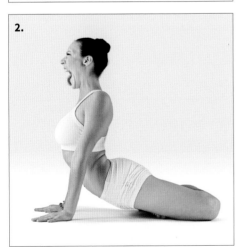

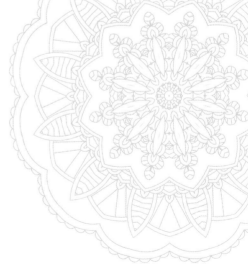

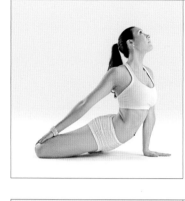

One Hand Lotus Cobra Pose

Eka Hasta Padma Bhujangasana

(EY-kuh HUH-stuh PUHD-muh buj-uhng-GAHS-uh-nuh)

Pose Type: prone, backbend

Drishti Point: Bhrumadhye or Ajna Chakra (third eye, between the eyebrows)

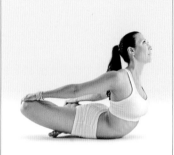

Lotus Cobra Pose

Padma Bhujangasana

(PUHD-muh buj-uhng-GAHS-uh-nuh)

Pose Type: prone, backbend

Drishti Point: Bhrumadhye or Ajna Chakra (third eye, between the eyebrows)

SAGE GHERANDA'S POSE: UNDER-HEAD GRIP

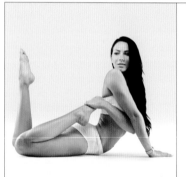

Revolved Pose Dedicated to Sage Gheranda 1

Parivritta Ardha Gherandasana 1

(puh-ri-VRIT-tuh UHR-duh gey-ruhn-DAHS-uh-nuh)

Pose Type: prone, backbend, twist

Drishti Point: Parshva Drishti (to the right), Parshva Drishti (to the left)

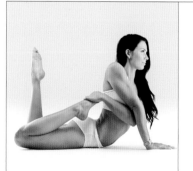

Half Pose Dedicated to Sage Gheranda 1

Ardha Gherandasana 1

(UHR-duh gey-ruhn-DAHS-uh-nuh)

Pose Type: prone, backbend

Drishti Point: Nasagrai or Nasagre (nose)

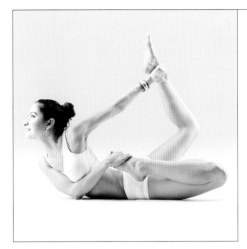

Pose Dedicated to Sage Gheranda 5B

Gherandasana 5 B

(gey-ruhn-DAHS-uh-nuh)

Modification: under-head grip, grabbing onto the ankle, elbow on the floor instead of the forearm
Pose Type: prone, backbend, twist
Drishti Point: Bhrumadhye or Ajna Chakra (third eye, between the eyebrows)

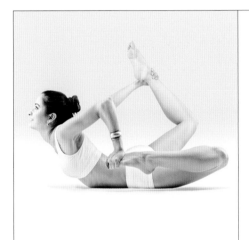

Pose Dedicated to Sage Gheranda 1B

Gherandasana 1 B

(gey-ruhn-DAHS-uh-nuh)

Modification: under-head grip
Pose Type: prone, backbend
Drishti Point: Bhrumadhye or Ajna Chakra (third eye, between the eyebrows)

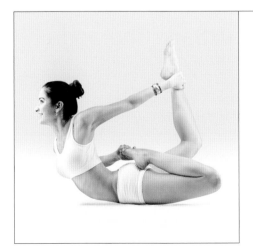

Pose Dedicated to Sage Gheranda 6

Gherandasana 6

(gey-ruhn-DAHS-uh-nuh)

Modification: under-head grip
Pose Type: prone, backbend, binding
Drishti Point: Bhrumadhye or Ajna Chakra (third eye, between the eyebrows)

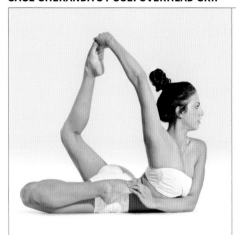

Pose Dedicated to Sage Gheranda 5

Gherandasana 5

(gey-ruhn-DAHS-uh-nuh)

Pose Type: prone, backbend, binding

Drishti Point: Nasagrai or Nasagre (nose), Bhrumadhye or Ajna Chakra (third eye, between the eyebrows)

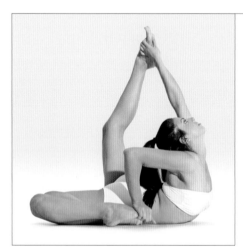

Pose Dedicated to Sage Gheranda 1

Gherandasana 1

(gey-ruhn-DAHS-uh-nuh)

Pose Type: prone, backbend

Drishti Point: Bhrumadhye or Ajna Chakra (third eye, between the eyebrows)

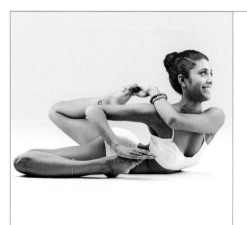

Pose Dedicated to Sage Gheranda 2

Gherandasana 2

(gey-ruhn-DAHS-uh-nuh)

Pose Type: prone, backbend, binding

Drishti Point: Bhrumadhye or Ajna Chakra (third eye, between the eyebrows)

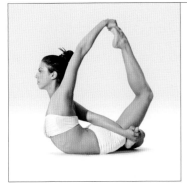

Pose Dedicated to Sage Gheranda 3

Gherandasana 3

(gey-ruhn-DAHS-uh-nuh)
Pose Type: prone, backbend, binding
Drishti Point: Nasagrai or Nasagre (nose), Bhrumadhye or Ajna Chakra (third eye, between the eyebrows)

Pose Dedicated to Sage Gheranda 4

Gherandasana 4

(gey-ruhn-DAHS-uh-nuh)
Modification: 1. back view
2. front view
Pose Type: prone, backbend, binding, twist
Drishti Point: Bhrumadhye or Ajna Chakra (third eye, between the eyebrows)

1.

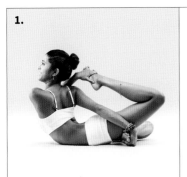

2.

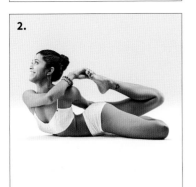

BACKBENDS: GARUDA LEGS: UNDER-HEAD GRIP

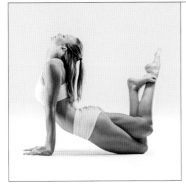

Twined Legs Cobra Pose

Parivitta Pada Bhujangasana

(puh-ri-VRIT-tuh PUH-duh buj-uhng-GAHS-uh-nuh)
Pose Type: prone, backbend
Drishti Point: Bhrumadhye or Ajna Chakra (third eye, between the eyebrows)

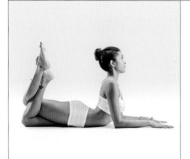

Supported Twined Legs Cobra Pose

Salamba Parivid Pada Bhujangasana

(SAH-luhm-buh PUH-ri-vid PUH-duh buj-uhng-GAHS-uh-nuh)

Also Known As: Supported Twined Legs Sphinx Pose
Pose Type: prone, backbend
Drishti Point: Bhrumadhye or Ajna Chakra (third eye, between the eyebrows)

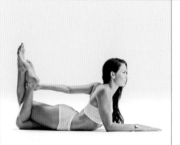

Leg Position of the Pose Dedicated to Garuda in One Hand Bow Pose

Pada Garudasana in Eka Hasta Dhanurasana

(PUH-duh guh-ru-DAHS-uh-nuh in EY-kuh HUH-stuh duh-nur-AHS-uh-nuh)

Modification: one forearm to the floor, one hand to the ankle, under-head grip
Pose Type: prone, backbend
Drishti Point: Bhrumadhye or Ajna Chakra (third eye, between the eyebrows)

BACKBENDS: GARUDA LEGS: OVERHEAD GRIP

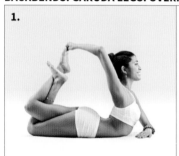

1.

Leg Position of the Pose Dedicated to Garuda in One Hand Big Toe Bow Pose

Pada Garudasana in Eka Hasta Padangushta Dhanurasana

(PUH-duh guh-ru-DAHS-uh-nuh in EY-kuh HUH-stuh puhd-ahng-GOOSH-tuh duh-nur-AHS-uh-nuh)

Modification: forearm to the floor
1. grabbing onto the top foot
2. grabbing onto the bottom foot
Pose Type: prone, backbend
Drishti Point: Bhrumadhye or Ajna Chakra (third eye, between the eyebrows)

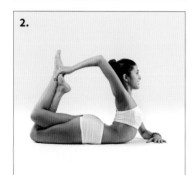

2.

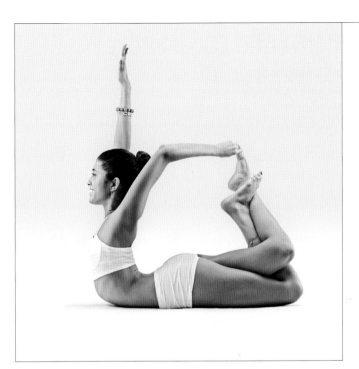

Unsupported Leg Position of the Pose Dedicated to Garuda in One Hand Big Toe Bow Pose

Niralamba Pada Garudasana in Eka Hasta Padangushta Dhanurasana

(nir-AH-luhm-buh puh-ri-vid-PUH-duh guh-ru-DAHS-uh-nuh in EY-kuh HUH-tuh puhd-ahng-GOOSH-tuh duh-nur-AHS-uh-nuh)

Also Known As: One Handed Twined Legs Bow Pose (Eka Hasta Parivid Pada Dhanurasana)

Pose Type: prone, backbend

Drishti Point: Bhrumadhye or Ajna Chakra (third eye, between the eyebrows)

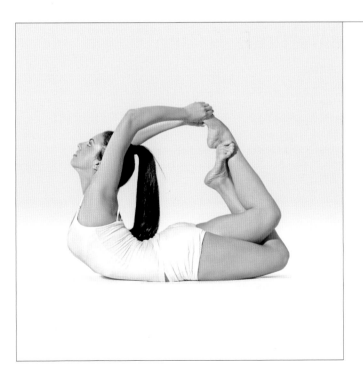

Leg Position of the Pose Dedicated to Garuda in Big Toe Bow Pose

Pada Garudasana in Padangushta Dhanurasana

(PUH-duh guh-ru-DAHS-uh-nuh in puhd-ahng-GOOSH-tuh duh-nur-AHS-uh-nuh)

Also Known As: Difficult Bow Pose (Dur Dhanurasana)

Pose Type: prone, backbend

Drishti Point: Bhrumadhye or Ajna Chakra (third eye, between the eyebrows)

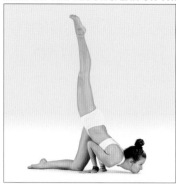

One-Legged Inverted Locust Pose

Eka Pada Viparita Shalabhasana

(EY-kuh PUH-duh vi-puh-REE-tuh shuh-luh-BAHS-uh-nuh)

Pose Type: prone, backbend, inversion

Drishti Point: Bhrumadhye or Ajna Chakra (third eye, between the eyebrows)

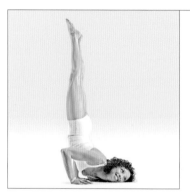

Ear Pressure Staff Formidable Face Pose

Karnapida Danda Ganda Bherundasana

(kuhr-nah-PEED-uh DUHN-duh GUHN-duh bey-run-DAHS-uh-nuh)

Pose Type: prone, backbend, inversion

Drishti Point: Bhrumadhye or Ajna Chakra (third eye, between the eyebrows)

CHEST ON THE FLOOR: BOTH LEGS STRAIGHT

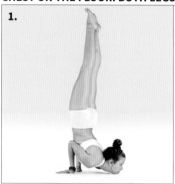
1.

Inverted Locust Pose

Viparita Shalabhasana

(vi-puh-REE-tuh shuh-luh-BAHS-uh-nuh)

Modification: 1. chin to the floor

2. chest to the floor, chin lifted off the floor

Pose Type: prone, backbend, inversion

Drishti Point: Bhrumadhye or Ajna Chakra (third eye, between the eyebrows)

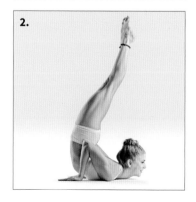
2.

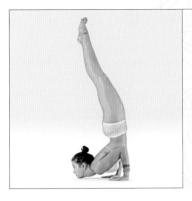

Formidable Face Staff Pose

Danda Ganda Bherundasana

(DUHN-duh GUHN-duh bey-run-DAHS-uh-nuh)

Also Known As: Intense Stretch Locust Pose A (Uttana Shalabhasana A)

Pose Type: prone, backbend, inversion

Drishti Point: Bhrumadhye or Ajna Chakra (third eye, between the eyebrows)

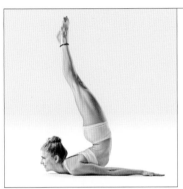

Inverted Locust Pose

Viparita Shalabhasana

(vi-puh-REE-tuh shuh-luh-BAHS-uh-nuh)

Also Known As: Raised Locust Pose—Urdhva Shalabhasana)

Modification: arms straight on the floor, palms down, chin lifted off the floor

Pose Type: prone, backbend, inversion

Drishti Point: Bhrumadhye or Ajna Chakra (third eye, between the eyebrows)

CHEST ON THE FLOOR: BOTH FEET TO HEAD

1.

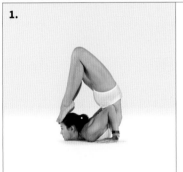

Formidable Face Pose

Ganda Bherundasana

(GUHN-duh bey-run-DAHS-uh-nuh)

Also Known As: Full Locust Pose (Purna Shalabhasana), Intense Stretch Locust Pose B (Uttana Shalabhasana B)

Modification: fingers pointing to the front of the body, feet to the head, chest on the floor

1. side view
2. front view

Pose Type: prone, backbend, inversion

Drishti Point: Bhrumadhye or Ajna Chakra (third eye, between the eyebrows)

2.

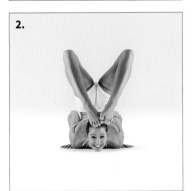

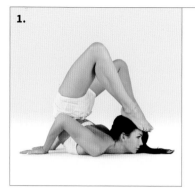

1.

Formidable Face Pose

Ganda Bherundasana

(GUHN-duh bey-run-DAHS-uh-nuh)

Modification: fingers pointing to the back

1. knees apart
2. knees together, chin lifted off the floor

Pose Type: prone, backbend, inversion

Drishti Point: Bhrumadhye or Ajna Chakra (third eye, between the eyebrows)

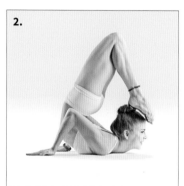

2.

Inverted Locust Pose

Viparita Shalabhasana

(vi-puh-REE-tuh shuh-luh-BAHS-uh-nuh)

Also Known As: Full Locust Pose (Purna Shalabhasana)

Modification: arms straight on the floor, palms down; feet to the head

Pose Type: prone, backbend, inversion

Drishti Point: Bhrumadhye or Ajna Chakra (third eye, between the eyebrows)

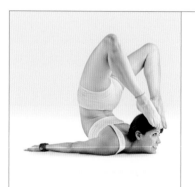

Formidable Face Pose

Ganda Bherundasana

(GUHN-duh bey-run-DAHS-uh-nuh)

Modification: feet to the head, grabbing onto both feet, chin off the floor

Pose Type: prone, backbend, inversion

Drishti Point: Bhrumadhye or Ajna Chakra (third eye, between the eyebrows)

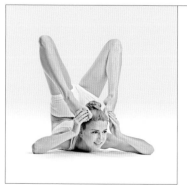

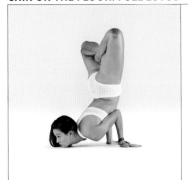

Inverted Lotus Peacock Pose

Viparita Padma Mayurasana

(vi-puh-REE-tuh PUHD-muh muh-yoor-AHS-uh-nuh)

Pose Type: prone, backbend, inversion

Drishti Point: Bhrumadhye or Ajna Chakra (third eye, between the eyebrows)

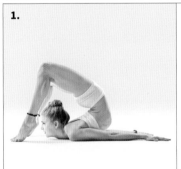

Inverted Locust Pose with Lotus Legs

Padma Viparita Shalabhasana

(PUHD-muh vi-puh-REE-tuh shuh-luh-BAHS-uh-nuh)

Pose Type: prone, backbend, inversion

Drishti Point: Bhrumadhye or Ajna Chakra (third eye, between the eyebrows)

CHEST ON THE FLOOR: FEET TO THE FLOOR

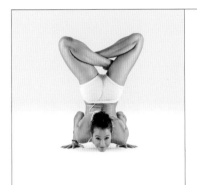

1.

Inverted Locust Pose

Viparita Shalabhasana

(vi-puh-REE-tuh shuh-luh-BAHS-uh-nuh)

Modification: arms straight on the floor, palms down; feet toward the floor over the head, legs bent

1. heels up

2. heels down

Pose Type: prone, backbend, inversion

Drishti Point: Bhrumadhye or Ajna Chakra (third eye, between the eyebrows)

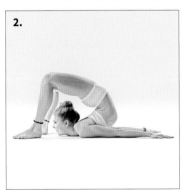

2.

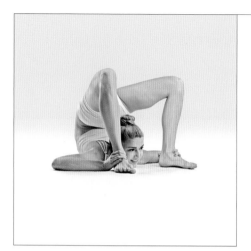

Formidable Face Pose

Ganda Bherundasana

(GUHN-duh bey-run-DAHS-uh-nuh)

Modification: feet on the floor, grabbing onto both ankles, chin off the floor
Pose Type: prone, backbend, inversion
Drishti Point: Bhrumadhye or Ajna Chakra (third eye, between the eyebrows)

CHEST AND KNEES ON THE FLOOR: KNEES UNDER THE HIPS

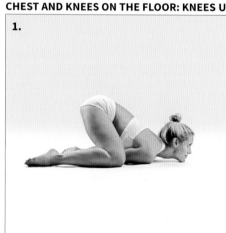

1.

Intense Extended Puppy Dog Pose

Uttana Shvanakasana

(ut-TAHN-uh shvuh-nuh-KAHS-uh-nuh)

Also Known As: Heart Pose (Anahatasana Modification), Extended Dog Pose
(Utthita Shvanasana)
Modification: 1. palms down to the floor
 2. grabbing onto the heels
Pose Type: prone, backbend
Drishti Point: Bhrumadhye or Ajna Chakra (third eye, between the eyebrows)

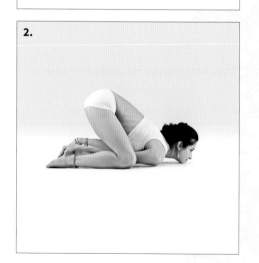

2.

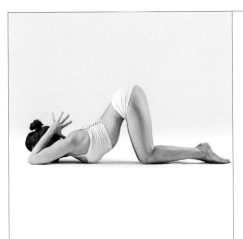

Intense Extended Puppy Dog Pose

Uttana Shvanakasana

(ut-TAHN-uh shvuh-nuh-KAHS-uh-nuh)

Also Known As: Prayer Heart Pose (Namaskar Anahatasana), Extended Dog Pose (Utthita Shvanasana)
Modification: thumbs to the upper back
Pose Type: prone, backbend
Drishti Point: Bhrumadhye or Ajna Chakra (third eye, between the eyebrows)

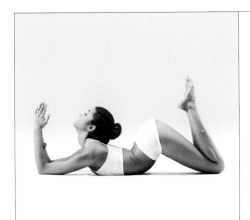

Water Grove Pose

Nirakunjasana

(neer-uh--kunj-AHS-uh-nuh)

Also Known As: Heart Pose (Anahatasana Modification)
Modification: arms in front, elbows bent; palms together; chin off the floor; heels toward the sitting bones
Pose Type: prone, backbend
Drishti Point: Bhrumadhye or Ajna Chakra (third eye, between the eyebrows), Angushtamadhye or Angushta Ma Dyai (thumbs)

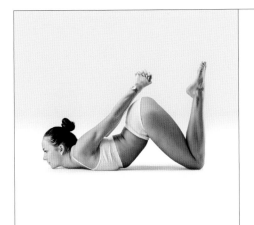

Hands Bound Water Grove Pose

Baddha Hasta Nirakunjasana

(BUH-duh HUH-stuh neer-uh-kunj-AHS-uh-nuh)

Also Known As: Heart Pose (Anahatasana Modification)
Modification: heels toward the sitting bones
Pose Type: prone, backbend
Drishti Point: Bhrumadhye or Ajna Chakra (third eye, between the eyebrows)

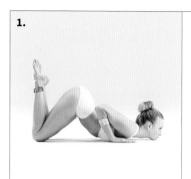

Pose Dedicated to Goddess Arani Prep.

Aranyasana Prep.

(uh-rah-NYAHS-uh-nuh)

Also Known As: Dragon Pose

Modification: 1. hands underneath the shoulders, elbows tucked in

2. arms reaching toward the knees, palms up

Pose Type: prone, backbend

Drishti Point: Bhrumadhye or Ajna Chakra (third eye, between the eyebrows)

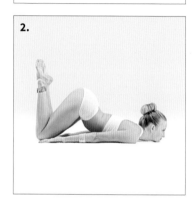

Pose Dedicated to Goddess Arani

Aranyasana

(uh-rah-NYAHS-uh-nuh)

Also Known As: Dragon Pose

Modification: 1. grabbing onto the shins

2. grabbing onto the hamstrings

Pose Type: prone, backbend

Drishti Point: Bhrumadhye or Ajna Chakra (third eye, between the eyebrows)

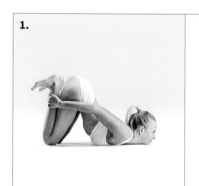

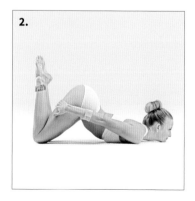

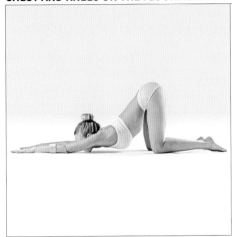

Intense Extended Puppy Dog Pose

Uttana Shvanakasana

(ut-TAHN-uh shvuh-nuh-KAHS-uh-nuh)

Also Known As: Heart Pose (Anahatasana Modification), Extended Dog Pose (Utthita Shvanasana)

Modification: arms extended to the front

Pose Type: prone, backbend

Drishti Point: Bhrumadhye or Ajna Chakra (third eye, between the eyebrows), Angushtamadhye or Angushta Ma Dyai (thumbs)

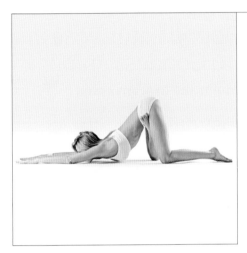

Half Lotus Intense Extended Puppy Dog Pose

Ardha Padma Uttana Shvanakasana

(UHR-duh PUHD-muh ut-TAHN-uh shvuh-nuh-KAHS-uh-nuh)

Also Known As: Half Lotus Heart Pose (Ardha Padma Anahatasana), Half Lotus Extended Dog Pose (Ardha Padma Utthita Shvanasana)

Pose Type: prone, backbend

Drishti Point: Bhrumadhye or Ajna Chakra (third eye, between the eyebrows), Angushtamadhye or Angushta Ma Dyai (thumbs)

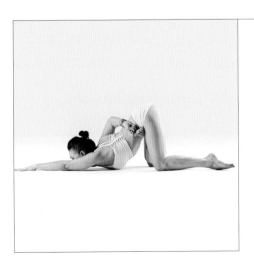

Half Bound Lotus Intense Extended Puppy Dog Pose

Ardha Baddha Padma Uttana Shvanakasana

(UHR-duh BUH-duh PUHD-muh ut-TAHN-uh shvuh-nuh-KAHS-uh-nuh)

Also Known As: Half Bound Lotus Heart Pose (Ardha Baddha Padma Anahatasana), Half Bound Lotus Extended Dog Pose (Ardha Baddha Padma Utthita Shvanasana)

Pose Type: prone, backbend, binding

Drishti Point: Bhrumadhye or Ajna Chakra (third eye, between the eyebrows), Angushtamadhye or Angushta Ma Dyai (thumbs)

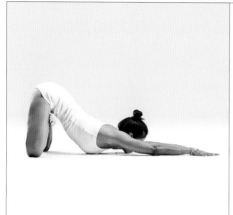

Lotus Intense Extended Puppy Dog Pose

Padma Uttana Shvanakasana

(PUHD-muh ut-TAHN-uh shvuh-nuh-KAHS-uh-nuh)

Also Known As: Lotus Heart Pose (Padma Anahatasana), Lotus Extended Dog Pose (Padma Utthita Shvanasana)

Pose Type: prone, backbend

Drishti Point: Bhrumadhye or Ajna Chakra (third eye, between the eyebrows), Angushtamadhye or Angushta Ma Dyai (thumbs)

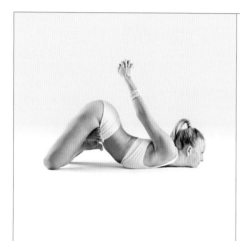

Upward Hands Bound Lotus Pose in Pose Dedicated to Goddess Arani

Urdhva Baddha Hasta Padmasana in Aranyasana

(OORD-vuh BUH-duh HUH-stuh puhd-MAHS-uh-nuh in uh-rah-NYAHS-uh-nuh)

Also Known As: Dragon Pose, Upward Bound Hand Lotus Heart Pose (Urdhva Baddha Hasta Padma Anahatasana)

Pose Type: prone, backbend

Drishti Point: Bhrumadhye or Ajna Chakra (third eye, between the eyebrows)

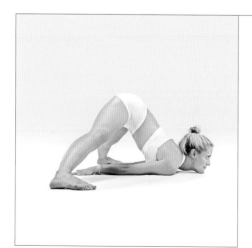

Feet Spread Wide Pose in Inverted Locust Pose

Prasarita Padottanasana in Viparita Shalabhasana

(pruh-SAH-ri-tuh puh-do-tahn-AHS-uh-nuh in vi-puh-REE-tuh shuh-luh-BAHS-uh-nuh)

Pose Type: prone, backbend

Drishti Point: Bhrumadhye or Ajna Chakra (third eye, between the eyebrows)

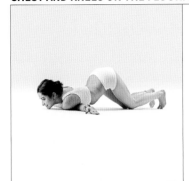

Water Grove Pose

Nirakunjasana

(neer-uh-kunj-AHS-uh-nuh)

Also Known As: Heart Pose (Anahatasana Modification)
Modification: arms straight and crossed in front
Pose Type: prone, backbend
Drishti Point: Bhrumadhye or Ajna Chakra (third eye, between the eyebrows)

1.

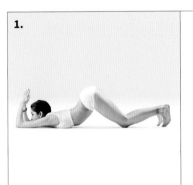

Water Grove Pose

Nirakunjasana

(neer-uh-kunj-AHS-uh-nuh)

Also Known As: Heart Pose (Anahatasana Modification)
Modification: chin and feet on the floor
1. knees on the floor
2. knees off the floor
Pose Type: prone, backbend
Drishti Point: Bhrumadhye or Ajna Chakra (third eye, between the eyebrows)

2.

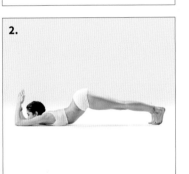

Eight Limbs Pose

Ashtangasana

(uhsh-tahng-AHS-uh-nuh)

Also Known As: Eight Point Bow Pose (Ashtanga Namaskara)
Pose Type: prone, backbend
Drishti Point: Bhrumadhye or Ajna Chakra (third eye, between the eyebrows)

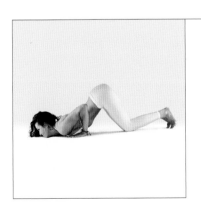

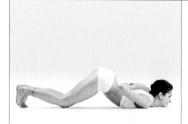

Reverse Prayer Water Grove Pose

Viparita Namaskar Nirakunjasana

(vi-puh-REE-tuh nuh-muhs-KAHR neer-uh-kunj-AHS-uh-nuh)

Also Known As: Back of the Body Prayer Water Grove Pose (Paschima Namaskara Nirakunjasana), Heart Pose Modification

Modification: toes curled in

Pose Type: prone, backbend

Drishti Point: Bhrumadhye or Ajna Chakra (third eye, between the eyebrows)

CHEST AND KNEES ON THE FLOOR: KNEES BEHIND HIPS—ARMS BEHIND THE BACK

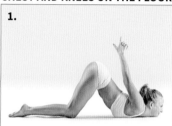

1.

Hands Bound Water Grove Pose

Baddha Hasta Nirakunjasana

(BUH-duh HUH-stuh neer-uh-kunj-AHS-uh-nuh)

Also Known As: Heart Pose (Anahatasana Modification)

Modification: 1. knees on the floor, toes pointed to the back

2. knees on the floor, toes curled in

3. knees off the floor

Pose Type: prone, backbend

Drishti Point: Bhrumadhye or Ajna Chakra (third eye, between the eyebrows)

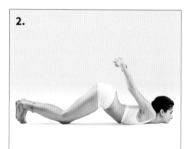

2.

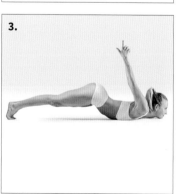

3.

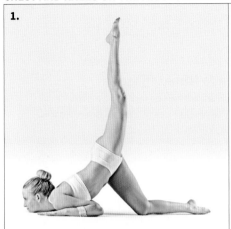

1.

One-Legged Water Grove Pose

Eka Pada Nirakunjasana

(EY-kuh PUH-duh neer-uh-kunj-AHS-uh-nuh)

Also Known As: Heart Pose (Anahatasana Modification)

Modification: 1. forearms on the floor, toes pointed

2. palms to the floor by the rib cage, elbows bent, toes curled in

Pose Type: prone, backbend

Drishti Point: Bhrumadhye or Ajna Chakra (third eye, between the eyebrows)

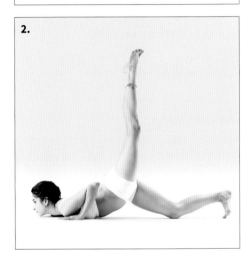

2.

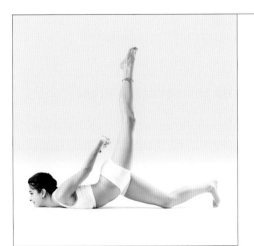

Hands Bound One-Legged Water Grove Pose

Baddha Hasta Eka Pada Nirakunjasana

(BUH-duh HUH-stuh EY-kuh PUHD-uh neer-uh-kunj-AHS-uh-nuh)

Also Known As: Heart Pose (Anahatasana Modification)

Pose Type: prone, backbend

Drishti Point: Bhrumadhye or Ajna Chakra (third eye, between the eyebrows)

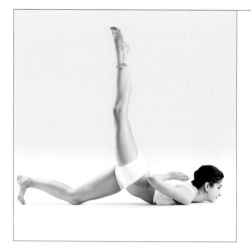

Reverse Prayer One-Legged Water Grove Pose

Viparita Namaskar Eka Pada Nirakunjasana

(vi-puh-REE-tuh nuh-muhs-KAHR EY-kuh PUH-duh neer-uh-kunj-AHS-uh-nuh)

Also Known As: Back of the Body Prayer One-Legged Water Grove Pose
(Paschima Namaskara Eka Pada Nirakunjasana), Heart Pose

Pose Type: prone, backbend

Drishti Point: Bhrumadhye or Ajna Chakra (third eye, between the eyebrows)

CHEST AND KNEES ON THE FLOOR: KNEES BEHIND HIPS—ONE LEG STRAIGHT AND LIFTED—BOTTOM KNEE BENT

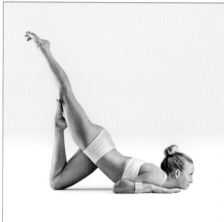

One-Legged Inverted Locust Pose Prep.

Eka Pada Viparita Shalabhasana Prep.

(EY-kuh PUH-duh vi-puh-REE-tuh shuh-luh-BAHS-uh-nuh)

Modification: forearms on the floor, knee of straight leg resting on the foot of the bottom leg

Pose Type: prone, backbend

Drishti Point: Bhrumadhye or Ajna Chakra (third eye, between the eyebrows)

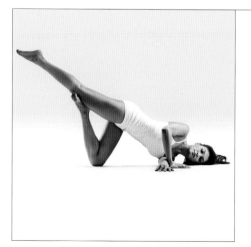

Revolved One-Legged Inverted Locust Pose Prep.

Parivritta Eka Pada Viparita Shalabhasana Prep.

(puh-ri-VRIT-tuh EY-kuh PUH-duh vi-puh-REE-tuh shuh-luh-BAHS-uh-nuh)

Modification: bottom leg bent, top leg straight, top knee resting on the sole of the bottom foot

Pose Type: forward bend, twist

Drishti Point: 1. Urdhva or Antara Drishti (up to the sky)
2. Hastagrai or Hastagre (hands)

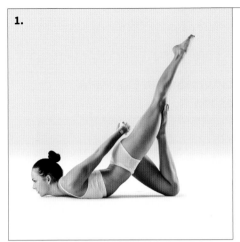

Upward Bound Hands One-Legged Inverted Locust Pose

Urdhva Baddha Hasta Eka Pada Viparita Shalabhasana

(OORD-vuh BUH-duh HUH-stuh EY-kuh PUH-duh vi-puh-REE-tuh shuh-luh-BAHS-uh-nuh)

Also Known As: Flying Locust Pose (Uddayate Shalabhasana)

Modification: 1. knee of the straight leg resting on the foot of the bottom leg
2. bottom foot away from the top leg

Pose Type: prone, backbend

Drishti Point: Bhrumadhye or Ajna Chakra (third eye, between the eyebrows)

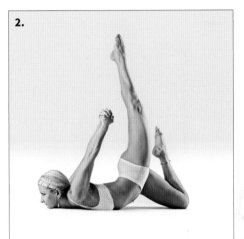

CHEST AND KNEES ON THE FLOOR: KNEES BEHIND HIPS—BOTH LEGS BENT—ARMS IN FRONT

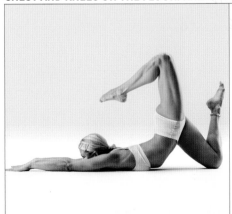

One-Legged Water Grove Pose

Eka Pada Nirakunjasana

(EY-kuh PUH-duh neer-uh-kunj-AHS-uh-nuh)

Also Known As: Heart Pose (Anahatasana Modification)

Modification: both knees bent; arms straight out in front, palms down

Pose Type: prone, backbend

Drishti Point: Bhrumadhye or Ajna Chakra (third eye, between the eyebrows), Angushtamadhye or Angushta Ma Dyai (thumbs)

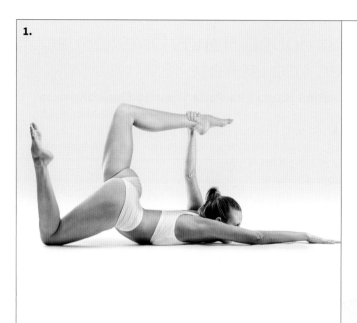

1.

Half Bow Pose in One-Legged Water Grove Pose

Ardha Dhanurasana in Eka Pada Nirakunjasana

(IUHR-duh duh-nur-AHS-uh-nuh in EY-kuh PUH-duh neer-uh-kunj-AHS-uh-nuh)

Also Known As: Heart Pose (Anahatasana Modification)
Modification: 1. right front side view
2. right back side view
Pose Type: backbend
Drishti Point: Bhrumadhye or Ajna Chakra (third eye, between the eyebrows), Angushtamadhye or Angushta Ma Dyai (thumbs)

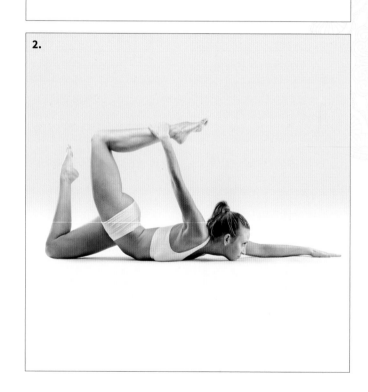

2.

1.

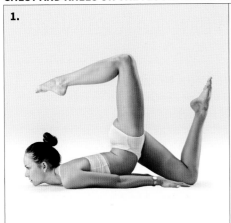

One-Legged Water Grove Pose

Eka Pada Nirakunjasana

(EY-kuh PUH-duh neer-uh-kunj-AHS-uh-nuh)

Also Known As: Heart Pose (Anahatasana Modification)

Modification: both knees bent

1. arms straight to the back, palms down

2. arms lifted off the floor

Pose Type: prone, backbend

Drishti Point: Bhrumadhye or Ajna Chakra (third eye, between the eyebrows)

2.

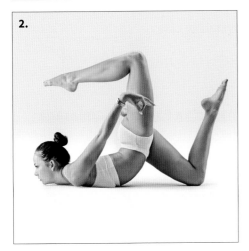

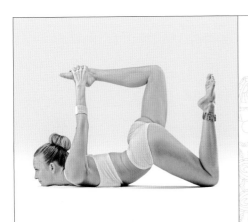

Bow Pose in One-Legged Water Grove Pose

Dhanurasana in Eka Pada Nirakunjasana

(duh-nur-AHS-uh-nuh in EY-kuh PUH-duh neer-uh-kunj-AHS-uh-nuh)

Also Known As: Heart Pose (Anahatasana Modification)

Modification: both hands grabbing the top foot with under-head grip; the knee of the bottom leg on the floor, toes pointing to the sky

Pose Type: prone, backbend

Drishti Point: Bhrumadhye or Ajna Chakra (third eye, between the eyebrows)

Prone Poses

627

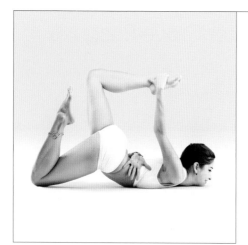

Half Bow Pose in One-Legged Water Grove Pose

Ardha Dhanurasana in Eka Pada Nirakunjasana

(UHR-duh duh-nur-AHS-uh-nuh in EY-kuh PUH-duh neer-uh-kunj-AHS-uh-nuh)

Also Known As: Heart Pose (Anahatasana Modification)

Modification: grabbing onto the foot on the opposite side, under-head grip; other hand to the lower back, palm up

Pose Type: prone, backbend, binding

Drishti Point: Bhrumadhye or Ajna Chakra (third eye, between the eyebrows)

CHEST AND KNEES ON THE FLOOR: KNEES BEHIND HIPS—BOTTOM KNEE BENT—OVERHEAD GRIP

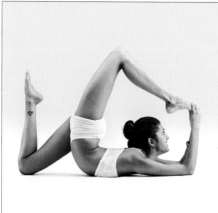

Big Toe Bow Pose in One-Legged Water Grove Pose

Padangushta Dhanurasana in Eka Pada Nirakunjasana

(puhd-ahng-GOOSH-tuh duh-nur-AHS-uh-nuh in EY-kuh PUH-duh neer-uh-kunj-AHS-uh-nuh)

Also Known As: Heart Pose (Anahatasana Modification)

Pose Type: prone, backbend

Drishti Point: Padayoragrai or Padayoragre (toes/feet), Bhrumadhye or Ajna Chakra (third eye, between the eyebrows)

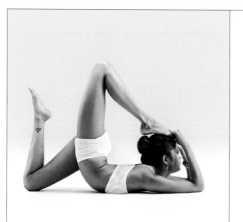

One Leg to the Head Water Grove Pose

Eka Pada Shirsha Nirakunjasana

(EY-kuh PUH-duh SHEER-shuh neer-uh-kunj-AHS-uh-nuh)

Also Known As: Heart Pose (Anahatasana Modification)

Pose Type: prone, backbend

Drishti Point: Bhrumadhye or Ajna Chakra (third eye, between the eyebrows)

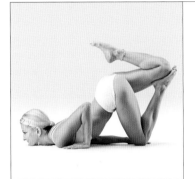

One-Legged Inverted Locust Pose

Eka Pada Viparita Shalabhasana

(EY-kuh PUH-duh vi-puh-REE-tuh shuh-luh-BAHS-uh-nuh)

Modification: one palm to the floor at the bottom of the ribs, other arm straight, palm down; both knees bent, knee of the top leg resting on the foot of the bottom leg

Pose Type: prone, backbend

Drishti Point: Bhrumadhye or Ajna Chakra (third eye, between the eyebrows)

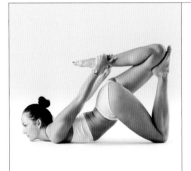

One Hand to Foot Inverted Locust Pose

Eka Hasta Pada Viparita Shalabhasana

(EY-kuh HUH-stuh PUH-duh vi-puh-REE-tuh shuh-luh-BAHS-uh-nuh)

Modification: grabbing onto the top foot with the opposite hand; other arm straight, palm down to the floor; both knees bent, knee of the top leg resting on the foot of the bottom leg

Pose Type: prone, backbend

Drishti Point: Bhrumadhye or Ajna Chakra (third eye, between the eyebrows)

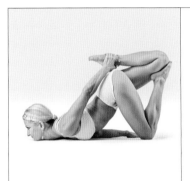

Both Hands to One Foot Inverted Locust Pose

Dwi Hasta Eka Pada Viparita Shalabhasana

(DWI-huh-stuh EY-kuh PUH-duh vi-puh-REE-tuh shuh-luh-BAHS-uh-nuh)

Modification: both hands grabbing the top foot with under-head grip; top knee resting on the sole of the bottom foot

Pose Type: prone, backbend

Drishti Point: Bhrumadhye or Ajna Chakra (third eye, between the eyebrows)

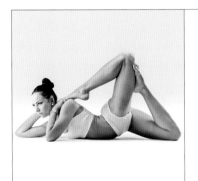

One Foot to the Shoulder Inverted Locust Pose

Eka Pada Bhuja Viparita Shalabhasana

(EY-kuh PUH-duh buj-uh vi-puh-REE-tuh shuh-luh-BAHS-uh-nuh)

Modification: grabbing onto the toes of the top foot; the quadriceps of the top leg resting on the sole of the bottom foot

Pose Type: prone, backbend

Drishti Point: Bhrumadhye or Ajna Chakra (third eye, between the eyebrows)

Supine Poses

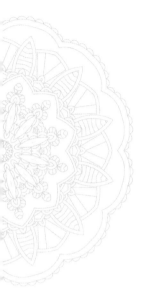

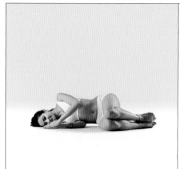

Sideways Wind Relieving Pose

Parshva Vayu Muktyasana

(PAHRSH-vuh VAH-yu muk-TYAHS-uh-nuh)

Modification: palms together in front of the face, knees together

Pose Type: supine (on the side)

Drishti Point: Angushtamadhye or Angushta Ma Dyai (thumbs)

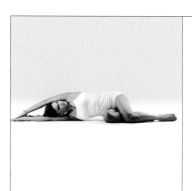

Arms Raised Sideways Wind Relieving Pose

Urdhva Hasta Parshva Vayu Muktyasana

(OORD-vuh HUH-stuh PAHRSH-vuh VAH-yu muk-TYAHS-uh-nuh)

Pose Type: supine (on the side)

Drishti Point: Urdhva or Antara Drishti (up to the sky)

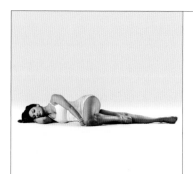

Sideways Wind Relieving Pose

Parshva Vayu Muktyasana

(PAHRSH-vuh VAH-yu muk-TYAHS-uh-nuh)

Modification: bottom leg straight; top knee bent, foot to the knee of the straight leg

Pose Type: supine (on the side)

Drishti Point: Nasagrai or Nasagre (nose)

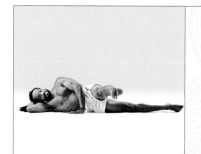

Infinity Pose

Anantasana

(uhn-uhnt-AHS-uh-nuh)

Also Known As: Sleeping Vishnu Pose

Modification: top leg lifted in front of the body, bottom leg straight

Pose Type: supine (on the side), forward bend

Drishti Point: Nasagrai or Nasagre (nose), Padayoragrai or Padayoragre (toes/feet)

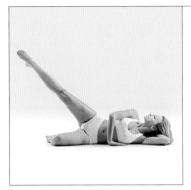

Infinity Pose

Anantasana

(uhn-uhnt-AHS-uh-nuh)

Also Known As: Sleeping Vishnu Pose
Modification: top leg straight and lifted; bottom leg bent, toes pointing to the back
Pose Type: supine (on the side)
Drishti Point: Padayoragrai or Padayoragre (toes/feet)

SHOULDER ON THE FLOOR: TWISTS AND BINDING

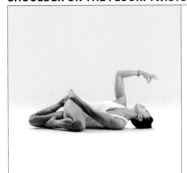

Svastika Legs in Twisted Stomach Pose

Pada Svastikasana in Jatara Parivartanasana

(PUH-duh svuh-sti-KAHS-uh-nuh in JAH-tuh-ruh puh-ri-vuhrt-ahn-AHS-uh-nuh)
Modification: grabbing onto the back foot, heel toward the glutes
Pose Type: supine (on the side), twist
Drishti Point: Hastagrai or Hastagre (hands)

Revolved One-Legged King Pigeon Pose 1

Parivritta Eka Pada Raja Kapotasana 1

(puh-ri-VRIT-tuh EY-kuh PUH-duh RAH-juh kuh-po-TAHS-uh-nuh)
Modification: back knee bent, both hands to the back foot; front foot to hip socket
Pose Type: supine (on the side), twist
Drishti Point: Urdhva or Antara Drishti (up to the sky)

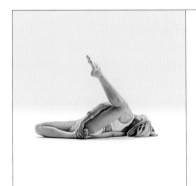

One-Legged Bound Infinity Pose

Eka Pada Baddha Anantasana

(EY-kuh PUH-duh BUH-duh uhn-uhnt-AHS-uh-nuh)
Also Known As: One-Legged Bound Sleeping Vishnu Pose
Modification: bottom leg bent, heel toward the glutes; top leg bent
Pose Type: supine (on the side), twist, binding
Drishti Point: Bhrumadhye or Ajna Chakra (third eye, between the eyebrows)

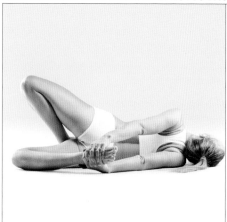

Sideways Half Lotus Bow Pose

Parshva Ardha Padma Dhanurasana

(PAHRSH-vuh UHR-duh PUHD-muh duh-nur-AHS-uh-nuh)

Modification: grabbing onto the bottom foot with both hands with under-head grip

Pose Type: supine (on the side), backbend

Drishti Point: Bhrumadhye or Ajna Chakra (third eye, between the eyebrows)

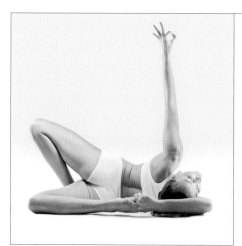

Sideways Half Lotus One-Handed Big Toe Bow Pose

Parshva Ardha Padma Eka Hasta Padangushta Dhanurasana

(PAHRSH-vuh UHR-duh PUHD-muh EY-kuh HUH-stuh puhd-ahng-GOOSH-tuh duh-nur-AHS-uh-nuh)

Modification: grabbing onto the bottom foot with overhead grip on the same side, top arm straight, fingertips to the sky

Pose Type: supine (on the side), backbend

Drishti Point: Bhrumadhye or Ajna Chakra (third eye, between the eyebrows)

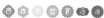

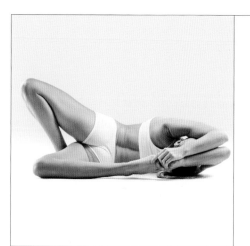

Sideways Half Lotus Two-Handed Big Toe Bow Pose

Parshva Ardha Padma Dwi Hasta Padangushta Dhanurasana

(PAHRSH-vuh UHR-duh PUHD-muh DWI-huh-stuh puhd-ahng-GOOSH-tuh duh-nur-AHS-uh-nuh)

Modification: overhead grip, both hands grabbing onto the foot

Pose Type: supine (on the side), backbend

Drishti Point: Bhrumadhye or Ajna Chakra (third eye, between the eyebrows)

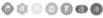

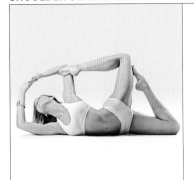

Mermaid Pose in Infinity Pose

Naginyasana in Anantasana

(nuh-gin-YAHS-uh-nuh in uhn-uhnt-AHS-uh-nuh)

Also Known As: Mermaid Pose in Sleeping Vishnu Pose

Pose Type: supine (on the side), backbend

Drishti Point: Bhrumadhye or Ajna Chakra (third eye, between the eyebrows)

1.

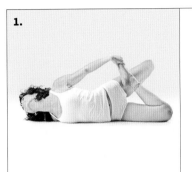

Sideways Half Lotus Bow Pose

Parshva Ardha Padma Dhanurasana

(PAHRSH-vuh UHR-duh PUHD-muh duh-nur-AHS-uh-nuh)

Modification: grabbing onto the top foot with the bottom hand; grabbing onto the bottom foot with top hand

1. front view
2. back view

Pose Type: supine (on the side), backbend

Drishti Point: Bhrumadhye or Ajna Chakra (third eye, between the eyebrows)

2.

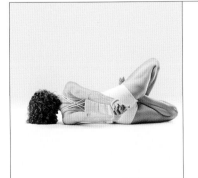

Hands Bound Lotus Pose in Infinity Pose
Baddha Hasta Padmasana in Anantasana

(BUH-duh HUH-stuh puhd-MAHS-uh-nuh in uhn-uhnt-AHS-uh-nuh)

Also Known As: Hands Bound Lotus Pose in Sleeping Vishnu Pose

Pose Type: supine (on the side), mild backbend

Drishti Point: Bhrumadhye or Ajna Chakra (third eye, between the eyebrows)

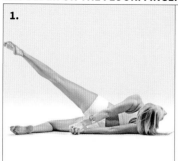

Hands Bound Infinity Pose

Baddha Hasta Anantasana

(BUH-duh HUH-stuh uhn-uhnt-AHS-uh-nuh)

Also Known As: Hands Bound Sleeping Vishnu Pose
Modification: 1. bottom leg bent, top leg straight and lifted; resting on the arms and the bent knee for support
2. bottom leg straight, top leg straight and lifted; arms lifted off the floor
Pose Type: supine (on the side), backbend
Drishti Point: Bhrumadhye or Ajna Chakra (third eye, between the eyebrows)

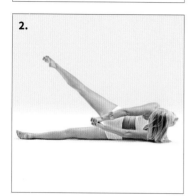

Hands Bound Half Lotus Pose in Infinity Pose

Baddha Hasta Ardha Padmasana in Anantasana

(BUH-duh HUH-stuh UHR-duh puhd-MAHS-uh-nuh in uhn-uhnt-AHS-uh-nuh)

Also Known As: Hands Bound Half Lotus Pose in Sleeping Vishnu Pose
Modification: 1. front view
2. back view
Pose Type: supine (on the side), backbend
Drishti Point: Bhrumadhye or Ajna Chakra (third eye, between the eyebrows)

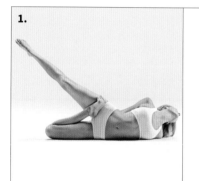

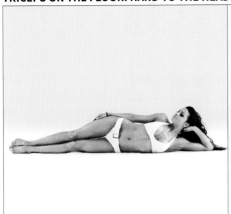

Infinity Pose

Anantasana

(uhn-uhnt-AHS-uh-nuh)

Also Known As: Sleeping Vishnu Pose
Modification: both legs straight and together; bottom leg on the floor
Pose Type: supine (on the side), side bend
Drishti Point: Padhayoragrai or Padayoragre (toes/feet)

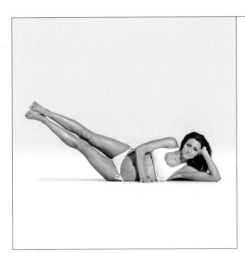

Infinity Pose

Anantasana

(uhn-uhnt-AHS-uh-nuh)

Also Known As: Sleeping Vishnu Pose
Modification: legs straight, together and lifted off the floor
Pose Type: supine (on the side), core, side bend
Drishti Point: Nasagrai or Nasagre (nose)

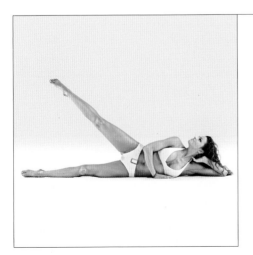

Infinity Pose

Anantasana

(uhn-uhnt-AHS-uh-nuh)

Also Known As: Sleeping Vishnu Pose
Modification: both legs straight, top leg lifted, bottom leg on the floor
Pose Type: supine (on the side), core, side bend
Drishti Point: Padayoragrai or Padayoragre (toes/feet), Urdhva or Antara Drishti (up to the sky)

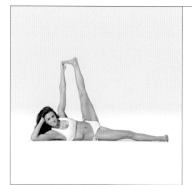

Extended Hand to Big Toe Pose in Infinity Pose

Utthita Hasta Padangushtasana in Anantasana

(UT-ti-tuh HUH-stuh puhd-ahng-goosh-TAHS-uh-nuh in uhn-uhnt-AHS-uh-nuh)

Also Known As: Extended Hand to Big Toe Pose in Sleeping Vishnu Pose
Pose Type: supine (on the side), forward bend, side bend
Drishti Point: Nasagrai or Nasagre (nose)

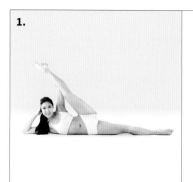

1.

Sundial Pose in Infinity Pose

Surya Yantrasana in Anantasana

(SOOR-yuh yuhn-TRAHS-uh-nuh in uhn-uhnt-AHS-uh-nuh)

Also Known As: Sundial Pose in Sleeping Vishnu Pose
Modification: 1. grabbing onto the heel on the outside of the calf
2. grabbing onto the heel on the inside of the calf
Pose Type: supine (on the side), forward bend, side bend
Drishti Point: Nasagrai or Nasagre (nose)

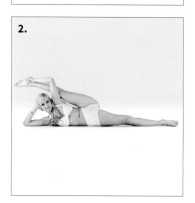

2.

TRICEPS ON THE FLOOR: BOTH KNEES BENT

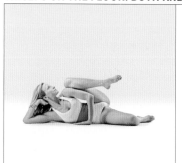

Infinity Pose

Anantasana

(uhn-uhnt-AHS-uh-nuh)

Also Known As: Sleeping Vishnu Pose
Modification: top knee to the top shoulder; both knees bent
Pose Type: supine (on the side), forward bend
Drishti Point: Bhrumadhye or Ajna Chakra (third eye, between the eyebrows) or
Padhayoragrai or Padayoragre (toes/feet)

1.

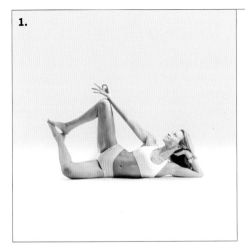

Bound Angle Pose in Infinity Pose

Baddha Konasana in Anantasana

(BUH-duh ko-NAHS-uh-nuh in uhn-uhnt-AHS-uh-nuh)

Also Known As: Bound Angle Pose in Sleeping Vishnu Pose

Modification: 1. top wrist on the top knee

2. top hand grabbing onto the top foot

Pose Type: supine (on the side), side bend

Drishti Point: Bhrumadhye or Ajna Chakra (third eye, between the eyebrows) or Hastagrai or Hastagre (hands)

2.

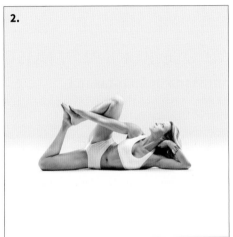

TRICEPS ON THE FLOOR: BOTTOM LEG STRAIGHT—BACKBENDS

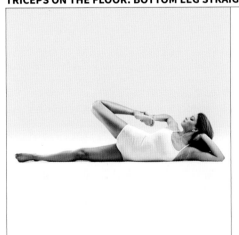

Half Frog Pose Prep. in Infinity Pose

Ardha Bhekasana in Anantasana

(UHR-duh bey-KAHS-uh-nuh in uhn-uhnt-AHS-uh-nuh)

Also Known As: Half Frog Pose Prep. in Sleeping Vishnu Pose

Modification: hand in beginner modification; neutral spine, top leg moving into a half-frog leg position

Pose Type: supine (on the side), mild backbend

Drishti Point: Padayoragrai or Padayoragre (toes/feet)

x

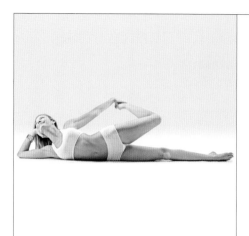

Half Bow Pose in Infinity Pose

Ardha Dhanurasana in Anantasana

(UHR-duh duh-nur-AHS-uh-nuh in uhn-uhnt-AHS-uh-nuh)

Also Known As: Half Bow Pose in Sleeping Vishnu Pose

Pose Type: supine (on the side), backbend

Drishti Point: Bhrumadhye or Ajna Chakra (third eye, between the eyebrows)

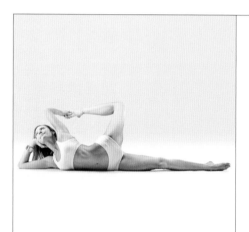

Half Big Toe Bow Pose in Infinity Pose

Ardha Padangushta Dhanurasana in Anantasana

(UHR-duh puhd-ahng-GOOSH-tuh duh-nur-AHS-uh-nuh in uhn-uhnt-AHS-uh-nuh)

Also Known As: Half Big Toe Bow Pose in Sleeping Vishnu Pose

Pose Type: supine (on the side), backbend

Drishti Point: Bhrumadhye or Ajna Chakra (third eye, between the eyebrows)

TRICEPS ON THE FLOOR: ONE LEG STRAIGHT, OTHER FOOT TO THE HIP SOCKET

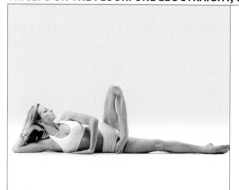

Infinity Pose

Anantasana

(uhn-uhnt-AHS-uh-nuh)

Also Known As: Sleeping Vishnu Pose

Modification: top foot to the hip socket, toes touching the floor; bottom leg straight on the floor

Pose Type: supine (on the side), side bend

Drishti Point: Padayoragrai or Padayoragre (toes/feet)

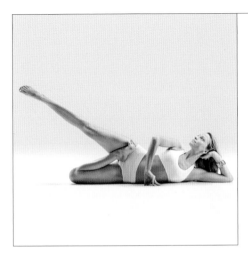

Half Lotus Pose in Infinity Pose

Ardha Padmasana in Anantasana

(UHR-duh puhd-MAHS-uh-nuh in anan-TAHS-annauhn-uhnt-AHS-uh-nuh)
Also Known As: Half Lotus Pose in Sleeping Vishnu Pose
Modification: bottom foot in half lotus, top leg lifted and straight
Pose Type: supine (on the side), side bend
Drishti Point: Padayoragrai or Padayoragre (toes/feet)

TRICEPS ON THE FLOOR: HALF LOTUS & FULL LOTUS

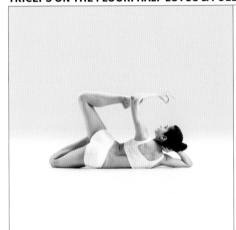

Half Lotus Mermaid Pose in Infinity Pose

Ardha Padma Naginyasana in Anantasana

(UHR-duh PUHD-muh nuh-gin-YAHS-uh-nuh in uhn-uhnt-AHS-uh-nuh)
Also Known As: Half Lotus Mermaid Pose in Sleeping Vishnu Pose
Pose Type: supine (on the side), backbend, side bend
Drishti Point: Hastagrai or Hastagre (hands)

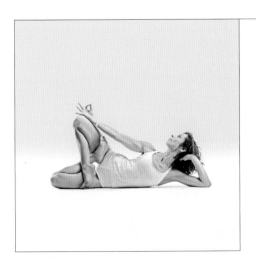

Lotus Pose in Infinity Pose

Padmasana in Anantasana

(puhd-MAHS-uh-nuh in uhn-uhnt-AHS-uh-nuh)
Also Known As: Lotus Pose in Sleeping Vishnu Pose
Pose Type: supine (on the side), side bend, knee, ankle opener
Drishti Point: Hastagrai or Hastagre (hands)

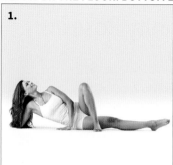

Infinity Pose

Anantasana

(uhn-uhnt-AHS-uh-nuh)

Also Known As: Sleeping Vishnu Pose

Modification: elbow to the floor, top knee bent, leg crossed over in front of the body; bottom leg straight

1. palm of the top hand on the floor
2. top hand on the top knee

Drishti Point: Urdhva or Antara Drishti (up to the sky)

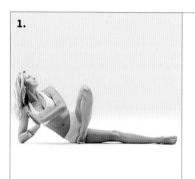

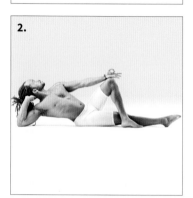

Infinity Pose

Anantasana

(uhn-uhnt-AHS-uh-nuh)

Also Known As: Sleeping Vishnu Pose

Modification: elbow to the floor, hands in Anjali Mudra (Hands in Prayer); top knee bent, foot by the hip, bottom leg straight

1. bottom leg on the floor
2. bottom leg lifted off the floor

Pose Type: 1. supine (on the side), side bend

2. supine (on the side), side bend, core

Drishti Point: Bhrumadhye or Ajna Chakra (third eye, between the eyebrows)

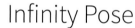

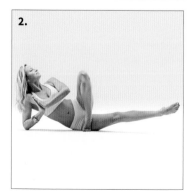

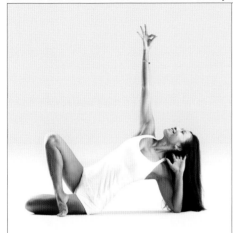

Infinity Pose

Anantasana

(uhn-uhnt-AHS-uh-nuh)

Also Known As: Sleeping Vishnu Pose
Modification: top leg crossed over in front, toes on the floor; bottom leg bent, toes to the back; elbow to the floor, other arm straight fingertips to the sky
Pose Type: supine (on the side)
Drishti Point: Hastagrai or Hastagre (hands)

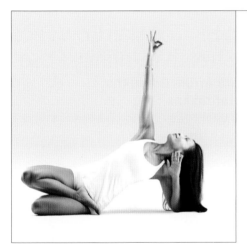

Half Lotus Pose in Infinity Pose

Ardha Padmasana in Anantasana

(UHR-duh puhd-MAHS-uh-nuh in uhn-uhnt-AHS-uh-nuh)

Also Known As: Half Lotus Pose in Sleeping Vishnu Pose
Modification: top leg in half lotus; bottom leg bent, heel to the sitting bone; elbow to the floor, other arm straight fingertips to the sky
Pose Type: supine (on the side)
Drishti Point: Hastagrai or Hastagre (hands)

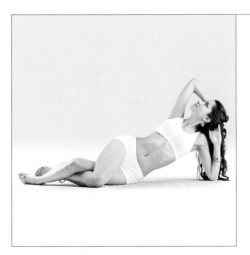

Leg Position of the Pose Dedicated to Garuda in Infinity Pose

Pada Garudasana in Anantasana

(PUH-duh guh-ru-DAHS-uh-nuh in uhn-uhnt-AHS-uh-nuh)

Also Known As: Leg Position of the Pose Dedicated to Garuda in Sleeping Vishnu Pose
Modification: elbow to the floor, hands behind the head
Pose Type: supine (on the side)
Drishti Point: Bhrumadhye or Ajna Chakra (third eye, between the eyebrows)

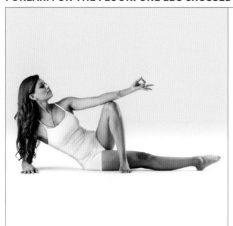

Infinity Pose

Anantasana

(uhn-uhnt-AHS-uh-nuh)

Also Known As: Sleeping Vishnu Pose

Modification: top leg crossed over; forearm to the floor, top elbow resting on the top knee

Pose Type: supine (on the side)

Drishti Point: Hastagrai or Hastagre (hands)

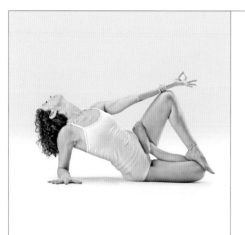

Extended Hand to Big Toe Half Cow Face Western Intense Stretch in Infinity Pose

Utthita Hasta Padangushta Ardha Gomukha Paschimottanasana in Anantasana

(UT-ti-tuh HUH-stuh puhd-ahng-GOOSH-tuh UHR-duh go-MUK-uh puhsh-chi-mo-tahn-AHS-uh-nuh in uhn-uhnt-AHS-uh-nuh)

Also Known As: Extended Hand to Big Toe Half Cow Face Forward Bend in Infinity Pose, Extended Hand to Big Toe Half Cow Face Western Intense Stretch in Sleeping Vishnu Pose

Modification: forearm to the floor; top leg crossed over; grabbing onto the big toe of the bottom foot, leg off the floor

Pose Type: supine (on the side), forward bend

Drishti Point: Hastagrai or Hastagre (hands)

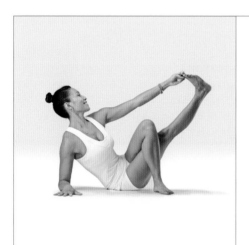

Half Lotus Pose in Infinity Pose

Ardha Padmasana in Anantasana

(UHR-duh puhd-MAHS-uh-nuh in uhn-uhnt-AHS-uh-nuh)

Also Known As: Half Lotus Pose in Sleeping Vishnu Pose

Modification: top foot to the bottom knee; top forearm to the top knee

Pose Type: supine (on the side), mild backbend

Drishti Point: Bhrumadhye or Ajna Chakra (third eye, between the eyebrows)

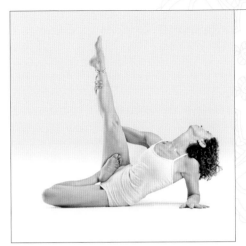

Half Lotus Extended Hand to Leg Pose in Infinity Pose

Ardha Padma Utthita Pada Hastasana in Anantasana

(UHR-duh PUHD-muh UT-ti-tuh PUH-duh huh-STAHS-uh-nuh in uhn-uhnt-AHS-uh-nuh)

Also Known As: Half Lotus Extended Hand to Leg Pose in Sleeping Vishnu Pose
Pose Type: supine (on the side), forward bend, mild backbend
Drishti Point: Bhrumadhye or Ajna Chakra (third eye, between the eyebrows)

FOREARM ON THE FLOOR: TOP LEG STRAIGHT, BOTTOM FOOT TO THE THIGH

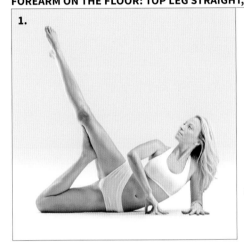

1.

Half Bound Angle Pose in Infinity Pose

Ardha Baddha Konasana in Anantasana

(UHR-duh BUH-duh ko-NAHS-uh-nuh in uhn-uhnt-AHS-uh-nuh)

Also Known As: Half Bound Angle Pose in Sleeping Vishnu Pose
Modification: forearm to the floor
1. finger tips of the top arm to the floor in front of the abdomen, elbow bent
2. top arm straight and parallel to the top leg
Pose Type: supine (on the side), side bend
Drishti Point: Padayoragrai or Padayoragre (toes/feet), Hastagrai or Hastagre (hands)

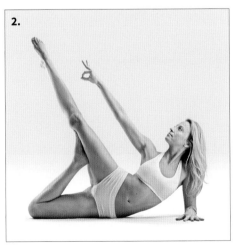

2.

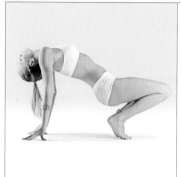

Tip Toe Half Eastern Intense Stretch Pose

Prapada Ardha Purvottanasana

(PRUH-puh-duh UHR-duh poor-vo-tahn-AHS-uh-nuh)

Also Known As: Tip Toe Half Reverse Plank Pose
Modification: prep—sitting bones below the knee level, on the fingertips
Pose Type: standing, backbend
Drishti Point: Bhrumadhye or Ajna Chakra (third eye, between the eyebrows)

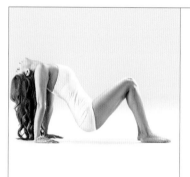

Half Eastern Intense Stretch Pose

Ardha Purvottanasana

(UHR-duh poor-vo-tahn-AHS-uh-nuh)

Also Known As: Half Reverse Plank
Modification: mild prep—sitting bones slightly off the floor, feet flat on the floor; palms flat on the floor, fingertips pointing to the heels
Pose Type: standing, backbend
Drishti Point: Bhrumadhye or Ajna Chakra (third eye, between the eyebrows)

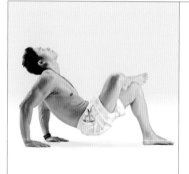

Half Fire Log Pose in Half Eastern Intense Stretch Pose

Ardha Agnistambhasana in Ardha Purvottanasana

(UHR-duh uhg-ni-stuhm-BAHS-uh-nuh in UHR-duh poor-vo-tahn-AHS-uh-nuh)

Also Known As: Half Firelog Pose in Half Reverse Plank
Modification: prep—sitting bones slightly off the floor; elbows bent, fingertips pointing to the heels
Pose Type: standing, forward bend
Drishti Point: Bhrumadhye or Ajna Chakra (third eye, between the eyebrows)

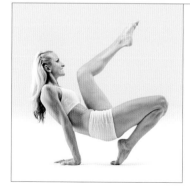

Intense Ankle Stretch Pose in One-Legged Half Eastern Intense Stretch Pose

Uttana Kulpasana in Eka Pada Ardha Purvottanasana

(ut-TAHN-uh kul-PAHS-uh-nuh in EY-kuh PUH-duh UHR-duh poor-vo-tahn-AHS-uh-nuh)

Also Known As: Intense Ankle Stretch Pose in One-Legged Half Reverse Plank
Modification: knee bent toward the chest, fingertips pointing away from the heels
Pose Type: standing, forward bend
Drishti Point: Padayoragrai or Padayoragre (toes/feet)

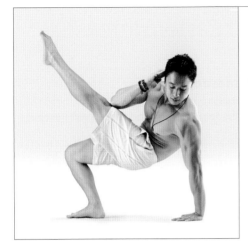

Revolved Half Eastern Intense Stretch Pose

Parivritta Ardha Purvottanasana

(puh-ri-VRIT-tuh UHR-duh poor-vo-tahn-AHS-uh-nuh)

Also Known As: Revolved Half Reverse Plank Pose
Modification: opposite elbow to knee of the straight leg
Pose Type: arm balance, forward bend, twist
Drishti Point: Hastagrai or Hastagre (hands)

EASTERN INTENSE STRETCH: KNEES BENT

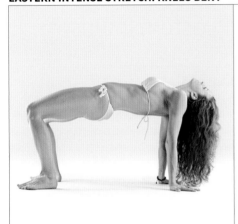

Half Eastern Intense Stretch Pose

Ardha Purvottanasana

(UHR-duh poor-vo-tahn-AHS-uh-nuh)

Also Known As: Reverse Table Top and Half Reverse Plank Pose
Modification: prep—knees bent and on top of the ankles, fingertips pointing away from the heels
Pose Type: standing, backbend
Drishti Point: Bhrumadhye or Ajna Chakra (third eye, between the eyebrows)

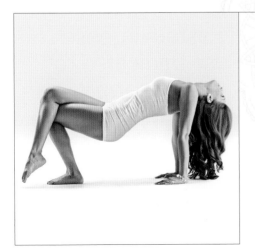

Uneven Leg Position of Cow Face Pose in Half Eastern Intense Stretch Pose

Vishama Pada Gomukhasana in Ardha Purvottanasana

(VISH-uh-muh PUH-duh go-muk-AHS-uh-nuh in UHR-duh poor-vo-tahn-AHS-uh-nuh)

Also Known As: Uneven Leg Position of Cow Face Pose in Reverse Table Top and Uneven Leg Position of Cow Face Pose in Half Reverse Plank
Modification: knees bent, fingertips pointing to the heels
Pose Type: standing, backbend
Drishti Point: Bhrumadhye or Ajna Chakra (third eye, between the eyebrows)

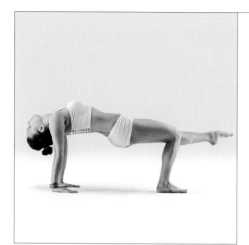

One-Legged Half Eastern Intense Stretch Pose

Eka Pada Ardha Purvottanasana

(EY-kuh PUH-duh UHR-duh poor-vo-tahn-AHS-uh-nuh)

Also Known As: One-Legged Reverse Table Top and One-Legged Half Reverse Plank Pose

Modification: prep—one knee bent, foot on the floor; other leg straight; knees in line, fingertips pointing to the heels

Pose Type: standing, backbend

Drishti Point: Bhrumadhye or Ajna Chakra (third eye, between the eyebrows)

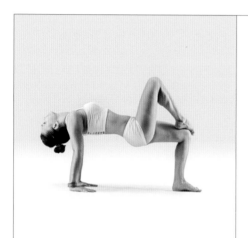

One-Legged Half Eastern Intense Stretch Pose

Eka Pada Ardha Purvottanasana

(EY-kuh PUH-duh UHR-duh poor-vo-tahn-AHS-uh-nuh)

Also Known As: One-Legged Reverse Table Top and One-Legged Half Reverse Plank

Modification: prep—both knees bent, top foot to the knee, fingertips pointing to the heels

Pose Type: standing, backbend

Drishti Point: Bhrumadhye or Ajna Chakra (third eye, between the eyebrows)

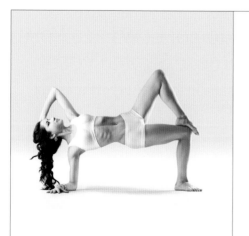

One-Legged Half Eastern Intense Stretch Pose in Pose Dedicated to Sage Vasistha on the Forearm

Eka Pada Ardha Purvottanasana in Vasishtasana

(EY-kuh PUH-duh UHR-duh poor-vo-tahn-AHS-uh-nuh in vuh-sish-TAHS-uh-nuh)

Also Known As: One-Legged Reverse Table Top in Pose Dedicated to Sage Vasistha on the Forearm, One-Legged Half Reverse Plank Top in Pose Dedicated to Sage Vasistha on the Forearm

Modification: both knees bent, foot to the knee

Pose Type: standing (on the forearm and the foot)

Drishti Point: Bhrumadhye or Ajna Chakra (third eye, between the eyebrows)

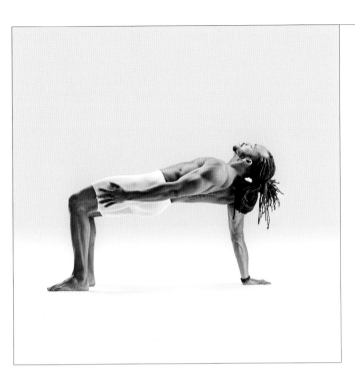

One Hand Half Eastern Intense Stretch Pose

Eka Hasta Ardha Purvottanasana

(EY-kuh HUH-stuh UHR-duh poor-vo-tahn-AHS-uh-nuh)

Also Known As: One Hand Reverse Table Top or One Hand Half Reverse Plank

Modification: knees bent, fingertips pointing away from the heels

Pose Type: standing, backbend

Drishti Point: Bhrumadhye or Ajna Chakra (third eye, between the eyebrows)

EASTERN INTENSE STRETCH: LEGS STRAIGHT

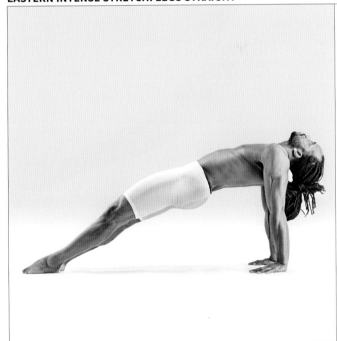

Eastern Intense Stretch Pose

Purvottanasana

(poor-vo-tahn-AHS-uh-nuh)

Also Known As: Reverse Plank and Upward Plank Pose

Modification: legs straight, fingertips pointing to the heels

Pose Type: standing, backbend

Drishti Point: Bhrumadhye or Ajna Chakra (third eye, between the eyebrows)

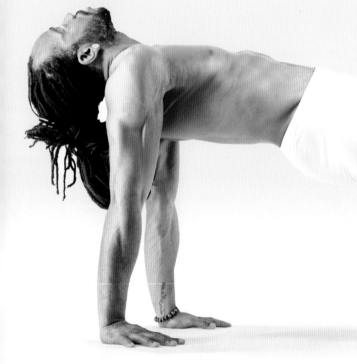
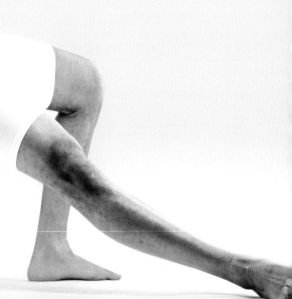

Half Eastern Intense Stretch Pose

Parshva Eka Pada Ardha Purvottanasana

(PAHRSH-vuh EY-kuh PUH-duh UHR-duh poor-vo-tahn-AHS-uh-nuh)

Also Known As: Foot to the Side Reverse Table Top, Foot to the Side Half Reverse Plank and Foot to the Side Half Upward Plank Pose

Pose Type: standing, backbend

Drishti Point: Bhrumadhye or Ajna Chakra (third eye, between the eyebrows)

How to Perform the Pose:

1. Begin by sitting on the floor with both your legs straight out in front of you. Keep your hands on the floor on the sides of your hips with fingertips pointing toward your feet. Engage your *mula bandha*, *uddhiyana bandha*, and *ujjayi* breathing.

2. Exhale, bend your knees, and slide your feet toward your sitting bones. Keep your feet and knees hip-width apart.

3. On the next exhale, press into your hands and feet and lift your sitting bones off the floor. Your shoulders should be on top of your wrists, your knees on top of your ankles, and your torso and thighs parallel to the floor.

4. Exhale, straighten your right leg, and bring it out to the side, flexing the toes of your right foot out to the side. Hold the pose for at least 30, and up to 90, seconds in order to receive full benefits.

5. Inhale and bring your right leg back to the center in line with your left leg. Repeat on the other side. Hold the pose for at least 30, and up to 90, seconds in order to receive the full benefits of the stretch.

6. Inhale and lower your hips to the floor, coming back to the starting position.

Modification: one knee bent, other leg straight out to the side, fingertips pointing to the heels

parshva = side
eka = one
pada = foot or leg
ardha = half
purva = east, the front of the body
ut = intense
tan = to stretch, to extend

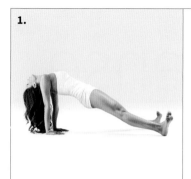

1.

Feet Wide Eastern Intense Stretch Pose

Prasarita Pada Purvottanasana

(pruh-SAH-ri-tuh PUH-duh poor-vo-tahn-AHS-uh-nuh)

Also Known As: Feet Wide Reverse Plank and Feet Wide Upward Plank Pose

Modification: legs straight, toes flexed in, fingertips pointing to the heels

1. side view

2. front view

Pose Type: standing, backbend

Drishti Point: Bhrumadhye or Ajna Chakra (third eye, between the eyebrows)

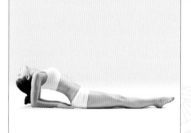

2.

EASTERN INTENSE STRETCH: FOREARMS ON THE FLOOR

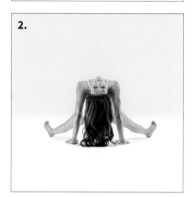

Easy Fish Pose

Sukha Matsyasana

(SUK-uh muhts-YAHS-uh-nuh)

Also Known As: Eastern Intense Stretch Pose Prep. (Purvottanasana Prep.), Reverse Plank Prep.

Modification: head off the floor, forearms on the floor, legs straight

Pose Type: seated, backbend

Drishti Point: Bhrumadhye or Ajna Chakra (third eye, between the eyebrows)

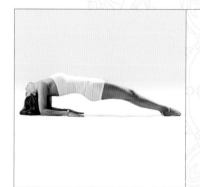

Eastern Intense Stretch Pose

Purvottanasana

(poor-vo-tahn-AHS-uh-nuh)

Also Known As: Reverse Plank on the Forearms and Upward Plank Pose on the Forearms

Modification: legs straight, forearms on the floor

Pose Type: standing (on the forearms), backbend

Drishti Point: Bhrumadhye or Ajna Chakra (third eye, between the eyebrows)

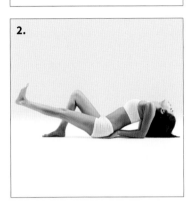

1.

2.

Easy Fish Pose

Sukha Matsyasana

(SUK-uh muhts-YAHS-uh-nuh)

Also Known As: Eastern Intense Stretch Pose Prep. (Purvottanasana Prep.), Reverse Plank Prep.

Modification: head off the floor, forearms to the floor; one leg straight, other knee bent, foot flat on the floor

1. straight leg on the floor

2. straight leg off the floor, toes flexed in

Pose Type: seated, backbend

Drishti Point: Bhrumadhye or Ajna Chakra (third eye, between the eyebrows)

EASTERN INTENSE STRETCH: FOREARMS TO FLOOR—ONE LEG OFF FLOOR

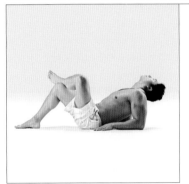

Half Fire Log Pose in Easy Fish Pose

Ardha Agnistambhasana in Sukha Matsyasana

(UHR-duh uhg-ni-stuhm-BAHS-uh-nuh in SUK-uh muhts-YAHS-uh-nuh)

Also Known As: Eastern Intense Stretch Pose Prep. (Purvottanasana Prep.), Reverse Plank Prep.

Modification: forearms to the floor, head off the floor

Pose Type: seated, backbend

Drishti Point: Bhrumadhye or Ajna Chakra (third eye, between the eyebrows)

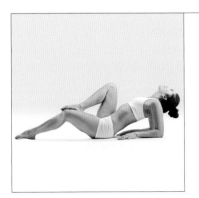

Easy Fish Pose

Sukha Matsyasana

(SUK-uh muhts-YAHS-uh-nuh)

Also Known As: Eastern Intense Stretch Pose Prep. (Purvottanasana Prep.), Reverse Plank Prep.

Modification: forearms to the floor, head off the floor, sole of the foot to the opposite knee

Pose Type: seated, backbend

Drishti Point: Bhrumadhye or Ajna Chakra (third eye, between the eyebrows)

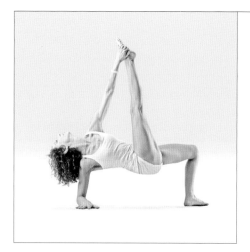

Revolved Hand to Foot Pose in Half Eastern Intense Stretch Pose on the Forearm

Parivritta Hasta Padasana in Ardha Purvottanasana

(puh-ri-VRIT-tuh HUH-stuh puh-DAHS-uh-nuh in UHR-duh poor-vo-tahn-AHS-uh-nuh)

Also Known As: Revolved Hand to Foot Pose in Reverse Table Top, Revolved Hand to Foot Pose in Half Reverse Plank

Modification: forearm on the floor; grabbing onto the outside edge of the foot, leg straight

Pose Type: standing (on the forearm and the foot), twist

Drishti Point: Bhrumadhye or Ajna Chakra (third eye, between the eyebrows)

EASTERN INTENSE STRETCH: FOREARMS TO FLOOR—GRABBING ONTO TRICEPS—KNEES BENT

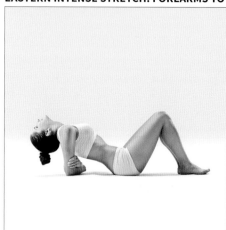

Hands Bound Easy Fish Pose

Baddha Hasta Sukha Matsyasana

(BUH-duh HUH-stuh SUK-uh muhts-YAHS-uh-nuh)

Modification: knees bent, feet to the floor

Pose Type: seated, backbend

Drishti Point: Bhrumadhye or Ajna Chakra (third eye, between the eyebrows)

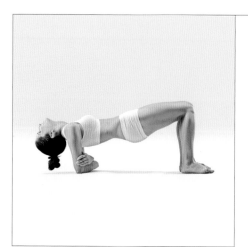

Hands Bound Half Eastern Intense Stretch Pose

Baddha Hasta Ardha Purvottanasana

(BUH-duh HUH-stuh UHR-duh poor-vo-tahn-AHS-uh-nuh)

Also Known As: Hands Bound Reverse Table Top, Hands Bound Half Reverse Plank

Pose Type: standing (on the forearms), backbend

Drishti Point: Bhrumadhye or Ajna Chakra (third eye, between the eyebrows)

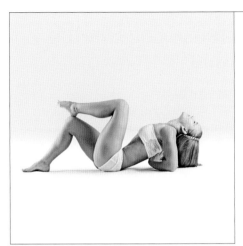

Reverse Prayer One-Legged Easy Fish Pose

Viparita Namaskar Eka Pada Sukha Matsyasana

(vi-puh-REE-tuh nuh-muhs-KAHR EY-kuh PUH-duh SUK-uh muhts-YAHS-uh-nuh)

Also Known As: Back of the Body Prayer One-Legged Easy Fish Pose (Paschima Namaskara Eka Pada Sukha Matsyasana)

Modification: both knees bent, heel to the knee

Pose Type: seated, backbend

Drishti Point: Bhrumadhye or Ajna Chakra (third eye, between the eyebrows)

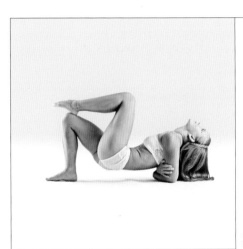

Hands Bound One-Legged Half Eastern Intense Stretch Pose

Baddha Hasta Eka Pada Ardha Purvottanasana

(BUH-duh HUH-stuh EY-kuh PUH-duh UHR-duh poor-vo-tahn-AHS-uh-nuh)

Also Known As: Hands Bound One-Legged Reverse Table Top, Hands Bound One-Legged Half Reverse Plank

Modification: heel to the knee; grabbing onto the triceps

Pose Type: standing (on the forearms), backbend

Drishti Point: Bhrumadhye or Ajna Chakra (third eye, between the eyebrows)

EASTERN INTENSE STRETCH: FOREARMS TO FLOOR—GRABBING ONTO THE TRICEPS

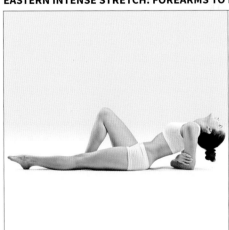

Hands Bound Easy Fish Pose

Baddha Hasta Sukha Matsyasana

(BUH-duh HUH-stuh SUK-uh muhts-YAHS-uh-nuh)

Modification: one leg straight to the floor; other knee bent, foot to the floor

Pose Type: seated, backbend

Drishti Point: Bhrumadhye or Ajna Chakra (third eye, between the eyebrows)

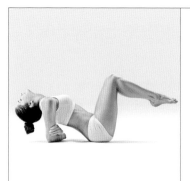

Hands Bound Easy Intense Leg Stretch

Baddha Hasta Sukha Uttana Padasana

(BUH-duh HUH-stuh SUK-uh ut-TAHN-uh puh-DAHS-uh-nuh)

Modification: knees bent at 90 degrees, feet off the floor

Pose Type: seated, backbend, core

Drishti Point: Bhrumadhye or Ajna Chakra (third eye, between the eyebrows)

EASTERN INTENSE STRETCH: ELBOWS ON THE FLOOR—HALF LOTUS

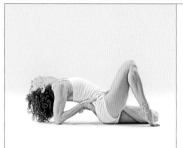

Half Lotus Easy Fish Pose

Ardha Padma Sukha Matsyasana

(UHR-duh PUHD-muh SUK-uh muhts-YAHS-uh-nuh)

Also Known As: Eastern Intense Stretch Pose Prep. (Purvottanasana Prep.), Reverse Plank Prep.

Modification: elbows to the floor, palms to the lower back; one leg in half lotus, other knee bent; heel up

Pose Type: seated, backbend

Drishti Point: Bhrumadhye or Ajna Chakra (third eye, between the eyebrows)

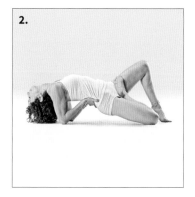

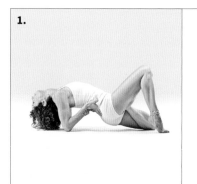

Half Lotus Half Eastern Intense Stretch Pose

Ardha Padma Ardha Purvottanasana

(UHR-duh PUHD-muh UHR-duh poor-vo-tahn-AHS-uh-nuh)

Also Known As: Half Lotus Reverse Table Top, Half Lotus Half Reverse Plank

Modification: elbows to the floor, palms to the lower back; one leg in half lotus, other knee bent; heel up

1. right side view
2. left side view

Pose Type: standing (on the elbows, knee and foot), backbend

Drishti Point: Bhrumadhye or Ajna Chakra (third eye, between the eyebrows)

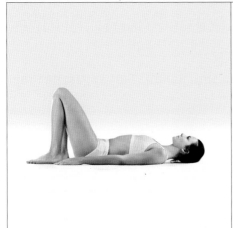

Bridge Whole Body Pose Prep.

Setu Bandha Sarvangasana Prep.

(SEY-tu BUHN-duh suhr-vuhng-GAHS-uh-nuh)

Modification: spine flat on the floor, palms down by the hips, heels down

Pose Type: supine

Drishti Point: Bhrumadhye or Ajna Chakra (third eye, between the eyebrows)

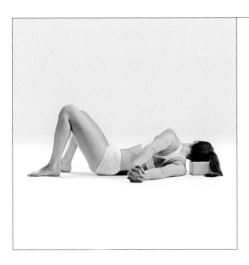

Reclined Hands Bound Twisted Stomach Pose in Bridge Whole Body Pose Prep.

Supta Baddha Hasta Jatara Parivartanasana in Setu Bandha Sarvangasana Prep.

(SUP-tuh BUH-duh HUH-stuh JAH-tuh-ruh puh-ri-vuhrt-uhn-AHS-uh-nuh in SEY-tu BUHN-duh suhr-vuhng-GAHS-uh-nuh)

Modification: ear resting on a yoga block

Pose Type: supine, twist

Drishti Point: Parshva Drishti (to the right), Parshva Drishti (to the left)

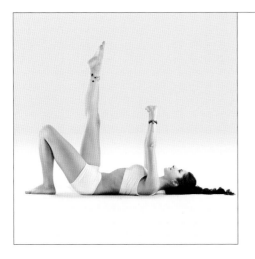

Reclined Hands Bound One Leg Extended Pose in Bridge Whole Body Pose Prep.

Supta Baddha Hasta Utthita Eka Padasana in Setu Bandha Sarvangasana Prep.

(SUP-tuh BUH-duh HUH-stuh UT-ti-tuh EY-kuh puh-DAHS-uh-nuh in SEY-tu BUHN-duh suhr-vuhng-GAHS-uh-nuh)

Modification: arms straight in front, palms facing up

Pose Type: supine

Drishti Point: Angushtamadhye or Angushta Ma Dyai (thumbs)

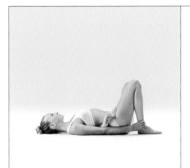

Reclined Half Bound Lotus Pose in Bridge Whole Body Pose Prep.

Supta Ardha Baddha Padmasana in Setu Bandha Sarvangasana Prep.

(SUP-tuh UHR-duh BUH-duh puhd-MAHS-uh-nuh in SEY-tu BUHN-duh suhr-vuhng-GAHS-uh-nuh)

Modification: grabbing onto the ankle
Pose Type: supine, binding
Drishti Point: Bhrumadhye or Ajna Chakra (third eye, between the eyebrows)

BRIDGE: HEELS DOWN, ARMS BEHIND THE BACK

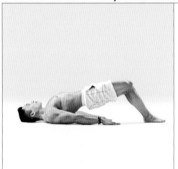

Bridge Whole Body Pose

Setu Bandha Sarvangasana

(SEY-tu BUHN-duh suhr-vuhng-GAHS-uh-nuh)

Modification: palms to the floor, arms straight; feet in front of the knees
Pose Type: supine, backbend
Drishti Point: Bhrumadhye or Ajna Chakra (third eye, between the eyebrows)

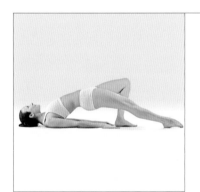

Uneven Bridge Whole Body Pose

Vishama Setu Bandha Sarvangasana

(VISH-uh-muh SEY-tu BUHN-duh suhr-vuhng-GAHS-uh-nuh)

Also Known As: Desk Pose Modification (Dwipadapitam)
Modification: palms down by the heel of the bent leg, other leg straight
Pose Type: supine, backbend
Drishti Point: Bhrumadhye or Ajna Chakra (third eye, between the eyebrows)

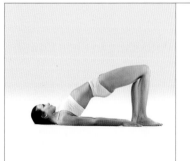

Bridge Whole Body Pose

Setu Bandha Sarvangasana

(SEY-tu BUHN-duh suhr-vuhng-GAHS-uh-nuh)

Also Known As: Shoulder Pose (Kandharasana)
Modification: palms down by the heels
Pose Type: supine, backbend
Drishti Point: Bhrumadhye or Ajna Chakra (third eye, between the eyebrows)

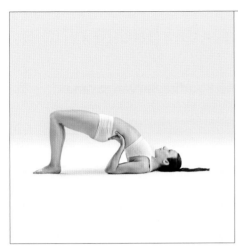

Bridge Whole Body Pose

Setu Bandha Sarvangasana

(SEY-tu BUHN-duh suhr-vuhng-GAHS-uh-nuh)

Modification: palms to the lower back

Pose Type: supine, backbend

Drishti Point: Bhrumadhye or Ajna Chakra (third eye, between the eyebrows)

BRIDGE: HEELS DOWN, ARMS OVERHEAD & BEHIND THE BACK

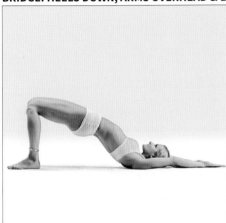

Bridge Whole Body Pose

Setu Bandha Sarvangasana

(SEY-tu BUHN-duh suhr-vuhng-GAHS-uh-nuh)

Also Known As: Desk Pose Modification (Dwipadapitam)

Modification: arms straight to the floor over the head, palms facing up

Pose Type: supine, backbend

Drishti Point: Bhrumadhye or Ajna Chakra (third eye, between the eyebrows)

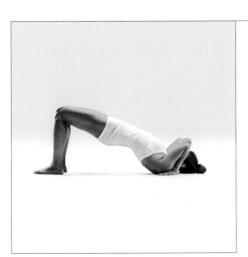

Bridge Whole Body Pose

Setu Bandha Sarvangasana

(SEY-tu BUHN-duh suhr-vuhng-GAHS-uh-nuh)

Also Known As: Upward Bow Pose Prep. (Urdhva Dhanurasana Prep.)

Modification: palms under the shoulders, fingertips pointing to the heels

Pose Type: supine, backbend

Drishti Point: Bhrumadhye or Ajna Chakra (third eye, between the eyebrows)

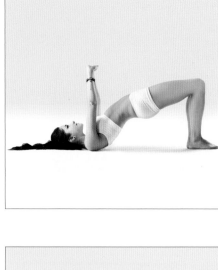

Upward Hands Bound Bridge Whole Body Pose

Urdhva Baddha Hasta Setu Bandha Sarvangasana

(OORD-vuh BUH-duh HUH-stuh SEY-tu BUHN-duh suhr-vuhng-GAHS-uh-nuh)

Also Known As: Desk Pose Modification (Dwipadapitam)
Pose Type: supine, backbend
Drishti Point: Angushtamadhye or Angushta Ma Dyai (thumbs)

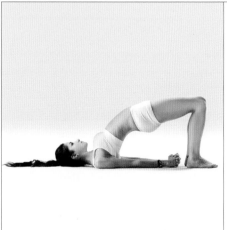

Hands Bound Bridge Whole Body Pose

Baddha Hasta Setu Bandha Sarvangasana

(BUH-duh HUH-stuh SEY-tu BUHN-duh suhr-vuhng-GAHS-uh-nuh)

Pose Type: supine, backbend
Drishti Point: Bhrumadhye or Ajna Chakra (third eye, between the eyebrows)

BRIDGE: HEELS DOWN, GRABBING ONTO THE ANKLES

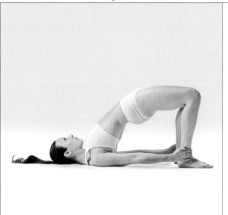

Hand to Ankle Bridge Whole Body Pose

Hasta Kulpa Setu Bandha Sarvangasana

(HUH-stuh KUL-puh SEY-tu BUHN-duh suhr-vuhng-GAHS-uh-nuh)

Also Known As: Desk Pose Modification (Dwipadapitam)
Pose Type: supine, backbend
Drishti Point: Bhrumadhye or Ajna Chakra (third eye, between the eyebrows)

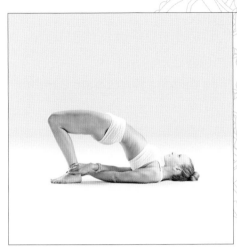

Hand to Ankle Bridge Whole Body Pose

Hasta Kulpa Setu Bandha Sarvangasana

(HUH-stuh KUL-puh SEY-tu BUHN-duh suhr-vuhng-GAHS-uh-nuh)

Also Known As: Desk Pose Modification (Dwipadapitam)
Modification: arms crossed
Pose Type: supine, backbend
Drishti Point: Bhrumadhye or Ajna Chakra (third eye, between the eyebrows)

BRIDGE: HEELS DOWN—ONE FOOT OFF THE FLOOR

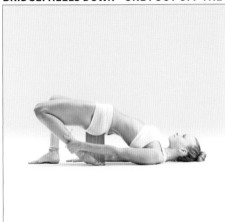

One Hand to Ankle Bridge Whole Body Pose

Eka Hasta Kulpa Setu Bandha Sarvangasana

(EY-kuh HUH-stuh KUL-puh SEY-tu BUHN-duh suhr-vuhng-GAHS-uh-nuh)

Modification: yoga block under the sitting bones; grabbing onto the ankle on the same side, top of the foot to the floor
Pose Type: supine, backbend
Drishti Point: Bhrumadhye or Ajna Chakra (third eye, between the eyebrows)

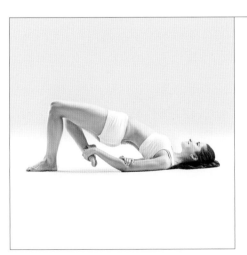

One Hand to Ankle Bridge Whole Body Pose

Eka Hasta Kulpa Setu Bandha Sarvangasana

(EY-kuh HUH-stuh KUL-puh SEY-tu BUHN-duh suhr-vuhng-GAHS-uh-nuh)

Modification: Arm 1: grabbing onto the ankle of the opposite leg
Arm 2: grabbing onto the opposite arm
Pose Type: supine, backbend, binding
Drishti Point: Bhrumadhye or Ajna Chakra (third eye, between the eyebrows)

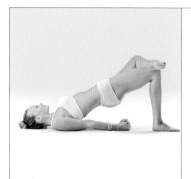

Half Fire Log Pose in One-Legged Hands Bound Bridge Whole Body Pose

Ardha Agnistambhasana in Eka Pada Baddha Hasta Setu Bandha Sarvangasana

(UHR-duh uhg-ni-stuhm-BAHS-uh-nuh in EY-kuh PUH-duh BUH-duh HUH-stuh SEY-tu BUHN-duh suhr-vuhng-GAHS-uh-nuh)

Modification: ankle on top of the knee heel down, toes of the top foot pointed
Pose Type: supine, backbend
Drishti Point: Bhrumadhye or Ajna Chakra (third eye, between the eyebrows)

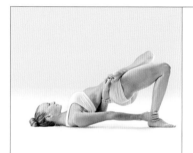

Half Bound Lotus One Hand to Ankle Bridge Whole Body Pose

Ardha Baddha Padma Eka Hasta Kulpa Setu Bandha Sarvangasana

(UHR-duh BUH-duh PUHD-muh EY-kuh HUH-stuh KUL-puh SEY-tu BUHN-duh suhr-vuhng-GAHS-uh-nuh)

Also Known As: Desk Pose Modification (Dwipadapitam)
Modification: heel down
Pose Type: supine, backbend, binding
Drishti Point: Bhrumadhye or Ajna Chakra (third eye, between the eyebrows)

BRIDGE: HEELS DOWN—ONE LEG TO THE SKY

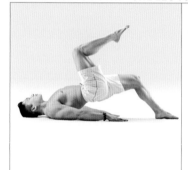

One-Legged Bridge Whole Body Pose

Eka Pada Setu Bandha Sarvangasana

(EY-kuh PUH-duh SEY-tu BUHN-duh suhr-vuhng-GAHS-uh-nuh)

Modification: palms down, arms straight on the floor; both knees bent
Pose Type: supine, backbend
Drishti Point: Bhrumadhye or Ajna Chakra (third eye, between the eyebrows)

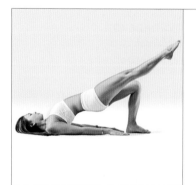

One-Legged Bridge Whole Body Pose

Eka Pada Setu Bandha Sarvangasana

(EY-kuh PUH-duh SEY-tu BUHN-duh suhr-vuhng-GAHS-uh-nuh)

Modification: palms down, arms straight on the floor; one leg up and straight, knees toward each other
Pose Type: supine, backbend
Drishti Point: Bhrumadhye or Ajna Chakra (third eye, between the eyebrows)

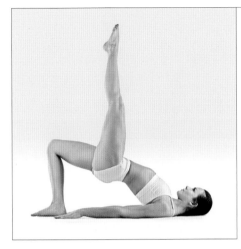

One-Legged Bridge Whole Body Pose

Eka Pada Setu Bandha Sarvangasana

(EY-kuh PUH-duh SEY-tu BUHN-duh suhr-vuhng-GAHS-uh-nuh)

Also Known As: Desk Pose Modification (Dwipadapitam)
Modification: palms down by the heel
Pose Type: supine, backbend
Drishti Point: Bhrumadhye or Ajna Chakra (third eye, between the eyebrows)

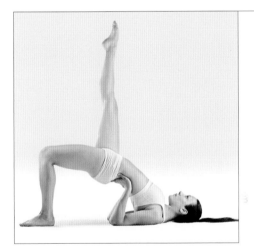

One-Legged Bridge Whole Body Pose

Eka Pada Setu Bandha Sarvangasana

(EY-kuh PUH-duh SEY-tu BUHN-duh suhr-vuhng-GAHS-uh-nuh)

Also Known As: Peacock Stretch Pose (Uttana Mayurasana)
Modification: palms to the lower back
Pose Type: supine, backbend
Drishti Point: Bhrumadhye or Ajna Chakra (third eye, between the eyebrows)

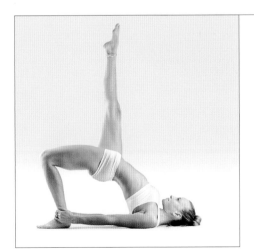

Both Hands to Ankle One-Legged Bridge Whole Body Pose

Dwi Hasta Kulpa Eka Pada Setu Bandha Sarvangasana

(DWI-huh-stuh KUL-puh EY-kuh PUH-duh SEY-tu BUHN-duh suhr-vuhng-GAHS-uh-nuh)

Modification: grabbing onto the ankle with both hands
Pose Type: supine, backbend
Drishti Point: Bhrumadhye or Ajna Chakra (third eye, between the eyebrows)

1.

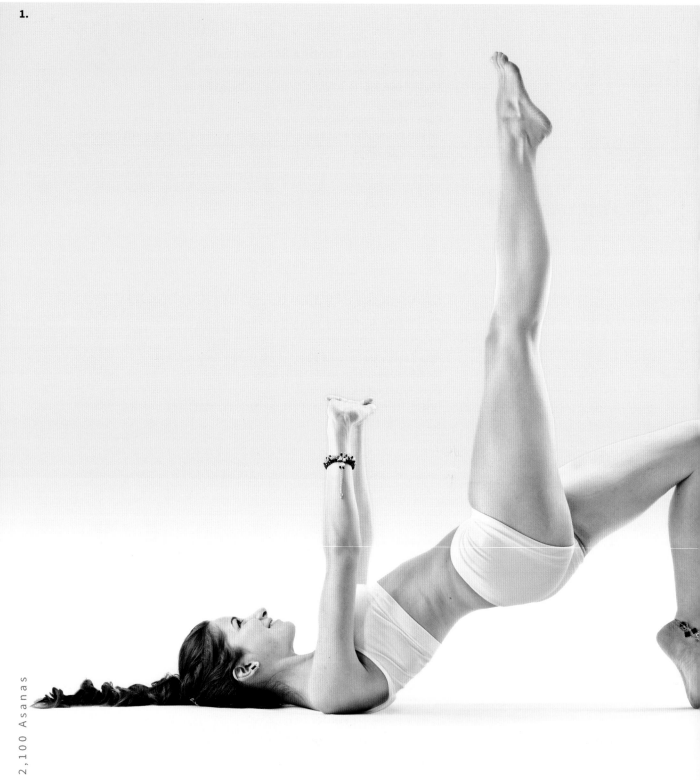

Bridge Whole Body Pose

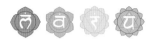

Eka Pada Urdhva Baddha Hasta Prapada Setu Bandha Sarvangasana

(EY-kuh PUH-duh OORD-vuh BUH-duh HUH-stuh PRUH-puh-duh SEY-tu BUHN-duh suhr-vuhng-GAHS-uh-nuh)

Pose Type: supine, backbend

Drishti Point: Angusthamadhye or Angustha Ma Dyai(thumbs)

How to Perform the Pose:

1. Begin by lying with your back flat on the floor. Keep your arms by the sides of your torso, hands by the sides of the hips, palms facing down. Engage your *mula bandha, uddhiyana bandha*, and *ujjayi* breathing.

2. Exhale, bend your knees, and slide your feet toward your sitting bones. Keep your feet flat on the floor, parallel to each other and in line with your sitting bones.

3. On the next exhale, push into your arms and feet and lift your hips off the floor until your thighs are parallel to the floor.

4. Inhale, interlock your fingers behind your back, and press your palms together. Exhale as you push through your chest and straighten the arms.

5. Exhale, bring your ankles and feet together. On the next exhale, lift your right leg, pointing your right toes up to the sky (Pose #2).

6. Exhale, bring your left heel up. Inhale, release your arms and bring them out in front of your chest. Exhale as you interlock your fingers, rotate your palms up to the sky and straighten the arms (Pose #1).

7. Hold the pose for at least 30, and up to 90, seconds in order to receive the full benefits of the stretch. Inhale, lower your right leg, and repeat on the opposite side.

8. On the next inhale, lower your spine to the floor and stretch the legs out in front of you, coming back to the starting position.

Modification: arms extended up to the sky, fingers interlocked, palms facing up, heel up

eka = one
pada = foot or leg
urdhva = upward
baddha = bound
hasta = hand
prapada = tip of the feet
setu = bridge, dam or dike
bandha = lock
sarvanga = the whole body

2.

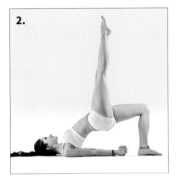

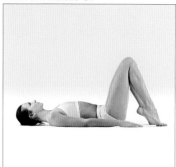

Tip Toe Bridge Whole Body Pose Prep.

Prapada Setu Bandha Sarvangasana Prep.

(PRUH-puh-duh SEY-tu BUHN-duh suhr-vuhng-GAHS-uh-nuh)

Modification: spine flat on the floor, palms down by the hips, heels up
Pose Type: supine
Drishti Point: Bhrumadhye or Ajna Chakra (third eye, between the eyebrows)

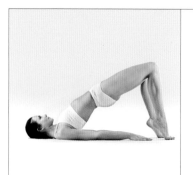

Tip Toe Bridge Whole Body Pose

Prapada Setu Bandha Sarvangasana

(PRUH-puh-duh SEY-tu BUHN-duh suhr-vuhng-GAHS-uh-nuh)

Modification: palms down
Pose Type: supine, backbend
Drishti Point: Bhrumadhye or Ajna Chakra (third eye, between the eyebrows)

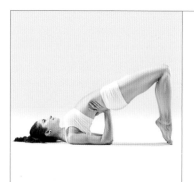

Tip Toe Bridge Whole Body Pose

Prapada Setu Bandha Sarvangasana

(PRUH-puh-duh SEY-tu BUHN-duh suhr-vuhng-GAHS-uh-nuh)

Modification: palms to the lower back
Pose Type: supine, backbend
Drishti Point: Bhrumadhye or Ajna Chakra (third eye, between the eyebrows)

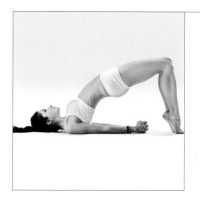

Hands Bound Tip Toe Bridge Whole Body Pose

Baddha Hasta Prapada Setu Bandha Sarvangasana

(BUH-duh HUH-stuh PRUH-puh-duh SEY-tu BUHN-duh suhr-vuhng-GAHS-uh-nuh)

Pose Type: supine, backbend
Drishti Point: Bhrumadhye or Ajna Chakra (third eye, between the eyebrows)

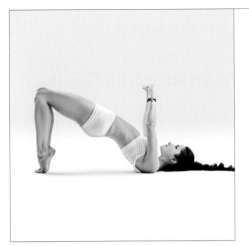

Upward Hands Bound Tip Toe Bridge Whole Body Pose

Urdhva Baddha Hasta Prapada Setu Bandha Sarvangasana

(OORD-vuh BUH-duh HUH-stuh PRUH-puh-duh SEY-tu BUHN-duh suhr-vuhng-GAHS-uh-nuh)

Pose Type: supine, backbend
Drishti Point: Angushtamadhye or Angushta Ma Dyai (thumbs)

BRIDGE: HEELS UP—ONE LEG CROSSED OVER

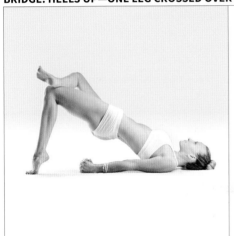

Half Fire Log Pose in One-Legged Hands Bound Tip Toe Bridge Whole Body Pose

Ardha Agnistambhasana in Eka Pada Baddha Hasta Prapada Setu Bandha Sarvangasana

(UHR-duh uhg-ni-stuhm-BAHS-uh-nuh in EY-kuh PUH-duh BUH-duh HUH-stuh PRUH-puh-duh SEY-tu BUHN-duh suhr-vuhng-GAHS-uh-nuh)

Modification: heel up; ankle on top of the knee, toes flexed in
Pose Type: supine, backbend
Drishti Point: Bhrumadhye or Ajna Chakra (third eye, between the eyebrows)

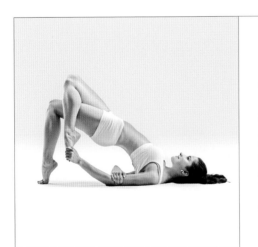

Uneven Leg Position of Cow Face Pose in One-Legged Tip Toe Bridge Whole Body Pose

Vishama Pada Gomukhasana in Eka Pada Prapada Setu Bandha Sarvangasana

(VISH-uh-muh PUH-duh go-muk-AHS-uh-nuh in EY-kuh PUH-duh PRUH-puh-duh SEY-tu BUHN-duh suhr-vuhng-GAHS-uh-nuh)

Modification: Arm 1: grabbing onto the foot of the opposite leg
Arm 2: grabbing onto the opposite arm
Pose Type: supine, backbend, binding
Drishti Point: Bhrumadhye or Ajna Chakra (third eye, between the eyebrows)

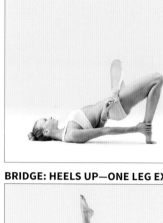

Half Bound Lotus One Hand to Ankle Tip Toe Bridge Whole Body Pose

Ardha Baddha Padma Eka Hasta Kulpa Prapada Setu Bandha Sarvangasana

(UHR-duh BUH-duh PUHD-muh EY-kuh HUH-stuh KUL-puh PRUH-puh-duh SEY-tu BUHN-duh suhr-vuhng-GAHS-uh-nuh)

Modification: heel up

Pose Type: supine, backbend, binding

Drishti Point: Bhrumadhye or Ajna Chakra (third eye, between the eyebrows)

BRIDGE: HEELS UP—ONE LEG EXTENDED TO THE SKY

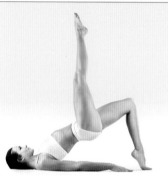

One-Legged Tip Toe Bridge Whole Body Pose

Eka Pada Prapada Setu Bandha Sarvangasana

(EY-kuh PUH-duh PRUH-puh-duh SEY-tu BUHN-duh suhr-vuhng-GAHS-uh-nuh)

Modification: palms down

Pose Type: supine, backbend

Drishti Point: Bhrumadhye or Ajna Chakra (third eye, between the eyebrows)

1.

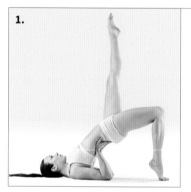

One-Legged Tip Toe Bridge Whole Body Pose

Eka Pada Prapada Setu Bandha Sarvangasana

(EY-kuh PUH-duh PRUH-puh-duh SEY-tu BUHN-duh suhr-vuhng-GAHS-uh-nuh)

Modification: palms to the lower back

1. fingertips pointing to the heel
2. fingertips pointing to the head

Pose Type: supine, backbend

Drishti Point: Bhrumadhye or Ajna Chakra (third eye, between the eyebrows)

2.

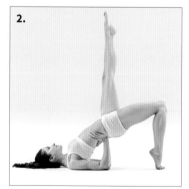

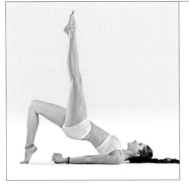

One-Legged Hands Bound Tip Toe Bridge Whole Body Pose

Eka Pada Baddha Hasta Prapada Setu Bandha Sarvangasana

(EY-kuh PUH-duh BUH-duh HUH-stuh PRUH-puh-duh SEY-tu BUHN-duh suhr-vuhng-GAHS-uh-nuh)

Modification: leg straight and extended to the sky, heel up

Pose Type: supine, backbend

Drishti Point: Bhrumadhye or Ajna Chakra (third eye, between the eyebrows)

BRIDGE: HEELS UP—ONE LEG EXTENDED TO THE SKY—"BALLET TOES"

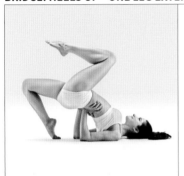

Intense Ankle Stretch One-Legged Bridge Whole Body Pose

Uttana Kulpa Eka Pada Setu Bandha Sarvangasana

(ut-TAHN-uh KUL-puh EY-kuh PUH-duh PRUH-puh-duh SEY-tu BUHN-duh suhr-vuhng-GAHS-uh-nuh)

Modification: palms to the lower back; both knees bent

Pose Type: supine, backbend

Drishti Point: Bhrumadhye or Ajna Chakra (third eye, between the eyebrows)

Intense Ankle Stretch One-Legged Bridge Whole Body Pose

Uttana Kulpa Eka Pada Setu Bandha Sarvangasana

(ut-TAHN-uh KUL-puh EY-kuh PUH-duh SEY-tu BUHN-duh suhr-vuhng-GAHS-uh-nuh)

Modification: palms to the lower back; top leg straight

Pose Type: supine, backbend

Drishti Point: Bhrumadhye or Ajna Chakra (third eye, between the eyebrows)

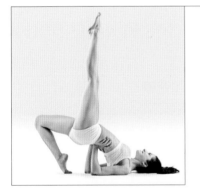

One Hand One-Legged Tip Toe Bridge Whole Body Pose

Eka Hasta Eka Pada Prapada Setu Bandha Sarvangasana

(EY-kuh HUH-stuh EY-kuh PUH-duh PRUH-puh-duh SEY-tu BUHN-duh suhr-vuhng-GAHS-uh-nuh)

Modification: lifted leg bent; palm to the lower back, heel up

Pose Type: supine, backbend

Drishti Point: Bhrumadhye or Ajna Chakra (third eye, between the eyebrows)

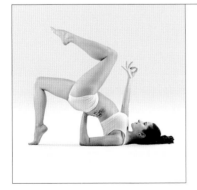

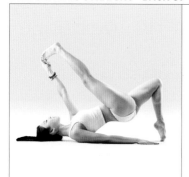

Extended Hand to Big Toe Pose Intense Ankle Stretch One-Legged Bridge Whole Body Pose

Utthita Hasta Padangushtasana in Uttana Kulpa Eka Pada Setu Bandha Sarvangasana

(UT-ti-tuh HUH-stuh puhd-ahng-goosh-TAHS-uh-nuh in ut-TAHN-uh KUL-puh EY-kuh PUH-duh SEY-tu BUHN-duh suhr-vuhng-GAHS-uh-nuh)

Pose Type: supine, backbend, forward bend

Drishti Point: Padayoragrai or Padayoragre (toes/feet)

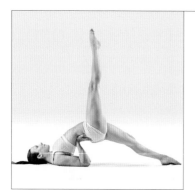

Complete Bridge Whole Body Pose

Paripurna Setu Bandha Sarvangasana

(puh-ri-POOR-nuh SEY-tu BUHN-duh suhr-vuhng-GAHS-uh-nuh)

Modification: palms to the lower back

Pose Type: supine, backbend

Drishti Point: Bhrumadhye or Ajna Chakra (third eye, between the eyebrows)

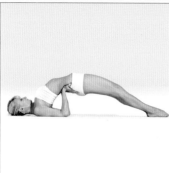

One-Legged Complete Bridge Whole Body Pose

Eka Pada Paripurna Setu Bandha Sarvangasana

(EY-kuh PUH-duh puh-ri-POOR-nuh SEY-tu BUHN-duh suhr-vuhng-GAHS-uh-nuh)

Modification: palms to the lower back

Pose Type: supine, backbend

Drishti Point: Bhrumadhye or Ajna Chakra (third eye, between the eyebrows)

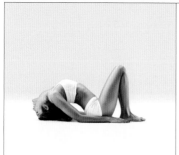

Half Fish Pose

Ardha Matsyasana

(UHR-duh muhts-YAHS-uh-nuh)

Modification: knees bent; feet flat on the floor, heels toward the sitting bones; palms down to the floor by the heels, elbows to the floor

Pose Type: seated, backbend

Drishti Point: Bhrumadhye or Ajna Chakra (third eye, between the eyebrows)

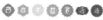

1.

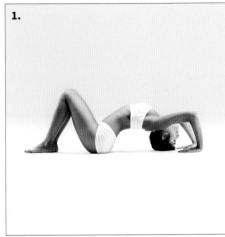

Half Fish Pose

Ardha Matsyasana

(UHR-duh muhts-YAHS-uh-nuh)

Modification: knees bent

1. arms over the head, feet flat on the floor

2. hands by the navel, palms pressed together, fingertips pointing up, both feet in the tip toe position

3. hands by the navel, palms pressed together, fingertips pointing up; one foot in the tip toe position, other leg raised

Pose Type: seated, backbend

Drishti Point: Bhrumadhye or Ajna Chakra (third eye, between the eyebrows)

2.

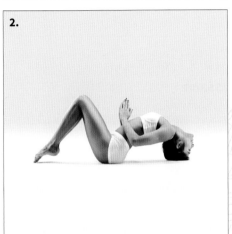

3.

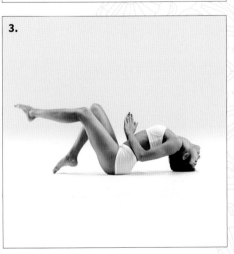

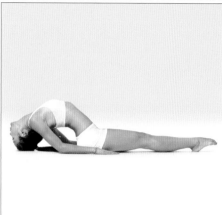

Fish Pose

Matsyasana

(muhts-YAHS-uh-nuh)

Modification: legs straight on the floor, elbows to the floor, palms down to the floor by the hips

Pose Type: seated, backbend

Drishti Point: Bhrumadhye or Ajna Chakra (third eye, between the eyebrows)

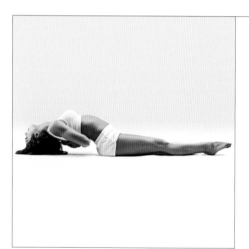

Reverse Prayer Fish Pose

Viparita Namaskar Matsyasana

(vi-puh-REE-tuh nuh-muhs-KAHR muhts-YAHS-uh-nuh)

Also Known As: Back of the Body Prayer Fish Pose (Paschima Namaskara Matsyasana)

Modification: legs straight to the floor

Pose Type: seated, backbend

Drishti Point: Bhrumadhye or Ajna Chakra (third eye, between the eyebrows)

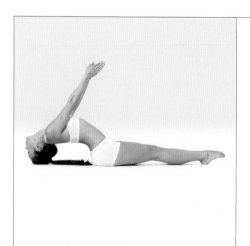

Intense Leg Stretch
Uttana Padasana

(ut-TAHN-uh puh-DAHS-uh-nuh)

Modification: legs straight on the floor, arms straight in front of the chest, palms pressed together

Pose Type: seated, backbend

Drishti Point: Bhrumadhye or Ajna Chakra (third eye, between the eyebrows)

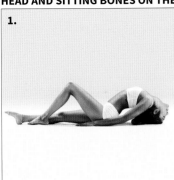

Fish Pose

Matsyasana

(muhts-YAHS-uh-nuh)

Modification: 1. one leg straight, other knee bent

2. one leg straight, other knee bent, bent leg crossed over

Pose Type: seated, backbend

Drishti Point: Bhrumadhye or Ajna Chakra (third eye, between the eyebrows)

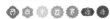

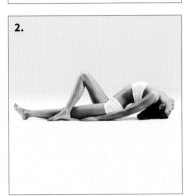

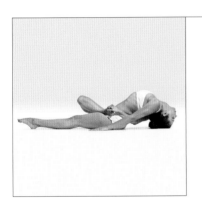

Half Bound Lotus Fish Pose

Ardha Baddha Padma Matsyasana

(UHR-duh BUH-duh PUHD-muh muhts-YAHS-uh-nuh)

Modification: sitting bones on the floor, palm to the floor by the hip

Pose Type: seated, backbend, binding

Drishti Point: Bhrumadhye or Ajna Chakra (third eye, between the eyebrows)

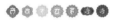

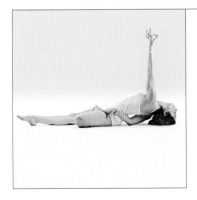

Half Bound Lotus Fish Pose

Ardha Baddha Padma Matsyasana

(UHR-duh BUH-duh PUHD-muh muhts-YAHS-uh-nuh)

Modification: one arm straight up to the sky, other arm grabbing onto the inside of the thigh behind the back; leg straight

Pose Type: seated, backbend, binding

Drishti Point: Bhrumadhye or Ajna Chakra (third eye, between the eyebrows)

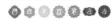

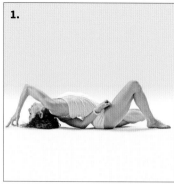

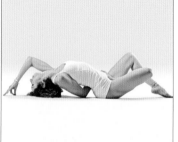

Half Bound Lotus Half Fish Pose

Ardha Baddha Padma Ardha Matsyasana

(UHR-duh BUH-duh PUHD-muh UHR-duh muhts-YAHS-uh-nuh)

Modification: grabbing onto the foot with arm behind the back, fingertips of the other arm touching the floor overhead, elbow bent; knee of the free leg bent

1. heel down
2. heel up

Pose Type: seated, backbend, binding

Drishti Point: Bhrumadhye or Ajna Chakra (third eye, between the eyebrows), Hastagrai or Hastagre (hands)

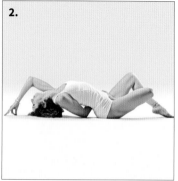

Intense Leg Stretch Pose Dedicated to Garuda

Uttana Pada Garudasana

(ut-TAHN-uh PUH-duh guh-ru-DAHS-uh-nuh)

Modification: fingertips and bottom foot to the floor

Pose Type: seated, backbend

Drishti Point: Angushtamadhye or Angushta Ma Dyai (thumbs)

RECLINED BOUND ANGLE POSE & FISH POSE

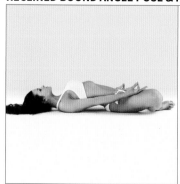

Reclined Bound Angle Pose

Supta Baddha Konasana

(SUP-tuh BUH-duh ko-NAHS-uh-nuh)

Modification: hands to the inner thighs, palms up

Pose Type: supine

Drishti Point: Bhrumadhye or Ajna Chakra (third eye, between the eyebrows)

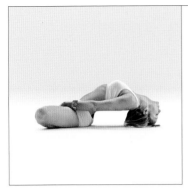

Reclined Bound Angle Pose

Supta Baddha Konasana

(SUP-tuh BUH-duh ko-NAHS-uh-nuh)

Also Known As: Bound Legs Fish Pose (Baddha Pada Matsyasana)
Modification: crown of the head to the floor, grabbing onto the shins, arms on top of the legs
Pose Type: seated, backbend
Drishti Point: Bhrumadhye or Ajna Chakra (third eye, between the eyebrows)

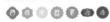

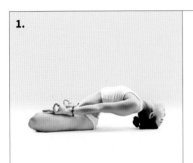
1.

Fish Pose

Matsyasana

(muhts-YAHS-uh-nuh)

Modification: 1. palms up on the inside of the thighs
2. grabbing onto the big toes, elbows to the floor
3. grabbing onto the forearms, arms up over the head
Pose Type: seated, backbend
Drishti Point: Bhrumadhye or Ajna Chakra (third eye, between the eyebrows)

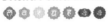

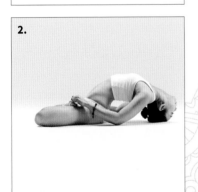
2.

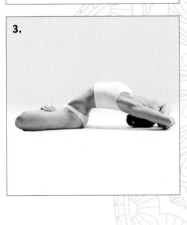
3.

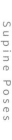

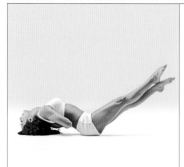

Reverse Prayer Intense Leg Stretch

Viparita Namaskar Uttana Padasana

(vi-puh-REE-tuh nuh-muhs-KAHR ut-TAHN-uh puh-DAHS-uh-nuh)

Also Known As: Back of the Body Prayer Intense Leg Stretch (Paschima Namaskara Uttana Padasana)

Modification: legs straight and off the floor, ankles crossed

Pose Type: seated, backbend, core

Drishti Point: Bhrumadhye or Ajna Chakra (third eye, between the eyebrows)

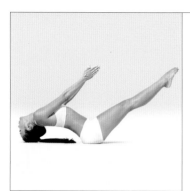

Intense Leg Stretch

Uttana Padasana

(ut-TAHN-uh puh-DAHS-uh-nuh)

Modification: legs straight and off the floor; arms straight in front of the chest, palms pressed together

Pose Type: seated, backbend, core

Drishti Point: Bhrumadhye or Ajna Chakra (third eye, between the eyebrows)

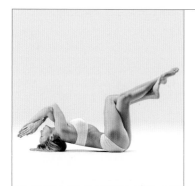

Intense Leg Stretch Pose Dedicated to Garuda

Uttana Pada Garudasana

(ut-TAHN-uh PUH-duh guh-ru-DAHS-uh-nuh)

Modification: legs and arms lifted off the floor

Pose Type: seated, backbend, core

Drishti Point: Angushtamadhye or Angushta Ma Dyai (thumbs)

BRIDGE POSE

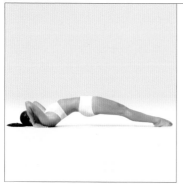

Complete Bridge Whole Body Pose

Paripurna Setu Bandha Sarvangasana

(puh-ri-POOR-nuh SEY-tu BUHN-duh suhr-vuhng-GAHS-uh-nuh)

Modification: palms to the floor under the shoulders, fingertips pointing to the heels; elbows tucked in, shoulder width apart

Pose Type: supine, backbend

Drishti Point: Bhrumadhye or Ajna Chakra (third eye, between the eyebrows)

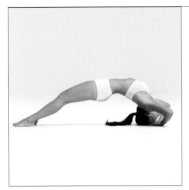

Vajra Cutter Sutra Bridge Pose

Vajracchedika Prajnaparamita Sutra Setu Bandhasana

(vahj-ruh-CHEY-di-kuh pruhj-NAH-puh-ruh-mi-TAH SU-truh SEY-tu buhn-DAHS-uh-nuh)

Modification: forehead to the floor, elbows splaying to the side, arms in "diamond" shape

Pose Type: standing (on the head and feet), backbend

Drishti Point: Bhrumadhye or Ajna Chakra (third eye, between the eyebrows)

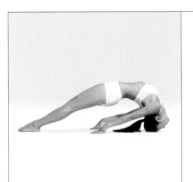

Bridge Pose

Setu Bandhasana

(SEY-tu buhn-DAHS-uh-nuh)

Modification: fingertips to the floor and pointing toward the heels

Pose Type: standing (on the head and feet), backbend

Drishti Point: Bhrumadhye or Ajna Chakra (third eye, between the eyebrows)

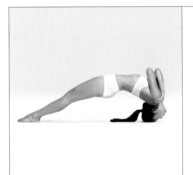

Bridge Pose

Setu Bandhasana

(SEY-tu buhn-DAHS-uh-nuh)

Modification: arms crossed in front of the chest, hands to the shoulders

Pose Type: standing (on the head and feet), backbend

Drishti Point: Bhrumadhye or Ajna Chakra (third eye, between the eyebrows)

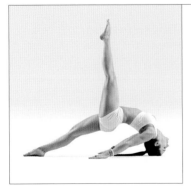

One-Legged Bridge Pose

Eka Pada Setu Bandhasana

(EY-kuh PUH-duh SEY-tu buhn-DAHS-uh-nuh)

Modification: fingertips pointing toward the heels, palms flat on the floor

Pose Type: standing (on the head and feet), backbend

Drishti Point: Bhrumadhye or Ajna Chakra (third eye, between the eyebrows)

1.

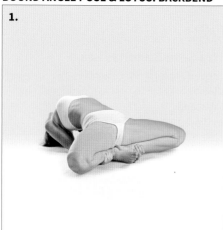

Reclined Bound Angle Pose
Supta Baddha Konasana
(SUP-tuh BUH-duh ko-NAHS-uh-nuh)
Also Known As: Bound Legs Fish Pose (Baddha Pada Matsyasana)
Modification: crown of the head to the floor, grabbing onto the shins under the legs
1. elbows to the floor
2. arms straight, elbows off the floor
Pose Type: backbend, standing (on the knees)
Drishti Point: Bhrumadhye or Ajna Chakra (third eye, between the eyebrows)

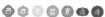

2.

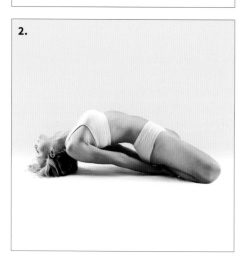

Intense Lotus Peacock
Uttana Padma Mayurasana
(ut-TAHN-uh PUHD-muh muh-yoor-AHS-uh-nuh)
Also Known As: Intense Front Body Stretching and Rejuvenating Lotus Pose (Purvottana Padma Sarvangasana), All Body Parts Lotus Pose (Sarvangasana Padmasana)
Modification: knees on the floor
Pose Type: supine, backbend
Drishti Point: Bhrumadhye or Ajna Chakra (third eye, between the eyebrows)

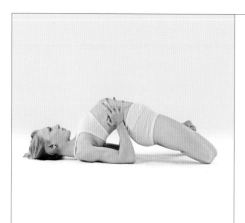

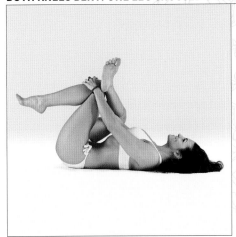

Eye of the Needle Pose

Sucirandrasana

(soo-chi-ruhn-DRAHS-uh-nuh)

Pose Type: supine, forward bend

Drishti Point: Bhrumadhye or Ajna Chakra (third eye, between the eyebrows)

1.

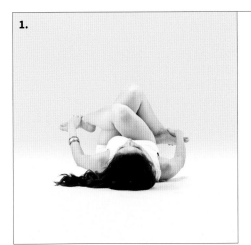

Reclined Leg Position of Cow Face Pose

Supta Pada Gomukhasana

(SUP-tuh PUH-duh go-muk-AHS-uh-nuh)

Modification: knees to the chest, grabbing onto both feet

1. front view
2. side view

Pose Type: supine, forward bend

Drishti Point: Bhrumadhye or Ajna Chakra (third eye, between the eyebrows)

2.

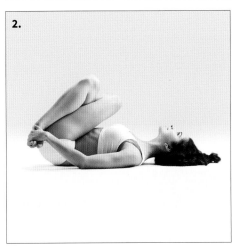

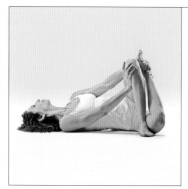

Reclined Twisting Fire Log Pose

Supta Parshva Agnistambhasana

(SUP-tuh PAHRSH-vuh uhg-ni-stuhm-BAHS-uh-nuh)

Pose Type: supine, forward bend, twist

Drishti Point: Bhrumadhye or Ajna Chakra (third eye, between the eyebrows)

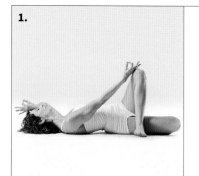

Reclined Leg Position of Half Cow Face Pose

Supta Pada Ardha Gomukhasana

(SUP-tuh PUH-duh UHR-duh go-muk-AHS-uh-nuh)

Modification: knees apart, top foot on the floor

1. one hand to the forehead, other hand on the top knee
2. grabbing onto the shoulders, arms crossed in front of the neck
3. one hand to the top ankle, other hand to the bottom foot

Pose Type: supine, forward bend, twist

Drishti Point: Bhrumadhye or Ajna Chakra (third eye, between the eyebrows)

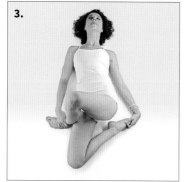

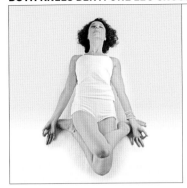

Reclined Leg Position of Cow Face Pose

Supta Pada Gomukhasana

(SUP-tuh PUH-duh go-muk-AHS-uh-nuh)

Modification: knees to the floor

Pose Type: supine

Drishti Point: Bhrumadhye or Ajna Chakra (third eye, between the eyebrows)

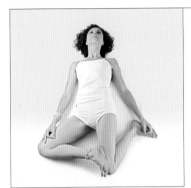

Universal All-Encompassing Diamond Pose

Vishvavajrasana

(vish-vuh-vuhj-RAHS-uh-nuh)

Also Known As: Double Diamond Pose

Modification: foot on top of the knee; hand to the sole of the back foot, other hand resting on the thigh of the front leg, looking straight ahead

Pose Type: supine, twist

Drishti Point: Bhrumadhye or Ajna Chakra (third eye, between the eyebrows)

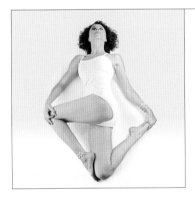

Revolved Universal All-Encompassing Diamond Pose

Parivritta Vishvavajrasana *(puh-ri-VRIT-tuh vish-vuh-vuhj-RAHS-uh-nuh)*

Also Known As: Revolved Double Diamond Pose

Modification: hand grabbing onto the foot; other hand grabbing onto the opposite knee, looking up to the sky

Pose Type: supine, forward bend, twist

Drishti Point: Bhrumadhye or Ajna Chakra (third eye, between the eyebrows)

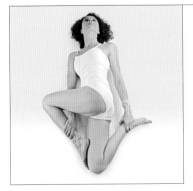

Revolved Universal All-Encompassing Diamond Pose

Parivritta Vishvavajrasana *(puh-ri-VRIT-tuh vish-vuh-vuhj-RAHS-uh-nuh)*

Also Known As: Revolved Double Diamond Pose

Modification: hand grabbing onto the ankle, arm under the thigh; other hand grabbing onto the ankle of the bottom leg, looking straight ahead

Pose Type: supine, forward bend, twist

Drishti Point: Bhrumadhye or Ajna Chakra (third eye, between the eyebrows)

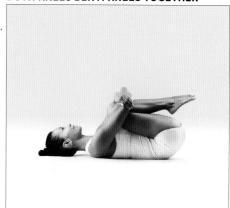

Reclined Child's Pose

Supta Balasana

(SUP-tuh bah-LAHS-uh-nuh)

Also Known As: Pelvic Pose (Apanasana)
Modification: binding arms, grabbing onto the triceps
Pose Type: supine, forward bend
Drishti Point: Bhrumadhye or Ajna Chakra (third eye, between the eyebrows)

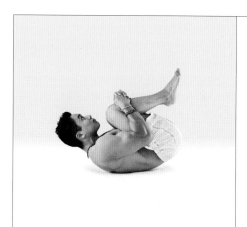

Wind-Relieving Pose

Vayu Muktyasana

(VAH-yuh muk-TYAHS-uh-nuh)

Also Known As: Wind Releaser Pose (Pavana Muktasana)
Modification: fingers interlocked on top of the shins
Pose Type: supine, forward bend, core
Drishti Point: Bhrumadhye or Ajna Chakra (third eye, between the eyebrows)

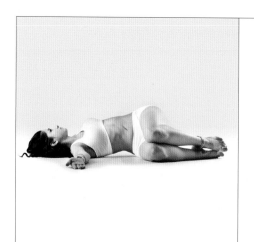

Twisted Stomach Pose

Jatara Parivartanasana

(JAH-tuh-ruh puh-ri-vuhrt-uhn-AHS-uh-nuh)

Also Known As: Reclining Waist Pose Prep.(Supta Madhyasana), Sideways Wind Releaser Pose (Pavana Muktasana)
Modification: knees bent, arms straight out to the sides
Pose Type: supine, forward bend, twist
Drishti Point: Bhrumadhye or Ajna Chakra (third eye, between the eyebrows)

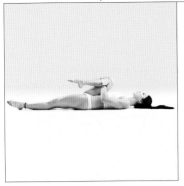

One-Legged Wind Relieving Pose

Eka Pada Pavana Muktasana

(EY-kuh PUH-duh puh-vuh-nuh muk-TAHS-uh-nuh)

Also Known As: Reclined Big Toe Pose A Prep. (Supta Padangushtasana A Prep.)

Modification: head on the floor, fingers interlocked on top of the shin

Pose Type: supine, forward bend

Drishti Point: Bhrumadhye or Ajna Chakra (third eye, between the eyebrows)

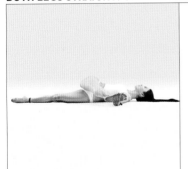

Reclining Tree Pose

Supta Vrikshasana

(SUP-tuh vrik-SHAHS-uh-nuh)

Also Known As: Reclined Big Toe Pose B Prep. (Supta Padangushtasana B Prep.)

Modification: hand to the bent knee, other hand along side of the torso, toes flexed in

Pose Type: supine

Drishti Point: Bhrumadhye or Ajna Chakra (third eye, between the eyebrows)

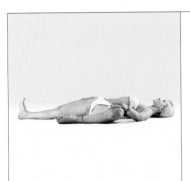

Revolved Reclining Hand to Foot Pose

Parivritta Supta Hasta Padasana

(puh-ri-VRIT-tuh SUP-tuh HUH-stuh puh-DAHS-uh-nuh)

Modification: legs straight, grabbing onto the inside arch of the foot

Pose Type: supine, forward bend, twist

Drishti Point: Bhrumadhye or Ajna Chakra (third eye, between the eyebrows)

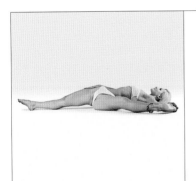

Reclining Big Toe Pose 2

Supta Padangushtasana 2

(SUP-tuh puhd-ahng-goosh-TAHS-uh-nuh)

Pose Type: supine, forward bend

Drishti Point: Bhrumadhye or Ajna Chakra (third eye, between the eyebrows)

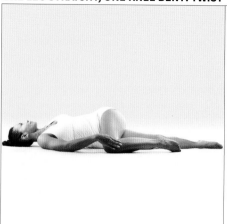

Reclined Lord of the Fishes Pose

Supta Matsyendrasana

(SUP-tuh muhts-yeyn-DRAHS-uh-nuh)

Also Known As: Revolving Reclined Big Toe Pose Prep. (Parivritta Supta Padan-gushtasana Prep.), Revolved Reclining Tree Pose (Parivritta Supta Vrikshasana)

Modification: knee bent at 90 degrees

Pose Type: supine, forward bend, twist

Drishti Point: Bhrumadhye or Ajna Chakra (third eye, between the eyebrows)

1.

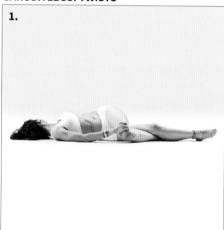

Sideways Reclining Leg Position of the Pose Dedicated to Garuda

Parshva Supta Pada Garudasana

(PAHRSH-vuh SUP-tuh PUH-duh guh-ru-DAHS-uh-nuh)

Modification: hand resting on the top knee, other arm to the floor along side the torso, looking to the side; arms straight out to the side, looking straight ahead

Pose Type: supine, twist

Drishti Point: Bhrumadhye or Ajna Chakra (third eye, between the eyebrows), Hastagrai or Hastagre (hands)

2.

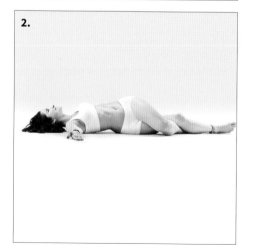

BOTH LEGS STRAIGHT AND TOGETHER: TWIST

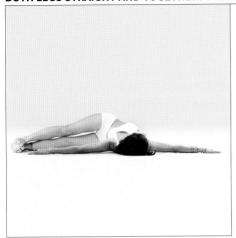

Twisted Stomach Pose

Jathara Parivartanasana

(JAH-tuh-ruh puh-ri-vuhrt-uhn-AHS-uh-nuh)

Also Known As: Reclining Waist Pose (Supta Madhyasana)
Modification: legs and arms straight
Pose Type: supine, forward bend, twist
Drishti Point: Hastagrai or Hastagre (hands)

ONE LEG STRAIGHT, ONE KNEE BENT: LEG CRADLE & HALF HAPPY BABY POSE

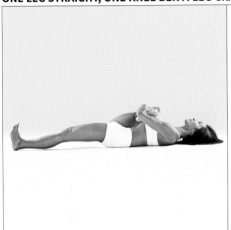

Reclined Baby Cradle Pose

Supta Hindolasana

(SUP-tuh hin-do-LAHS-uh-nuh)

Modification: back leg straight
Pose Type: supine, forward bend
Drishti Point: Bhrumadhye or Ajna Chakra (third eye, between the eyebrows)

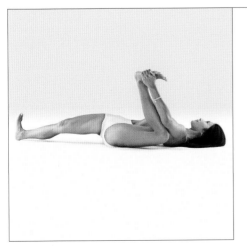

Reclined One Hand to Foot Pose

Supta Eka Hasta Padasana

(SUP-tuh EY-kuh HUH-stuh puh-DAHS-uh-nuh)

Pose Type: supine, forward bend
Drishti Point: Bhrumadhye or Ajna Chakra (third eye, between the eyebrows)

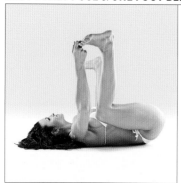

Happy Baby Pose

Sukha Balasana

(SUK-uh bahl-AHS-uh-nuh)

Also Known As: Happy Baby Pose (Ananda Balasana)
Modification: grabbing onto the big toes of the feet
Pose Type: supine, forward bend
Drishti Point: Bhrumadhye or Ajna Chakra (third eye, between the eyebrows)

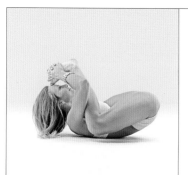

Reclined Star Pose

Supta Tarasana

(SUP-tuh tah-RAHS-uh-nuh)

Pose Type: supine, forward bend
Drishti Point: Bhrumadhye or Ajna Chakra (third eye, between the eyebrows), Padayoragrai or Padayoragre (toes/feet)

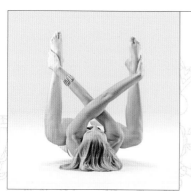

Happy Baby Pose

Sukha Balasana

(SUK-uh bahl-AHS-uh-nuh)

Also Known As: Happy Baby Pose (Ananda Balasana)
Modification: arms crossed, grabbing onto the outside edges of the feet
Pose Type: supine, forward bend
Drishti Point: Bhrumadhye or Ajna Chakra (third eye, between the eyebrows)

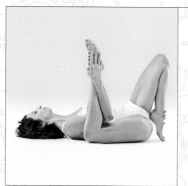

Reclined One Hand to Foot Pose

Supta Eka Hasta Padasana

(SUP-tuh EY-kuh HUH-stuh puh-DAHS-uh-nuh)

Modification: grabbing onto the back foot, heel to the sitting bone, toes pointed to the floor
Pose Type: supine, forward bend
Drishti Point: Bhrumadhye or Ajna Chakra (third eye, between the eyebrows)

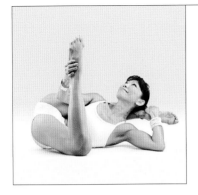

Reclined One Hand to Foot One Leg Behind the Head Pose in Infinity Pose

Supta Eka Hasta Pada Eka Pada Shirshasana in Anantasana

(SUP-tuh EY-kuh-HUH-stuh PUH-duh EY-kuh PUH-duh sheer-SHAS-uh-nuh in uhn-uhnt-AHS-uh-nuh)

Modification: bottom knee to the floor, toes pointing up to the sky

Pose Type: supine, forward bend

Drishti Point: Bhrumadhye or Ajna Chakra (third eye, between the eyebrows)

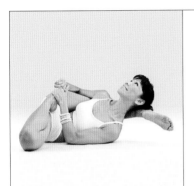

One Leg Behind the Head in Infinity Pose

Eka Pada Shirshasana in Anantasana

(EY-kuh PUH-duh sheer-SHAHS-uh-nuh in uhn-uhnt-AHS-uh-nuh)

Modification: bottom heel toward the hip

Pose Type: supine, forward bend

Drishti Point: Bhrumadhye or Ajna Chakra (third eye, between the eyebrows)

ONE AND BOTH FEET BEHIND THE HEAD

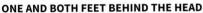

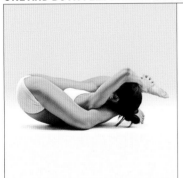

Pose Dedicated to Bhairava in Half Upward Facing Western Intense Stretch 2

Bhairavasana in Ardha Urdhva Mukha Paschimottanasana 2

(b-eye-ruh-VAHS-uh-nuh in UHR-duh OORD-vuh MUK-uh puhsh-chi-mo-tahn-AHS-uh-nuh)

Also Known As: Pose Dedicated to Bhairava in Half Upward Facing Forward Bend 2

Modification: 1. front view

2. back view

Pose Type: supine, forward bend

Drishti Point: Bhrumadhye or Ajna Chakra (third eye, between the eyebrows)

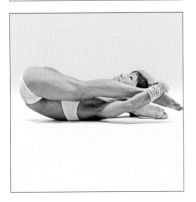

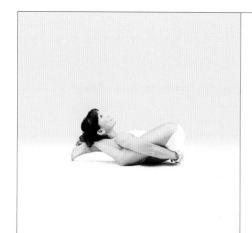

Hands Bound Yogic Sleep Pose

Baddha Hasta Yoganidrasana

(BUH-duh HUH-stuh yo-guh-ni-DRAHS-uh-nuh)

Modification: hands bound
Pose Type: supine, forward bend
Drishti Point: Bhrumadhye or Ajna Chakra (third eye, between the eyebrows)

HORIZONTAL SPLITS

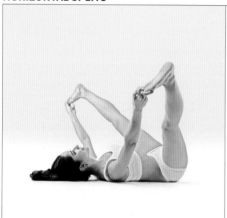

Reclined Angle Pose

Supta Konasana

(SUP-tuh ko-NAHS-uh-nuh)

Modification: back flat on the floor, feet lifted off the floor, grabbing onto the big toes
Pose Type: supine, forward bend
Drishti Point: Bhrumadhye or Ajna Chakra (third eye, between the eyebrows)

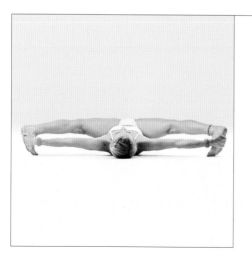

Reclined Angle Pose

Supta Konasana

(SUP-tuh ko-NAHS-uh-nuh)

Modification: back flat on the floor, toes to the floor, grabbing onto the outside edges of the feet
Pose Type: supine, forward bend
Drishti Point: Bhrumadhye or Ajna Chakra (third eye, between the eyebrows)

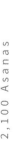

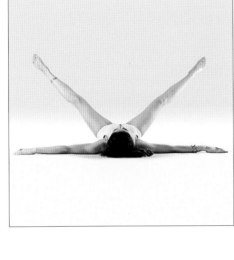

Reclined Angle Pose

Supta Konasana

(SUP-tuh ko-NAHS-uh-nuh)

Modification: back flat on the floor, feet lifted off the floor, arms straight out to the sides, palms down to the floor

Pose Type: supine

Drishti Point: Bhrumadhye or Ajna Chakra (third eye, between the eyebrows)

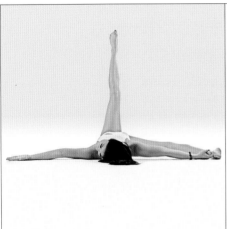

Sideways Reclined Angle Pose

Parshva Supta Konasana

(PAHRSH-vuh SUP-tuh ko-NAHS-uh-nuh)

Modification: back flat on the floor, head turning to side

Side 1: leg in the air; arm straight on the floor, palm facing up

Side 2: leg on the floor, grabbing onto the big toe

Pose Type: supine, twist

Drishti Point: Hastagrai or Hastagre (hands)

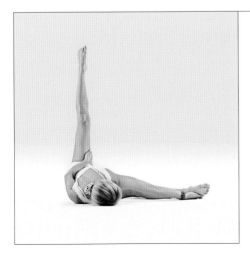

Revolved Half Bound Reclined Angle Pose

Parivritta Ardha Baddha Supta Konasana

(puh-ri-VRIT-uh UHR-duh BUH-duh SUP-tuh ko-NAHS-uh-nuh)

Modification: both legs straight

Side 1: leg pointing to the sky; arm wrapping around the back, hand to the inside of the hip on the opposite side

Side 2: leg on the floor, opposite hand grabbing onto the foot

Pose Type: supine, twist, binding

Drishti Point: Hastagrai or Hastagre (hands), Padayoragrai or Padayoragre (toes/feet)

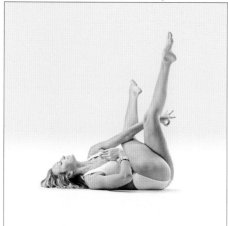

Upward Facing Western Intense Stretch

Urdhva Mukha Paschimottanasana

(OORD-vuh MUK-uh puhsh-chi-mo-tahn-AHS-uh-nuh)

Also Known As: Upward Facing Forward Bend

Modification: legs crossed, one arm threaded through the legs, other hand to the center of the chest

Pose Type: supine, forward bend, twist

Drishti Point: Bhrumadhye or Ajna Chakra (third eye, between the eyebrows), Padayoragrai or Padayoragre (toes/feet)

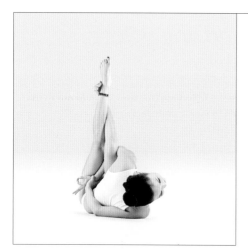

Reclined Hands Bound Pose Dedicated to Astavakra

Supta Baddha Hasta Ashtavakrasana

(SUP-tuh BUH-duh HUH-stuh uhsh-tuh-vuh-KRAHS-uh-nuh)

Also Known As: Reclined Hands Bound Eight Angle Pose

Modification: ankles crossed

Pose Type: supine, forward bend, twist, binding

Drishti Point: Bhrumadhye or Ajna Chakra (third eye, between the eyebrows)

ONE KNEE BENT TO THE BACK, OTHER LEG STRAIGHT

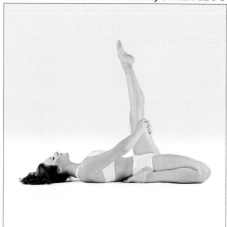

One-Legged Reclined Hero Pose

Eka Pada Supta Virasana

(EY-kuh PUH-duh SUP-tuh veer-AHS-uh-nuh)

Modification: straight leg lifted, fingers interlocked on the back of the thigh

Pose Type: supine, forward bend

Drishti Point: Bhrumadhye or Ajna Chakra (third eye, between the eyebrows)

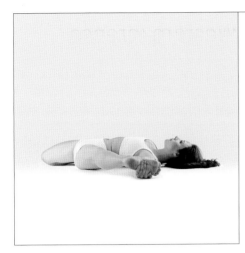

One-Legged Reclined Hero Pose

Eka Pada Supta Virasana

(EY-kuh PUH-duh SUP-tuh veer-AHS-uh-nuh)

Modification: leg straight out to the side, grabbing onto the outside edge of the foot

Pose Type: supine, forward bend

Drishti Point: Bhrumadhye or Ajna Chakra (third eye, between the eyebrows)

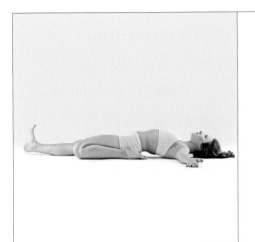

One-Legged Reclined Hero Pose

Eka Pada Supta Virasana

(EY-kuh PUH-duh SUP-tuh veer-AHS-uh-nuh)

Modification: leg straight on the floor, toes flexed in; arms straight out to the sides, palms facing up

Pose Type: supine

Drishti Point: Bhrumadhye or Ajna Chakra (third eye, between the eyebrows)

ONE KNEE BENT TO THE BACK, OTHER LEG BENT

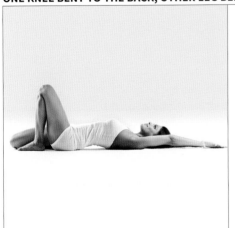

One-Legged Reclined Hero Pose

Eka Pada Supta Virasana

(EY-kuh PUH-duh SUP-tuh veer-AHS-uh-nuh)

Modification: Leg 1: in Hero Pose (Virasana)

Leg 2: knee up to the sky, heel to the sitting bones; arms up over the head, palms facing up

Pose Type: supine

Drishti Point: Bhrumadhye or Ajna Chakra (third eye, between the eyebrows)

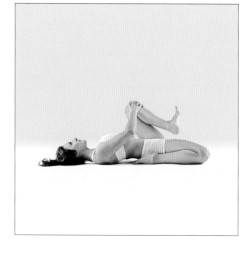

One-Legged Reclined Hero Pose

Eka Pada Supta Virasana

(EY-kuh PUH-duh SUP-tuh veer-AHS-uh-nuh)

Modification: Leg 1: in Hero Pose (Virasana)

Leg 2: knee toward the chest, toes flexed in; fingertips interlocked on top of the knee

Pose Type: supine, forward bend

Drishti Point: Bhrumadhye or Ajna Chakra (third eye, between the eyebrows)

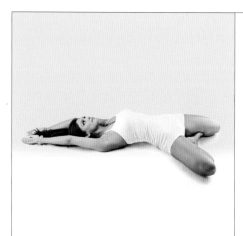

Half Bound Angle Pose in One-Legged Reclined Hero Pose

Ardha Baddha Konasana in Eka Pada Supta Virasana

(UHR-duh BUH-duh ko-NAHS-uh-nuh in EY-kuh PUH-duh SUP-tuh veer-AHS-uh-nuh)

Modification: arms up over the head, palms facing upward

Pose Type: supine

Drishti Point: Bhrumadhye or Ajna Chakra (third eye, between the eyebrows)

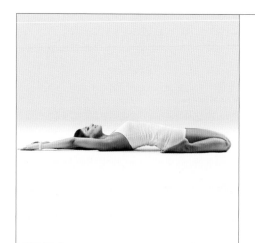

Reclined Hero Pose

Supta Virasana

(SUP-tuh veer-AHS-uh-nuh)

Also Known As: Bed Pose B (Paryankasana B)

Modification: arms up over the head, palms facing upward

Pose Type: supine

Drishti Point: Bhrumadhye or Ajna Chakra (third eye, between the eyebrows)

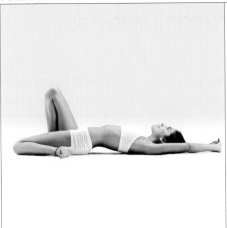

Reclined One-Legged Thunderbolt Pose

Supta Eka Pada Vajrasana

(SUP-tuh EY-kuh PUH-duh vuhj-RAHS-uh-nuh)

Modification: Leg 1: in Thunderbolt Pose (Vajrasana)

Leg 2: knee up to the sky, heel to the sitting bones; arms up over the head, fingers interlocked, palms facing out

Pose Type: supine

Drishti Point: Bhrumadhye or Ajna Chakra (third eye, between the eyebrows)

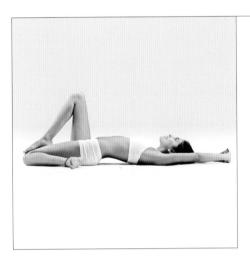

Reclined One-Legged Thunderbolt Pose

Supta Eka Pada Vajrasana

(SUP-tuh EY-kuh PUH-duh vuhj-RAHS-uh-nuh)

Modification: Leg 1: in Thunderbolt Pose (Vajrasana)

Leg 2: knee up to the sky, sole of the foot to the thigh; arms up over the head, fingers interlocked, palms facing out

Pose Type: supine

Drishti Point: Bhrumadhye or Ajna Chakra (third eye, between the eyebrows)

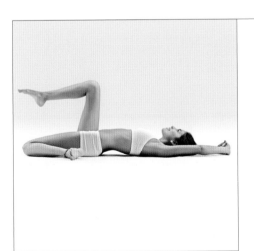

Reclined One-Legged Thunderbolt Pose

Supta Eka Pada Vajrasana

(SUP-tuh EY-kuh PUH-duh vuhj-RAHS-uh-nuh)

Modification: Leg 1: in Thunderbolt Pose (Vajrasana)

Leg 2: knee bent at 90 degrees, heel off the floor; arms up over the head, fingers interlocked, palms facing out

Pose Type: supine

Drishti Point: Bhrumadhye or Ajna Chakra (third eye, between the eyebrows)

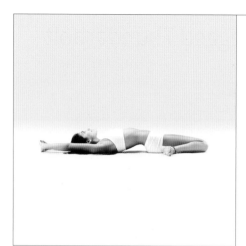

Reclined Complete Thunderbolt Pose

Supta Paripurna Vajrasana

(SUP-tuh puh-ri-POOR-nuh vuhj-RAHS-uh-nuh)

Modification: arms up over the head, fingers interlocked, palms facing out
Pose Type: supine
Drishti Point: Bhrumadhye or Ajna Chakra (third eye, between the eyebrows)

TOES TURNED OUT TO THE SIDE: ONE KNEE BENT TO THE BACK, OTHER LEG STRAIGHT & FOREARM POSES

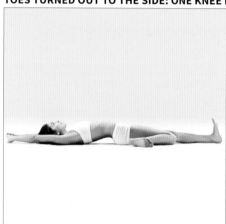

Reclined One-Legged Thunderbolt Pose

Supta Eka Pada Vajrasana

(SUP-tuh EY-kuh PUH-duh vuhj-RAHS-uh-nuh)

Modification: leg straight to the floor, toes flexed in; arms up over the head, fingers interlocked, palms facing out
Pose Type: supine
Drishti Point: Bhrumadhye or Ajna Chakra (third eye, between the eyebrows)

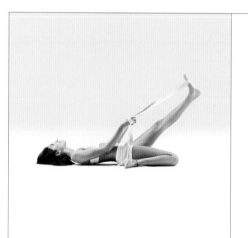

Reclined One-Legged Thunderbolt Pose

Supta Eka Pada Vajrasana

(SUP-tuh EY-kuh PUH-duh vuhj-RAHS-uh-nuh)

Modification: leg straight and lifted off the floor by using a Yoga strap
Pose Type: supine
Drishti Point: Bhrumadhye or Ajna Chakra (third eye, between the eyebrows)

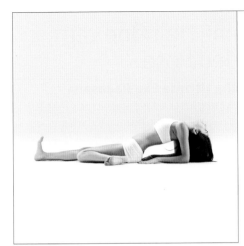

Reclined One-Legged Thunderbolt Pose

Supta Eka Pada Vajrasana

(SUP-tuh EY-kuh PUH-duh vuhj-RAHS-uh-nuh)

Modification: forearms to the floor in a backbend, one leg straight to the floor, toes flexed in, other leg in Thunderbolt Pose (Vajrasana)
Pose Type: seated, backbend
Drishti Point: Bhrumadhye or Ajna Chakra (third eye, between the eyebrows)

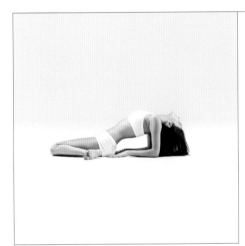

Reclined Complete Thunderbolt Pose

Supta Paripurna Vajrasana

(SUP-tuh puh-ri-POOR-nuh vuhj-RAHS-uh-nuh)

Modification: forearms to the floor in a backbend
Pose Type: seated, backbend
Drishti Point: Bhrumadhye or Ajna Chakra (third eye, between the eyebrows)

VERTICAL SPLITS: SCISSOR LEGS—BOTH KNEES BENT & ONE KNEE BENT, ONE LEG STRAIGHT

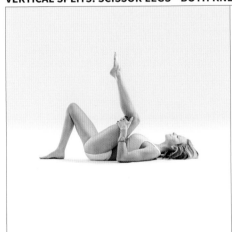

Reclining Both Hands to the Leg Pose

Supta Dwi Hasta Padasana

(SUP-tuh DWI-huh-stuh puh-DAHS-uh-nuh)

Modification: elbows bent, triceps on the floor, fingers interlocked behind the back of the thigh
Leg 1: slight knee bend, foot flat on the floor
Leg 2: knee bent at 90 degrees, knee toward the chest
Pose Type: supine, forward bend
Drishti Point: Bhrumadhye or Ajna Chakra (third eye, between the eyebrows) or Padayoragrai or Padayoragre (toes/feet)

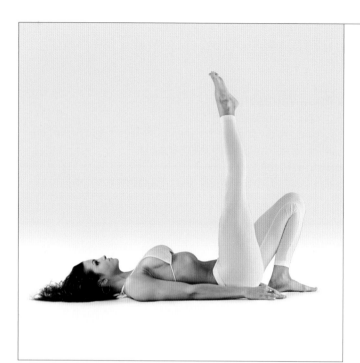

Reclining Half One Leg Extended Pose

Supta Ardha Utthita Eka Padasana

(SUP-tuh UHR-duh UT-ti-tuh EY-kuh puh-DAHS-uh-nuh)

Modification: palms flat to the floor on the sides.

Leg 1: straight up to the sky

Leg 2: knee bent, foot flat to the floor, heel to the sitting bones

Pose Type: supine, forward bend

Drishti Point: Bhrumadhye or Ajna Chakra (third eye, between the eyebrows), Padayoragrai or Padayoragre (toes/feet)

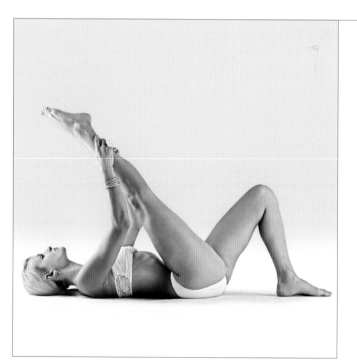

Reclining Both Hands to the Leg Pose

Supta Dwi Hasta Padasana

(SUP-tuh DWi-huh-stuh puh-DAHS-uh-nuh)

Modification: grabbing onto the calf muscle, elbows bent

Leg 1: straight and toward the chest

Leg 2: knee bent, foot flat to the floor

Pose Type: supine, forward bend

Drishti Point: Bhrumadhye or Ajna Chakra (third eye, between the eyebrows), Padayoragrai or Padayoragre (toes/feet)

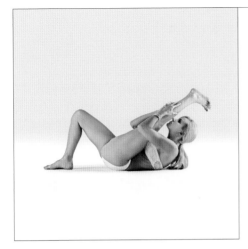

Reclining Both Hands to the Leg Pose

Supta Dwi Hasta Padasana

(SUP-tuh DWI-huh-stuh puh-DAHS-uh-nuh)

Modification: grabbing onto the calf muscle, elbows bent at 90 degrees, nose toward the shin

Leg 1: straight and toward the chest

Leg 2: knee bent, foot flat to the floor

Pose Type: supine, forward bend, core

Drishti Point: Padayoragrai or Padayoragre (toes/feet), Nasagrai or Nasagre (nose)

VERTICAL SPLITS: SCISSOR LEGS—BOTH LEGS STRAIGHT

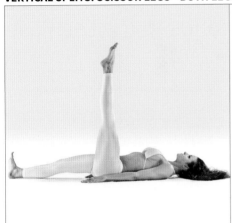

Reclining One Leg Extended Pose

Supta Utthita Eka Padasana

(SUP-tuh UT-ti-tuh EY-kuh puh-DAHS-uh-nuh)

Modification: palms flat to the floor on the sides

Leg 1: straight up to the sky

Leg 2: straight out on the floor, toes flexed in

Pose Type: supine, forward bend

Drishti Point: Bhrumadhye or Ajna Chakra (third eye, between the eyebrows), Padayoragrai or Padayoragre (toes/feet)

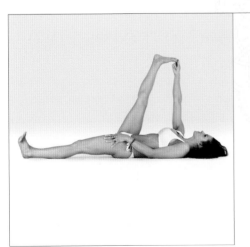

Reclining Big Toe Pose 1

Supta Padangushtasana 1

(SUP-tuh puhd-uhng-goosh-TAHS-uh-nuh)

Modification: back flat on the floor

Pose Type: supine, forward bend

Drishti Point: Bhrumadhye or Ajna Chakra (third eye, between the eyebrows), Padayoragrai or Padayoragre (toes/feet)

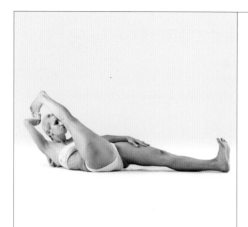

Reclining Big Toe Pose 1

Supta Padangushtasana 1

(SUP-tuh puhd-uhng-goosh-TAHS-uh-nuh)

Modification: head and shoulders off the floor, nose to the shin

Pose Type: supine, forward bend

Drishti Point: Bhrumadhye or Ajna Chakra (third eye, between the eyebrows), Nasagrai or Nasagre (nose)

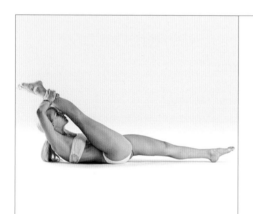

Reclining Both Hands to the Leg Pose

Supta Dwi Hasta Padasana

(SUP-tuh DWI-huh-stuh puh-DAHS-uh-nuh)

Modification: head and shoulders off the floor, nose to the shin, toes pointed

Pose Type: supine, forward bend, core

Drishti Point: Nasagrai or Nasagre (nose), Bhrumadhye or Ajna Chakra (third eye, between the eyebrows)

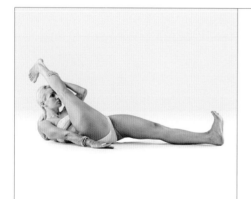

Reclining One Hand to the Leg Pose

Supta Eka Hasta Padasana

(SUP-tuh EY-kuh HUH-stuh puh-DAHS-uh-nuh)

Modification: hand to opposite leg, head and shoulders off the floor, nose to the shin, toes flexed in

Pose Type: supine, forward bend, core

Drishti Point: Nasagrai or Nasagre (nose), Bhrumadhye or Ajna Chakra (third eye, between the eyebrows)

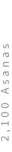

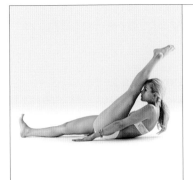

Reclining One Leg Extended Pose

Supta Utthita Eka Padasana

(SUP-tuh UT-ti-tuh EY-kuh puh-DAHS-uh-nuh)

Modification: palms flat to the floor on the sides, head and shoulders off the floor, nose to the knee, bottom toes flexed in

Pose Type: supine, forward bend

Drishti Point: Nasagrai or Nasagre (nose)

BOTH LEGS STRAIGHT AND TOGETHER

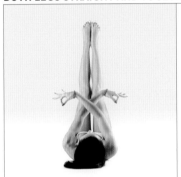

Reclining Legs Extended Pose

Supta Utthita Padasana

(SUP-tuh UT-ti-tuh puh-DAHS-uh-nuh)

Modification: arms crossed in front of the chest

Pose Type: supine

Drishti Point: Bhrumadhye or Ajna Chakra (third eye, between the eyebrows), Padayoragrai or Padayoragre (toes/feet)

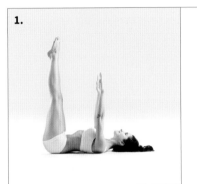

Reclining Legs Extended Pose

Supta Utthita Padasana

(SUP-tuh UT-ti-tuh puh-DAHS-uh-nuh)

Modification: arms straight up to the sky

1. arms and legs perpendicular to the floor

2. arms and legs slightly lowered toward the floor

Pose Type: supine

Drishti Point: Bhrumadhye or Ajna Chakra (third eye, between the eyebrows), Padayoragrai or Padayoragre (toes/feet), Hastagrai or Hastagre (hands)

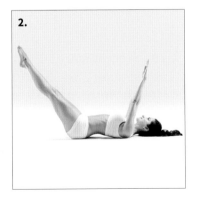

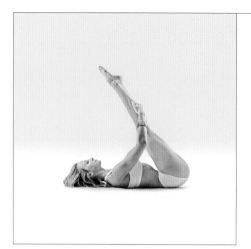

Half Upward Facing Western Intense Stretch 2

Ardha Urdhva Mukha Paschimottanasana 2

(UHR-duh OORD-vuh MUK-uh puhsh-chi-mo-tahn-AHS-uh-nuh)

Also Known As: Half Upward Facing Forward Bend, Upward Facing Western Intense Stretch Pose 2 Prep. (Urdhva Mukha Paschimottanasana 2 Prep.)

Modification: grabbing onto the calf muscles

Pose Type: supine, forward bend

Drishti Point: Bhrumadhye or Ajna Chakra (third eye, between the eyebrows), Padayoragrai or Padayoragre (toes/feet)

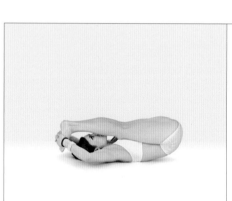

Upward Facing Western Intense Stretch 2

Urdhva Mukha Paschimottanasana 2

(OORD-vuh MUK-uh puhsh-chi-mo-tahn-AHS-uh-nuh)

Also Known As: Upward Facing Forward Bend 2

Pose Type: supine, forward bend

Drishti Point: Bhrumadhye or Ajna Chakra (third eye, between the eyebrows), Padayoragrai or Padayoragre (toes/feet)

SUPINE LOTUS & CORPSE POSE

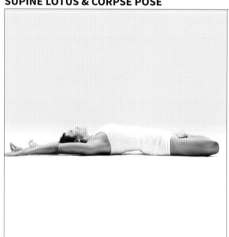

Reclining Lotus Pose

Supta Padmasana

(SUP-tuh puhd-MAHS-uh-nuh)

Also Known As: Fish Pose (Matsyasana)

Modification: back flat on the floor; arms up over the head, palms facing up

Pose Type: supine

Drishti Point: Bhrumadhye or Ajna Chakra (third eye, between the eyebrows)

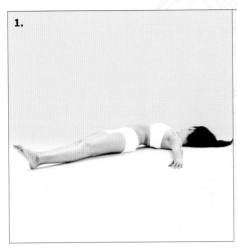

Side Corpse Pose

Parshva Shavasana

(PAHRSH-vuh shuh-VAHS-uh-nuh)

Also Known As: Belly Twist (Jataraparivritti)
Modification: 1. head turned to the opposite side of feet
2. looking straight ahead
Pose Type: supine, side bend
Drishti Point: Bhrumadhye or Ajna Chakra (third eye, between the eyebrows), Hastagrai or Hastagre (hands)

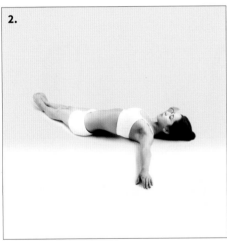

Corpse Pose

Shavasana

(shuh-VAHS-uh-nuh)

Also Known As: Dead Pose (Mrtasana)
Pose Type: supine
Drishti Point: Bhrumadhye or Ajna Chakra (third eye, between the eyebrows)

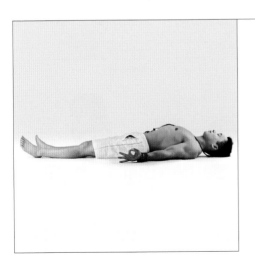

ACKNOWLEDGMENTS

Meet the talented people of Mr. Yoga, Inc. who have contributed their energy, passion, and skills to this project.

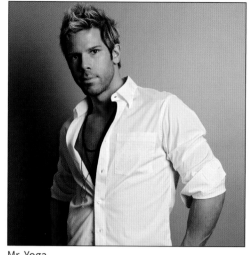

Mr. Yoga

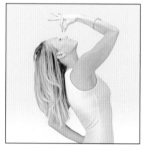

Victoria B.

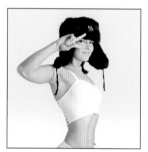

Tatiana U.

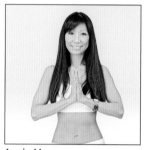

Aggie M.

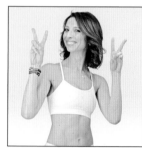

Susan M.

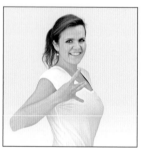

Olga Q. B.

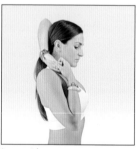

Laura Lisa

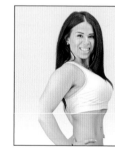

Vanessa D. S.

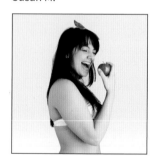

Snow W.

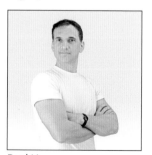

Paul M.

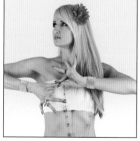

Kat D.

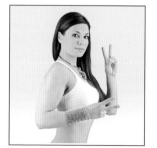

Paula O.

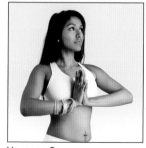

Venessa S.

Additional special thanks to: Adrienne Yau, Silvia Bogers, Antoine Bogers, Evelyn Lacerda, Chris Morino, Scott Mendel, Black Dog & Leventhal Publishers, Hachette Book Group

Welcome to the Mr. Yoga, Inc. global family. All of the models selected to appear in this book are students of Daniel Lacerda, aka Mr. Yoga.

 Frances L.

 Cristine C.

 Carolyn L.

 Tatiana U.

 Elena B.

 Stephanie M. & Iva M.

 Matthew B.

 Shriya M. D.

 Mariah A.

 Erin B.

 Valeryia G.

 Michael C.

 Brent J.

 Kristen S.

 Christina D. F.

 Laura M.

 Victoria B.

 Eva M.

 Jemma B.

 Menaka I.

 Hagar E.

 Kellys E.

 Diana M.

 Alessandra F.

 Neelam P.

 Katerina D.

 Crio C.

 Paula O.

 Dasha C.

 Elissa R.

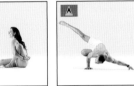 Eli M.

 Josiah B.

 Nicki B.

 Rachel M.

 Hue N.

 Deanna D.

 Aggie M.

 Corrado R. M.

 Taylor K.

 Susan M.

 Neil F.

 Justin L.

Thank you to special guest, Danny Paradise.

GLOSSARY

A

adho mukha = having the face downward

agni = fire

ahimsa = nonviolence; the word has not merely the negative and restrictive meaning of "nonkilling or nonviolence," but the positive and comprehensive meaning of "love embracing all creation" ; one of the *yamas*

ajna = to command

ajna chakra = energy or command *chakra*, energy center/the nerve plexus located between the eyebrows, the third eye, the seat of command, the sixth *chakra*

akarna = near the ear

akuncha = contraction or bend

alamba = a prop or support

anahata = unstruck

anahata chakra = spiritual heart *chakra*, energy center situated near the heart, the nervous plexus situated in the cardiac region, the fourth *chakra*

ananda = joy, happiness, bliss, ecstasy

ananta = infinite, without end; a name of Vishnu and also of Vishnu's couch, the serpent Sesa

anga = limb, points, step, the body; a limb or a part of the body; a constituent part

angushta (angula) = finger or digit, the thumb

anjali = hands held together as in prayer

anjali-mudra = the gesture of *anjali*

Anjaneya = son of Anjani (Hanuman's mother's maiden name is Anjani)

antara = within, interior

apanasana = pelvic floor yoga pose

aparigraha = non-greediness, freedom from greed, desire, hoarding or collecting; one of the *yamas*

Arani = Hindu Goddess of Fire

aranya = wild animal

asana = a physical posture, the third limb or stage of yoga, originally this meant "meditation posture" or "seat"

ashta (asta, astau) = eight

Ashtavakra = one having eight bends (crooked in eight places), in reference to a Hindu Sage who was born with eight physical deformities in his body, and went on to become a spiritual preceptor of King Janaka of Mitila

ashva (asva) = horse

ashva sanchala = horse, riding posture

asteya = nonstealing, freedom from avarice; one of the *yamas*

atman = individual soul, the true self, consciousness; the term Vedanta uses instead of *purusha*

avabhinna = broken

avatara = divine manifestation, descent, advent or incarnation of God. There are ten avataras of Vishnu: Matsya (the Fish), Kurma (the Tortoise), Varaha (the Boar), Narasimha (the Man-Lion), Vamana (the Dwarf), Parasurama, Rama (hero of the epic *Ramayana*), Krishna (hero of the epic *Mahabharata*, who related the *Bhagavad Gita*), Balarama, and Kalki

B

baddha = bound

baka = crane, heron, a wading bird

bala = young, childish, not fully grown

bandha = a bond, tying, energetic lock, contraction, bondage, or fetter; a posture in which certain organs or body parts are contracted and controlled

Benu = the mythological bird of ancient Egypt symbolic of rebirth and creation, also associated with the Sun

bhaga = strength

Bhagavad Gita = one of India's most beloved and sacred texts, the divine song of the Lord, the most influential of all *shastras*; the epic story of Arjuna, a warrior prince who confronts moral dilemmas through sacred dialogues with Krishna (one of Lord Vishnu's Avatars) and is led to a better understanding of reality by learning the teachings of Samkhya, Yoga, and Vedanta

Bhagavata Purana = also called Shrimad Bhagavatam, a *purana* that deals with devotion to the Supreme Being in the form of Lord Vishnu and describes some of the avatars of Vishnu, including Krishna

bhairava = terrible, gruesome, formidable; one of the fierce manifestations of Shiva

bhakti = devotion, worship or love; from *bhaj*, (to divide), the belief that there is an eternal divide between the Supreme Being and the world that cannot be overcome through knowledge, hence the Supreme Being must be met with an attitude of devotion

bhangi = position

Bharadvaja (Bharadwaja) = a Vedic *rishi*, great warrior described in the *Mahabharata*,

Pindola Bharadvaja was one of four *arhats* asked by Buddha to stay on earth to propagate Buddhist law, or *dharma*

bharman = load, nourishment, care, burden, maintenance load

bheka = a frog

bherunda = terrible, frightful; it also means a species of a bird or a name of a yogi

bhuja = arm or shoulder

bhujanga (bhujagga) = serpent, snake

bhuja-pida = pressure on the arm or shoulder

bidala = cat

bija-mantra = a mystical syllable with a sacred prayer repeated mentally during *pranayama*, and the seed thus planted in the mind germinates into one-pointedness

bindu (bindhu) = seed, point, dot, the creative potency of anything where all energies are focused, the third eye

bitila = cow

Brahma = a five-headed first deity of the Hindu Trinity; the Supreme Being, the creator; responsible for the creation of the world, he is the first being to appear at the dawn of each universe to create it based on its subconscious conditioning: the Brahma of the present universe is called Prajapati (progenitor), the predecessor of humankind

brahmachari = a religious student vowed to celibacy and abstinence; one who is constantly moving (*charin*) in *brahman* (The Supreme Spirit); one who sees divinity in all

brahmacharya = chastity or teacher of the soul, abstinence, a life of celibacy, religious study and self-restraint, recognition of Brahma in everything; one of the *yamas*

Brahman = the absolute, or divinity itself, infinite consciousness, universal soul, deep reality, the reality that cannot be reduced to a deeper layer; the Supreme Being, the cause of the Universe, the all-pervading spirit of the Universe

Buddha = enlightened one

C

chakora = a type of bird like a partridge (Greek partridge), moonbeam bird, said to feed on moonbeams

chakra = literally, a wheel or circle, the wheel of a wagon; metaphorically, psycho-energetic subtle centers of the subtle body in which energy flows, located along the spine, believed to transform cosmic energy into spiritual energy when activated. Energy (prana) is said to flow in the human body through three main channels (nadis), namely, sushumna, pingala, and ida; sushumna is situated inside the spinal column. Pingala and ida start respectively from the right and the left nostrils, move up to the crown of the head, and course downward to the base of the spine. These two nadis intersect with each other and also the sushumna. These junctions of the nadis are known as chakras of the flywheels, which regulate the body mechanism. The important chakras are: (a) muladhara (mula = root, source; adhara = support, vital part) situated in the pelvis, above the anus; (b) svadhishtana (sva = vital force, soul; adhishtana = seat of abode) situated above the organs of gestation; (c) manipuraka (manipura = navel) situated in the navel; (d) manas (mind) and (e) surya (the sun) which are situated between the navel and the heart; (f) anahata (= unbeaten) situated in the cardiac area; (g) vishuddha (= pure) situated in the pharyngeal region; (h) ajna (= command) situated between the eyebrows; (i) sahasrara (= a thousand) which is called a thousand-petaled lotus in the cerebral cavity; and (j) lalata (= forehead) which is at the top of the forehead.

chalana = to churn

chamatkara = delight or savoring; the refined pleasure that a connoisseur takes in a lovely poem, painting, or fine wine. Chamatkarasana is translated as "Wild Thing Pose" probably because the posture looks like someone who has just seen something so amazing and beautiful that they are "bowled over" or "blown away."

chandra (candra) = moon

chapa = bow, rainbow, arc

chatur (chatuari, chatura) = four

chatush = four times

chatushpada = quadruped

chikitsa = therapy

chitta = consciousness that comprises mind, intellect, the restraint of consciousness; a mind in its total or collective sense, being composed of three categories: (a) mind, having the faculty of attention, selection, and rejection; (b) reason, the decisive state which determines the distinction between things; and (c) ego, the I-maker, the aggregate of intellect (buddhi), egoity (ahamkara) and thinking agent (manas)

chittavritti (chitta-vritti, chitta vritti) = an imbalance of the mental state, fluctuations of the mind, movement of the consciousness; a course of behavior, mode of being, condition, or mental state

cibi = chin

D

dakshina = the right side

danda = stick, staff (refers to the spine)

dasha = ten

dhanu (dhanura) = bow

dharana = concentration, sixth limb of Ashtanga yoga, orienting the mind toward a single point

dhyana = generally translated as meditation, freedom from attachments, an ongoing stream of awareness from the meditator toward the object of meditation, and of information from the object toward the meditator; the seventh limb of Ashtanga yoga

dhyana-yoga = yoga of meditation

Diti = the mother of the demons, also called Daityas

drishti = focal point, perception or looking place, "view" or "sight": yogic gazing, such as at the tip of the nose or the spot between the eyebrows

dur = difficult

Durvasa = a very irascible, notoriously angry sage

dvija = twice-born

dwi (dve) = two

dwihasta = two hands

dwipada = two feet or legs

E

eka (ekam) = one

eka-pada (ekapada) = one leg, one-legged, one-footed

G

gaja = elephant

Galava = the pupil or son of Viswamitra

ganda = the cheek or side of the face including the temple

gandha = subtle earth element; quantum of (tanmatra) earth; smell

gandha-bherunda = a species of bird, also a two-headed mythological bird that embodies immense powers and destructive forces

garbha = an infant, womb, fetus

garbha kosha = uterus

garbha pinda (garbha-pinda) = fetus, embryo in the womb

Garuda = Hindu deity, half-man half-eagle, fierce bird of prey, vehicle (vahana) of Lord Vishnu, king of birds; Garuda is represented as a vehicle of Vishnu and as having a white face, an aquiline beak, red wings, and a golden body

gava = cow

Gheranda = author of Gheranda Samhita, an important text on Hatha Yoga which he taught to Chanda Kapali

Gheranda Samhita = a Tantric treatise describing Hatha Yoga written by the sage Gheranda in the 15th century

Gitananda = a well-known yogi, living in the 20th century CE

go = cow

godha = iguana

gomukha = cow face, face resembling a cow, cow head; it is also a kind of musical instrument, narrow at one end and broad at the other, like the face of a cow

Goraksha (Goraksha, Gorakshanath) = an 11th to 12th Century Hindu Nath yogi, one of Matsyendranath's two most important disciples; tending to or breeding cattle, cowherd

graiva = a chain worn around the neck of an elephant; necklace or collar

guru = "he who is heavy, weighty," a spiritual teacher or preceptor, one who illuminates the darkness of spiritual doubt, one who hands down a system of knowledge to a disciple; heavy one or dark/light, dispeller of darkness, one who helps to gain knowledge

guru-shishya parampara = the tradition of teaching dating back centuries, where a guru imparts his knowledge to his students

H

ha = first syllable of the word hatha, which is composed of the syllables ha (= sun) and tha (= moon); the object of Hatha Yoga is to balance the flow of solar and lunar energy in the human system

hala = plow

hamsa (hansa) = a swan; a metaphor for the soul; a vehicle of Lord Brahma; the name of the mantra by which prakriti permeates the universe; also refers to the breath as it moves within the body

Hanuman = a powerful monkey chief, a mythological entity, of extraordinary strength and prowess, whose exploits are celebrated in the epic Ramayana; he was the son of Anjana and Vayu, the god of wind, monkey-god, hero of *Ramayana*, egoless superhero and perfect devotee, who resembles a monkey leaping

hasta = hand

hastasana = forward stretch of the arms

hatha = force; the word *hatha* is used adverbially in the sense of "forcibly" or "against one's will"; Hatha Yoga is so called because it prescribes rigorous discipline in order to find union with the Supreme

hatha-vidya = the science of Hatha Yoga

Hatha Yoga = "Forceful Yoga," a major branch of yoga, developed by Goraksha and other adepts c. 1000–1100 CE, emphasizing the physical aspects of the transformative path, notably postures (*asana*), cleansing techniques (*shodhana*) and breath (*pranayama*); literally, sun/moon yoga (*ha* = sun, *tha* = moon), it emphasizes balancing the solar and lunar energy channels in the body. Hatha Yoga shifted the focus away from the mysticism and philosophy of the older Upanishadic types of yoga toward using the body as a tool; combines opposing forces to achieve balance, sighting the soul through the restraint of energy, yoga concerned with mastering control over the physical body as a path to enlightenment (self-realization)

Hatha Yoga Pradipika = a celebrated treatise on yoga compiled in the 12th century by the sage Svatmarama

himsa = violence, killing

Hindola = cradle or swing; also Hindu Religious Festival associated with baby Krishna being rocked in a decorated swing

I

ida = a *nadi*, a channel through which *prana* moves, starting from the left nostril, then moving to the crown of the head and then descending to the base of the spine on the left side; in its course it conveys lunar energy and so is called *chandra nadi,* "channel of the lunar energy"; associated with pale or blue (left/feminine)

Indra = ruler, lord of thunder, king of the heavens

indudala = crescent moon

Ishvara = God, the Supreme Being, Brahman, with form

ishvara pranidhana = one of the *niyamas*; centering on the divine, devotion or surrender to God, dedication to the Lord of one's actions and one's will

J

jalandhara bandha (jalandharabandha) = a *bandha* that locks the throat, chin lock; straightening the back of the neck by keeping your head straight while slightly receding your chin; a yoga pose where the neck and throat are contracted and the chin is rested in the notch between the collarbones at the top of the breast-bone

janu = knee

jatara = stomach, belly, or the interior of anything

jatara-parivartana = an action of an *asana* (yoga pose) in which the abdomen is made to move to and fro

Jnana Yoga = the emphasis is on questioning, contemplation, and meditation as a path to enlightenment, yoga that seeks to teach the identity of the individual self (*atman*) and the infinite consciousness (*brahman*)

K

kaka = crow

Kala Bhairava = Shiva in his terrible or gruesome form as Destroyer of the Universe

Kali = Hindu Goddess of Time and Change

Kamala = Hindu Goddess of Wealth, "One of the Lotus"

Kamalamuni = one of the 18 Siddhars believed to be over 4,000 years old

kanda = a bulbous root, a knot, egg, stem, stalk, trunk; the *kanda* is a round shape of about four inches situated twelve inches above the anus and near the navel, where the three main *nadis* (*sushumna, ida,* and *pingala*) unite and separate; it is covered as if with a soft white piece of cloth

kapala = skull

kapalabhati = bellow-like breathing technique with sharp, quick inhalations and exhalations; a cleansing ritual for the respiratory tract, lungs, and sinuses; skull shining

kapila = a sage or *rishi*, the founder of the Samkhya system, one of the six orthodox systems of Hindu philosophy, noted in the *Bhagavad Gita* and *Bhagavata Purana* as a manifestation of the Supreme Being

kapinjala = a kind of partridge, the *chataka* bird, which is supposed to drink only raindrops

kapota = dove, pigeon

kapya = monkey

karanda = duck

karani = making, doing

karma (karma law) = action, activity of any kind, including ritual acts; said to be binding only so long as engaged in a self-centered way; the law of cause and effect, or the movement toward balanced consciousness: everything that you do, say, or think has an immediate effect on the universe that will reverberate back to you in some way

karma yoga (karma-yoga) = yoga of action, path to enlightenment is through selfless acts and service to others, the achievement of union with the Supreme Universal Soul through action; in its original Vedic sense, Karma Yoga is any yoga that employs ritualistic action, such as *asana*, meditation, or *mantra*, to produce spiritual gain. The term excludes Jnana Yoga and Bhakti Yoga, which are thought to operate beyond spiritual gain

karna = the ear; also one of the heroes in the *Mahabharata*

karna-pida = pressure around the ear, blocked ears

Kashyapa = an ancient Hindu sage, husband of Aditi and Diti; he is one of the lords or progenitors of living things

khaga = bird

khanjana = a wagtail bird

Khimi Karani = mythological pond of milk in which Garuda drowned a snake to give birth to the Shami Tree

kona = angle

Konganar = one of the Siddhars, student of Siddhar Bogar

Koormamuni = Hindu Sage

Korakar = one of the 18 Siddhars, a well-known sage, author of works on philosophy, medicine, and alchemy

Koundinya (Kaundinya) = Hindu sage, Vedic scholar, and a descendant of Vasishta

kriya = act, action, cleansing

kriya yoga = the yoga of action and participation in life, preliminary yoga consisting of simplicity (*tapas*), the reading of sacred texts (*svadhyaya*), and acceptance of the existence of a Supreme Being (*ishvarapranidhana*); also, a Tantric mode of yoga using breath, *mantra*, and visualization.

krakacha = a saw

krounch (krouncha, krauncha) = heron

kukkuta = rooster, cock

kulpa = ankle

kundalini = a coiled female serpent; the divine cosmic energy, the obstacle that closes the mouth of *sushumna*; the rising of *shakti* in the *sushumna*; this force or energy is symbolized as a coiled and sleeping serpent lying dormant in the lowest nerve center at the base of the spinal column, the *muladhara-chakra*. This latent energy has to be aroused and made to ascend the main spinal channel, the *sushumna* piercing all the *chakras* right up to the *sahasrata*, the thousand-petaled lotus in the head. Then the *yogi* is in union with the Supreme Universal Soul.

Kundalini Yoga = a mode of yoga that focuses on the raising of the life force

kunja = grove, alcove

kunta = spear, lance

kurma (koorma) = a tortoise, it is also the name of one of the subsidiary vital airs whose function is to control the movements of the eyelids to prevent foreign matter or light that is too bright going into the eyes

L

laghu = little, small, simple; it also means "handsome"

lasya = beauty, happiness, and grace; also a dance performed by Goddess Parvati in response to her husband Shiva's *tandava*

Linga (Lingam, Shivalinga) = symbol of union and origin of all life associated with Lord Shiva and Goddess Shakti

lola = tremulous, dangling, pendant; charm, swing; swinging like a pendulum, moving to and fro

M

madhya (madya) = middle of the body, central

maha = great, mighty, powerful, lofty, noble

maha bandha = the great lock

maha mudra = the great seal

Mahabharata = the celebrated epic, the largest piece of literature created by humankind, authored by Rishi Vyasa and containing the *Bhagavad Gita*, dating to the first century BCE; *dharma shastra* (scripture dealing with right action), which comes to the conclusion that however hard you try, you can never be completely right

makara = a mythological sea creature, who is the vehicle of the river Goddess Ganga; a crocodile

makshika = fly

mala = a garland or a wreath, often of prayer beads or flowers

manas-chakra = nervous plexus situated between the navel and the heart

mandala = a circle ambulation, a circular drawing or design that exemplifies sacred geometry that draws your eye to the center and is used as a focal point while meditating; it also means a "collection," a division of Rig Veda

manduka = frog

manipuraka = a nervous plexus situated in the region of the navel; the third *chakra*, the navel *chakra*, the fire energy center, site of the sense of fear and apprehension

mantra = a mystical syllable designed to create and alter reality by influencing the vibrational patterns that make up creation; a sacred sound or phrase that has a transformative effect

Marichi = a sage, son of Brahma, the great-grandfather of Manu, the Vedic Adam and the father of humanity, the creator of the universe, and the father of Kasyapa

marjarai = cat

matsya = fish

Matsyendra = a Hindu sage and one of the first teachers of Hatha Yoga; a legend, king or lord of the fish

mayura = peacock

moksha (moksa) = liberation from bondage, final emancipation of the soul from recurring births

mrita (mrta, mritra) = dead, corpse

mudra = a seal; a pleasant hand gesture or seal posture; directs the life current (life energy) through the human body, usually a combination of *asana*, *pranayama*, and *bandha*

mukha = face

mukta = free, unbound, liberated

mukti = release, liberation, final absolution of the soul from the chain of birth and death

mula = root, foundation, bottom; a yoga pose where the body from the anus to the navel is contracted and lifted toward the spine

mula bandha (mula-bandha) = rectal lock, root lock; contraction of the pubococcygeus, a yoga pose where the body from the anus to the navel is contracted and lifted up and toward the spine

muladhara = root foundation, the name of the first *chakra*

muladhara chakra = the first *chakra*, the base *chakra*, the earth energy center situated at the root of the spine, nervous plexus situated in the pelvis above the anus at the base or root of the spine, the main support of the body that controls sexual energy

mushti = fist

mutra kosa = bladder

N

nabi = navel

nadi = river; nerve or conduit, channels that distribute energy from the *chakras* throughout the body, a tubular organ of the subtle body through which energy flows, subtle vibratory passages of psychospiritual energy; it consists of three layers, one inside the other, like insulation of an electric wire. The innermost layer is called the *sira* and the middle layer, *damani*. The entire organ as well as the outer layer is called *nadi*; they connect at special points of intensity (*chakras*).

naga = great mythological snake; one of the subsidiary vital airs that relieves abdominal pressure, causing one to belch

Nahusha = Hindu King of Aila Dynasty

nakra = crocodile

namaskar = greeting, worship, salutation with hands in prayer

namaste mudra = a *mudra* in which the hands are placed together in a prayerlike fashion to honor the inner light

nantum = to bow with respect

nara = a man

Narasimha = an avatar of the Hindu god Vishnu in his fourth incarnation, often visualized as half-man, half-lion

nasika = nose

nata = actor, dancer, mime

Nataraj = name of Shiva as a cosmic dancer, the lord of the dancers

natya = dancing

nauka = boat

nava = boat

nava = nine

nidra = deep, dreamless sleep; the third state listed in the *Mandukya Upanishad*. The others are waking state (*jagrat*), dream (*susupt*), and consciousness (*turiya*); also the fourth fluctuation of the mind listed by Patanjali in *Yoga Sutra* I.6 (the others are correct cognition, wrong cognition, perceptualization, and memory).

nindra (nantra) = sage, praise, wonder

nindra (nitara) = standing firm, standing

nir = without

nira = water

niralamba = self-supported, independent, without support

niyama = self-restraint, personal observances, self-purification by discipline, the Vedic system of logic; the second stage or limb of Ashtanga Yoga mentioned by Patanjali; five personal disciplines, as defined by Patanjali in his *Yoga Sutras*: *shaucha, santosha, tapas, svadhyaya,* and ishvarapranidhana

O

om (aum) = the original *mantra* symbolizing the ultimate reality, the sacred syllable emitted by the Supreme Being, the sound that produces all other sounds and into which all other sounds return. Like the Latin word *omne*, the Sanskrit work *aum* means "all" and conveys concepts of Omnipotence, Omnipresence, and Omniscience.

P

pada = foot or leg; also a part of a book or text

pada-hasta = hand(s)-to-feet

padangushta = big toe

padma = lotus

pakshaka = wing

pakshi = bird

pancha = five

parampara = tradition, uninterrupted series, convention, a succession

parigha = iron bar used for locking, bolting, or shutting a gate

parigraha = hoarding, possessiveness

paripurna = full, entire, complete

parivartana = turning around, revolving

parivartana-pada = with one leg turned around

parivid = twined, twisted around

parivritta = revolved, turned around

parivritti = crossed or with a twist, turning, rolling

parshva = the side, flank, lateral

parshvaika = *parsva* (side) + *eka* (one)

parshvaika-pada = with one leg turned sideways

parvata = mountain

paryanka = a bed, a couch

pasa (pasha) = snare, trap, noose, fetter

paschima = the back of the whole body from head to heels, west side, western

paschimatana = intense stretch of the back side of the body from the nape to the heels

pakshya = being in or belonging to the wings

patan = to collapse

Patanjali = a sage, the author of the *Yoga Sutras*, a treatises on Sanskrit and Ayurveda; the founder of yoga, most likely lived between 200 BCE and 300 CE; a manifestation of the serpent of infinity

pavanamuktasana = wind release pose

perineum = the area between the thighs, behind the genitals, and in front of the anus

pichamayura = peacock with stretched feathers

pid = squeeze

pida = pain, discomfort, pressure

pincha = a feather of a tail, the chin

pinda = a fetus, an embryo in an early stage of gestation, ball, the body

pingala = a channel on the right side of the spine through which *prana* moves, associated with reddish color, a *nadi* or channel of masculine energy starting from the right nostril, then moving to the crown of the head and then downward to the base of the spine; as the solar energy flows through it, it is also called *surya-nadi*

pitam = stool, chair

plavana = jump through

pliha = the spleen

poorna = full

prana = breath, life, vitality, wind, energy, strength; connotes the soul, life force or inner breath; sometimes refers to anatomical or outer breath; vital upward energy current

pranayama = breath control, energy control through breathing, consisting of conscious inhalation (*puraka*), retention (*kumbhaka*), and exhalation (*rechaka*), breath extension, breathing exercises to harmonize the flow of life force; the fourth stage or limb of Ashtanga Yoga

prapada = tip of the feet

prasarita = spread, stretched out

pratyahara = internalization of the senses, independence from sensory stimuli; the fifth stage or limb of Ashtanga Yoga, withdrawal and emancipation of the mind from the domination of the senses and sensual objects; withdrawal of the mind, mental detachment from the external world

prishta = back

Punakeesar (Punnakeesar) = one of the Siddhars, a *guru* of Machamuni (also referred to as Matsyendra)

pungu = Telugu word for "wounded"

purna = complete

purva = eastern

purvottana = intense stretch of the front side of the body

R

raja = king, royal

raja yoga (raja-yoga) = royal yoga; a term generally applied to the three higher limbs of Ashtanga Yoga, that is *dharana, dhyana,* and *samadhi*; the royal road to self-realization through the control of the mind. The achievement of union with the Supreme Universal Spirit by becoming the ruler of one's own mind by defeating its enemies, sighting the soul through a restraint of consciousness

raja-kapota (rajakapota) = king pigeon

Ramayana = literally, Rama's way; a famous ancient epic (*itihasa*) authored by Sage Valmiki that describes the life of Rama, an *avatar* of Lord Vishnu

Rig Veda = literally "Knowledge of Praise," it consists of 1,028 hymns and is the oldest known reference to *yoga* and possibly the oldest known text in the world

rishi = a Vedic seer, a liberated sage or saint, one who through suspension of the mind can see to the bottom of his heart

Ruchika (Richika, Ruschika) = name of a Hindu sage, dedicated to the grandfather of an incarnation of Vishnu

S

sa = with

sahaja = easy, natural

sahasrara chakra = energy center situated at the crown of the head, the thousand-petaled lotus in the cerebral cavity, the most important seventh *chakra* which, when uncoiled, brings the seeker to freedom

St. Brighid = known for establishing numerous monasteries

sakti = power

salamba = with support

sama = same, equal, even, upright

samadhi = "putting together": the ecstatic or state in which the mediator becomes one with the object of meditation, forgetting him/herself completely (the Supreme Spirit pervading the universe) where there is a feeling of unutterable joy and peace, absorption, ecstasy, enlightenment, self-realization; the state of meditation in which ego disappears and all becomes one; a state of absolute bliss; the eighth limb or stage of Ashtanga Yoga

samadhi yoga = yoga of absorption

samastiti = a state of balance

Sankarar = yogi from the eighth century BC

Sanskrit = the programming language used to write the operating system of the subtle body; the language of the gods

santosha (santosa) = contentment; one of the *niyamas*

sapta = seven

sarpa = serpent, snake

sarva = all, whole

sarvanga = all parts, the whole body

sasanga = rabbit

satya = truth; one of the yamas

Shesha = a celebrated serpent, said to have a thousand heads; Sesa is represented as the couch of Vishnu, floating on the cosmic ocean, or as supporting the world on his hoods; other names of Shesha are Ananta and Vasuki

setu = a bridge, dam, dike

setu-bandha = the construction of a bridge; name of an *asana* in which the body is arched

shalabha = grasshopper, locust

Shankara, Adi = world teacher, yoga master, propounder of Jnana Yoga and Advaita Vedanta; author of commentaries on the *Brahma Sutra*, the *Upanishads*, the *Bhagavad Gita* and thirty other texts; founder of ten monk orders and four large monasteries whose abbots today still carry the title Shankaracharya. His dates are disputed. Western academics often place him at 800 CE. Tradition places him at 1800 BCE. Also known as Shankaracharya or Shankara Bhagavatpada

shanti = peace

shat = six

shaucha = purity or inner and outer cleanliness; one of the *niyamas*

shava (shava) = corpse

shayana = bed, couch, sleeping

shirsha = head

Shiva (Siva) = the most Powerful God in Hinduism, the Destroyer, a name of the Supreme Being, pure consciousness, Brahman with form

shvana (swana) = dog; inspiration

shvnaka = puppy dog

siddha = accomplished, fulfilled, perfected; a sage, seer, or prophet; also a semi-divine being of great purity and holiness, a perfected being, a yoga master who has become an immortal, ethereal being

siddhi = divine attribute, perfection, supernatural power, proof

simha = lion

Skanda = a name of Kartikeya, the god of war, general of the celestial army, Lord of War, second son of Lord Shiva and Godmother Uma Parvat

stamba = transition

steya = theft, robbery

sucirandra = threading the needle

sukha = ease, lightness, comfort, happiness, delight, joy, pleasure; literally, agreeable mental space

Sundaranandar = one of the eighteen Siddhars, author of numerous works on medicine

supta = lying down or sleeping, reclining, supine

surya = sun

surya yantra = sun dial

surya-chakra = nervous plexus situated between the navel and the heart

surya-nadi = the *nadi* of the Sun; another name for *pingala-nadi*

sushumna = the main *nadi* channel situated inside the spinal column, a hollow passageway between *pingala nadi* and *ida nadi* that runs through the spinal cord, and through which *kundalini* can travel once it is awakened

sutra = thread: a work consisting of aphoristic statements such as Patanjali's *Yoga Sutra*

sva = one's own, innate, vital force; soul, self

svadhyaya = education of self by study of divine literature, self-study, to study one's body, mind, intellect, and ego; one of the *niyamas*

svarga = heaven

svastika = good fortune

Svatmarama = the author of *Hatha-yoga-pradipika*, a classical textbook on Hatha Yoga

swadhishtana chakra = site of worldly desires, energy center located above the organ of generation

Swami Sivananda = a well-known *yogi* of the 20th century, founder of Sivananda Yoga

Swami Vishnu Devananda = a close disciple of Swami Sivananda

T

taal-vrksa = palm tree

tada = mountain, straight tree

tadasana-samasthiti = a state of balance; an even distribution of weight while standing

tan = stretch, lengthen out or extend

tana = to stretch out, extend

Tandava (Thandava) = sacred frantic dance representing the cosmic cycles of creation and destruction performed by the Hindu Deity Lord Shiva

tantra = thread on the loom

Tantra (Tantric) Yoga = this yoga is characterized by certain rituals designed to awaken the *kundalini*

tap = to burn, to blaze, to shine, to suffer pain, to be consumed by heat

tapa = austerity

tapas = a burning effort, glow, heat; austerity gained through the committed practice of yoga, self-discipline; practice with discipline, devotion and religiosity; one of the *niyamas*

tara = star

Taraka = a demon slain by Kartikeya, the god of war

tha = the second syllable of the word *hatha*; the first syllable *ha* stands for the sun, while the second syllable *tha* stands for the moon; the union of these two is represented in Hatha Yoga

thavali = frog in Tamil

tirieng = horizontal, oblique, transverse, reverse, upside down

tiryak = horizontally, sideways, obliquely, across

tiryang-mukha = backward facing

tittibha = a small bird living along the coastline; firefly; or insect

tola = balance, scale

tolana = weighing

tri (tri, tra) = three

tryanga = three limbs

trikona = three angle or triangle

Trivikrama = Vishnu in his fifth incarnation, The Dwarf *avatar* of Lord Vishnu, who with his three steps (*krama*) filled the earth, heaven and hell, the conqueror of three worlds

tulya = equilibrium, balance

U

ubhaya = both

uddayate = fly, soar, fly up

uddiyana = a fetter or bondage, a yogic abdominal lock; here the diaphragm is lifted high up the thorax and the abdominal organs by tilting your pelvic floor up and pulling your belly button back toward your spine; the *uddiyana-bandha,* the great bird *prana* (life), is forced to fly up through the *shushumna-nadi*; to fly up

ujjayi = a *pranayama* that produces sound in the throat with the inhalation, literally meaning "extended victory"; the lungs are fully expanded and the chest is puffed out, slow throat breathing

Upanishad = the word is derived from the prefixes *upa* (near) and *ni* (down) added to the root *shad* (to sit); it means sitting down near a *guru* to receive spiritual instruction. The *Upanishad* scriptures of ancient Hindu philosophy are the philosophical portion of the Vedas, the most ancient sacred literature of the Hindus, dealing with the nature of man and the universe and the union of the individual or self with the Universal Soul

upavishta (upavistha) = seated, sitting, with legs spread

urdhva (urdhwa) = upward, raised, elevated, inverted

urdhva-mukha = face upward

ushtra (ustra) = camel

ut = intense, a particle denoting intensity

utkata = fierce, powerful, exceeding the usual measure, excessive, squat

utpluti = lifting or pumping up

utripada = upright tripod

uttana = an intense stretch, upright

utthita = extended, risen or rising, raised up, stretched

V

Vaasamuni Siddhar = a disciple of Shiva

vadivu = old form; Gaja Vadivu is an animal posture from Kalari Yoga, a mystical tantric form of *yoga*, which stems from Kalarippayat

vajra = thunderbolt, Indra's weapon

Vajracchedika Prajnaparamita Sutra = Diamond Cutter Sutra, one of the *sutras* of Mahayana Buddhism focusing on non-attachment

vakra = bent, curved, crooked

Valakhilya = flying wise and virtuous companions, celestial beings; a class of divine personages of the size of a thumb, produced from the Creator's body, and said to precede the chariot of the sun

Valmiki = known as the father of Sanskrit classical poetry

vama = left side

Vamadeva = the name of the preserving aspect of the God Shiva

vamana = Vishnu in his fifth incarnation, when he was born as a dwarf to humble the demon king Bali

Vasishta = a celebrated sage, author of Yoga Vasistha; several Vedic hymns, most excellent, best, richest

vatayana = horse

vayu = air, vital force, wind, vital air

Vedas = the sacred scriptures of the Hindus, revealed by the Supreme Being

vibhuti = might, power, greatness

vimshati = twenty

vini = single movement

vinyasa = a steady flow of connected yoga *asanas* linked with breath, work in a continuous movement, going progressively, variation

viparita = reversed, inverted, turned

vira = a brave or eminent man, heroic, chief, hero

virabhadra = a legendary warrior, a powerful hero created out of Shiva's matted hair

Virancha (Viranchi) = one of the names of Lord Brahma

vishama = uneven, unequal

Vishnu (Vishnu, Narayana, Hari) = the second deity of the Hindu Trinity, All-Pervading essence of all beings, one who supports, Preserver God

vishuddhi chakra = seat of intellectual awareness, energy center situated behind the throat, the nervous plexus in the pharyngeal region

vishva = entire, whole

Vishvamitra = a celebrated Hindu Sage, ruler so impressed with Vasistha's knowledge and contentment that he became his disciple

vrischika = scorpion

vriksha = tree

vrishta = fallen or dropped as rain

vyaghra = tiger

Y

yajna = Hindu Sacrificial Ceremony

yama = ethical codes for daily life, self-restraint

Yama = the god of death; Yama is also the first of the eight limbs or means of attaining yoga. Yamas are universal ethical codes for daily life, self-restraint, and moral commandments or ethical disciplines transcending creeds, countries, age, and time. The five mentioned by Patanjali are: non-violence, truth, non-stealing, continence, and non-coveting

yantra = to sustain

yoga = union, communion, the path which integrates the body, senses, mind, and the intelligence with the self, derived from "yuj", meaning to join or to yoke, to concentrate one's attention on. It is the union of our will to the will of God, a poise of the soul which enables one to look evenly at life in all its aspects. The chief aim of yoga is to teach the means by which the human soul may be completely united with the Supreme Spirit pervading the universe and thus secure absolution

yoga-mudra = a posture, a seal

yoga-nidra = the sleep of yoga, where the body is at rest as if in sleep while the mind remains fully conscious, though all its movements are stilled; *yoga-nidra* is also the name of an *asana*

Yogananda = a great yogi of the twentieth century

yogasana = yogic posture

Yoga Sutra (yoga-sutra) = a classical collection of aphorisms on the practice of yoga, attributed to the sage Patanjli. It consists of 185 terse aphorisms on yoga and it is divided into four parts dealing respectively with *samadhi*, the means by which yoga is attained, the powers the seeker comes across in his quest, and the state of absolution

yogi or yogini = one who follows the path of *yoga*, a student, a seeker of truth

yogic = an adjective describing things that are associated with *yoga*

yoni = the womb

yoni-mudra = womb or female seal or awakened *kundalini*, the sealing; the breeding place, and *mudra* is a seal; *yoni-mudra* is a sealing posture where the apertures of the head are closed and the aspirant's senses are directed within to enable him to find out the source of his being

yudha = from Yudhisthira, a legendary warrior mentioned in the ancient Hindu epic *Mahabharata*

yuj = to join, to yoke, to use, to concentrate one's attention on

yukti = union

INDEX

POSES INDEXED BY SANSKRIT NAME

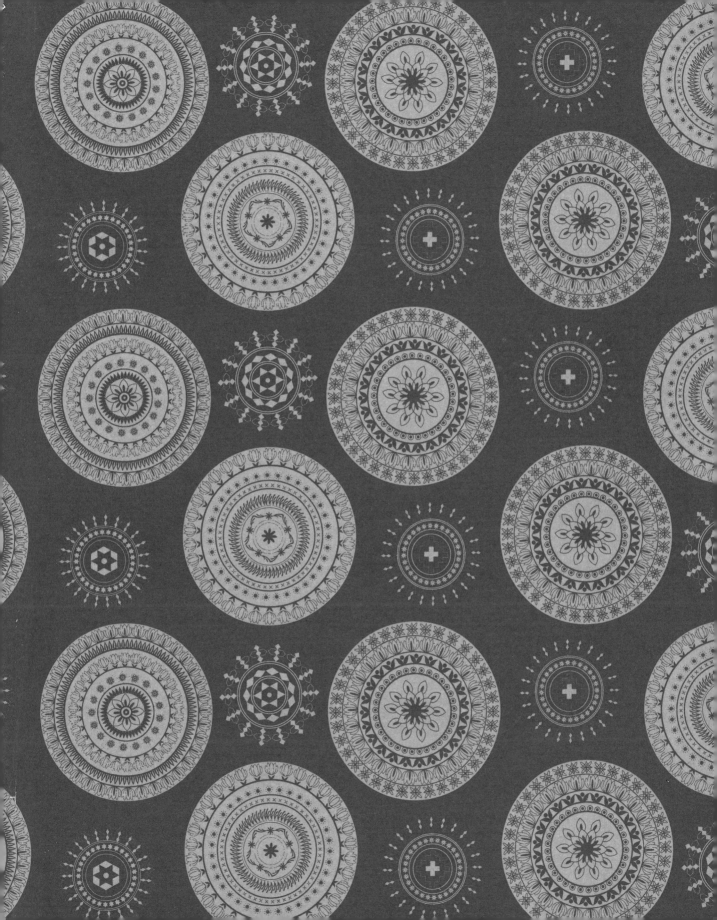

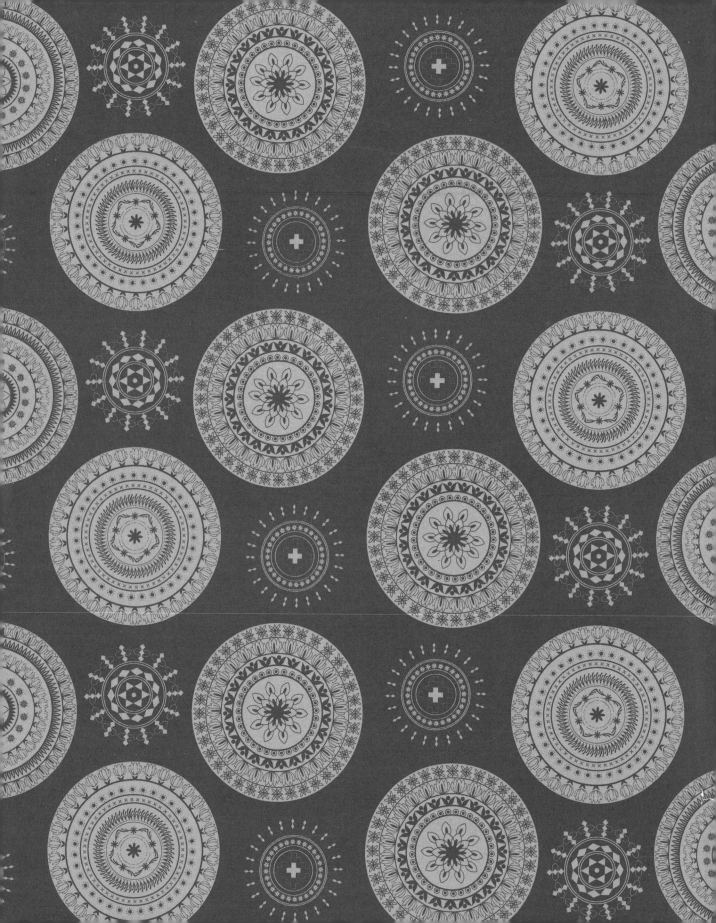